Manual of Nutritional Therapeutics

Fourth Edition

David H. Alpers, M.D.
William B. Kountz Professor of Geriatrics in Medicine
Assistant Director, Center for Human Nutrition
Washington University School of Medicine
St. Louis, Missouri

William F. Stenson, M.D.
Professor of Medicine
Washington University School of Medicine
St. Louis, Missouri

Dennis M. Bier, M.D.
Professor of Pediatrics
Baylor College of Medicine
Director
USDA/ARS Children's Nutrition Research Center
Houston, Texas

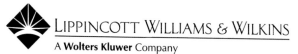
LIPPINCOTT WILLIAMS & WILKINS
A **Wolters Kluwer** Company
Philadelphia · Baltimore · New York · London
Buenos Aires · Hong Kong · Sydney · Tokyo

Acquisitions Editor: Beth Barry
Developmental Editor: Kerry B. Barrett
Production Editor: Emily Lerman
Manufacturing Manager: Colin J. Warnock
Cover Illustrator: Kevin Kall
Compositor: Circle Graphics
Printer: R. R. Donnelley, Crawfordsville

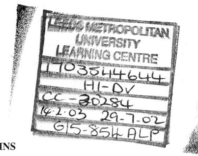

© 2002 by **LIPPINCOTT WILLIAMS & WILKINS**
530 Walnut Street
Philadelphia, PA 19106 USA
LWW.com

Printed in the USA

Library of Congress Cataloging-in-Publication Data

Alpers, David H.
    Manual of nutritional therapeutics / David H. Alpers, William F. Stenson, Dennis M. Bier.—4th ed.
        p. ; cm.
    Includes bibliographical references and index.
    ISBN 0-7817-3122-4 ✓
        1. Diet therapy—Handbooks, manuals, etc. I. Stenson, William F. II. Bier, Dennis M. III. Title.
        [DNLM: 1. Diet Therapy. 2. Nutrition. WB 400 A456m 2001]
    RM217.2 .A41 2001
    615.8′54—dc21

                                                                        2001029923

10 9 8 7 6 5 4 3 2 1

Manual of Nutritional Therapeutics

Fourth Edition

To our fathers, who taught us both respect for knowledge and concern for the individual

CONTENTS

APPENDIXES

PREFACE

In the six years since the publication of the third edition of the *Manual of Nutritional Therapeutics*, the amount of factual information relating to the use of nutritional therapy has greatly increased. Single Recommended Dietary Allowance values have been largely replaced by more encompassing Dietary Reference Intakes (DRI), which now also allow for estimates on the content of nutrients in available supplements and the need for certain supplements in disease prevention. The amount of new information concerning vitamins, minerals, and disease prevention has been impressive. Many advances have been made in the assessment of micronutrient deficiencies. To keep pace with this information, each chapter has been fully updated. To make this increased amount of information more accessible, we have retained the outline format of each chapter, and have referenced the manual more extensively. In addition, the chapter on AIDS has been extended to include the other major wasting illness, malignancy, and a chapter on alternative medicines related to nutrition has been added.

This manual is designed as a reference source to therapy-related nutritional facts that are difficult to find gathered together in one place. The presentation is designed for such healthcare workers as physicians, nurses, and dietitians in various disciplines and for students at all levels in each of the disciplines. It is assumed that the healthcare worker has some knowledge of the underlying disease processes that might be benefited by nutritional intervention and of the uses to which the information can be applied. This edition of the *Manual of Nutritional Therapeutics*, like its predecessors, is not meant as a general textbook of disease diagnosis or treatment. Although the focus of the book remains management of nutritional problems in adult patients, much of the information is applicable to adolescents and older children. As before, the information offered is meant to be practical, without being a *cookbook* for managing patients. Explanations for the recommendations are provided as fully as space has allowed.

The organization of material in nutritional categories (e.g., vitamins, minerals, enteral nutrition, and parenteral nutrition) rather than disease states has been largely continued. This organization allows users freedom to plan nutritional therapy for individual patients, while still providing the information needed to pursue *standard* therapies, such as the use of enteral or parenteral nutrition, or the treatment of individual nutrient deficiencies. Certain key nutrition-related disorders such as diabetes, hyperlipidemia, chronic renal disease, and obesity are still covered in separate chapters.

The information is as up-to-date as it can possibly be at the time of publication. However, preparations of nutrients often change rapidly, as has been the case for enteral supplements or multivitamin preparations. Thus, the reader should always check the local availability of any given preparation. Because the nutrient content of fast foods is now available in many commercial publications, this particular appendix has been removed. The URLs for many web sites providing nutritional information have been included, and these can be consulted for information that is updated after the publication of this book.

The authors express their gratitude to Beth Taylor, R.D., M.S., C.N.S.D. for help with the chapter on enteral nutrition, to Ms. Taylor and to Way Huey, PHARM.D. for assistance with the chapter on parenteral nutrition, and to the reviewers of all the chapters, particularly Dr. Samuel Klein for his insights regarding the chapter on obesity. The authors are indebted to Nina Branscum and Christina Burleson for secretarial and formatting assistance, and to Leslie Loddeke for editorial assistance. Our colleagues at Lippincott Williams & Wilkins, particularly Kerry B. Barrett, have provided editorial assistance and advice of the highest quality, and have made our task much easier. Once again, we thank our wives and families whose indulgent support has made possible all our efforts in producing this book.

David H. Alpers, M.D.
William F. Stenson, M.D.
Dennis M. Bier, M.D.

I. GENERAL CONCEPTS OF NUTRITION

1. APPROACH TO NUTRIENT DEFICIENCY

The medical use of nutrients to rectify states of deficiency depends on an appropriate knowledge base. This chapter outlines some general areas that involve both macronutrients (energy, protein, lipids) and micronutrients (vitamins, minerals). The subjects covered include (a) definitions of the nutrient requirement, (b) the concept of dietary goals and guidelines, along with food composition and preparation, (c) the identification of individual nutrient deficiency, (d) the medical use of nutrition support, and (e) the interaction of other medical therapies (drugs) with components of nutritional therapy. Subsequent chapters expand on many of these topics in more detail, and the reader is referred to these chapters when appropriate. This discussion is not meant to include all possible variants on these themes but rather highlights some common examples.

I. **Definitions of nutrient sufficiency**
   A. **Recommended dietary allowance (RDA).** The RDA is still the most widely publicized of the definitions of nutrient sufficiency in the United States. It is based on available scientific knowledge, is the result of deliberation by experts, and is approved by the Food and Nutrition Board of National Academy of Sciences Committee on Dietary Allowances. The RDA outlines the levels of intake of essential nutrients judged to be adequate to meet the known nutritional needs of practically all healthy persons. The RDA is set two standard deviations above the estimated mean, and so exceeds the requirements of most persons. It is important to remember that the RDA cannot be relied on for a precise estimate of the needs of patients with medical illness, particularly if malabsorption is present. The RDA was revised most recently in 1989. Values quite similar to the RDA have been developed for the basal requirements of the inhabitants of many other countries (1,2).

   Nonetheless, these guidelines have been deemed insufficient for many reasons. New understanding has been acquired of nutrient requirements and of the role of food components in reducing the risk for chronic diseases (e.g., cancer, heart disease, osteoporosis) and preventing classic deficiency syndromes. RDAs were previously developed with only the latter goal in mind. Moreover, RDAs were formerly based on the assumption that all nutrients are derived from natural foods; currently, however, dietary tablets, fortified foods, and food supplements are important sources of some nutrients. Thus, the governments of the United States and Canada together have formulated the dietary reference intake (Appendix B).

   B. **Dietary reference intake (DRI).** The DRI is now a collective term that includes the estimated average requirement (EAR), recommended dietary allowance (RDA), adequate intake (AI), and tolerable upper intake level (UL). The DRI is newly developed and has replaced the periodically revised RDA. It is the undertaking of the Standing Committee on the Scientific Evaluation of Dietary Reference Intakes of the Food and Nutrition Board, Institute of Medicine, National Academy of Sciences (www.nas.edu), in collaboration with Health Canada. It is being developed for 12 life stages, and four volumes have appeared thus far, covering calcium, vitamin D, magnesium, and phosphorus (3); the B vitamins niacin, biotin, and choline (4); antioxidant micronutrients, including vitamins C and E, selenium, and carotenoids (5); and vitamins A and K, iron, zinc, and trace minerals (6). Subsequent volumes will address macronutrients, trace elements, electrolytes and water, and other food components (e.g., fiber).

   The EAR is the daily intake value estimated to meet the requirements of 50% of persons in a normal life stage and gender group. It is used to set the RDA and plan recommendations for intake in various groups. The RDA is the intake level sufficient to meet the daily requirements of most people in a specific life stage and gender group and is set at two standard deviations above the EAR. This estimate also includes a coefficient of variation of 10% if the data do not permit the calculation of standard deviations. If not enough data are available to calculate an EAR, adequate intake (AI) is used. AI is based on approximations of average nutrient intake by an age- and/or gender-defined subgroup. The tolerable upper intake level (UL) is the maximum amount of a daily nutrient intake that is unlikely to pose a health threat for persons within an age and gender subgroup. This new term was deemed important because so many nutrients are now ingested from supplements at levels far exceeding those possible in the diet. Compromises within the DRI recommendation must be made, both because these values are often not precisely known and because the new recommendation may be used to prevent onset of disease (e.g., fracture risk) rather than clinical deficiency (rickets). Table 1-1 outlines some of the suggested population-based

Table 1-1. Population reference intakes/guidelines of dietary constituents for prevention of chronic diseases in adults, ages 20 to 50

	WCRF[a]	NAS[b]	WHO[c]	AHA[d]	PRI/goal[e]
Constituent					
macronutrients					
CHO (% kcal)	55–75	>55	55–75	55–60	45–55
Starch (%)	50–70	—	50–70	55–60	—
Sugar, nonmilk (%)	<10	—	<10	Low	10
Nonsoluble fiber (g/d)	20–35	—	16–24	20–25	39
Fats (% kcal)	15–30	<30	15–30	≤30	20–30
Polyunsaturated	2–10	≤10	3–7	≤10	2.5
Monosaturated	3–10	—	—	≤15	—
Saturated	0–10	<10	<10	8–10	10
Cholesterol (mg/d)	100–130	<300	<300	<300	—
Protein (% kcal)	9–12	—	10–15	—	—
Vegetable	6–12	—	—	—	—
Animal	0–3	—	—	—	—
Alcohol (% kcal)	<2	<2 oz	—	<2 oz	—
Micronutrients					
Carotenoids (mg/d)	9–18	—	—	—	—
Vitamin C (mg/d)	175–400	—	30	—	40–45
Folate (μg/d)	250–450	—	200	—	200
Vitamin D (μg/d)	0 (sun)–10	—	2.5	—	0–15
Vitamin E (mg/d)	4–7	—	—	—	<4
Calcium (mg/d)	500–750	—	400–500	—	700
Selenium (μg/d)	75–125	—	30–40	—	55
Iodine (μg/d)	125–150	—	120–150	—	130
Iron (mg/d)	15–25	—	16	—	9–21
Potassium (g/d)	1.6–3.2	—	—	—	3.1
Sodium (g/d)	<4	<4	<4	<6	0.58–3.5
Zinc (mg/d)	11–13	—	7.1–9.5	—	7.1–9.5

[a] WCRF, World Cancer Research Fund/American Institute for Cancer Research. *Food, nutrition, and the prevention of cancer: a global perspective, 1997.* Provides estimates of probable range of dietary constituents consumed as result of following recommendations of the report.
[b] NAS, National Academy of Sciences Food and Nutrition Board, 1989 recommendations for individuals.
[c] WHO, World Health Organization, 1990.
[d] AHA, American Heart Association, dietary guidelines for healthy American adults. Krauss RM, et al. *Circulation* 1996;94:1795–1800.
[e] PRI/goal, population reference intake ranges (female–male) for young European adults (ages 19 to 50), Commission of the European Community. Report of the Scientific Commission for Food (31st Series): Nutrient and energy intakes, 1993, or ultimate European goals (James WPT. Healthy nutrition, European series 24. Copenhagen: WHO Regional Office for Europe: 1988).

reference intakes that have been recommended to prevent cancer and heart disease, and those levels recommended by the World Health Organization and the Commission of the European Community for young, healthy adults.

C. **Daily reference values (DRVs).** The RDAs were standards set by the U.S. Food and Drug Administration in 1973 for purposes of food labeling. *Daily value* and *percent daily value* are the new reference terms on the nutrition label. The term *daily value* encompasses two sets of reference values: daily reference values (DRVs) and the old reference daily intakes (RDIs), now called *dietary reference intakes* (DRI). DRVs are provided for total and saturated fat, cholesterol, total carbohydrates, dietary fiber, sodium, potassium, and protein. They are based on current nutritional recommendations for adults and children age 4 or older. RDIs are the same as the current U.S. RDAs for 19 vitamins and minerals. The terms *DRV* and *RDI* do not appear on the nutrition label. What do appear are daily values, reflecting DRVs and RDIs for a 2,000-cal reference diet (Table 1-2). (See Appendix C for further details.)

D. **Reference weights.** These will be based on the Third National Health and Nutrition Examination Survey (NHANES III) in the United States. Table 1-3 shows the body mass index (BMI) calculated from such reference data for young adults.

E. **Estimated minimum requirements for healthy persons.** For some nutrients (Na, Cl, K), the daily requirements appear to be much lower than the

Table 1-2. Daily values for adults and children age 4 or older

Food component	Daily value[a]	Percentage of total caloric intake
Total fat	65 g[b]	30
Saturated fat	20 g[b]	10
Cholesterol	300 mg	—
Sodium	2,400 mg	—
Potassium	3,500 mg	—
Total carbohydrate	300 g[b]	60
Dietary fiber	25 g[c]	—
Protein	50 g[b]	10
Vitamin A	5,000 IU	—
Vitamin C	60 mg	—
Calcium	1 g	—
Iron	18 mg	—
Vitamin D	400 IU	—
Vitamin E	30 IU	—
Thiamine	1.5 mg	—
Riboflavin	1.7 mg	—
Niacin	20 mg	—
Vitamin B_6	2.0 mg	—
Folate	0.4 mg	—
Vitamin B_{12}	6.0 mg	—
Biotin	0.3 mg	—
Pantothenic acid	10 mg	—
Phosphorus	1 g	—
Iodine	150 µg	—
Magnesium	400 mg	—
Zinc	15 mg	—
Copper	2.0 mg	—

[a] Based on daily reference values and reference daily intakes.
[b] Daily value based on a 2,000-cal reference diet.
[c] Daily value based on 11.5 g/1,000 cal.

Table 1-3. Reference heights and weights for children and adults in the United States, NHANES III, 1997

Male (y)	Median BMI (kg/m²)	Female (y)	Median BMI (kg/m²)
4–8	15.8	4–8	15.8
9–13	18.5	9–13	18.3
14–18	21.3	14–18	21.3
19–30[a]	24.4	19–30	22.8

NHANES, National Health and Nutrition Examination Survey; BMI, body mass index.
[a] Because no evidence indicates that weights should change with aging, provided that activity is maintained, the reference weights of this group are applicable to all adults.
From Dietary reference intakes. *Nutr Rev* 1997;55:319–326.

content in an average U.S. diet. Thus, the concept of RDA is replaced by that of a minimum requirement (Table 1-4). These will remain in place until the DRIs are developed.

F. **Estimated safe and adequate daily dietary intakes of selected minerals.** With some micronutrients, the information is insufficient for actual recommendations to be made. Moreover, a high intake of rare earth metals may lead to toxic systemic levels. Thus, for these nutrients, ranges of intake, to be met but not exceeded, are provided (Table 1-5). Many vitamins and minerals have been reported to cause toxicity when taken in excess (Table 1-6). This concern is the major reason for the new UL recommendations (Appendix B). Most cases of nutrient toxicity are associated with supplementation, not food intake. Estimated toxic levels range from as low as five times (selenium) to 25 to 50 times (folate, vitamins C and E) the recommended dietary intake. The best-documented toxicities from nutrients involve vitamins A, B_3 (niacin), B_6, and D, iron, and selenium. Besides direct toxicity, significant problems can arise when high doses of some nutrients interact with other nutrients. For example, high doses of calcium can interfere with iron absorption, high doses of zinc can impair copper absorption, and high doses of vitamin E can impair vitamin K action.

Table 1-4. Estimated *minimum* requirements for healthy persons for sodium, chloride, and potassium

Age	Weight kg	Weight lb	Sodium (mg)	Chloride (mg)	Potassium (mg)
Up to 5 months	4.5	10	120	180	500
6–11 months	8.9	20	200	300	700
1 year	11	24	225	350	1,000
2–5 years	16	35	300	500	1,400
6–9 years	25	55	400	600	1,600
10–18 years	50	110	500	750	2,000
Over 18 years	70	154	500[a]	750	2,000[a]

[a]The minimum requirement does not allow for prolonged losses by vomiting, diarrhea, or excessive dieting. The Food and Nutrition Board of the National Academy of Sciences has recommended a daily salt intake of 6 g or less, or a sodium intake of 2.4 g, 4.8 times the minimum requirement. The National Research Council recommends a high intake of potassium-containing fruits and vegetables, even though the average U.S. adult diet contains 3.5 g of potassium, nearly twice the minimum requirement. This recommendation takes into account the supposed benefits of increased dietary potassium in hypertension and of dietary fiber in preventing colonic malignancy.
From National Research Council. *Recommended dietary allowances*, 10th ed. Washington, DC: National Academy Press, 1989, with permission.

Table 1-5. Estimated safe and adequate dietary intakes of selected trace elements

Category	Age (y)	Copper	Manganese	Fluoride	Chromium	Molybdenum
		(mg)			(µg)	
Infants	0–0.5	0.4–0.6	0.3–0.6	0.1–0.5	10–40	15–30
	0.5–1	0.6–0.7	0.6–1.0	0.2–1.0	20–60	20–40
Children	1–3	0.7–1.0	1.0–1.5	0.5–1.5	20–80	25–50
	4–6	1.0–1.5	1.5–2.0	1.0–2.5	30–120	30–75
	7–10	1.0–2.0	2.0–3.0	1.5–2.5	50–200	50–150
Adolescents	11+	1.5–2.5	2.0–5.0	1.5–2.5	50–200	75–250
Adults		1.5–3.0	2.0–5.0	1.5–4.0	50–200	75–250

Adapted from National Research Council. *Recommended dietary allowances*, 10th ed. Washington, DC: National Academy Press, 1989.

II. Dietary guidelines and properties of available foods for healthy persons

A. Guidelines. Based in part on the nutritional assessments listed above, guidelines have been developed for average normal persons and for persons with special needs (Table 1-1; see also Chapter 2). These guidelines generally advise that a normal weight be achieved and maintained. In addition, total fat intake should be limited to about 30% of calories, cholesterol intake decreased, intake of complex carbohydrates and fiber increased, excess intake of salt avoided, and alcohol ingested only in moderation.

The U.S. guidelines emerged after compromises were made between various lobbying groups and the U.S. Department of Agriculture and Department of Health and Human Services. This advice can be roughly quantified so that foods from four groups (cereal grains, fruits and vegetables, dairy products, protein-rich foods) are consumed in recommended proportions of 4:4:2:2. The guidelines should be considered a means of achieving the U.S. National Nutrition Objectives for the year 2000, outlined in 1991 (Table 1-7).

B. Food composition. Practical application of the dietary guidelines is based on a knowledge of food composition. Many guides are available, some of which are listed in Table 1-8. These sources differ in the type of information offered. All cover most vitamins and minerals and macronutrients (water, proteins, lipids, and carbohydrate, including total or crude fiber). McNance and Widdowson also cover total dietary fiber, oligosaccharides, selenium, manganese, iodine, nonstarch polysaccharides, and fatty acids for every food. The *Eurofood Monitor* is designed as a loose-leaf binder to accommodate yearly updates. It provides information on European Community legislation regarding food labeling, advertising, additives, composition, ingredients, and methods of analysis of specific products. *Nutrients in Food* categorizes food content by individual nutrients. All these sources list the nutrient contents of foods by different food groups (fats and oils, meats, nuts, legumes). Each book can be valuable depending on the clinical need.

The U.S. Department of Agriculture *Handbook 8-20* provides information on the content of raw and processed foods. The sections are updated individually. These now include new values for dairy and egg products, species and herbs, cereal grains and pasta, baby foods, and fast foods, in addition to updated information for a wide variety of other food products. The handbook is now available online from the U.S. Department of Agriculture, and is an enormous wealth of nutrition-related information. Table 1-9 lists some sources of information.

C. Food processing. The data included in the *Handbook 8-20* document the differences in the composition of raw and processed foods, but the enormous variety of changes that occur during processing cannot be covered. Foods are affected by the type of processing (freezing, canning, concentration),
(*text continues on page 11*)

Table 1-6. Vitamin and mineral toxicity

Nutrient	Symptoms of toxicity	Minimal intake
Vitamin B$_1$	Headache, irritability, insomnia	?, probably >50 mg/d
	Fast heart rate, weakness, occasional severe allergic reaction (anaphylaxis)	
Vitamin B$_2$	Yellow-orange color of urine	Safe up to 10 mg/d
Vitamin B$_6$	Peripheral sensory neuropathy (numbness)	2–6 g/d
Niacin	Flushing, burning of hands and face	>1 g/d
	Nausea, vomiting, diarrhea, abnormal heart rhythm, exacerbation of gout, rash, itching, glucose intolerance, abnormal liver blood chemistries	>3 g/d
Folate	Convulsions if on phenytoin (Dilantin)	>40 mg
	In pregnancy can compete with Zn and Fe for absorption, rare allergy (rash, itching, fever, wheezing)	
Vitamin B$_{12}$	None	
Vitamin C	False-positive sugar in urine, false low sugar in blood, false-negative test for blood in stool, diarrhea	2–6 g/d
	Dental erosions, increased oxalate, kidney stones, interference with anticoagulation from warfarin (Coumadin)	4–9 g/d
Biotin	None	
Pantothenic acid	Diarrhea	10–20 mg/d
Vitamin A	Nausea, vomiting, skin desquamation	50,000–100,000 IU/d Chronic ingestion
	Fatigue, hair loss, bone pain, anorexia, irritability	
	Vomiting, bulging fontanelles, growth failure, optic atrophy, sixth nerve palsy	>4,000 IU/kg/d
	Newborn microcephaly, dilated ventricles	15,000 IU/d if taken between 14 and 40 days of gestation
Vitamin D	Increased calcium in blood and urine, nausea, anorexia, itching, increased urine, thirst, abdominal pain, constipation, bone pain, kidney stones, weight loss, pancreatitis, hypertension, abnormal heart rhythm	>400 IU/d in non-growing adults, depends on Ca intake
Vitamin E	? Any symptoms, occasional weakness, fatigue, hypertension, nausea, increased effect of warfarin (Coumadin)	800–900 IU/d
Vitamin K	Jaundice in newborn	>10 mg/d to infant or pregnant mother
Na	Edema	If retaining sodium (heart, liver disease)
	Confusion	If very excessive intake

Table 1-6. (*Continued*)

Nutrient	Symptoms of toxicity	Minimal intake
K	Weakness, confusion, abnormal heart rhythm	If renal function low and 50–100 mEq/d in supplements, drugs
Ca	Nausea, vomiting, weakness, constipation, dry mouth, increased urine, abnormal heart rhythm, kidney stones	Especially if vitamin D >400 IU/d and supplement >1–2 g/d
Mg	Nausea, vomiting, hypertension, drowsiness	If renal function low and Mg given IV
P	? Symptoms not related to low calcium	Only in renal failure
Fe	Nausea, vomiting, diarrhea, abdominal pain	>20 mg/kg per day
Zn	Copper deficiency (anemia), ? decreased immune function, nausea, vomiting, rash, dehydration, gastric ulceration	>450 mg/d
Cu	Nausea, vomiting, diarrhea, cramps	>15 mg/d
I	Decreased thyroid function	>2,000 μ>g/d
F	Spine and muscle pain, weakness	20–80 mg/d
Mn	None	Up to 10 mg/d
Cr	None recognized	
Se	Hair and nail loss, skin lesions, tooth decay	>5 mg/d
	Nausea, vomiting, fatigue, hair loss, diarrhea, irritability	>20 mg/d

Table 1-7. U.S. national nutrition objectives for the year 2000

Health status	Risk reduction
↓ CAD deaths to <1/1,000 ↓ Cancer deaths to <1.3/1,000 ↓ Overweight from 24% to <20% in men 27% to <20% in women 15% to <15% in adolescents ↓ Growth retardation in low-income children <5 y from 16% to <10% ↓ Iron deficiency from 4–9% to <3%, ages 1–4 from 5% to <3% in pregnancy	↓ Fat intake from 36% to <30% of kcal ↓ Saturated fat intake from 13% to <10% of kcal ↑ Complex CHO/fiber from 2.5 to 5 servings (vegetables) and from 3 to 6 servings (grains) ↑ Persons adopting sound dietary practices and regular exercise from 25–30% to 50% ↑ Intake of Ca^{++}-rich foods to 3 servings per day to 50% from 24% of pregnant/lactating women to 50% from 7% of women ages 19–24 to 50% from 14% of men ages 19–24 ↑ Intake of Ca^{++}-rich foods to 2 servings per day to 50% from 15% of women ages 25–50 to 50% from 23% of men ages 25–50 ↓ Added Na^+ in prepared food from 54% to <35% Added Na to food from 68% to <20% ↑ Breast-feeding from 54% to 75% after birth from 21% to >50% at 6 months ↑ Use of food labels for nutritious choice from 74% to >85% in adults

From Nutrition in healthy people 2000. In: *National health promotion and disease prevention objectives.* Washington, DC: U.S. Government Printing Office, 1991.

Table 1-8. Selected food composition guides

Authors	Title	Year, edition	Publisher
Pennington, Jea	Bowes & Church, Food Values of Portions Commonly Used	1998, 7th	Lippincott Williams & Wilkins
Jackson, Rita	Nutrition & Food Servings Integrated	1997, 1st	Aspen Publishers
Sizer, Louise	Diet Analysis Win / Mac	1995, 6th	Wadsworth
ESHA Research	Diet Analysis Plus Version 5.0 Win / Mac	1999, 1st	Wadsworth
McNance and Widdowson	The Composition of Foods	1991, 5th	CRC Press
Souci SW, Fachmann W, Kraut H	Food Composition and Nutrition Tables	1999, 6th	CRC Press
Dobbs, J, Novotny R, Titchenal A	Computer Nutrient Analysis Handbook For Food, Culinary, and Health Professionals	1998, 1st	CRC Press
European Community Legislation on Food Stuffs	Eurofood Monitor	1992, 1st	Agra Europe
USDA, Human Nutrition Information Service	Composition of Foods—Raw, Processed, Prepared	1989–91, supplements	U.S. Government Printing Office
American Dietetic Association	Manual of Clinical Dietetics	2000, 6th	American Dietetic Association
Nelson, Jennifer	Mayo Clinic Diet Manual	1994, 7th	Mosby–Year Book

Table 1-9. Nutrition-related Internet sites

Organization	Internet address
American Council on Science and Health (consumer education consortium)	*www.acsh.org/nutrition/ index.html*
American Dietetic Association	*www.eatright.org*
American Institute of Nutrition	*nutrition.org*
Council for Responsible Nutrition (trade organization for supplement industry)	*www.crnusa.org*
Food and Drug Administration	*www.fda.gov*
FDA, Center for Food Safety and Applied Nutrition	*vm.cfsan.fda.gov*
FDA, *Report Adverse Effects of Supplements* Healthcare professionals Consumers	*www.fda.gov/medwatch/ report/hcp.htm report/consumer/consumer.htm*
International Food Information Council	*ificinfo.health.org*
National Center for Complementary and Alternative Medicine	*nccam.nih.gov*
National Health Information Center	*nhic-nt.health.org*
National Products Alert Database, University of Illinois	*pcog8.pmmp.uic.edu/mcp/ nap1.html*
Office of Dietary Supplements	*dietary-supplements.info.nih.gov*
Office of Disease Prevention & Health Promotion	*odphp.osophs.dhhs.gov*
ODPHP, *Nutrition & Your Health,* 4th ed.	*odphp.osophs.dhhs.gov/pubs/ dietguid/default.htm*
Rosenthal Center for Alternative/ Complementary Medicine, Columbia University	*cpmcnet.columbia.edu/ dept/rosenthal*
Tufts Nutrition Navigator (reference for sites)	*navigator.tufts.edu*
USDA, Dietary Guidelines Advisory Commission	*www.usda.gov/dgac*
USDA, *Food Composition Handbook 8-20*	*www.nal.usda.gov/fmic/ foodcomp*
United States Pharmacopoeia	*www.usp.org*
World Health Organization	*www.who.ch*

the length of the processing procedure, during which nutrients can be lost or inactivated, and the effects of storage. The factors most likely to render nutrients unstable in food are heating, oxidation, and pH (Table 1-10).

Most processed foods are usually less stable than dry foods because of a lesser degree of oxidation and the possibility of microbial contamination. Fresh produce must be kept moist to prevent wilting and loss of nutrients through cell damage. In modern practice, the characteristics of a controlled environment maintained to retard ripening (as for apples, pears, tomatoes) can play a major role in nutrient stability. The percentage of nutrients lost can be significant, and also varies for enriched versus unenriched foods. Examples are given in Table 1-11.

Other specific examples of the effects of food processing are provided in Chapters 6 and 7 in the sections on individual vitamins and minerals. For the most part, water-soluble vitamins and minerals are lost when foods are boiled and are better preserved when foods are broiled, sautéed, or steamed.

Table 1-10. Factors rendering nutrients unstable in foods or having little effect

Nutrients	Heat	Oxygen or air	Light	Acid	pH Neutral	pH Alkaline	Moisture[a]
Vitamins							
Vitamin A or carotenes	U	U	U	U	S	S	U
Ascorbate (C)	U	U	U	S	U	U	U
Biotin	U	S	S	S	S	S	—
Choline	S	U	S	S	S	S	—
Cobalamin (B_{12})	S	U	U	S	S	S	—
Vitamin D	U	U	U	S	S	U	U
Folic acid	U	U	U	U	U	S	—
Inositol	U	S	S	S	S	S	—
Vitamin K	S	S	U	U	S	U	—
Niacin	S	S	S	S	S	S	—
Pantothenate	U	S	S	S	S	U	—
Pyridoxine (B_6)	U	S	U	S	S	S	—
Riboflavin	U	S	U	S	S	U	U
Thiamine	U	U	S	S	U	U	U
Tocopherols (E)	U	U	U	S	S	S	U
Amino acids							
Isoleucine	S	S	S	S	S	S	—
Leucine	S	S	S	S	S	S	—
Lysine	U	S	S	S	S	S	—
Methionine	S	S	S	S	S	S	—
Phenylalanine	S	S	S	S	S	S	—
Threonine	U	S	S	U	S	U	—
Tryptophan	S	S	U	U	S	S	—
Valine	S	S	S	S	S	S	—
Fatty acids polyunsaturated	S[b]	U	U	S	S	U	—

[a] Moist processed foods are always less stable than dry because of greater risk of oxidation, effects of heat, and possibilities for microbial growth. In fresh produce, however, adequate moisture to prevent wilting is important in nutrient stability.
[b] If not excessive, such as when dripped on hot coals.
Modified from Harris RS, Karmas E. *Nutritional evaluation of food processing,* 2nd ed. Westport, CT: AVI, 1975.

D. Food supplements, fortifiers, and additives. A particular nutrient can be added to the diet of a population in several ways. These include (a) providing supplements containing the nutrient, (b) fortifying food samples with the nutrient, and (c) increasing the intake of foods rich in the nutrient. The benefit of supplements is that only appropriate groups are targeted. The consumption of table foods is more natural and conducive to a good diet, but if the nutrient is needed in doses close to or exceeding the upper limit of the DRI (e.g., folic acid to prevent neural tube defects), diet alone may be inadequate. The advantage of fortification is that the nutrient reaches many more people. Although supplements, fortifiers, and additives are defined separately, it is sometimes difficult to distinguish between them, as all are added to foods (Table 1-12). In fact, the U.S. Department of Agriculture brochure on food additives (7) categorizes food additives as outlined in Table 1-12 and defines them broadly as "any substance the intended use of which results or may reasonably be expected to result—directly or indirectly—in its becoming a component or otherwise af-

Table 1-11. Retention of nutrients in cooked vegetables[a]

	Ascorbic acid (%)	Thiamine (%)	Riboflavin (%)	Niacin (%)	Vitamin B_6 (%)	Folacin (%)	Vitamin A (%)
Potatoes							
Prepared from raw							
Baked in skin	80	85	95	95	95	90	—
Boiled in skin	75	80	95	95	95	90	—
Boiled without skin	75	80	95	95	95	75	—
Fried	80	80	95	95	95	75	—
Hashed-brown[b]	25	40	85	80	—	65	—
Mashed	75	80	95	95	95	75	—
Scalloped and au gratin	80	80	95	95	95	75	—
Prepared from frozen							
French fried, heated	50	75	95	95	95	75	—
Baked, stuffed, heated	80	85	95	95	95	80	—
Hashed-brown	80	80	95	95	95	80	—
Other vegetables[c]							
Prepared from raw, drained							
Greens, dark and leafy	60	85	95	90	90	65	95
Roots, bulbs, other vegetables of high starch and/or sugar content[d]	70	85	95	95	95	70	90
Other[e,f]	80	85	95	90	90	70	90
Prepared from frozen, drained							
Greens, dark and leafy[c]	60	90	95	90	90	55	95
Roots, bulbs, other vegetables of high starch and/or sugar content[d]	70	90	95	95	95	70	90
Other[e,f]	80	90	95	90	90	70	90

[a] % True retention = nutrient content per gram of cooked food × grams of food after cooking/ nutrient content per gram of raw food × grams of food before cooking × 100.
[b] Potatoes were pared, boiled, and held overnight before hash-browning.
[c] Cooked in small or moderate amount of water until tender.
[d] Vegetables such as beets, carrots, green peas, lima beans, onions, parsnips, rutabagas, salsify, turnips, summer and winter squash, and other immature seeds of the legume group.
[e] Vegetables such as asparagus, bean sprouts, broccoli, brussels sprouts, cabbage, cauliflower, eggplant, kohlrabi, okra, and sweet peppers.
[f] Because of limited data, values are based on nutrient retention data from other cooked plant products.
From *Composition of foods—raw, processed, prepared, 1990 supplement*. Washington, DC: U.S. Department of Agriculture, Human Nutrition Information Service, Agriculture Handbook No. 8, 1990.

fecting the characteristics of any food." By this definition, a nutrient fortifier is considered an additive. However, each category is regulated differently and should be considered separately.

  1. **Food/nutrient supplements.** The U.S. Food and Drug Administration first regulated supplements as foods "for special dietary use" (1938), and vitamins, minerals, and other dietary substances were included. In

Table 1-12. Common food additives

Additive function	Nutrient type	Nutrient form	Foods likely used
Maintain nutrition	B vitamins	Thiamine, ribo-flavin, niacin, pyridoxine, folate, B_{12}	Cereals, pasta, flour, breads, corn meals, rice
	Fat-soluble vitamins	Vitamins A, D	Milk, milk products
	Minerals	FeEDTA, Zn oxide Ca citrate, carbon-ate iodide	Cereals, breads Juices, flour, cereal Salt, premature infant formulas
Enhance flavor, desirability	Sweeteners	Aspartame, saccharine, acesulfame K, sucralose, fructose, sugar alcohols, honey, cane juice, molasses	Beverages, yogurt, gelatin desserts, candies, chewing gum
	Fat substitute	Egg white/milk protein blend (Simplesse)	Frozen desserts
		Sucrose-triglyceride (Olestra)	Potato/corn chips
	Glutamates	MSG	Soups
	Stimulants	Caffeine	Soft drinks
Maintain palatability	Preservatives	Ascorbate, BHA, BHT, benzoates, Na nitrite, Na sulfite	Bread, cheese, meat, frozen/dried fruit, mar-garine, chips
Control pH	Acids/bases	NaHCO$_3$, citric acid, phosphoric acid, tartrazine	Soft drinks, cakes, chocolates, butter
Improve consistency	Bulk agents	Lecithin, mono- and di-glycerides, pectin, car-rageenan, guar gum, alginates	Baked goods, salad dressing, ice cream, processed cheese

EDTA, ethylenediamine-tetraacetic acid; MSG, monosodium glutamate; BHA, butylated hydrox-yanisole; BHT, butylated hydroxytoluene.

1994, the Dietary Supplement Health and Education Act (DSHEA) be-came law and provided for some regulation of supplements, while pro-hibiting their regulation as drugs or food additives. A dietary supplement was defined as a product intended to supplement the diet that contains a vitamin, mineral, herb, amino acid, a substance meant to increase the total dietary intake, or any metabolites, constituents, or combinations of the above. Like conventional foods, they are not sub-ject to premarket approval by the Food and Drug Administration and are exempt from food additive regulations. In other words, clinical studies are not required to demonstrate their efficacy, safety, or possible interactions. Safety issues are handled by public warnings or recalls. Because the law separated supplements from additives,, ingredients on the market before 1994 were considered safe. Supplements introduced after 1994 must be accompanied by evidence that the ingredient is "reasonably expected to be safe." Hundreds of supplements have not been approved (8); individual micronutrient supplements are discussed in Chapters 6 and 7, and other types of nutrient supplements in Chapter 11.

2. Nutrient fortification. The addition of nutrients during processing to improve the nutritional qualities of foods is initiated legislatively and regulated by the Food and Drug Administration. The most common nutrients in the United States that are regulated as additives are thiamine, niacin, riboflavin, iron (all in fortified flour since the 1950s), and folate (in cereal grain products and ready-to-eat cereals since 1998) (Table 1-13). The increased intake of these nutrients, documented in the 1997 report *Nutrient Content of the U.S. Food Supply* (U.S. Department of Agriculture Center for Nutrition Policy and Promotion), is a consequence of the fortification of grains. The increased intake of vitamins A and C and carotene is the result of the consumption of larger amounts of fruits and vegetables. These changes reflect a shift from animal fat to vegetable oils and other plant products. Increased intake of calcium and phosphorus is largely a consequence of greater cheese consumption.

Food fortification also prevents the deficiency of nutrients whose major dietary contribution is from only selected foods (e.g., iron or vitamin D), exemplified by the principles used in iron fortification (U.S. Department of Agriculture, *Food Technology,* April 1989). A need for the

Table 1-13. FDA-recommended fortification levels based on a caloric standard

Nutrient	U.S. RDA	Level of nutrients per 100 kcal
Vitamin A, IU	5,000	250
Vitamin C, mg	60	3
Thiamine, mg	1.5	0.075
Riboflavin, mg	1.7	0.085
Niacin, mg	20	1.0
Calcium, g	1	0.05
Iron, mg	18	0.9
Vitamin D, IU	400	20[a]
Vitamin E, IU	30	1.5
Vitamin B_6, mg	2.0	0.1
Folic acid, mg	0.4	0.02
Vitamin B_{12}, µg	6	0.3
Phosphorus, g	1	0.05
Iodine, µg	150	7.5[a]
Magnesium, mg	400	20
Zinc, mg	15	0.75
Copper, mg	2.0	0.1
Biotin, mg	0.03	0.015
Pantothenic acid, mg	10	0.5
Potassium, g	—[b]	0.125
Manganese, mg	—[b]	0.2

IU, international unit; RDA, recommended daily allowance.
[a] Optional.
[b] No U.S. RDA has been established for these nutrients.
Data from Miller SA, Stephenson MF. Food fortification. *Bibl Nutr Dieta* 1987;40:82.

nutrient must be demonstrated in a defined population (e.g., vitamin D in milk for infants and the elderly), use of the product must not lead to toxicity, the vehicle to which nutrients are added must be appropriate (e.g., addition of iron to cereal to prevent deficiency in children), and use of the product must not be confusing to consumers.

3. Food additives. Additives are becoming nearly ubiquitous in processed foods. Although some of these substances have no nutrient value *per se,* they carry the potential for toxicity and thus can affect the acceptance or availability of a prepared food to which they have been added. The original Food and Agriculture Organization (FAO)/World Health Organization definition of an additive (1955) was "non-nutritive substances added intentionally to food, generally in small quantities, to improve its appearance, flavor, texture, or storage properties." Now the definition of the Codex Alimentarius (sponsored by the World Health Organization) includes "any substance not normally consumed as a food by itself and not normally used as a typical ingredient of the food, whether or not it has nutritive value, the intentional addition of which to food for a technological purpose in the manufacturing, processing, preparation, treatment, packing, packaging, transport, or holding of such food results . . . in it or its by-products becoming a component of . . . such foods."

The use of additives is governed by the Food and Drug Act of 1906, which prevented the manufacture of adulterated foods; the Food, Drug, and Cosmetic Act of 1938, which allowed the government to remove adulterated foods from the market but did not regulate food additives; and by the Food Additives Amendment to the Federal Food, Drug, and Cosmetic Act of 1958. This amendment required that a new preservative or new use or amount of preservative be approved by the Food and Drug Administration before use, and that the compound be safe for humans. The preservative may not be used to make a product appear other (e.g., fresher) than it is. This is the rationale for not allowing sulfites to be added to meats. The additive must also be of food grade. Nearly 3,000 additives are used in food processing. Most recently, the Food Additives Amendment (Delaney clause) has provided that "no additive shall be deemed to be safe if it is found to produce cancer in man or animal."

Additives are used (a) to improve nutritional value (vitamin D in milk, vitamin A in margarine, iodine in table salt, B vitamins and iron in refined breads and cereals); (b) to make food more appealing (colors, flavor enhancers, and sweeteners, most often sugar, salt, and corn syrup or their substitutes); (c) to maintain palatability and freshness (sodium nitrates to protect cured foods, vitamin C to prevent uncooked fruit from browning); (d) to control pH (in baking mixes, soft drinks), and (e) to improve consistency or aid in processing (carrageenan to give consistency to peanut butter, leavening agents to make baked goods rise) (Table 1-12).

Two major categories are exempt from testing and approval. About 700 additives are "generally recognized as safe" (GRAS) because past experience indicates that they have no known harmful effects. "Prior sanctioned substances," approved for use in food before 1958, also are exempt. New evidence can reopen testing on an additive, however. Most recently, butylated hydroxyanisole (BHA) and sulfites have been reviewed and approval continued (Food and Drug Administration, June 1998).

Similar regulations have been applied by the Joint Expert Committee for Food Additives of the FAO/World Health Organization. Additives are classified for safety by acceptable daily intake (ADI) from 0 mg/kg to some upper limit (World Health Organization, 1987). The ADI is calculated by dividing the highest dose with no observable adverse effect in animals by a safety factor, usually 100. This improved approach to safety factor determination has been validated in a number of cases, including BHA, saccharine, and the coloring agent erythrosine (9).

III. Signs and symptoms of nutrient deficiency

A. General assessment. A person's nutritional status can be altered by any ill-ness that affects nutrient intake, absorption, or utilization, and it should be a part of any general medical examination or evaluation for a medical disor-der. The assessment comprises a history, physical examination, and labora-tory tests. Many of the details of these components are covered in subsequent chapters, but the general outline is considered here.

1. Nutritional history. The history should be focused on identifying pos-sible causes of altered nutrient intake or absorption and of increased losses or requirements (Table 1-14).

Special attention should be paid to changes in body weight (see Chapters 5 and 14), alcohol intake, causes of nutrient loss (bleeding, di-arrhea), intercurrent illness, and medication that might affect intake or nutrient losses. Key questions should become a routine part of the history, including the following: (a) Has the patient's weight changed recently? By how much and how rapidly? (b) Has the patient's appetite changed? (c) Is the appetite change caused by altered taste or smell, problems with chew-ing or swallowing, poorly fitting dentures, or depression? (d) Who pre-pares meals for the patient, and has that changed recently? (e) Who shops and pays for food? (f) Are symptoms of gastrointestinal disease present? (g) Does the patient consume alcohol, medications, or dietary supplements or herbal remedies? (h) Is the patient on a restricted diet of any sort? Decreased or altered taste is a common symptom that often is overlooked or incompletely assessed. Many common causes are not related to nutri-ent status, such as menopause, depression, or poor dental hygiene. Deficiencies of vitamin A, vitamin B_{12}, and perhaps zinc may also alter taste. Medications are among the most common causes of decreased or al-tered taste, especially chloride salts, which are secreted by salivary glands (see list of drugs in Table 1-23) and drugs with anticholinergic effects, which produce xerostomia (see list of drugs in Table 1-18).

2. Physical examination. Tissues that proliferate rapidly (skin, oral and gastrointestinal mucosa, hair, bone marrow) are most likely to manifest signs of nutrient deficiency. Some are accessible to the physical examina-tion, some (gastrointestinal mucosa) are manifested by history (diarrhea), and others (bone marrow failure) present indirectly. The examination can be approached in one of four ways: assessment of the physical findings to identify the nutrient deficiency, a search for relevant signs of nutrient de-ficiency suspected from the history, oral examination (a neglected area of the physical examination), or, in selected cases, anthropomorphic measurements.

a. Dehydration. Deficiencies of Na, Cl, and H_2O lead to dehydration (see also discussion of sodium in Chapter 7). In adult patients, the manifestations of dehydration (including sunken eyeballs, mucosal xerosis, low blood pressure, and mental confusion) are less striking and specific than in children and infants. One or none may be pre-sent in any individual case.

b. Nutrient deficiency. An important part of the physical examina-tion is the search for signs of nutrient deficiency. Table 1-15 lists the most common signs and the nutrient deficiencies frequently associ-ated with them. Table 1-16 lists physical examination findings ac-cording to the individual vitamin that is lacking.

c. Oral mucosa. Because the oral mucosa regenerates rapidly, it can be a sensitive indicator of nutrient deficiency. Table 1-17 lists the oral manifestations commonly associated with individual nutrient defi-ciencies. Oral manifestations are not specific for nutrient deficiency, and the same conditions can be caused in particular by medication. Table 1-18 lists some of the more important drug-induced oral pre-sentations.

(*text continues on page 24*)

Table 1-14. Nutritional history screen

Mechanism of deficiency	If history of	Suspect deficiency of
Inadequate intake	• All foods, ask about alcoholism, weight loss, poverty, dental disease, AIDS, taste changes	Calories, protein, thiamine, niacin, folate, pyridoxine, riboflavin
	• Fruit, vegetables, grains	Vitamin C, thiamine, niacin, folate, dietary fiber
	• Meat, dairy products, eggs	Protein, vitamin B_{12}
	• Food idiosyncrasies, allergy	Lactose
Inadequate absorption	• Drugs (especially antacids, anticonvulsants, cholestyramine, laxatives, neomycin, alcohol)	Selected vitamins and minerals
	• Malabsorption (diarrhea, weight loss, steatorrhea)	Vitamins A, D, and K, calories, protein, iron, calcium, magnesium, zinc
	• AIDS	Vitamin B_{12}
	• Surgery	
	Gastrectomy	Vitamin B_{12}, iron
	Resection of small intestine	Vitamin B_{12}, bile salts (if >100 cm of distal ileum), all others (if jejunal)
Increased losses	• Alcohol abuse	Magnesium, zinc, phosphorus
	• Blood loss	Iron
	• Diabetes, poorly controlled	Calories
	• Diarrhea	Protein, zinc, electrolytes
	• Draining abscesses, wounds	Protein
	• Peritoneal dialysis or hemodialysis	Protein, water-soluble vitamins, zinc
	• Drugs (especially diuretics, laxatives)	Potassium, magnesium
Increased requirements	• Fever	Calories
	• Hyperthyroidism	Calories
	• Increased physiologic demands (infancy, adolescence, pregnancy, lactation)	Various nutrients
	• Surgery, trauma, burns, infection	Calories, protein

Table 1-15. Signs and symptoms of nutritional deficiency in adult patients

Sign or symptom	Possible nutrient deficiency
General	
Wasted, skinny (especially temporal muscles)	Protein–calorie
Abdomen	
Distension	Protein–calorie
Hepatomegaly	Protein–calorie
Extremities	
Edema	Protein, thiamine
Decubitus ulcers, poor wound healing	Protein, vitamin C, zinc
Bone tenderness	Vitamin D
Bone ache, joint pain	Vitamin C
Muscle wasting and weakness	Protein, calorie, vitamin D
Muscle tenderness, muscle pain	Thiamine
Skin	
Pallor	Folate, iron, vitamin B_{12}
Follicular hyperkeratosis	Vitamins A and C
Perifollicular petechiae (especially after raised venous pressure	Vitamin C
Flaking dermatitis, scaling	Protein, calories, niacin, riboflavin, zinc, vitamin A
Bruising, purpura	Vitamin C, vitamin K, essential fatty acids
Pigmentation changes, desquamation of semiexposed areas	Niacin, protein–calorie
Scrotal dermatosis	Riboflavin
Cellophane appearance	Protein (also corticosteroid use, aging)
Hair	
Sparse and thin	Protein, zinc, biotin
Easy to pull out	Protein
Corkscrew hairs, coiled hair	Vitamin C, vitamin A
Nails	
Spooning	Iron
Transverse lines	Protein
Eyes	
History of night blindness (especially impaired visual recovery after glare)	Vitamin A
Photophobia, blurring, conjunctival inflammation	Riboflavin, vitamin A
Mouth	
Glossitis (slick red tongue)	Riboflavin, niacin, folic acid, vitamin B_{12}, protein
Gums—bleeding, receding, spongy, ulcers, hypertrophic	Vitamins C, A, and K; folic acid, niacin
Cheilosis (dry, cracking, ulcerated lips)	Riboflavin, pyridoxine, niacin
Angular stomatitis	Riboflavin, pyridoxine, niacin
Hypogeusia	Zinc, vitamin A, vitamin B_{12}
Tongue fissuring	Niacin
Burning, sore mouth and tongue	Vitamins B_{12} and B_6, niacin, vitamin C, folic acid, iron
Leukoplakia	Vitamins A, B_{12}, and B complex; folic acid, niacin

continued

Table 1-15. (*Continued*)

Sign or symptom	Possible nutrient deficiency
Neck	
Goiter	Iodine
Parotid enlargement	Protein (also alcohol excess, starch chewing)
Neurologic	
Tetany	Calcium, magnesium
Peripheral neuropathy (paresthesias)	Thiamine, pyridoxine
Loss of reflexes, wrist drop, foot drop (loss of vibratory and position sense)	Vitamin B_{12}, vitamin E
Dementia, disorientation	Niacin, vitamin B_{12}
Confabulation	Thiamine
Ophthalmoplegia	Thiamine, vitamin E
Depression	Biotin, folic acid, vitamin B_{12}

Table 1-16. Clinical manifestations of vitamin deficiency states

Vitamin	Major causes of deficiency	Clinical deficiency symptoms
Thiamine	Inadequate intake, alcoholism	*Neurologic*—mental confusion, irritability, sensory loss and paresthesias (peripheral neuropathy), weakness, anorexia *Eyes*—ophthalmoplegia *Cardiac*—tachycardia, cardiomegaly, congestive heart failure *Other*—constipation, sudden death, muscle tenderness and pain
Riboflavin	Inadequate intake	*Skin*—nasolabial seborrhea, fissuring and redness around eyes and mouth, magenta tongue, genital dermatosis *Eyes*—corneal vascularization
Pyridoxine	Inadequate intake, old age, alcoholism	*Skin*—nasolabial seborrhea, glossitis, cheilosis *Neurologic*—paresthesias, peripheral neuropathy *Other*—anemia
Niacin	Inadequate intake, alcoholism, carcinoid syndrome	*Skin*—nasolabial seborrhea, fissuring eyelid corners, angular fissures around mouth, papillary atrophy, pellagrous dermatitis (sun-exposed areas), burning mouth or tongue *Neurologic*—mental confusion *Other*—diarrhea
Folic acid	Inadequate intake, alcoholism, malabsorption, pregnancy, hemolysis, drugs (anticonvulsants, sulfasalazine, methotrexate)	*Skin*—pallor *Oral*—glossitis, hyperpigmentation of tongue *Neurologic*—depression *Other*—diarrhea, anemia

Table 1-16. (*Continued*)

Vitamin	Major causes of deficiency	Clinical deficiency symptoms
Cobalamin (B$_{12}$)	Malabsorption, pernicious anemia, vegetarian diets	*Skin*—hyperpigmentation, pallor *Oral*—glossitis *Neurologic*—ataxia, optic neuritis, paresthesias, peripheral neuropathy, mental disorders *Other*—anemia, anorexia, diarrhea
Vitamin C	Alcoholism, inadequate intake	*Skin*—petechiae, purpura, swollen bleeding gums, delayed wound healing, flaking dermatosis *Other*—bone pain, depression, anorexia
Biotin	Total parenteral nutrition (TPN)	*Skin*—pluckable sparse hair, pallor, seborrheic dermatitis *Neurologic*—depression *Other*—anemia, fatigue
Vitamin A	Fat malabsorption, alcoholism	*Eyes*—Bitot's spots, conjunctival and corneal xerosis (dryness), keratomalacia, poor dark adaptation *Skin*—follicular hyperkeratosis, xerosis *Hair*—coiled, keratinized
Vitamin D	Fat malabsorption, lack of sunlight, breast-fed newborn	*Bone*—bowlegs, beading of ribs, bone pain, epiphyseal deformities, vertebral fractures, muscle pain
Vitamin E	Premature infants, fat malabsorption, cystic fibrosis, chronic biliary obstruction	*Neurologic*—peripheral neuropathy, ophthalmoplegia
Vitamin K	Fat malabsorption, excessive warfarin dose	*Skin*—subcutaneous hemorrhage, ecchymoses

Table 1-17. Nutritional deficiencies and related oral manifestations

Nutrient deficiency	Oral manifestations
Vitamin A	Candidiasis *Gingivae*—hypertrophy, inflammation *Oral mucosa*—keratosis, leukoplakia Periodontal disease
Vitamin B complex	*Lips*—angular cheilosis *Oral mucosa*—leukoplakia Periodontal disease *Tongue*—papillary hypertrophy, magenta color, fissuring, glossitis
Vitamin B$_2$ (riboflavin)	Filiform papillae—atrophic Fungiform papillae—enlarged *Lips*—shiny, red, angular cheilosis *Tongue*—magenta color, soreness

continued

Table 1-17. (*Continued*)

Nutrient deficiency	Oral manifestations
Vitamin B$_3$ (niacin)	*Lips*—angular cheilosis *Oral mucosa*—intense irritation/inflammation, red, painful, denuded, ulcerated, mucositis/stomatitis *Tongue*—glossitis; tip/borders—red, swollen, beefy; dorsum—smooth, dry Ulcerative gingivitis
Vitamin B$_6$ (pyridoxine)	*Oral mucosa*—burning/sore mouth *Lips*—angular cheilosis *Tongue*—glossitis, glossodynia
Vitamin B$_{12}$ (cobalamin)	*Lips*—angular cheilosis Burning/sore mouth *Oral mucosa*—ulcerations (aphthous type), mucositis/stomatitis *Tongue*—beefy red, glossy, smooth, glossitis, glossodynia, loss of papillae
Vitamin C (megavitamin C withdrawal)	Burning/sore mouth Candidiasis *Gingivae*—friability, raggedness, swelling, redness Hemorrhagic tendency—petechiae, subperiosteal Periodontal disease *Teeth*—marked mobility, spontaneous exfoliation
Vitamin D	Periodontal disease
Vitamin K	*Gingivae*—bleeding
Folic acid	*Oral mucosa*—mucositis/stomatitis, ulcerations (aphthous type) Burning/sore mouth Candidiasis Filiform/fungiform papillae—atrophic *Gingivae*—inflammation *Lips*—angular cheilosis *Tongue*—glossitis; tip/borders—red swollen; dorsum—slick, bald, pale, or fiery red
Iron	Dental caries—increased susceptibility Filiform papillae—atrophic *Lips*—angular cheilosis, pallor *Oral mucosa*—pallor, sore mouth, ulcerations (aphthous type) Oral parethesias, burning *Tongue*—atrophic, pale; glossitis Xerostomia
Protein	*Oral mucosa*—fragility, burning sensation *Lips*—angular cheilosis Periodontal disease

Modified from Chernoff R. *Geriatric nutrition*. Gaithersburg, MD: Aspen Publishers, 1991.

Table 1-18. Common drug-induced oral manifestations

Candidiasis
  Antibiotics
  Antineoplastics
  Corticosteroids
  Immunosuppressives
  Steroid inhalers
Contact hypersensitivity
  Iodine
  Menthol
  Thymol
  Topical analgesics
  Topical antibiotics
Erythema multiforme
  Anticonvulsants
  Antimalarials
  Barbiturates
  Busulfan
  Chlorpropamide
  Isoniazid
  Meprobamate
  Minoxidil
  Penicillins
  Phenolphthalein
  Phenylbutazone
  Propylthiouracil
  Salicylates
  Sulfonamides
  Tetracyclines
Fixed drug eruptions
  Barbiturates
  Chlordiazepoxide
  Sulfonamides
  Tetracyclines
Gingival hyperplasia
  Cyclosporine
  Nifedipine
  Phenytoin sodium
Hairy tongue
  Antibiotics
  Corticosteroids
  Sodium peroxide
Intraoral bleeding, petechiae, purpura
  Antiarrhythmics
  Phenylbutazone
  Potassium chloride
  Sulfonamides
  Thiocyanate
  Thiouracil
  Warfarin sodium
Ulcerations, mucositis, stomatitis
  Antiarrhythmics
  Antineoplastics

  Aspirin
  D-Penicillamine
  Gold salts
  Indomethacin
  Lithium
  Meprobamate
  Mercurial diuretics
  Methotrexate
  Methyldopa
  Naproxen
  Phenylbutazone
  Potassium chloride
  Propranolol
  Spironolactone
  Thiazide diuretics
  Tolbutamide
Xerostomia
  Anorexiants
  Antiarrhythmics
  Antibiotics (broad-spectrum)
  Anticholinergics
  Anticoagulants
  Anticonvulsants
  Antidepressants
  Antidiarrheals
  Antihistamines
  Antihypertensives
  Antinauseants
  Antineoplastics
  Antiparkinsonism agents
  Antispasmodics
  Aspirin
  Benzodiazepines
  Bronchodilators
  CNS stimulants
  Decongestants
  Diuretics
  Ganglion-blocking agents
Salivary gland enlargement
  Antipsychotics
  Iodides
  Isoproterenol
  Methyldopa
  Hypnotics
  Lithium
  Monoamine oxidase inhibitors
  Muscle relaxants
  Narcotics
  Nonsteroidal antiinflammatory
    agents
  Sympathomimetics
  Tranquilizers

Modified from Chernoff R. *Geriatric nutrition.* Gaithersburg, MD: Aspen Publishers, 1991.

   d. **Anthropomorphic measurements** most useful include body weight and height, but the latter is overlooked in many cases by physicians. These measurements are important in estimating the general nutritional status by a comparison with weight guidelines (see Chapter 5), and height is also important in assessing energy needs and determining body mass index.
3. **Laboratory tests.** When the history and physical examination findings suggest a deficiency, it is often appropriate to assess the status of individual nutrients by specific tests. One must be careful to use the proper test, depending on whether one is assessing total body stores or recent intake (Tables 1-19 and 1-20). Each of these tests is discussed in detail in Chapters 6 and 7.

   Many of the tests listed in Tables 1-19 and 1-20 measure static nutrient content. A few tests measure actual function and allow a direct assessment of nutrient status (Table 1-21). Unfortunately, these tests are less often available than those that sample only fasting blood or urine.

IV. Diet therapy. Diets are used for many purposes, only some of them therapeutic. Some diets are recommended to prevent the onset of chronic diseases, such as atherosclerosis or obesity (see Chapters 12 and 13). The data regarding the efficacy of such diets are incomplete. Other diets are used to manage medical illnesses, such as diabetes, hyperlipidemia, and renal disease (see Chapter 12). Still others are used for one specific aspect of overall management, such as the addition of calcium-containing foods for osteopenia (see Chapter 7). A few diets are used to eliminate or treat specific disorders, such as low-fat, low-lactose, low-sodium, or gluten-free diets (see Chapter 11).

Some diets are advertised commercially as providing nutritional remedies (usually unproven) for serious illness (most commonly cancer) and preventing cancer or obesity. One must keep in mind the strong placebo effect of all treatments, including diets. The greatest caution must be exercised in regard to unproven nutritional remedies for cancer because of the highly charged emotional situation in which these treatments are undertaken (1). Dietary supplements have included laetrile; wheat germ (also administered as an enema); megadoses of vitamins E, C, and A, singly or in combination; and megadoses of selenium. In some cases, not just supplements but whole diet programs are offered, but their efficacy in cancer prevention or management is unproven. The claims made for these diets can best be countered by promoting the diet recommended for cancer prevention (1) (see Chapter 14), which is very similar to that recommended for all healthy adults (Chapter 2). In both these diets, the primary goal is achieving and maintaining a normal weight.

Following a U.S. Court of Appeals decision (Pearson v Shalala), the Food and Drug Administration revoked the regulations codifying its policy not to allow health claims for four substances and their relationship to disease to appear on food labels. These claims are for dietary fiber and cancer, antioxidant vitamins and cancer, ω-3 fatty acids and coronary artery disease, and 0.8-mg folate supplements to reduce neural tube defects versus lower amounts of folate in conventional food. However, reversal of the Food and Drug Administration policy is not the equivalent of claims by the Food and Drug Administration regarding substance–disease relationships. Such claims must now be individually assessed.

V. Drugs and nutrients

   A. **Effects of drugs on micronutrient metabolism** (see Table 3-2). The clinical importance of many such effects is often not apparent because the drugs are used for only a limited time.
   B. **Effect of vitamins and minerals on drug action** (Table 1-22). Although large doses of micronutrients are usually required to produce a clinical effect, the mechanism by which some sources of vitamins (e.g., grapefruit juice) affect drug metabolism (decreasing the area under the curve following absorption) differs from that of nutrient provision.

(text continues on page 29)

Table 1-19. Clinical laboratory tests for detection of vitamin deficiency

Vitamin	Test	Fluid	Reference range (units)[a]		Usefulness
			Marginal	Deficient	
B_1	Transketolase ratio	RBC	1.16–1.24	>1.25	+ when severe
	Thiamine	Serum		<12.7 (nmol/L)	Direct measure
	Thiamine	Urine		<27 (µg/g creat.)	Body stores
B_2	GSH reductase ratio	Serum	1.20–1.40	>1.40	Recent intake
	Riboflavin	Urine	27–79	<27 (µg/g creat.)	Body stores
B_6	AST activity ratio	RBC	1.70–1.85	>1.85	Body stores
	Pyridoxal-5-PO_4	Plasma	20–30	<20 (nmol/L)	Stores, sensitive
	4-pyridoxic acid	Urine		<3.0 (µmol/d)	Recent intake
	Total vitamin B_6	Urine		<0.5 (µmol/d)	Recent intake
Niacin	N-methylnicotinamide	Urine	0.5–2.5	<0.5 (mg/g creat.)	Recent intake
	2-pyridone	Urine	2.0–3.9	<2.0 (mg/g creat.)	Recent intake
Folate	Folic acid	Plasma	3.0–5.9	<3.0 (ng/mL)	Stores + intake
	Folic acid	RBC	140–159	<140 (ng/mL)	Body stores
Folate or B_{12}	Homocysteine	Plasma	12–15	>15 (µmol/L)	Function
	Cobalamin	Serum	150–200	<150 (pg/mL)	Body stores
	Methylmalonic acid	Serum		>376 (nmol/L)	Function
	Holotranscobalamin II	Serum	40–60	>60 (pg/mL)	Stores, sensitive
C	Ascorbic acid	Serum	11–23	<11 (µmol/L)	Recent intake
	Ascorbic acid	WBC	10–20	<10 (µg/10^8 cells)	Stores
A	Retinol	Plasma	10–19	<10 (µg/dL)	Stores + intake
	Retinol-binding protein	Plasma		<50 (mg/L)	Function
D	25-OH vitamin D	Serum	12–25	<12 (nmol/L)	Body stores
	1,25-$(OH)_2$ vitamin D	Serum	48–65	<48 (pmol/L)	Function
E	α-tocopherol	Serum	5.0–7.0	<5 (µg/mL)	Body stores
	α-tocopherol/total lipid	Serum	0.8–1.0	<0.8	Preferred
	H_2O_2 hemolysis	RBC	10–20	>20 (%)	Function
K	Prothrombin time	Plasma	1.5–2.0	>2.0 (sec. over function control)	Function
	Phylloquinone			<0.35 (nmol/L)	Recent intake

GSH, glutathione; AST, aspartate amino transferase. [a] Check local laboratory for variations from ranges.

Table 1-20. Clinical laboratory detection of micronutrient mineral deficiency

Nutrient	Test	Method	Reference range (units)[a]	Usefulness
Iron	Iron (serum)	Colorimetric	50–200 (mg/dL)	Poor measure of body stores
	Total iron binding (serum)	Colorimetric	245–400 (mg/dL)	
	Iron-binding capacity (TIBC)	Calculation	15–50 (%)	Insensitive for iron status
	Transferrin (serum)	Immunoturbidimetric	200–400 (mg/dL)	Preferred over TIBC if available
	Ferritin (serum)	Immunoturbidimetric	18–300 (ng/mL)	Measures body stores: high specificity when low, poor sensitivity
Zn	Zinc (plasma)	Flame atomic absorption	20–130 (mg/dL)	Poor specificity for body stores
	Zinc tolerance test (plasma Zn)	Flame atomic absorption	>2-fold increase over baseline at 2 h	For malabsorption
Cu	Copper (serum)	Flame atomic absorption	55–175 (mg/dL)	Insensitive for body stores
	Ceruloplasmin (plasma)	Immunoturbidimetric	10–60 (mg/dL)	Independent of body stores
Selenium	Selenium (serum)	Fluorometry	100–340 (ng/mL)	Insensitive for body stores
	Glutathione peroxidase (plasma)	Spectrophotometric	455–800 (U/L)	More sensitive for body stores

[a] Check local laboratory for variation from ranges.

Table 1-21. Classification of functional indices of vitamin status

Index	Nutrient tested
In vitro tests of in vivo function	
Capillary fragility	C
Enzyme stimulation	B_1, B_2, B_6
Red blood cell fragility	E
Lipid peroxidation (breath ethane/pentane)	E
Prothrombin time	K
Platelet aggregation	E
D-Uridine suppression	B_{12}, folic acid
Methylmalonic acid, homocysteine (urine, blood)	B_{12}, folic acid
Induced responses in vivo	
Histidine loading	Folic acid
Tryptophan loading	B_6
[^{14}C]Histidine or [^{14}C]serine (breath $^{14}CO_2$)	Folic acid
Relative dose response	A
Glucose loading followed by exercise	B_1
Oxygen/ozone loading (lipid peroxidation)	E
Urinary 3-OH-isovaleric acid after leucine loading	Biotin
Spontaneous in vivo response	
Abducens (cranial nerve VI) function	B_1
Central scotoma	A
Color discrimination	A
Dark adaptation/night blindness	A
Host defense	B_6
Nerve function	B_1, B_{12}
Neutrophilic hypersegmentation	B_{12}, folic acid
Olfactory acuity	A, B_{12}
Physical performance/endurance	B_1, B_2, B_6
Taste acuity	A
Vasopressor response	C

Modified from Shrijven J. Indices of vitamin status in men: an urgent need of functional markers. *Food Rev Int* 1991;7:1–32.

Table 1-22. Vitamins and minerals that affect drug action

Supplement	Drug	Effect
Vitamins		
Vitamin A	Alcohol	Hypervitaminosis A may enhance hepatotoxicity of alcohol.
	Isotretinoin	Additive toxic effects may result from combination therapy with vitamin A or other supplements containing vitamin A.
	Tetracycline	Combination therapy may enhance drug-induced intracranial hypertension (severe headache).
Vitamin D	Digoxin	Vitamin D-induced hypercalcemia may potentiate the effects of the drug and result in cardiac arrhythmias.
Vitamin E	Warfarin	May enhance anticoagulant response to warfarin.
Vitamin K	Warfarin	Vitamin K in liquid food supplements may inhibit the hypoprothrombic effect of drug.
Ascorbic acid	Fluphenazine	Large doses may interfere with drug absorption and result in a return of manic behavior.
	Warfarin	Megadoses may decrease prothrombin time.
Folacin	Methotrexate	Folacin or its derivatives in vitamin preparations may alter responses to drug.
	Phenytoin	May decrease anticonvulsant action of drug.
Pyridoxine	Levodopa	Reverses antiparkinsonism effect of drug.
	Phenytoin	Large doses may reduce phenytoin levels.
	Hydralazine, isoniazid, penicillamine	May correct drug-induced peripheral neuropathy.
Minerals		
Calcium, iron	Tetracycline	Concurrent use may decrease drug absorption.
Magnesium, zinc, iron	Penicillamine	Concurrent use may decrease drug effectiveness.

Modified from Pemberton CM. *Mayo Clinic diet manual,* 6th ed. Toronto: Decker, 1988.

Table 1-23. Examples of drug-induced alteration of food intake

Hypophagic drugs	Hyperphagic drugs	Drugs producing hypogeusia/dysgeusia
Alcohol	Amitriptyline hydrochloride	Amphetamines
Amphetamines	Anabolic steroids	Benzodiazepines
Cisplatin	Benzodiazepines	Captopril
Cocaine	Buclizine hydrochloride	Carbimazole
Diethylpropion	Chlortetracycline	Carbimazole
hydrochloride	Cyproheptadine hydrochloride	Chlorhexidine
Fenfluramine	Glucocorticoids	Chlorpromazine
hydrochloride	Phenothiazines	Clofibrate
Hydroxyurea	Reserpine	D-Penicillamine
Methotrexate	Sulfonylureas	Encainide
Metformin	Tricyclic antidepressants	Ethionamide
Phenmetrazine		5-Fluorouracil
hydrochloride		Gold salts
SSRIs		Griseofulvin
		Levodopa
		Lincomycin
		Lithium carbonate
		Methimazole
		Methocarbamol
		Methylthiouracil
		Oxyfedrine
		Penicillin
		Phenindione
		Propranolol
		Psychotropic agents
		Quinidine
		Vitamins (high-dose)

SSRI, selective serotonin reuptake inhibitor.

C. Drug-induced alterations of food intake. Many drugs (including alcohol) decrease appetite, especially in persons with chronic illness. Some drugs, especially tricyclic antidepressants, increase appetite in depressed and also nondepressed persons. Amitriptyline is the most active of this group and causes weight gain, perhaps in part through hyperphagia. Drugs are the most common cause of dysgeusia. Most chloride salts (or other halides) are secreted in saliva and may affect taste. Drugs with anticholinergic effects cause dry mouth and may affect appetite. Table 1-23 lists some drugs that commonly affect food intake.

References
1. World Cancer Research Fund/American Institute for Cancer Research. *Food, nutrition, and the prevention of cancer: a global perspective.* Washington, DC: WCRF/AICR 1997.
2. World Health Organization. *Trace elements in human nutrition and health.* Prepared in collaboration with the Food and Agriculture Organization of the United Nations and the International Atomic Energy Agency. Geneva: WHO, 1996.
3. Standing Committee on the Scientific Evaluation of Dietary Reference Intakes, Food and Nutrition Board, Institute of Medicine. *Dietary reference intakes for calcium, phosphorus, magnesium, vitamin D, and fluoride.* Washington, DC: National Academy Press, 1997.
4. Standing Committee on the Scientific Evaluation of Dietary Reference Intakes, Food and Nutrition Board, Institute of Medicine. *Dietary reference intakes for thiamin, riboflavin, niacin, vitamin B₆, folate, vitamin B₁₂, pantothenic acid, biotin, and choline.* Washington, DC: National Academy Press, 2000.

5. Standing Committee on the Scientific Evaluation of Dietary Reference Intakes, Food and Nutrition Board, Institute of Medicine. *Dietary reference intakes for vitamin E, vitamin C, selenium, and carotenoids.* Washington, DC: National Academy Press, 2000.
6. Standing Committee on the Scientific Evaluation of Dietary Reference Intakes, Food and Nutrition Board, Institute of Medicine. *Dietary reference intakes for vitamin A, vitamin K, arsenic, boron, chromium, copper, iodine, iron, manganese, molybdenum, nickel, silicon, vanadium, and zinc.* Washington, DC: National Academy Press, 2001. File available online at *http://www.nap.edu/books/0309072794/html.* Accessed January 14, 2001.
7. U.S. Department of Agriculture, Food and Drug Administration. *Food additives.* Washington, DC: U.S. Government Printing Office, 1992.
8. Sarubin A. *The health professional's guide to popular dietary supplements.* Chicago: The American Dietetic Association, 1999.
9. Pascal G. Safety assessment of food additives and flavoring substances. In: van der Heijden K, Younes M, Fishbein L, Miller S, eds. *International food safety handbook.* New York: Marcel Dekker Inc, 1999:239.

2. RECOMMENDATIONS FOR HEALTHY YOUNG ADULTS

I. Introduction. Despite the extensive array of volumes on nutrition, diet, and health displayed in bookstores today, virtually all expert scientific panels reporting guidelines for good nutritional practice have devised remarkably simple and consistent recommendations for healthy adults. The most widely disseminated general recommendations for healthy adults are included in two reports. The first, which represents the combined recommendations of the U.S. Department of Agriculture and the U.S. Department of Health and Human Services, is called *Nutrition and Your Health: Dietary Guidelines for Americans, 2000* (1); the second, *AHA Dietary Guidelines Revision 2000: a Statement for Health Care Professionals from the Nutrition Committee of the American Heart Association,* reflects the recommendations of the American Heart Association (2).

A. Dietary Guidelines for Americans, 2000. *Dietary Guidelines for Americans, 2000* (1) offers 10 guidelines for a healthy diet grouped under three principal themes: Aim for Fitness, Build a Healthy Base, and Choose Sensibly. The Aim for Fitness theme encompasses two recommendations, one for healthy weight maintenance and one for regular daily physical activity. The Build a Healthy Base theme provides four guidelines directed at choosing a variety of grains daily, choosing a variety of fruits and vegetables daily, using the U.S. Department of Agriculture Food Guide Pyramid as an aid in food selection (Fig. 2-1), and developing habits that minimize the risk for food-borne illness. The Choose Sensibly aim develops three guidelines for maintaining a diet low in saturated fat and cholesterol, with moderate amounts of sugars and a lesser amount of salt, and a fourth guideline for limiting the intake of alcoholic beverages.

B. American Heart Association Dietary Guidelines Revision 2000. The *AHA Dietary Guidelines Revision 2000* (2) recommends four population goals: A Healthy Eating Pattern Including Foods from All Major Food Groups, A Healthy Body Weight, A Desirable Blood Cholesterol and Lipoprotein Profile, and A Desirable Blood Pressure. The Healthy Eating Pattern goal is based on recommendations for consuming a variety of fruits, vegetables, and grain products and including low-fat or nonfat dairy products, fish, legumes, poultry, and lean meats in the diet. The Healthy Body Weight goal recommends matching energy intake with energy needs, limiting the consumption of foods with a high caloric density or poor nutritional quality, and maintaining a level of physical activity that is compatible with fitness and balances energy intake. The Desirable Blood Cholesterol and Lipoprotein Profile goal recommends limiting the intake of foods high in saturated fatty acids and cholesterol, and substituting grains and unsaturated fatty acids derived from vegetables, fish, legumes, and nuts. The Desirable Blood Pressure goal recommends limiting dietary intake of salt and consumption of alcohol while reinforcing the need for maintaining a healthy body weight and consuming the dietary pattern detailed in the other aims.

II. Consolidated recommendations. From the brief summary presented above, the common guiding principles and overall similarity of the recommendations outlined by the two expert committees should be readily apparent. Further, both sets of guidelines emphasize consuming adequate amounts of the known essential nutrients and incorporating healthy dietary practices into lifestyle patterns to be maintained throughout life. Together, these two sets of dietary recommendations can be consolidated as follows:

A. Do not become obese. Obesity is the most significant form of malnutrition in the United States today. Data obtained in the third National Health and Nutrition Examination Survey (NHANES III), completed in 1994, show that 55% of adults, 11% of adolescents, and 14% of children are overweight (3,4). During approximately the last 30 years, the prevalence of overweight adults

31

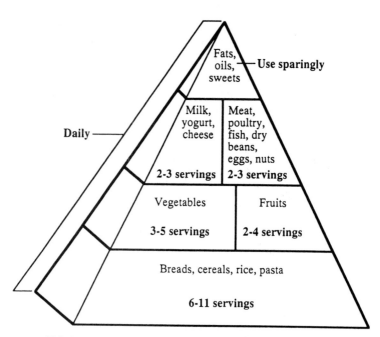

FIG. 2.1. U.S. Department of Agriculture food guide pyramid.

has increased about 12%, overweight adolescents about 6%, and overweight children about 8.5% (3,4). Obesity is associated with an increased risk for morbidity and mortality from coronary heart disease, hypertension, type II non–insulin-dependent diabetes, arthritis, gallstones, and endometrial cancer. In the Framingham Heart Study, the risk for death within 26 years increased by 1% for *each* extra pound gained between 30 and 42 years of age, and increased by 2% for *each* pound gained between 50 and 62 years of age (5).

The first step in devising a dietary plan is to set one's energy intake at a level to maintain a body mass index (BMI), which is one's weight in kilograms divided by the square of one's height in meters, within the normal adult range of 19 to 25. Remember, however, that all initial estimates of dietary energy intake for an individual person are just that, crude estimates, and must be refined upward or downward based on that person's body weight response to the initial approximation.

The resting energy expenditure (in kilocalories per day) for adult men can be estimated from body weight (in kilograms) according to the following equations (see also Chapter 5 for other methods of estimation) (6):

$$REE = (15.3 \times weight) + 679 \text{ for } 18\text{- to } 30\text{-year-olds}$$

$$REE = (11.6 \times weight) + 879 \text{ for } 30\text{- to } 60\text{-year-olds}$$

Similar estimates for adult women can be obtained from the following equations:

$$REE = (14.7 \times weight) + 496 \text{ for } 18\text{- to } 30\text{-year-olds}$$

$$REE = (8.7 \times weight) + 829 \text{ for } 30\text{- to } 60\text{-year-olds}$$

Very light physical activity requires 1.5 times the REE, light physical activity uses 2.5 REE, moderate physical activity burns 5.5 REE, and heavy physical activity 7.0 REE. For the purposes of estimating a daily dietary energy intake for young adult men, the National Academy of Sciences Food and Nutrition Board set an average overall daily activity level of 1.60 REE for young men and 1.55 REE for young women (6). For a 79-kg man and 63-kg woman, then, the average daily energy allowances are 2,900 kcal (37 kcal/kg) and 2,200 kcal (36 kcal/kg), respectively. The normal intersubject variation of approximately ±20% shows that the algorithms above are crude estimates only and must be tailored to the individual person.

B. **Be physically active on a daily basis.** Avoid a sedentary lifestyle. Regular physical activity burns calories. In addition, it is conducive to cardiovascular fitness; reduces the risk for heart disease, colon cancer, and type II diabetes; maintains muscle and bone health; enhances muscle strength and endurance; helps control blood pressure; and promotes psychological well-being. At least 30 minutes of moderate physical activity is recommended on most days of the week (7). Physical activity in this context should be interpreted to include not only activities traditionally considered to be "exercise," but also the routine activities of daily life, such as walking, bicycle riding, gardening, mowing the lawn, climbing stairs, cleaning the house, and others.

C. **Enjoy a wide variety of foods.** No single food can supply all the known essential nutrients in sufficient amounts. For this reason, it is imperative to consume a wide variety of foods, both within and among the different food groups. Additionally, variety enhances the enjoyment of eating. Nonetheless, in our society, where an abundance of affordable food is readily available, persons who expend relatively low amounts of energy on a daily basis are at increased risk for becoming obese. To maintain a healthy weight, particular attention must also be paid to portion size and to the energy and nutrient densities of the foods consumed. In these circumstances, foods that are low in energy but relatively nutrient-dense (e.g., fruits and vegetables) are preferable to energy-dense foods that are relatively nutrient-poor (e.g., fats, oils, and alcohol.)

D. **Consume a variety of fruits, vegetables, and grain products daily.** Dietary patterns characterized by the consumption of large amounts of fruits, vegetables, and grains (especially whole grains) have been associated with decreased risks for cardiovascular disease, stroke, hypertension (2), and certain cancers (8) (see also Tables 14-1, 14-2, and 14-3). That these food components should form the basis of a healthy diet is indicated by their position in the bottom two tiers of the food guide pyramid (Fig. 2-1). In addition, because they are rich in nutrients but low in caloric density, these foods help one to maintain a healthful weight, and because they are high in fiber, they may promote satiety, enhance bowel function, and modestly lower blood cholesterol levels. On average, at least two to four servings of fruit, three to five servings of vegetables, and six to 11 servings of grains should be consumed daily.

Vegetables, fruits, and grains are significant sources of vitamins A, C, and K, folate, niacin, and riboflavin; of the minerals potassium, magnesium, and manganese; and of dietary fiber. The dietary reference intakes (DRIs) and recommended dietary allowances (RDAs) for these nutrients are shown in Appendix B. No dietary requirement for fiber has been established, although it has a variety of beneficial effects in the gastrointestinal tract and may reduce the incidence of colon cancer and cardiovascular disease. The average daily fiber intake in the United States is estimated to be about 12 g/d.

Fresh fruits and vegetables should be included. When vegetables are cooked, a minimal amount of water should be used and the vegetables cooked only until tender to limit the loss of vitamins and nutrients. Whole grains should be consumed whenever possible because the plant endosperm and bran are rich in nutrients and fiber. Legumes are good sources of vegetable protein in addition to fiber. Because most fruits, vegetables, and grains are also low in fat, they are good alternatives to high-fat foods.

E. Choose a diet low in saturated fats and cholesterol. More than 30 years of extensive epidemiologic research have shown that heart disease is increased in populations and persons who consume diets high in saturated fats and, to a lesser extent, cholesterol (2,9). Likewise, recent evidence indicates that the *trans* fatty acids present in processed foods containing partially hydrogenated vegetable oils act like saturated fatty acids in that they increase serum low-density-lipoprotein (LDL) cholesterol. For these reasons, it is prudent to limit one's combined intake of dietary saturated and *trans* fatty acids to less than 10% of total energy intake, and to limit dietary cholesterol intake to less than 300 mg/d. Until recently, these recommendations were part of a general recommendation to reduce the total dietary intake of fat. However, current guidelines recommend a moderate total intake of fat of approximately 30% of dietary energy. In part, this recommendation reflects the currently large data sets showing that blood lipoprotein patterns are favorable in persons who consume moderate total amounts of fat when the fats consist predominantly of polyunsaturated fatty acids rather than saturated fatty acids (9). Additionally, ω-3 fatty acids, particularly the long-chain ω-3 fatty acids found in fish oils [docosahexanoic acid (DHA) and eicosapentenoic acid (EPA)], may have the specific beneficial effects of diminishing the risk for coronary artery disease (2). Finally, although reducing the total fat intake may aid in preventing excessive consumption of dietary energy and help maintain body weight, the evidence that low-fat diets reduce the risk for various forms of cancer is now less than compelling (9).

Beef, pork, liver and other organ meats, processed meats and cold cuts, whole milk, nondairy creamers, cheese, ice cream, eggs, butter, margarine, mayonnaise, lard, shortening, salad and cooking oils, deep-fried foods of all types, pastries, doughnuts, cookies, pie crusts, and cakes represent the major sources of fat, saturated fat, and cholesterol in the American diet. Further, various prepared foods often contain significant amounts of "hidden" fat. An informed consumer *always* reads the label. A good rule of thumb for reducing cholesterol and total and saturated fat intake is to limit one's daily intake of meat, fish, and poultry to 2 to 3 servings (cooked weight of no more than about 5 to 7 oz).

F. Exercise moderation in salt and sugar consumption. These two dietary recommendations are the subject of more conflicting data and therefore of more ongoing debate than all the others combined. The debate about salt does not focus on the generally agreed-on importance of limiting salt to control blood pressure in hypertensive persons. Rather, the issue centers on the need to restrict sodium intake in the general population (9), in which, most would agree, far more salt is consumed than is physiologically necessary. Based on recent clinical studies and metaanalyses of earlier studies, the consensus view is that moderate salt intake is a prudent approach. For adults, a daily intake of 6 g of salt (2.4 g of sodium) is considered an approachable goal. However, achieving this goal can be very difficult because the principal sources of salt are processed and prepared foods, over which the consumer has little control other than nonconsumption.

The debate about sugar intake is no less vocal, although the data indicating that dietary sugars are harmful to health are far less compelling than those for salt. In fact, the only convincing medical consequence of excessive sugar intake is the development of dental caries and, even here, sugar intake is only one of many contributing factors. No evidence is available to indicate that sugars *per se* cause many of the problems commonly attributed to them, such as hyperactivity, obesity, and diabetes. Additionally, no evidence indicates that "added sugars" produce effects different from those of intrinsic sugars, and absolutely no controlled data have demonstrated beneficial effects of low-sugar diets at any level. Because dietary sugars are often consumed in foods that have a lower density of other nutrients, the principal reason for recommending moderate sugar consumption is to prevent the consumption of unnecessary calories, or "dilution" of the intake of other essential nutrients in the diet (1,9). Nonetheless, this argument also applies to selective overconsumption of the other macronutrients and is not unique to sugars. In controlled feeding studies, diets with a high sugar content do not promote weight gain if energy intake is maintained at the isocaloric level. One unsettled concern about dietary sugar intake is the development of hypertriglyceridemia, decreased concentrations of high-density lipoproteins, and increased concentrations of low-density lipoproteins in some persons consuming a high-carbohydrate diet, a lipoprotein pattern that is associated with atherogenesis. The implications of these observations for the general population remain unresolved at this time.

G. **Drink alcoholic beverages in moderation, if at all, and don't smoke.** The evidence for the detrimental effects of smoking on health is overwhelming. Although data now suggest that one and two alcoholic drinks daily for women and men, respectively, may reduce the risk for cardiovascular disease, far more ample evidence indicates that excessive consumption of alcohol has significant detrimental effects on health, including increased risks for hypertension, stroke, liver disease, some cancers (10), accidents, violent behavior, and suicide. For these reasons, one should consider whether any consumption of alcoholic beverages is prudent. Further, because the risks of alcohol consumption during embryogenesis and fetal development are well established (9), pregnant women and women of childbearing age who may become pregnant should not consume alcohol.

H. **Moderate your protein intake.** The RDA for protein in young adults of both sexes is 0.8 g/kg per day (6). The RDA for protein represents about 10% of dietary energy intake for young adults. The average protein intake of young American adults is significantly greater than 1 g/d (4,6). No evidence indicates that intake above the RDA has any benefit, although modest increments above this level, representing 12% to 15% of total energy intake, are more likely to be consistent with current lifestyle habits. These increments should be plant rather than animal protein; sources of animal protein are more expensive as a rule and are also generally high in fat calories, saturated fat, and cholesterol. Additionally, prolonged high intake of animal protein is suspected to contribute to renal failure, reduced bone density, and cancers of the breast and colon. However, elimination of all animal sources of protein is not necessarily desirable because these foods are the only source of vitamin B_{12}, the best source of readily absorbable iron, and a good source of zinc.

I. **Maintain an adequate intake of calcium.** Adequate cellular function, skeletal growth, and proper bone and dental mineralization require the essential nutrient calcium. All but about 1% of total body calcium is found within bones and teeth. Accelerated rates of calcium deposition occur at or near the onset of puberty and continue during the adolescent growth spurt. The net gain of bone calcium during early adolescence is a critical determinant in the prevention of osteoporosis much later in life. After menarche, net bone calcium deposition rates fall, and by the age of about 20, bone calcium accretion is essentially complete. Thus, consumption of adequate dietary calcium intake is especially important for teenagers, particularly girls. Similarly, maintaining optimal bone mineralization during young adult life is equally important. An adequate intake (AI) of calcium is 1,300 mg daily for adolescent boys and girls 9 to 18 years of age (11). For adult men and women between the ages of 19 and 50, the calcium AI is 1,000 g/d (11). Pregnancy or lactation does not alter these values for adolescent or adult women (11).

The principal dietary sources of calcium are milk and milk products. To maintain the dietary objective of reduced saturated fat intake, the best approach to achieving adequate calcium intake is consumption of low-fat or nonfat milk and milk products in addition to fruit juices and soy products with added calcium. Although calcium is also found in various dark green leafy vegetables, the oxalic acid in some of these vegetables (e.g., spinach) makes the calcium less bioavailable. Although inadequate calcium intake is associated with an increased incidence of fractures, and although some (albeit debatable) evidence suggests that inadequate calcium intake may contribute to hypertension, thus far evidence is unconvincing that additional protective effects are conferred by the consumption of calcium above AI levels in supplements and by other means. The tolerable upper intake level (UL) of calcium is 2.5 g/d for children and adults (11).

J. Do not take unnecessary dietary supplements in excessive amounts.
Except for selected persons in special circumstances, nutritional needs can be met with ordinary foods (6). Approximately half of adults in the United States take a vitamin or mineral supplement with some regularity. A single daily multivitamin and mineral supplement containing 100% of the RDA is not known to be harmful, but neither is it known to be beneficial for the vast majority of persons already meeting their nutritional needs by consuming a regular diet. By and large, persons who take supplements are those who are more likely to consume an adequate diet. Little evidence is available to indicate that such persons will reap a sizable health "dividend" from this form of nutrition "insurance." At the present time, no convincing direct evidence indicates that the consumption of "pharmacologic" amounts of vitamins, minerals, antioxidants, and other food constituents of unknown or dubious function has any direct, long-term effect of preventing chronic disease in persons who consume a balanced diet containing essential nutrients at the RDA level (1,2,9,11–14).

III. Implementation guidance. Figure 2-1 shows the U.S. Department of Agriculture food guide pyramid, a schematic illustration designed to facilitate visualization of the U.S. Department of Agriculture and U.S. Department of Health and Human Services recommendations for dietary health and to aid the consumer in planning meals. The relative sizes of the blocks of the pyramid are meant to reflect the relative proportions of the constituents within each block to be maintained in overall daily energy intake. (See also Chapter 11, Section IA, for further details on use of the food guide pyramid.)

At the base of the pyramid are grain foods, breads, cereals, rice, and pasta, which form the foundation of a healthy diet. Six to 11 servings are recommended daily. Within this group, a serving is equivalent to one slice of bread, one cup of ready-to-eat cereal, or one-half cup of cooked cereal, rice, or pasta.

The second level of the pyramid includes the fruits (two to four servings daily) and vegetables (three to five servings daily). A vegetable serving is the equivalent of one cup of raw leafy vegetables, three-fourths cup of vegetable juice, or one-half cup of other cooked or raw vegetables. Correspondingly, a fruit serving consists of one medium apple, banana, orange, pear, or similar fruit; three-fourths cup of fruit juice; or one-half cup of other raw, cooked, or canned fruits.

The third level of the pyramid reflects primarily animal foods, including meat, poultry, fish, eggs, and milk and milk products, of which two or three daily servings of each class are recommended. In the dairy group, one cup of milk or yogurt constitutes a serving, as does 1.5 oz of natural cheese and 2 oz of processed cheese. In the "meat" group, one serving consists of 2 to 3 oz of cooked lean meat, poultry, or fish. One-half cup of cooked dry beans, one-half cup of tofu, one-third cup of nuts, or two tablespoons of peanut butter are considered the equivalent of 1 oz ounce of meat.

The apex of the pyramid includes fats, oils, and sweets, which are important components of a healthy diet when consumed in moderation according to the guidelines presented above.

Figure 2-2 depicts the *Mediterranean diet pyramid,* an alternative schematic illustration devised by the Harvard School of Public Health, the European office of the World Health Organization, and the Oldways Preservation and Exchange Trust. The goal of this formulation is to emulate the diet of those Mediterranean regions where life expectancy is high and rates of chronic diseases are low. In many ways, the Mediterranean and U.S. Department of Agriculture diet pyramids are similar. Both aim for consumption of a largely plant-based diet. In both, the foundation of the diet is grain products, with lib-

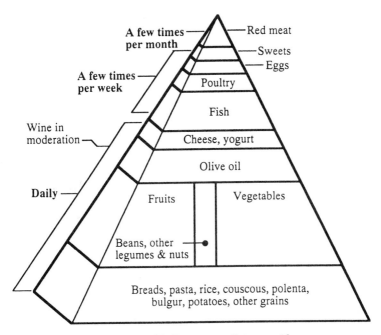

FIG. 2.2. The Mediterranean diet pyramid.

eral consumption of fruits and vegetables. Furthermore, beans, nuts, eggs, fish, and poultry, on the whole, occupy similar fractions of overall energy intake over time. Each diet more than adequately meets vitamin requirements. On the other hand, dairy products, particularly milk, comprise a smaller fraction of the Mediterranean diet, so that marginal calcium intakes are provided according to the current U.S. recommendations. Also, although both diets recommend consumption of unsaturated rather than saturated fats, the Mediterranean pyramid includes a more liberal amount of oils than the U.S. Department of Agriculture pyramid; however, recent dietary recommendations (1,2) more closely approach those of the Mediterranean pyramid. A significantly smaller intake of red meat is recommended in the Mediterranean pyramid, which can lead to a marginal intake of zinc or iron, particularly if phytate intake is high. Finally, the U.S. Department of Agriculture pyramid does not include alcohol, and the *Dietary Guidelines for Americans, 2000* recommend moderate ingestion, if any, as discussed above. The Mediterranean pyramid recommends daily wine consumption in moderation, and it is conceivable that the recommendation for moderate alcohol consumption may be applied more sensibly in European countries, where wine consumption is part of the traditional lifestyle. This recommendation, however, remains controversial in the United States. Nonetheless, if persons actually consume alcohol "in moderation," according to the quantities specified in both schemes, the recommendations are not seriously disparate.

In any case, rather than confuse the basic issues by highlighting differences between the two pyramid approaches, it is important to emphasize that both aim to maximize plant foods, minimize animal sources of saturated fat and cholesterol, and provide dietary fat in the form of monounsaturated or polyunsaturated oils. Consumers' attention to adequate intakes of calcium, iron, and zinc and a truly sensible approach to alcohol intake will reduce any remaining disparities between these dietary guidelines.

IV. Suggestions for implementation. The following are various practical suggestions for achieving the dietary guidelines outlined earlier.

  A. Cook at home as frequently as possible. At home, you can best control the composition of your diet. Restaurant food, particularly "fast food," tends to be high in fat, cholesterol, and salt. If you eat out, ask the chef to prepare food the way you want it. After all, that's his or her job, and you're paying the bill.

  B. Start shopping in the supermarket produce department. Continue around the perimeter of the store, where fresh foods, unprocessed foods, fish, poultry, and dairy products are generally located. Avoid processed foods, and be careful not to consume too many foods that can contribute more calories to your diet than nutrients.

  C. Always read the label. *Repeat,* always read the label. With the present vast array of food technologies and the plethora of foods prepared accordingly and obtainable in today's supermarket, it is impossible to know the actual composition of a processed food without reading the label. Virtually all processed foods must carry the new food label described in Appendix C. The information on the label provides a good guide to the calories in a product, in addition to the content of fat, protein, carbohydrate, sodium, calcium, iron, and vitamins A and C. Reading the label will help you identify hidden sources of dietary fat.

  D. Understand the difference between grams of fat and percentage of calories from fat. The dietary guidelines discussed earlier include moderating total fat intake to about 30% of total calorie intake. For example, while 8 oz of plain yogurt made from whole milk contains 8 g of fat and 150 calories, nearly 50% of the calories in the yogurt come from fat because 8 g of fat provides 72 cal.

  E. Steam, broil, bake, or microwave foods to avoid increasing the fat content. Stir-frying is an additional acceptable alternative because proper stir-frying techniques require intense heat but almost no fat. Use nonstick cookware and very little oil when sautéeing.

  F. Slowly **wean yourself from adding salt** while cooking or eating. Proper seasoning with herbs and spices helps reduce the need for salt. The taste for salt is largely acquired, and once you adapt to the taste of unsalted food, you will find salted food "too salty."

  G. Maintain calcium intake by consuming low-fat or nonfat dairy products. Although regular dairy products are the best source of dietary calcium, they are also the second-largest source of saturated fats after meats, the leading source. However, a very large array of reduced-fat or nonfat dairy products of all descriptions is now available in supermarkets, in addition to a variety of calcium-fortified juices and other products. These facilitate attaining the adult AI for calcium without jeopardizing the goals for fat reduction.

  H. Avoid fads and "magic bullets." Excellent nutritional health can be achieved by following the sensible dietary guidelines discussed previously. No fad diet has ever been shown to provide better nutrition, and many have been shown to provide less than adequate nutrition. Similarly, no individual plant, animal, biochemical, or chemical "magic bullet" has ever been shown to achieve effects beyond those provided by a nutritionally adequate diet alone.

References

1. U.S. Department of Health and Human Services, U.S. Department of Agriculture. *Nutrition and your health: dietary guidelines for Americans, 2000* 5th ed. Washington, DC: U.S. Government Printing Office, 2000. Booklet online, available at *http://www.usda.gov/cnpp/DietGd.pdf.* Accessed December 11, 2000.
2. Krauss RM, Eckel RH, Howard B, et al. AHA dietary guidelines revision 2000: a statement for healthcare professionals from the nutrition committee of the American Heart Association. *Circulation* 2000;102:2284.

3. Flegal KM, Carroll MD, Kuczmarski RJ, et al. Overweight and obesity in the United States: prevalence and trends, 1960–94. *Int J Obes Relat Metab Disord* 1998;6:51S.
4. U.S. Department of Health and Human Services, Centers for Disease Control and Prevention, National Center for Health Statistics. Third National Health and Nutrition Examination Survey (NHANES III) public use data files, 2000. File online available at *http://www.cdc.gov/nchs/products/catalogs/subject/nhanes3/nhanes3.htm*. Accessed December 11, 2000.
5. Hubert HB. The importance of obesity in the development of coronary risk factors and disease: the epidemiological evidence. *Annu Rev Public Health* 1986;7:493.
6. National Research Council. *Recommended dietary allowances,* 10th ed. Washington, DC: National Academy Press, 1989.
7. Pate RR, Pratt M, Blair SN, et al. Physical activity and public health: a recommendation from the Centers for Disease Control and Prevention and the American College of Sports Medicine. *JAMA* 1995;273:402.
8. Jacobs DR Jr, Marquart L, Slabin J, et al. Whole grain intake and cancer: an expanded review and meta-analysis. *Nutr Cancer* 1998;30:85.
9. U.S. Department of Health and Human Services, U.S. Department of Agriculture. Dietary Guidelines Advisory Committee. *Report of the Dietary Guidelines Advisory Committee on the Dietary Guidelines for Americans, 2000,* 5th ed. Washington, DC: U.S. Government Printing Office, 2000. Report online available at *http://www.usda.gov/cnpp/Pubs/DG2000/Full%20Report.pdf*. Accessed December 11, 2000.
10. Smith-Warner SA, Spiegelman D, Yaun S, et al. Alcohol and breast cancer in women: a pooled analysis of cohort studies. *JAMA* 1996;279:535.
11. Standing Committee on the Scientific Evaluation of Dietary Reference Intakes, Food and Nutrition Board, Institute of Medicine. *Dietary reference intakes for calcium, phosphorus, magnesium, vitamin D, and fluoride.* Washington, DC: National Academy Press, 1997.
12. Standing Committee on the Scientific Evaluation of Dietary Reference Intakes, Food and Nutrition Board, Institute of Medicine. *Dietary reference intakes for thiamin, niacin, vitamin B_6, folate, vitamin B_{12}, pantothenic acid, biotin, and choline.* Washington, DC: National Academy Press, 1998.
13. Standing Committee on the Scientific Evaluation of Dietary Reference Intakes, Food and Nutrition Board, Institute of Medicine. *Dietary reference intakes for vitamin C, vitamin E, selenium, and carotenoids.* Washington, DC: National Academy Press, 2000.
14. Standing Committee on the Scientific Evaluation of Dietary Reference Intakes, Food and Nutrition Board, Institute of Medicine. *Dietary reference intakes for vitamin A, vitamin K, arsenic, boron, chromium, copper, iodine, iron, manganese, molybdenum, nickel, silicon, vanadium, and zinc.* Washington, DC: National Academy Press, 2001.

3. RECOMMENDATIONS FOR HEALTHY ELDERLY ADULTS

I. Introduction

A. Definitions. Aging is a continuous function, and one does not suddenly pass from young to elderly at a precise age. Furthermore, chronologic age alone is not a particularly precise measure of biologic or functional age because individual characteristics, such as physical ability and mental health, vary widely as people become older. No uniform legal criteria exist. At age 60, a person can participate in the benefits of the Older Americans Act, but the same person does not receive Medicare or full Social Security benefits until age 65. Society has its own arbitrary definition. Age 60 defines an old age pensioner in the United Kingdom. Many banks, theaters, shops, and service organizations in the United States offer discounts or special services to senior citizens, but the eligibility criteria for " senior citizen" vary widely. At age 50, a person can join the largest service and lobbying group for the elderly in the United States, the American Association of Retired Persons, whether the person is retired or not. Only recently, the U.S. Census Bureau recognized the demographic heterogeneity of the elderly by classifying them into three groups: ages 65 through 74, 75 through 84, and 85 or older.

B. Population trends. In 1998, 42 million Americans (15.7% of the population) were 60 or more years of age, and 3 million Americans (6.9% of the population) were 85 or more years of age (1,2). Projections estimate that 69 million Americans (20% of the population) will be over the age of 65 in the year 2030. Even more importantly, the elderly population is getting older. From 1980 to 1990, the number of American women age 85 years or older increased by 43%, and the corresponding number of American men increased by 24%. The number of Americans age 85 years or older is expected to double by 2025 and to increase fivefold by 2050, when the last cohort of "baby boomers" will enter this category. The data in this chapter refer to the U.S. population. Similar trends occur in aging populations in other developed countries.

C. Life expectancy. During the twentieth century, the average life expectancy of an American increased 56%, from a mean of 47 years at the beginning of the century to 73.8 years for men and 79.7 years for women in 1999 (3,4). At the same time, the age-adjusted death rate declined 74%, and the leading causes of death changed from infections to consequences of chronic diseases. Approximately 60% of the gain in life span, however, represents improved survival in infancy and childhood because of immunization, treatment of infectious diseases, and public health sanitary measures, including safe food and water supplies. Another 15% to 20% gain in life span represents reductions in young adult mortality. Once a person reaches maturity, the gain is less. The average 65-year-old man today lives 3 years longer and the average 65-year-old woman today lives an average of 6 years longer than corresponding adults who reached age 65 in 1990. Overall, women live about 7 years longer than men. Current trends in mortality lead to the conclusion that more than half of the elderly population will be older than 75 years by the turn of the century, and about half will live to age 85 in the year 2010. By the middle of the twenty-first century, half the *entire* U.S. population will be over the age of 50 years.

D. Dietary intakes. The third National Health and Nutrition Examination Survey (NHANES III) collected data on the health and nutritional status of representative adults from across the nation between 1988 and 1994. In persons over the age of 50, dietary energy intake declined with increasing age and was below the recommended dietary allowance (RDA) for both men and women. Calcium intake was well below RDA levels. These data are consistent with various other surveys of dietary energy and calcium intake in elderly adults. Vitamin D levels tend to be low in elderly adults who do not consume vitamin D-fortified dairy products. Vitamin E intakes were low, but this was likely the result of underreporting (see below). On the other hand, according to the NHANES data, the dietary intakes of protein, iron, niacin, thiamine, riboflavin, and vitamin C in elderly adults were within acceptable ranges. Information from assorted other studies on dietary intakes of folate and vitamin B_{12} support the fact that a significant minority of elderly adults do not consume these vitamins in adequate amounts or do not absorb them adequately, as in the case of impaired B_{12} absorption secondary to atrophic gastritis. Nonetheless, one of the considerations in interpreting the adequacy of nutrient intake levels based on the RDAs is the fact that adults should be consuming less than the RDAs because these are set at the upper end of the normal distribution curve to ensure adequacy in nearly all persons. A convenient, conventional population index of potential nutrient inadequacies is the fraction of the population consuming less than two-thirds of the RDA. Nonetheless, the amount of a nutrient necessarily adequate for an individual elderly adult is not known accurately or precisely without specific biochemical testing. By and large, elderly persons are more likely to be nutritionally deficient as they advance in age and if they are poor or institutionalized.

II. Pathobiology of aging

A. Theories of aging. Aging has no known cause. A variety of currently popular theories are shown in Table 3-1. These include the following: inexorable results of damage caused by the continuous generation of free radicals during aerobic metabolism; consequences of the accumulation of altered proteins resulting from oxidative damage; glycosylation and other posttranslational modifications; additive effects of the imperfect repair of damaged DNA; conclusion of a finite number of absolute cell divisions as a consequence of telomere shortening; cumulative effects of impaired immunologic competence or autoimmune destruction; accelerated apoptosis; winding down of an internal chronobiologic clock; and consequences of accumulated inadequacies of energy metabolism.

Recent intriguing recent data in this area have provided support for the fact that diminished proteosome function may contribute to accumulation of oxidatively damaged proteins (5), that accelerated apoptosis may play an important role in the aging process (6), that circulating humoral factor(s) may act as "antiaging" hormones (7), that telomere length may be an important determinant in aging and carcinogenesis (8,9), and that alterations in genes that limit energy metabolism may provide mechanisms for the long-observed extension of the life span in calorie restriction models of aging (10).

B. Pathophysiologic consequences of aging

  1. Body composition. Lean body mass declines approximately 6% per decade after age 30. To a significant extent, this decrement is a consequence of diminished physical activity rather than of the aging process itself.

Table 3-1. Selected theories of aging

Free radical damage

Accumulation of damaged proteins
  Oxidized, glycosylated, and cross-linked protein
  Diminished proteosome activity

Defective protein synthesis

Enhanced apoptosis

Faulty DNA repair

Finite capacity for cell divisions
  Telomere attrition

Impaired immunocompetence and autoimmune destruction

"Winding down" of biologic clock

Defect in energy metabolism

     a. Obesity. One consequence of the decline in lean body mass is a corresponding increase in fat mass. Many elderly persons are overweight and frankly obese. Others who fit within normal weight-for-height ranges are relatively obese–that is, they have a disproportionate increase in adipose tissue.

     b. Protein metabolism. Rates of whole body protein turnover (synthesis and breakdown) decline slightly with age. When corrected for the age-related changes in lean body mass, however, protein turnover rates are relatively constant throughout adult life. No evidence indicates that protein needs are altered by aging; the net nitrogen balance (the difference between the slower protein synthesis and slower protein breakdown rates) is achieved at the same levels of dietary protein intake in aging persons.

  2. Energy expenditure. Energy is expended principally by the metabolically active lean tissues. Because lean body mass declines with age, energy expenditure declines correspondingly. Thus, to maintain energy balance, an elderly person must consume fewer calories. This is the most uniform and consistent nutritional consequence of aging.

  3. Gastrointestinal function. During aging, a generalized decline in organ function involves the gastrointestinal system, but not its absorptive or nutrient assimilation properties. Aging is associated with diminished smell and taste, particularly the loss of sweet and salty tastes. A reduction in salivary flow, loss of teeth, and disturbances of swallowing and esophageal dysfunction may be noted. Many persons experience various forms of discomfort in associated with eating, including heartburn, gas, and constipation. Approximately 10% to 30% of persons over age 60 have atrophic gastritis, and its prevalence reaches about 40% over age 80. Although originally thought to be a consequence of aging, atrophic gastritis appears to be caused by infection with *Helicobacter pylori*. Reductions in gastric acid, pepsin, and intrinsic factor lead to slower emptying of mixed meals and diminished absorption of iron, folate, and vitamin B_{12}. Bacterial overgrowth in the proximal small bowel is sometimes an accompanying feature. Pancreatic secretion is usually normal, but some people have a reduced hepatic function that is secondary to reduced blood flow, not altered hepatocyte function. Nonetheless, except for the vitamins and iron mentioned above, absorption of macronutrients, vitamins, and minerals is generally normal.

  4. Function of other systems. Aging is also associated with declining cardiac, pulmonary, and renal function and with diminished secretion of growth hormone, which some feel contributes to the decline in lean body and muscle mass (sarcopenia) that accompanies aging. Furthermore, a decrease in cell-mediated immunity is manifested by decreased numbers of circulating T cells and defective cell-mediated immune responses, which may contribute to the morbidity associated with aging. Humoral immunity is generally less severely affected, but the incidence of autoimmune disorders is increased. Atherosclerosis, arthritis, osteoporosis, diabetes, assorted cancers, and diminished sight and hearing are all commonly present. To varying degrees, these conditions can limit mobility and access to food, affect mood, and diminish appetite.

III. Nutritional issues in elderly persons
  A. Food access and selection
    1. Economics. A reduced income generally accompanies aging. This reduction often entails alterations in dietary habits, including the elimination of relatively high-priced items such as meat.

    2. Mobility. Because of their physical infirmities, various illnesses, and loss of means of transportation, the mobility of elderly adults is often limited. Such limitation can directly or indirectly restrict access to food purchase.

    3. Psychosocial and neurologic problems, such as depression and mental deterioration, may lead to loss of the desire to shop, a diminished appetite, forgetfulness about meals, or frank inability to eat.

B. Calcium. Osteopenia secondary to osteoporosis and osteomalacia is a significant problem in the elderly, particularly elderly women. The resultant increased incidence of fractures is responsible for a very high level of physical and psychosocial disabilities in addition to substantial financial costs. Calcium intake and absorption decline with age. Reduced absorption may be a consequence of decreased vitamin D function, in turn caused by the combined effects of reduced dietary intake, decreased exposure to sunlight and capacity of the aged skin to synthesize vitamin D, reduced intestinal absorption of the vitamin, and reduced hepatic and renal ability to hydroxylate vitamin D to its active form. The average calcium intake in women over age 51 is only about 50% of the adequate intake (AI) level. The calcium intake of men over age 51 is somewhat better, but the mean is still only about 60% of the AI, which has been set at 1,200 mg for persons over 51 years of age because of increasing evidence that calcium intake is a factor in maintaining body density (11). Nonetheless, conclusive evidence for the effects of calcium intake on maintenance of bone density and prevention of the consequences of osteoporosis have not been uniformly observed across studies, and dietary calcium intake recommendations for elderly adults remain a topic of debate.

C. Antioxidants. The theory that highly reactive free radicals, generated during normal oxidative metabolic processes, contribute to the tissue deterioration of aging is highly popular. The free radicals damage tissue through membrane lipid peroxidation, oxidation of proteins and carbohydrates, and abnormal DNA cross-linking. Considerable experimental evidence indicates that these events occur at the cellular level during normal metabolism, Therefore, many people consume increased quantities of antioxidants: vitamins E and C, β-carotene, selenium (a cofactor for glutathione peroxidase), and cofactors of the superoxide dismutase system, including copper, zinc, and manganese. However, compelling *in vivo* data to support a decline in cancer incidence, a decrease in morbidity from other causes, and prolongation of life in elderly human beings have not been forthcoming. A recent, extensive review of the role of antioxidant supplementation in the prevention of the chronic diseases associated with aging concluded that no convincing evidence is available to support the recommendations for antioxidant supplementation in humans (12). (See also the sections on vitamins C, A, and E in Chapter 6.)

D. Fiber. Increasing the intake of dietary fiber is an important adjunct in the treatment of constipation in the elderly, although abdominal discomfort, flatulence, and potentially decreased absorption of iron and zinc may be the unwanted side effects of excess consumption. The mechanism by which dietary fiber improves gastrointestinal mobility is unknown. A high intake of dietary fiber is also associated with a modest reduction in serum cholesterol and may reduce the risk for colorectal, gastric, and endometrial cancers. However, the latter beneficial effects may be derived from other components of the consumed fruits, vegetables, and whole grains and cannot definitely be attributed to fiber alone. (See also Chapters 11 and 14.) Nonetheless, improving the intake of foods high in dietary fiber is a healthful nutritional option for elderly adults because these foods contain important vitamins and minerals.

E. Drugs. Elderly adults use almost 25% of the over-the-counter drugs sold in the United States, and the vast majority of elderly adults take at least one prescription drug daily. Many adults take multiple medications daily (polypharmacy). Some common drugs known to affect nutritional status are listed in Table 3-2. Conversely, nutrients affect drug absorption, as shown in Table 3-3. Thus, both physicians and the elderly adults under their care are responsible for assessing potential nutrient–drug interactions. The physician must be alert to potentially detrimental nutritional effects of the prescribed therapeutic regimen. Likewise, the patient must pay close attention to the package insert and physician's instructions regarding the timing of drug

Table 3-2. Effects of drugs on nutrients

Drug	Effect
Antiinfective agents	
Amikacin, gentamicin, sisomicin, tobramycin	Hypokalemia, hypomagnesemia, and hypocalcemia; increased urinary potassium and magnesium loss
Aminosalicylic acid	Decreased vitamin B_{12} and fat absorption
Amphotericin B	Increased urinary excretion of potassium and decreased serum potassium and magnesium levels
Capreomycin	Hypokalemia, hypomagnesemia, and hypocalcemia
Cycloserine	Decreased serum folate
Isoniazid	Pyridoxine deficiency
Neomycin	Decreased absorption of carotene, iron, vitamin B_{12}, and cholesterol
Rifampin	Decreased serum 25-hydroxycholecalciferol level
Sulfasalazine	Folate deficiency
Tetracycline	Decreased absorption of Ca, Mg, Fe, Zn
Anticoagulants	
Warfarin	Decreased vitamin K-dependent coagulation factors
Cardiovascular drugs	
Colestipol	Decreased absorption of fat-soluble vitamins and folic acid
Hydralazine	Pyridoxine deficiency
Sodium nitroprusside	Decreased total serum vitamin B_{12}
Thiazides, ethacrynic acid	Increased urinary loss of Na, K, Mg, Zn, P
Triamterene, spironolactone	Increased urinary loss of K, Ca, Mg, Zn
CNS drugs	
Alcohol	Increased urinary loss of Mg, Zn, Ca
Aspirin	Decreased serum folate
	Decreased leukocyte and platelet ascorbic acid levels
	Increased iron loss
Monoamine oxidase inhibitors	
Isocarboxazid	Increased sensitivity to tyramine-containing foods; possible development of hypertensive crisis
Pargyline	
Phenelzine	
Tranylcypromine	Pyridoxine deficiency
Phenobarbital	Decreased serum vitamin K_1
Phenytoin	Decreased serum folate, calcium, 25-hydroxycholecalciferol levels
Electrolyte drugs	
Potassium chloride, slow-release	Decreased vitamin B_{12} absorption
Gastrointestinal drugs	
Aluminum hydroxide	Decreased absorption of iron, phosphate, vitamin B_{12}
Cholestyramine	Decreased absorption of vitamins A, D, E, K, and B_{12} and folate along with decreased absorption of inorganic phosphate and fat

Table 3-2. (*Continued*)

Drug	Effect
H$_2$-receptor antagonists, proton pump inhibitors	Decreased absorption of protein-bound vitamin B$_{12}$
Laxatives	Increased fecal loss of Na, K, Ca, Mg
Mineral oil	Decreased absorption of vitamins A, D, E, and K
Hormones	
Glucocorticoids	Increased urinary loss of K, Ca; increased Na absorption
Oral contraceptives	Decreased serum folate, pyridoxine deficiency, riboflavin deficiency
Other agents	
Colchicine	Decreased absorption of vitamin B$_{12}$, sodium, potassium, fat, nitrogen
Penicillamine	Pyridoxine deficiency

From Weinsier RL, Morgan SL. *Fundamentals of clinical nutrition.* St. Louis: Mosby, 1993:186, with permission.

ingestion relative to the consumption of food and drink (see Table 1-22 for the effect of vitamins and minerals on drug action, and Table 1-23 for the effect of drugs on food intake).

IV. **Nutrient requirements and nutritional recommendations.** The principal biologic factor underlying the altered nutrient needs of the elderly adult is the decline in energy expenditure secondary to a reduction of lean body mass. Because of this decline, less macronutrient intake is needed to satisfy energy needs; concomitantly, the intake of various vitamin and mineral constituents of the diet is diminished. Additional physical infirmities, dentures, neuropsychological disorders, social conditions, and economic constraints may aggravate further the inability to consume diets adequate in quantity or quality. In this context, then, elderly individuals should consume foods that are nutrient-dense–that is, that have a high ratio of nutrients to energy.

Until recently, dietary intake recommendations for persons older than 51 years were largely extrapolated from data obtained in healthy young adults. Furthermore, nutritional needs were not stratified as a function of age over 51, and the Food and Nutrition Board of the Institute of Medicine at the National Academy of Sciences traditionally included only a single set of RDAs for all persons 51 years of age or older. Within the last several years, the Food and Nutrition Board standing committees on the scientific evaluation of dietary reference intakes (DRIs) has divided older persons into those between the ages of 51 and 70 years and those older than 70 years for the purposes of establishing intake recommendations (11–14). To date, however, the defined DRI values in each age range have been identical except for vitamin D, for which the AI level increases from 10 to 15 µg daily above the age of 70.

Although it is clear that significant biologic, physical, and psychosocial differences exist between very old (> 85 years of age) and moderately old (between 70 and 85 years of age) persons, no specific dietary standards for the very old, who often have special needs because of physical disabilities or mental infirmity, have been agreed on. However, recent assessments have focused on the special metabolic and nutritional needs of the elderly (11–18), and if elderly adults remain physically and mentally capable of following the dietary guidelines outlined in Chapter 2 for young adults, with the relatively minor adjustments discussed below, it is unlikely that they will become malnourished. Finally,

Table 3-3. Effects of nutrients on drugs

Food can change the absorption characteristics of certain drugs. The mechanisms for the effect include physicochemical interactions with food in the intestinal lumen, changes in gastric emptying, competition between drug and food components for absorption, and altered first-pass hepatic kinetics. These effects can decrease the efficacy of the drug or increase the absorption of the drug, so that a greater response to the drug or a side effect results. There can be large differences from one formulation to another, and no drug class effects can be assumed. The reader should check carefully with the literature and the manufacturer's information concerning individual formulations, especially when the therapeutic window is narrow. Listed below are some of the drugs commonly used that can be affected by food and instructions on how to minimize the effects of food on the drug.

Decreased absorption (Avoid taking these drugs with food. Take at least 1 hour before or 2 hours after a meal.)

Ampicillin	Erythromycin stearate	Levodopa/carbidopa	Quinidine
Atenolol	Ferrous salts	Lisinopril	Sotalol
Calcium carbonate	Folic acid	Methotrexate	Sulfamethoxazole
Captopril	Furosemide	Omeprazole	Tetracycline
Cephalexin	Iron	Penicillin G	Trimethoprim
Cloxacillin	Isoniazid	Penicillin V	Zinc sulfate
Digitalis	Isosorbide	Phenytoin	
Disopyramide	Lansoprazole	Propantheline	

Increased absorption (Food will alter the amount of the drug absorbed; therefore, the drug should be taken at the same time(s) each day relative to meals.)

Buspirone	Gemfibrozil	Methoxsalen	Propranolol
Carbamazepine	Griseofulvin	Metoprolol	Spironolactone
Chlorothizide	Labetalol	Nifedipine	Sulfadiazine
Diazepam	Lithium	Nitrofurantoin	Trazodone
Dicumarol	Lovastatin	Phenytoin	

Delayed absorption (Food will delay the absorption of these drugs but not the overall amount absorbed. These drugs should be taken at least 1 hour before or 2 hours after a meal.)

Acetaminophen	Hydrochlorothiazide	Pentobarbital	Suprofen
Aspirin	Hydrocortisone	Pentoxifylline	Tocainide
Cimetidine	Indomethacin	Sulfisoxazole	
Doxycycline	Ketoprofen		

From Weinsier RL, Morgan SL. *Fundamentals of clinical nutrition.* St. Louis: Mosby, 1993:188, with permission, and Utermohlen V. In: Shils ME, Olson JA, Shike M, et al., eds., *Modern nutrition in health and disease,* 9th ed. Baltimore: Williams & Wilkins, 1998:1621.

regular physical exercise and a balanced diet do more to promote and preserve health in elderly adults than all other so-called health supplements, "nutritional" or otherwise. The desire and ability of elderly adults to prepare and consume a wide variety of foods are often enhanced by simple companionship during grocery shopping and meals.

A. **Energy.** Resting energy expenditure declines as a function of age and lean body mass after age 50. Regular exercise, particularly resistance exercise, can help preserve strength and lean mass. Reduced physical activity further contributes to the loss of lean mass and decline in energy expenditure seen in the elderly. Therefore, setting a single recommended energy intake level for the elderly is not entirely appropriate, but a daily energy intake of about 30 kcal/kg is typical. However, as with all calorie intake recommendations at any age, the value initially estimated for an individual person must be tailored to the value that maintains body weight within a desirable range. Major nutritional intake surveys show consistently that healthy elderly persons consume fewer calories than the RDA for energy (19) shown in Table 3-4. For example, NHANES III data show that men between the ages of 50 and 59 consume energy at the level recommended in Table 3-4, but that women consume about 250 to 300 calories less than the recommended level daily. Above the age of 80, however, both men and women consume approximately 500 calories less than the RDA on a daily basis. For persons who are physically inactive, either as a result of advanced age or physical incapacity, the energy intakes must be reduced correspondingly.

B. Protein. No systematic body of evidence indicates that protein needs are increased in elderly adults. The current RDA is set at the same level as the RDA for young adults, 0.8 g/kg per day (19). Healthy elderly adults generally consume this amount of protein. However, because dietary protein intake is linked closely to dietary energy intake, elderly adults with low dietary

Table 3-4. Recommended nutrient intakes for persons 51 years of age and older

	Recommended dietary allowances*	
	Men	Women
Energy (kcal)	2,300	1,900
Protein (g)	63	50
Vitamin A (µg RAE)[a]		700
Vitamin C (mg)	90	75
Vitamin E (mg)[c]	15	15
Vitamin K (µg)	120	90
Thiamin (mg)	1.2	1.1
Riboflavin (mg)	1.3	1.1
Niacin (mg)[d]	16	14
Vitamin B_6 (mg)	1.7	1.5
Folate (µg)	400	400
Vitamin B_{12} (µg)[e]	2.4	2.4
Iron (mg)	10	10
Zinc (mg)	15	12
Phosphorus (mg)	700	700
Magnesium (mg)	420	320
Selenium (µg)	55	55
Iodine (µg)	150	150
Adequate Intakes[#]		
Calcium (mg)	1,200	1,200
Vitamin D (µg)[b]	10	10

[a] Retinol activity equivalents: 1 RAE = 1 µg all-*trans*-retinol or 6 µg β-carotene = 24 µg α-carotene and β-cryptoxanthin.
[b] As cholecalciferol: 1 µg cholecalciferol = 40 IU of vitamin D. Above the age of 70 years, the daily recommended intake for vitamin D increases to 15 µg/d.
[c] As α-tocopherol, including *RRR*-α-tocopherol, the natural food form, and the 2R-stereoisomeric forms that occur in fortified foods and supplements, but not the 2S-stereoisomers that are also found in fortified foods and supplements.
[d] As niacin equivalents: 1 NE = 1 mg niacin or 60 mg dietary tryptophan
[e] Because elderly individuals may malabsorb food-bound vitamin B_{12}, it is advisable for the elderly to meet the requirement by consuming foods fortified with vitamin B_{12} or with a supplement containing vitamin B_{12}.
*From National Research Council, Food and Nutrition Board. *Recommended dietary allowances,* 10th ed. Washington, DC: National Academy Press, 1989.
[#] From references 11 through 14.

energy intakes are also at risk for insufficient protein intakes. The physician and other caregivers should be alert to this possibility.

C. **Fat-soluble vitamins.** (See Chapter 6 for more details.) Vitamin A status appears adequate in the majority of elderly men and women, although about one-third of Americans older than 70 questioned in NHANES III reported that they consume less than two-thirds of the current RDA for vitamin A. This apparent contradiction is explained by the fact that the RDA may be excessive for elderly adults, as vitamin A absorption appears to be increased and plasma clearance of vitamin A decreased in elderly persons. In any case, hepatic vitamin A stores do not decrease with age in humans. Thus, the RDAs of 900 µg of retinol activity equivalents for men and 700 µg of retinol activity equivalents for women are certainly adequate (14) (Table 3-4).

Vitamin D is not a vitamin in the classic sense because it can be synthesized in the skin. Because the ability of the skin to synthesize vitamin D is reduced in elderly persons, and because elderly adults often spend less time in the sun, they are potentially more dependent on the consumption of exogenous vitamin D. Unfortunately, elderly adults often reduce rather than increase their consumption of dairy products fortified with vitamin D, and more than three-fourths of elderly adults have a vitamin D intake that is less than two-thirds of the RDA. Additionally, evidence suggests that bone mineral density is better preserved in elderly women who supplement their intake of vitamin D. For these reasons, the AI of vitamin D has been set at 10 µg/d for persons between the ages of 51 and 70, and at 15 µg/d for those above the age of 70 (11) (Table 3-4).

Vitamin E metabolism is not influenced by age. Vitamin E deficiency does not occur in persons consuming a usual American diet, and no evidence indicates that vitamin E intake is inadequate in elderly adults, although NHANES III reported that in about 75% of Americans older than 70 years, vitamin E intake is less than two-thirds the RDA. Nonetheless, this observation is likely the result of underreporting because of the inability to estimate the amounts and types of fats and oils used in food preparation and the incomplete determination of the vitamin E content of food sources in available databases (12). Because of the currently increased use of polyunsaturated oils, which contain vitamin E, the intake of this vitamin is almost certainly more than sufficient in most persons. Although the potential advantages of further increasing vitamin E intake for its antioxidant actions have been hotly debated, no benefits of this course of action have yet been confirmed (12). The current RDA for vitamin E (Table 3-4) is 15 mg of α-tocopherol daily for elderly men and women (12). In this context, α-tocopherol includes *RRR*-α-tocopherol, the form occurring naturally in foods, and the 2*R*-stereoisometric forms found in fortified foods and supplements, but it does not include the inactive 2*S*-stereoisomers that are also found in fortified foods and supplements.

Vitamin K is found widely in food and is manufactured by intestinal bacteria. Therefore, vitamin K deficiency is rare. Although experimental evidence indicates a slight age-related decline in plasma vitamin K metabolites, no clinical consequences of this observation are known. Current daily AIs for vitamin K are 120 and 90 µg for elderly men and women, respectively (14) (Table 3-4).

D. **Water-soluble vitamins.** (See Chapter 6 for more details). The levels of *vitamin C* in plasma and leukocyte levels decline with age, apparently as a function of intake, as absorption, metabolism, and excretion do not change consistently with age. Additional data indicate that saturation of the vitamin C body pool in the elderly requires a daily intake at approximately the RDA of 75 mg/d in women, but at more than the RDA of 90 mg/d in men (12). Approximately 25% of elderly men and women consumed less than the RDA for vitamin C in NHANES III. Fewer than 10% consumed less than two-thirds of the RDA.

Thiamine status, measured by the erythrocyte transketolase assay, has been highly variable and reported to be low in small to significant fractions of elderly adults. In NHANES III, only about 10% of elderly Americans consumed less than the RDA of thiamine. The most significant clinical cause of thiamine deficiency in aging adults is alcohol consumption coupled with decreased dietary intake. The current RDAs for thiamine are 1.2 mg/d for elderly men and 1.1 mg/d for elderly women (13) (Table 3-4).

Riboflavin absorption and metabolism are unaffected by aging, and riboflavin status appears to be normal in most aging adults, although various surveys report low riboflavin intakes in 20% to 25% of Americans and Western Europeans and a higher prevalence in some developing countries. In NHANES III, approximately 10% of elderly Americans consumed less than the riboflavin RDA of 1.3 mg/d for elderly men and 1.1 mg/d for elderly women (13) (Table 3-4). Milk and other dairy products (except butter) are convenient dietary sources of both calcium and riboflavin for elderly adults.

Niacin requirements do not change with age. In NHANES III, about 10% of elderly Americans consumed less than the RDA of niacin, which has been set at 16 mg/d for elderly men and 14 mg/d for elderly women(13) (Table 3-4).

Vitamin B_6 intake values appear to vary widely, although incomplete vitamin B_6 food composition data limit our ability to quantify them with any precision. The current RDAs for vitamin B_6 are estimated as 1.7 mg/d for men over the age of 51 and 1.5 mg/d for women in the same age category (13).Various nutrition surveys, including NHANES III, and biochemical assessments of vitamin B_6 status (e.g., age-related declines in plasma pyridoxal phosphate levels, various transaminase activities, and plasma homocysteine levels) suggest that vitamin B_6 intake may be inadequate in 10% to 25% of elderly men and 25% to 50% of elderly women (13), although clinical evidence of vitamin B_6 deficiency is rare.

Folate is widely distributed in foods, although the amount and bioavailability of the various forms of folate in food are the subject of some debate because analytic methods are inadequate. Serum and, more representatively, red cell levels of folate reflect folate status, and various dietary surveys suggest that about 5% of elderly adults have low serum levels of folate. However, according to data collected in NHANES III, approximately 50% to 60% of elderly men and women consume less than the RDA for folate. The prevalence of low folate nutriture is higher in persons with a low income, whose intake of foods high in folate is reduced. Although folate absorption is limited by the atrophic gastritis often found in elderly adults, a compensatory increase in folate production occurs in bacterial overgrowth in the proximal small bowel. Both folate and vitamin B_{12} are required to convert homocysteine to methionine, and folate intakes below 400 µg/d appear to be associated with elevated homocysteine levels, an independent risk factor for coronary artery and cerebrovascular disease (20). For this reason, the RDAs for folate have recently been revised upward to 400 µg of dietary folate equivalents in elderly men and women (13,21). Dietary folate equivalents take into account the fact that folic acid is more bioavailable than dietary food folates, particularly when taken without food. Thus, one dietary folate equivalent equals 1 µg of food folate, 0.6 µg of folic acid from fortified foods or from a folic acid supplement taken with food, or 0.5 µg of a folic acid supplement taken on an empty stomach (13,21).

Vitamin B_{12} levels are often low in elderly adults. No evidence has been found that aging *per se* alters vitamin B_{12} absorption. However, B_{12} malabsorption is more frequent in elderly adults because of an increased prevalence of pernicious anemia and atrophic gastritis. The absorption of vitamin B_{12} is altered in atrophic gastritis not because of any abnormal intrinsic factor, but because dissociation of the vitamin from food proteins is limited by inadequate acid digestion (22,23). Additionally, because of bacterial overgrowth in the proximal small intestine secondary to atrophic gastritis, some vitamin B_{12} that reaches the small bowel is metabolized by bacteria rather than absorbed. Vitamin B_{12} is found only in animal products, and some elderly adults have low levels of B_{12} because of their decreased consumption of animal products. Often, this is for economic reasons, although the prevalence of B_{12} deficiency is not increased in the low-income elderly. Elderly vegetarians are particularly at risk for vitamin B_{12} deficiency. The current RDA for vitamin B_{12} is 2.4 mg/d for elderly men and women (13), and nearly all elderly Americans consumed this level in NHANES III. Because atrophic gastritis is present in 10% to 30% of the elderly population (23), vitamin B_{12} requirements in the elderly are best met by the consumption of fortified food products or a supplement containing vitamin B_{12}, one of the very few circumstances in human nutrition in which supplements are recommended in preference to foods to satisfy requirements.

E. **Minerals.** (See also Chapter 7 for more details.) *Calcium* intakes in elderly women and men above age 70 are consistently well below the recommended AIs. As discussed earlier, this deficit is further compounded by abnormalities in vitamin D metabolism in aging persons. Although most bone calcium is laid down during adolescence and young adult life, growing evidence that increasing the dietary calcium intake may be beneficial in reducing bone mineral loss in older adults has led to recent recommendations that the AI of dietary calcium be set at 1,200 mg for both women and men over the age of 51 years (11) (Table 3-4). For some persons with very low dietary calcium intakes, supplementation to achieve the AI appears prudent.

Phosphorus intake is generally higher than calcium intake, and most diets provide ample phosphorus. Data from the various NHANESs show that elderly adults meet the current RDA of 700 mg/d for phosphorus (11).

Magnesium intake in about 50% of elderly adults is generally below two-thirds of the current RDA levels of 420 mg/d for men and 320 mg/d for women (11) (Table 3-4). Because magnesium occurs in many foods and in drinking water (albeit at highly variable concentrations), and because clinical magnesium deficiency is rare, the RDA may be set at a very generous level, particularly in light of the fact that the RDAs were based on the results of magnesium balance studies in a limited number of elderly men and the results of a single study in young adult women extrapolated to elderly women (11). In elderly persons, however, one must be aware that digoxin, diuretics, and impaired renal tubular function may enhance magnesium loss. Laxatives also can augment intestinal magnesium loss, but magnesium-containing laxatives and antacids are common sources of excessive magnesium intake in the elderly.

Iron absorption does not diminish with age, and iron status understandably improves in women following the cessation of menses. When iron deficiency occurs in the elderly, one must first eliminate possible causes of chronic occult blood loss and the reduction of nonheme iron absorption associated with atrophic gastritis, which account for most cases, before searching for reasons for inadequate dietary iron intake. The NHANESs show that iron intake averages about 13 to 14 mg/d in elderly men and about 9 to 10 mg/d in elderly women. The current RDA for iron is 8 mg/d in elderly men and women (14) (Table 3-4).

Zinc absorption declines with age, but endogenous zinc losses also decline, so zinc balance is preserved. Various dietary intake surveys, including the NHANESs, show that many elderly adults generally consume less than two-thirds the current RDA levels for zinc, set at 11 mg/d for men and 8 mg/d for women (14) (Table 3-4). Nonetheless, normal plasma zinc levels are generally maintained, and only 3% of elderly adults in NHANES II had plasma zinc levels in a deficient range. Little clinical evidence of zinc deficiency has been found in elderly adults, although some have questioned whether a lowered zinc status may contribute to the altered immune competence of the elderly, as zinc is important to maintaining immune function (18). Given this consideration, it appears prudent to aim for the current zinc RDA intake level.

Iodine has only a single essential function, which is thyroid hormonogenesis. Iodine levels in the United States have declined slightly during the last decade. However, since the introduction of iodized salt in 1924, the use of iodate dough oxidizers in bread making, and recent patterns of increased

Table 3-5. Selected sources of reliable information for elderly adults

Administration on Aging
Wilbur J. Cohen Bldg.
330 Independence Ave., SW
Washington, DC 20201
www.aoa.gov

Alzheimer's Association
919 North Michigan Ave., Suite 1100
Chicago, IL 60611
www.alz.org

American Association of Retired
 Persons
601 E St., NW
Washington, DC 20049
www.aarp.org

American Cancer Society
1599 Clifton Road, NE
Atlanta, GA 30329
www.cancer.org

American Diabetes Association
1701 North Beauregard St.
Alexandria, VA 22311
www.diabetes.org

American Federation for Aging Research
1414 Avenue of the Americas, 18th floor
New York, NY 10019
www.afar.org

American Geriatrics Society
Empire State Building, Suite 801
New York, NY 10118
www.americangeriatrics.org

American Heart Association
7272 Greenville Ave.
Dallas, TX 75231
www.americanheart.org

American Society for Nutritional Sciences
9650 Rockville Pike
Bethesda, MD 20814
www.faseb.org/asns/

American Society for Clinical Nutrition
9650 Rockville Pike
Bethesda, MD 28014
www.faseb.org/ascn/

Department of Agriculture
Office of Information
14th St. and Independence Ave., SW
Washington, DC 20250
www.usda.gov

Gerontology Research Center, National
 Institute on Aging
Baltimore City Hospitals
4940 Eastern Ave.
Baltimore, MD 21224
www.grc.nia.nih.gov

National Resource Center for Health
 Promotion and Aging
c/o National Council on the Aging
600 Maryland Ave., SW, West Wing 100
Washington, DC 20024
*www.athealth.com/Consumer/rcenter/
 resource_data.cfm?TopicCF=Aging*

National Institute on Aging
National Institutes of Health
Bldg. 31, Room 5C27
31 Center Drive, MSC 2292
Bethesda, MD 20892
www.nih.gov/nia

USDA Human Nutrition Research
 Center on Aging
Tufts University
711 Washington St.
Boston, MA 02111
www.hnrc.tufts.edu

seafood consumption, little evidence of clinical iodine deficiency has been seen. The current RDA for iodine in elderly men and women is 150 µg/d. One gram of iodized salt provides 76 µg of iodine.

Selenium is an essential cofactor for the antioxidant enzyme glutathione peroxidase. No evidence has been found that selenium requirements or biochemical markers of selenium status are affected by age (12). Selenium intake varies enormously among populations according to the selenium content of the soils. Although various surveys have reported low selenium intakes in elderly adults, NHANES III, which evaluated more than 6,000 persons over the age of 51, showed a mean selenium intake of 134 μg in men between the ages of 51 and 70, and 112 μg in men over the age of 70. Corresponding values for women were 94 μg and 83 μg. The fifth percentile intake levels in all groups were at or above the current RDA of 55 μg/d for men and women over the age of 50 years (12). There is also no reason to suspect selenium deficiency on the basis of dietary intake information, food composition data, or available metabolic indices. Selenium deficiency is a problem only in areas of the world where food is grown in soil with an extremely low selenium content and in patients undergoing long-term parenteral nutrition with selenium- deficient solutions. Thus far, no compelling reasons have been found to consume excess dietary selenium to improve cardiovascular function or prevent cancer (12). Because selenium is stored in the body, excessive consumption can result in toxicity, and a UL of 400 μg has been established (12).

The RDAs of *other micronutrients* are the same as in younger adults. These are copper (900 μg) and molybdenum (45 μg) (14). AIs for manganese (2.3 mg in men and 1.8 mg in women) are likewise the same as those in younger adults (14).

V. Resources. Because of the ever-growing elderly population, a wide variety of public and private societal resources have become available. A selected small number of these are listed in Table 3-5.

References

1. Rogers CC. *Changes in the older population and implications for rural areas.* U.S. Department of Agriculture, Economic Research Service, Rural Development Research Report No:90, Washington, DC, 1999:

2. U.S. Department of Commerce, Bureau of the Census:Population projections of the United States by age, sex, race, and Hispanic origin: 1995 to 2050. *Current Population Reports,* Series P-25-1130, Washington, DC, 1996:

3. World Health Organization. *The world health report 2000—health systems: improving performance.* Geneva: World Health Organization, 2000. Report online available at *http://www.who.int/whr.* Accessed December 16, 2000.

4. Guyer B, Freedman MA, Strobino DM, et al. Annual summary of vital statistics: trends in the health of Americans during the 20th century. *Pediatrics* 2000;106,1307.

5. Friguet B, Bulteau A-L, Chondrogianni N, et al. Protein degradation by the proteosome and its implications in aging. *Ann N Y Acad Sci* 2000;908:143.

6. Higami Y, Shimokawa I. Apoptosis in the aging process. *Cell Tissue Res* 2000; 301:125.

7. Takahashi Y, Kuro-o M, Ishikawa F. Aging mechanisms. *Proc Natl Acad Sci USA* 2000;97:12407.

8. Lansdorp PM. Repair of telomeric DNA prior to replicative senescence. *Mech Ageing Dev* 2000;118:23.

9. Aragona M, Maisano R, Panetta S, et al. Telomere length maintenance in aging and carcinogenesis. *Int J Oncol* 2000;17:981.

10. Rogina B, Reenan RA, Nilsen SP, et al. Extended life-span conferred by cotransporter gene mutations in *Drosophila. Science* 2000;290:2137.

11. Standing Committee on the Scientific Evaluation of Dietary Reference Intakes, Food and Nutrition Board, Institute of Medicine. *Dietary reference intakes for calcium, phosphorus, magnesium, vitamin D, and fluoride.* Washington, DC: National Academy Press, 1997.

12. Standing Committee on the Scientific Evaluation of Dietary Reference Intakes, Food and Nutrition Board, Institute of Medicine. *Dietary reference intakes for vitamin C, vitamin E, selenium, and carotenoids.* Washington, DC: National Academy Press, 2000.

13. Standing Committee on the Scientific Evaluation of Dietary Reference Intakes, Food and Nutrition Board, Institute of Medicine. *Dietary reference intakes for thiamin, niacin, vitamin B₆, folate, vitamin B₁₂, pantothenic acid, biotin, and choline.* Washington, DC: National Academy Press, 1998.

14. Standing Committee on the Scientific Evaluation of Dietary Reference Intakes, Food and Nutrition Board, Institute of Medicine. *Dietary reference intakes for vitamin A, vitamin K, arsenic, boron, chromium, copper, iodine, iron, manganese, molybdenum, nickel, silicon, vanadium, and zinc.* Washington, DC: National Academy Press, 2001.
15. Russell RM. New views on the RDAs for older adults. *J Am Diet Assoc* 1997; 97:515.
16. Russell RM, Rasmussen H, Lichtenstein AH. Modified food guide pyramid for people over seventy years of age. *J Nutr* 1999;129:751.
17. Russell RM:The aging process as a modifier of metabolism. *Am J Clin Nutr* 2000;72[Suppl]529S.
18. Ausman LM, Russell RM. Nutrition in the elderly. In: Shils ME, Olson JA, Shike M, et al., eds. *Modern nutrition in health and disease,* 9th ed. Baltimore: Williams & Wilkins, 1999.
19. National Research Council. *Recommended dietary allowances,* 10th ed. Washington, DC: National Academy Press, 1989.
20. Selhub J, Jacques PF, Wilson PW, et al. Vitamin status and intake as primary determinants of homocysteinemia in an elderly population. *JAMA* 1993;270:2693.
21. 21:Suitor CW, Bailey LB. Dietary folate equivalents: interpretation and application. *J Am Diet Assoc* 2000;100:88.
22. Carmel R. *In vitro* studies of gastric juice in patients with food-cobalamin malabsorption. *Dig Dis Sci* 1994;39;2516.
23. Hurwitz A, Brady DA, Schaal ES, et al. Gastric acidity in older adults. *JAMA* 1997;278:659.

4. PREGNANCY AND LACTATION

Studies in humans and animals indicate that nutrition during pregnancy influences not only the health and neurologic development of the newborn, but also the subsequent morbidity and mortality of the grown adult offspring. Low maternal weight before pregnancy, inadequate weight gain during pregnancy, and inadequate intake of protein and calories by the expectant mother are all associated with the delivery of low-birth-weight infants. Low birth weight is, in turn, associated with increased perinatal mortality, impaired neurologic development, and a retarded growth pattern. Furthermore, compelling evidence is now available to indicate that infants born small, as a consequence of nutritional or other negative influences on fetal growth, are at increased risk for the development of hypertension, coronary artery disease, diabetes, and possibly other conditions during adult life (1,2). Current recommendations for nutrition during pregnancy stress the importance of a proper pattern of weight gain and an adequate intake of calories, protein, vitamins, and minerals to allow for optimal fetal development and the preservation of maternal health. These recommendations also stress evaluation of the mother, either before conception or early in pregnancy, for the presence of nutritional risk factors that might jeopardize the outcome of the pregnancy.

I. Energy and protein requirements

A. Energy requirements are minimally increased during most of the first trimester, but they rise rapidly at the end of this period and remain elevated until after delivery (3). The recommended dietary allowance (RDA) of calories during the second and third trimesters is 300 kcal above basal requirements, corresponding to a 15% increase over nonpregnancy requirements (4,5). These recommendations presume a moderate level of activity; a woman who is considerably less active during pregnancy than before may not require any additional caloric intake.

B. Protein requirements. The RDA for protein in the mature nonpregnant woman is 50 g/d (approximately 0.8 g/kg per day) (4) (Table 4-1). The calculated additional intakes of dietary protein required to support the deposition of new tissue are 1.3, 6.1, and 10.7 g/d during the first, second, and third trimesters of pregnancy, respectively. Because of the uncertainties in these calculated figures, the RDA for protein is increased by 10 g/d throughout pregnancy (4,5) (Table 4-1). This level of protein intake is achieved easily on the standard middle class Western diet. However, women from lower socioeconomic groups or women who by preference eat a diet low in meat and dairy products may require dietary counseling to achieve this level of protein intake.

II. Maternal weight gain

A. Previous recommendations. Recommendations for weight gain during pregnancy have fluctuated during the past several decades (5). Severe restriction of weight gain during pregnancy (total weight gain of 16 to 18 lb) was recommended widely until several decades ago in an attempt to prevent preeclampsia and eclampsia. Because these conditions were associated with marked weight gain (largely edema), it was thought that restriction of weight gain would prevent them. It now appears that eclampsia causes weight gain in the form of edema rather than that weight gain causes eclampsia. Restricted weight gain does not reduce the incidence of preeclampsia and eclampsia. Therefore, in the 1970s and 1980s, recommended weight gains of 24 lb or more gradually became the common obstetric advice (5).

Restricted weight gain may affect pregnancy adversely, resulting in an infant with a low or very low birth weight. Limited weight gain during pregnancy, especially when the mother's weight is low before pregnancy, increases the risk for fetal growth retardation. The risk for mortality is markedly increased in infants with a low birth weight, especially in those with a very low

Table 4-1. Estimates of dietary needs for nonpregnant, pregnant, and lactating women

Nutrient	Recommended intake for nonpregnant teenager (ages 11–13 y)	Recommended intake for nonpregnant teenager (ages 14–18 y)	Recommended intake for nonpregnant adult	Recommended increment for pregnancy	Recommended increment for lactation
Calories	2,200	2,200	2,200	+300	+500
Protein (g)	46	44	50	+10	+15
Vitamin A (μg RAE)[a]	600	700	700	+70	+600
Vitamin D (μg)	5*	5*	5*	0	0
Vitamin E (mg)[b]	11	15	15	0	+4
Vitamin C (mg)	45	65	75	+10	+35
Folate (μg)[c]	300	400	400	+200	+100
Niacin (mg NE)[d]	12	14	14	+4	+3
Riboflavin (mg)	0.9	1.0	1.1	+0.3	+0.5
Vitamin B_6 (mg)	1.0	1.2	1.3	+0.6	+0.7
Vitamin B_{12} (μg)	1.8	2.4	2.4	+0.2	+0.4
Calcium (mg)	1,300*	1,300*	1,000*	0	0
Magnesium (mg)	240	360	315 ± 5	+40	0
Iron (mg)	8	15	18	+9[e]	0
Zinc (mg)	8	9	8	+3	+4

[a] Retinol activity equivalent: 1 μg RAE = 1 μg all-*trans*-retinol or 12 μg β-carotene or 24 μg α-carotene and β-cryptoxanthin.
[b] α-Tocopherol.
[c] As dietary folate equivalents (DFE). 1 DFE = 1 μg food folate = 0.6 μg of folic acid from fortified food or as a supplement consumed with food = 0.5 μg of a supplement taken on an empty stomach.
[d] Niacin equivalent: 1 NE = 1 mg of niacin or 60 mg of dietary tryptophan.
[e] A supplement usually is recommended. The increased requirement during pregnancy often cannot be met by the iron content of the maternal diet or by the existing iron stores of many women; therefore, the use of 30 to 60 mg of supplemental iron is often recommended. Iron needs during lactation are not substantially different from those of nonpregnant women, but continued supplementation of the mother for 2 to 3 months after parturition is advisable to replenish stores depleted by pregnancy.
*Values followed by an asterisk are adequate intakes (AI). The other values are recommended dietary allowances (RDA).
From *Dietary reference intakes: applications in dietary assessment*. Washington, DC: National Academy Press, 2000, with permission.

birth weight. Similarly, in low-birth-weight infants who survive, an inverse relationship is noted between birth weight and degree of neonatal morbidity and between birth weight and adverse neurologic outcomes.

B. **Current recommendations.** In 1990, the Institute of Medicine published a comprehensive reassessment of the available information on weight gain during pregnancy and, based on these data, issued its recommendations in *Nutrition during Pregnancy* (5). These recommendations (Table 4-2) differed in several important ways from prior recommendations in recognizing that healthy, normal infants are delivered to mothers whose gestational weight gains vary by as much as 30 lb. The report also recognized that weight accretion during pregnancy is affected by the mother's prepregnancy body mass index (BMI), which is the ratio of weight in kilograms to height in square meters (kg/m^2). Thus, mothers with a low BMI before pregnancy gain more weight during pregnancy than mothers with a high BMI before pregnancy. Based on this information, the *Nutrition during Pregnancy* report recommends a set of target ranges of weight gain according to the mother's prepregnancy BMI (2) (Table 4-2). Other aspects of maternal nutrition in pregnancy have also been reviewed (6).

C. **The pattern of weight gain** is also important. Weight gain during the *first trimester* is usually slight, averaging 0.2 to 0.3 kg weekly. Weight gain during the *second trimester* averages about 0.45 kg (1 lb) weekly, and during the *third trimester* about 0.40 kg (0.9 lb) weekly. During the second and third trimesters, weight gains of more than 3 kg/mo or increments of less than 1 kg/mo require further evaluation by the physician.

D. **Fluid retention.** The most common cause of excessive weight gain is excessive fluid retention. Moderate fluid retention and slight edema are now considered to be normal physiologic changes of pregnancy. The normal fluid retention of pregnancy is a gradual process; sudden retention of large amounts of fluid, especially late in pregnancy, is a premonitory sign of toxemia.

E. **The components of weight gain in a typical pregnancy** are listed in Table 4-3. The pregnancy illustrated resulted in a 24-lb weight gain and the delivery of a 7.7-lb infant. Weight gained during the second trimester largely represents expansion of the maternal blood volume, increases in the size of the mother's uterus and breasts, and deposition of maternal fat. Weight gain during the third trimester reflects growth of the fetus and placenta, production of amniotic fluid, and retention of salt and water in the mother's legs and pelvis.

III. **Requirements for specific nutrients**
   A. **Iron**
      1. **Iron requirements are markedly increased during pregnancy.** Hematologic changes during pregnancy profoundly affect iron home-

Table 4-2. Recommended total weight gain ranges for pregnant women[a] by prepregnancy body mass index[b]

Pregnancy weight-for-height category	Recommended total gain	
	kg	lb
Low (BMI <19.8)	12.5–18	28–40
Normal (BMI of 19.8–26.0)	11.5–16	25–35
High (BMI >26.0–29.0)[c]	7–11.5	15–25

[a] Young adolescents and black women should strive for gains at the upper end of the recommended range. Short women (<157 cm, or 62 in) should strive for gains at the lower end of the range.
[b] BMI is calculated in metric units.
[c] The recommended target weight gain for obese women (BMI >29.0) is at least 6.0 kg (15 lb).
From Institute of Medicine, Food and Nutrition Board, Committee on Nutritional Status During Pregnancy and Lactation. *Nutrition during pregnancy,* part I: *weight gain;* part II, *nutrient supplements.* Washington, DC: National Academy Press, 1990, with permission.

Table 4-3. Identifiable components of weight gained at 40 weeks' gestation

Tissue or fluid	Weight	
	g	lb
Fetus	3,500	7.7
Placenta	650	1.4
Amniotic fluid	800	1.8
Uterus	900	2.0
Breasts	405	0.9
Interstitial fluid	1,200	2.7
Maternal blood	1,800	4.0
Total weight identifiable	9,255	20.5
Total weight gained during average pregnancy	10,986	24.0
Weight gained but not accounted for	1,641	3.5

From Jacobson HN. Weight and weight gain in pregnancy. *Clin Perinatol* 1976;2:233, with permission.

ostasis (6). The maternal red cell volume increases 20% to 30%, so that the delivery of an extra 450 mg of iron to the maternal marrow is required for erythropoiesis. An additional 350 mg of iron is transferred to the fetus and placenta. About 250 mg of iron is lost in blood at delivery. Of the total 1,000 mg of extra iron required during a pregnancy, almost all is used during the latter half of gestation. This amounts to an extra 5 to 6 mg/d above the nonpregnant requirement of 1 mg/d required to compensate for the normal basal iron turnover losses that continue during pregnancy, amounting to about another 250 mg.

2. **Absorption.** Only about 10% of dietary iron is absorbed in before pregnancy or during the first trimester. Efficiency of absorption increases to about 20% in iron deficiency and may increase up to 15% to 20% during the third trimester. The typical American diet provides only about 1 to 2 mg of absorbed iron each day. Even a diet carefully selected for foods rich in iron may not satisfy the increased iron requirements of the last half of pregnancy. An attempt to provide all the iron requirement with dietary iron is likely to result in excessive calorie intake.

3. **Iron stores.** The average woman has iron stores of only 300 to 1,000 mg; in comparison, the average man has 500 to 1,500 mg. Iron stores may be even lower in a woman with a history of heavy menstrual blood flow or multiple pregnancies. The total of absorbed dietary iron plus maternal stores may be less than the iron requirements of pregnancy. When this occurs, the result is maternal iron deficiency.

The most sensitive indicator of maternal iron depletion is a reduction of *iron stores in the bone marrow.* (See Chapter 7 for a discussion of the determination of iron stores.) Somewhat less sensitive but more practical indicators are reductions of maternal red blood cell distribution width, hemoglobin levels, mean corpuscular volume, and serum ferritin levels. Serum transferrin and iron-binding capacity should not be used because transferrin levels rise during pregnancy in the absence of iron deficiency. Many pregnant women have a low serum iron level despite a normal hemoglobin level and hematocrit. However, serum iron measures a transport compartment, and concentrations can change rapidly, falling especially during acute infections. If anemia is defined as a hemoglobin level below 11 g/dL, then about one-third to one-half of pregnant women who do not take iron supplements are anemic. The percentage with depleted iron reserves, as determined by low serum iron, is even higher. Most studies indicate that moderate maternal iron deficiency is not associated with significant fetal morbidity. However, reports from India suggest an increased incidence of spontaneous abortion, stillbirths, and prenatal mortality in the pregnancies of moderately to severely anemic women.

4. Because it may be difficult to meet the iron requirements of pregnancy by diet alone, *iron supplementation* is recommended by obstetricians. The standard recommendation is a daily supplement of 30 mg of elemental iron in the form of simple iron salts (ferrous gluconate, ferrous sulfate, ferrous fumarate) beginning at about the twelfth week of pregnancy. This amount is recommended for women whose hemoglobin and iron stores are normal before pregnancy. Women pregnant with more than one fetus or those already anemic from menstrual blood loss or multiple pregnancies should take 60 to 100 mg of supplemental elemental iron per day until the hemoglobin concentration becomes normal, at which time the supplementation can be reduced to 30 mg/d. The commonly used prenatal vitamin and mineral supplements contain 45 to 60 mg of elemental iron per tablet; a 320-mg ferrous sulfate tablet contains 64 mg of elemental iron. (See Chapter 7 and Table 7-36 for a discussion of iron supplements.)

5. Oral iron supplements can cause *gastrointestinal side effects,* including heartburn, nausea, constipation or diarrhea, abdominal cramps, and change in stool color.

   a. **Postponement of supplementation until second trimester.** Nausea is a problem for many women early in pregnancy and may be exacerbated by iron supplements. Because iron requirements do not increase until the second trimester, it is reasonable to defer iron supplementation until the second trimester for women whose nausea is worsened by iron supplements.

   b. **Timing of dose.** The unpleasant gastrointestinal side effects of iron can be minimized by taking the iron supplement after a meal rather than on an empty stomach. Unfortunately, iron ingested with or after a meal is not absorbed as well as iron taken during fasting.

   c. **Constipation** is commonly associated with oral iron supplementation and can be treated with bulk "laxatives," such as psyllium preparations.

   d. **Changed stool color.** Patients given iron supplements should be warned that their stools will turn black.

   e. Pregnant women with small children should be warned to keep iron supplements out of reach. Ingestion of maternal prenatal iron supplements is a common cause of significant *iron intoxication in children.*

   f. **Antacids** impair the absorption of iron, and the two should not be taken together. This is of some importance because gastroesophageal reflux with heartburn develops frequently in late pregnancy.

6. **Pica,** the craving for unnatural foods, develops occasionally in pregnant women and is often associated with iron-deficiency anemia. In the past, the consumption of starch, clay, and dirt was thought to be a cause of iron deficiency because these substances bind iron in the gut, preventing absorption. More recently, an alternative view has been expressed that *iron deficiency is a cause of pica.* The precise craving induced by iron deficiency may be determined by social and cultural factors; the craving is not always for unnatural foods. Pregnant women with iron-deficiency anemia should be asked about pica, and those with pica should be tested for iron-deficiency anemia.

B. **Folic acid depletion** is the most common vitamin deficiency of pregnancy. Folate is required for the synthesis of the thymidylate moiety and thus for DNA synthesis. The major reason for the markedly increased folate requirement in pregnancy is increased maternal erythropoiesis. During the last two trimesters, the total erythrocyte volume increases 20% to 30%.

1. The primary maternal manifestation of severe folate deficiency is **megaloblastic anemia.** Severe folate deficiency is not commonly seen as a complication of pregnancy in the United States. If **depletion of folate stores** rather than clinical deficiency is used to define folate deficiency, then the incidence is much higher. Several surveys have revealed incidences of folate deficiency of 25% to 30% among pregnant women when folate deficiency is defined as a reduction of serum or red cell folate levels.

   The *clinical significance* of moderately diminished serum folate levels in the second and third trimesters of pregnancy is not clear. Ill effects for the mother are not well defined. However, inadequate folate availability (because of deficient intake or defective metabolism) during embryogenesis, organogenesis, and early fetal life is known to have profound consequences. At least one of these, incomplete closure of the neural tube, is largely preventable, as discussed below.

   Folic acid antagonists, such as the commonly prescribed drugs phenobarbital, phenytoin, primidone, carbamazepine, trimethoprim, and triamterene, when taken during the second or third month after the last menstrual period, double the relative risk for fetal cardiovascular defects, urinary tract defects, or oral clefts (95% confidence intervals ranging from 1.2–1.5 to 3.0–3.7) (7). Folic acid antagonists taken either before or after this 2-month window appear to have no deleterious effects on fetal development (7). The use of folic acid supplements during pregnancy diminished the effects of dihydrofolate reductase inhibitors, but not the teratogenic effects of antiepileptic drugs (7).

   Some surveys have indicated higher incidences of recurrent abortion, abruptio placentae, toxemia, impaired fetal growth, and limb defects in association with diminished maternal red cell folate levels. However, these are *unproven consequences* because it is difficult in such surveys to separate low folate levels from other manifestations of poor nutrition and low socioeconomic status.

2. **Neural tube defects.** Overwhelming evidence is now available to indicate that the incidence of neural tube defects (anencephaly, spina bifida) in the offspring of women who take folic acid supplements of at least 400 mg/d before and during the first 4 weeks of pregnancy is approximately one-fourth to one-half the incidence in the offspring of women who do not (8,9). The effect of supplemental folic acid is lost after the first month of gestation because embryonic neural tube closure is complete by then. Only about 5% of neural tube defects are recurrences. Approximately half the women of childbearing age who become pregnant do not plan to do so. In addition, by the time most women realize they are pregnant, they are halfway through the first 4 weeks of gestation. For these reasons, in September of 1992, the Centers for Disease Control and Prevention issued the recommendation that *all women of childbearing age* take supplemental folic acid (9). Further, to help ensure adequate levels of folate in women of childbearing age, cereal grain products in the United States are now fortified with 140 µg of folic acid per 100 g of grain (10).

3. **Folate requirements.** Few studies of folate balance in adult nonpregnant women have been performed, and the results of these differ according to the endpoints used to define adequacy and according to whether the subjects were studied at maintenance intakes or following dietary depletion and repletion. Based on a careful analysis of the limited data, the Food and Nutrition Board has set the estimated average requirement (EAR) for folate in women of childbearing age at 320 µg of folate equivalents per day and the RDA for folate at 400 µg/d (11,12). For pregnant women, approximately 200 µg of *additional* folate is required daily, so that the RDA for folate in pregnant women is set at 600 µg of folate equivalents per day (11,12). The latter recommendation, however, does not cover the issue of neural tube defect prevention (see below)

because the neural tube is substantially formed before most women know that they are pregnant and seek professional advice.

A *healthful diet* contains approximately 700 µg of food folates, of which about half is bioavailable. Thus, this diet nearly meets the recent recommendations for women of childbearing age, but a slightly substandard diet that is more typical of the current American diet would be deficient in folate. Good dietary sources of folate are dark green leafy vegetables, green and lima beans, orange juice, fortified cereals, yeast, mushrooms, liver, and kidneys. Root vegetables, eggs, and most dairy products are poor sources of folate. Remember too that dietary folate is markedly influenced by food storage and methods of food preparation. Folate is destroyed by boiling and other food-processing methods, including canning.

Normal body stores of folate are in the range of 12 to 18 mg. A pregnant woman consuming a folate-deficient diet could deplete her normal folate stores in a few weeks to a few months, depending on the level of her prior stores and the degree of dietary deficiency. Women consuming a diet chronically deficient in folate (including alcoholics and many from lower socioeconomic groups) have small folate stores that would be depleted even more rapidly.

4. **Folate supplementation.** In September 1992, because of the accumulating data on the efficacy of folic acid supplementation in significantly decreasing the incidence of neural tube defects, the U.S. Public Health Service through the Centers for Disease Control and Prevention issued the following recommendation: *"All women of childbearing age in the United States who are capable of becoming pregnant should consume 0.4 mg of folic acid per day for the purposes of reducing their risk of having a pregnancy affected with spina bifida and other neural tube defects. Because the effects of high intakes are not well-known but include complicating the diagnosis of B_{12} deficiency, care should be taken to keep total folate consumption under 1 mg/d, except under the supervision of a physician. Women who have a prior NTD-affected pregnancy are at high risk of having a subsequent affected pregnancy. When these women are planning to become pregnant, they should consult their physician for advice"* (9).

It is important to realize that the current RDA of 400 µg of folate equivalents for nonpregnant women does not strictly conform to the Centers for Disease Control recommendation; in clinical studies of the prevention of neural tube defects, folic acid, not food folates, was used, and in the Centers for Disease Control recommendation, as written, supplementation is in the form of folic acid. Thus, an operational recommendation for *"women capable of becoming pregnant is to take 400 µg of folate per day from fortified foods and/or a supplement as well as food folate from a varied diet."* (11).

The *effects of oral contraceptives on folate metabolism* are not completely defined. Some surveys have indicated that red cell levels of folate are diminished in long-time users of oral contraceptives. Oral contraceptives have variously been described to interfere with folate absorption and accelerate folate degradation in the liver. Whatever the mechanism, it appears that folate stores may be depleted in women who have used oral contraceptives, and that folate deficiency is more likely to develop in these women during pregnancy.

C. **Calcium and vitamin D**
1. The added *calcium* requirement of pregnancy is about 25 to 30 g—the amount of calcium in the fetus at term. Almost all the fetal calcium is added during the last trimester, when the fetus takes up an average of 300 mg/d. In the first half of pregnancy, fetal calcium accretion is only about 50 mg/d.

Unlike maternal iron stores, which are relatively small, *maternal calcium stores are large.* Almost all the maternal stores are in the skeleton, some of which can be mobilized easily if needed. The 30-g calcium requirement of a single pregnancy represents 2.5% of the total maternal stores. Further increased maternal absorption of dietary calcium easily fulfills the small additional need, and no evidence has been found that maternal bone mineral density changes during pregnancy in relation to calcium intake. Therefore, the recommended adequate intake (AI) of calcium during pregnancy, 1,000 mg/d, remains unchanged from the corresponding recommendation for nonpregnant adult women (13) (Table 4-1). Some evidence indicates that adolescents may need to increase their calcium intake during pregnancy, but this issue requires more study.

An adequate intake of *dietary calcium* is easily achieved by women who consume dairy products (1 qt of milk contains 1,000 mg of calcium). Even women who avoid dairy products because of lactose intolerance may be able to achieve an adequate dietary calcium intake. Those who are relatively lactose-deficient may substitute hard cheese for milk. For example, 2 oz of Swiss cheese has twice as much calcium as 8 oz of milk but only one-eleventh as much lactose. Rare cases of osteomalacia have been reported in multiparous women in underdeveloped countries, who have very low levels of dietary calcium. This has not been a problem in the United States. The calcium intakes recommended for pregnancy are sometimes not achieved with dietary sources alone in some groups having special or selective food preferences and in some black, Hispanic, and Native American populations. These groups should be encouraged to increase their intake of calcium from acceptable food sources or, less preferably, be given a calcium supplement.

When *calcium supplementation* is needed, calcium carbonate, gluconate, or lactate can be given to provide 600 mg of calcium daily and make up the difference between the calcium requirement and dietary intake. (See Table 7-19 for a list of available calcium preparations.) A good calcium supplement is calcium carbonate; a 500-mg tablet contains 200 mg of calcium. However, it is less soluble than some other preparations, such as calcium gluconate, so that it is not universally useful. One must exercise caution with supplements, and a tolerable upper intake limit (UL) for calcium during pregnancy has been set at 2,500 mg/d, a value no different from that advised for nonpregnant women (13). When supplements are necessary to treat deficiency, the degree of replacement can be followed by measuring the 24-hour urinary excretion of calcium.

2. **Vitamin D** regulates calcium and phosphorus metabolism. It increases calcium absorption from the gut and potentiates bone resorption induced by parathyroid hormone. Maternal vitamin D is transported across the placenta to the fetus. In the United States, significant vitamin D deficiency is rare, and routine vitamin D supplementation during pregnancy is not required. The RDA for vitamin D in pregnant women is 5 μg (200 IU), the same as in nonpregnant women (13).

Evidence suggests that *maternal vitamin D deficiency* can result in fetal vitamin D deficiency, manifested by neonatal hypocalcemia. Vitamin D deficiency is usually the result of a very low dietary intake combined with minimal exposure to sunlight. Daily supplementation with 5 μg of vitamin D should be considered for complete vegetarians and for persons who avoid sunlight or vitamin D-fortified milk.

Excessive maternal intake of vitamin D may result in severe infantile hypercalcemia. The tolerable UL for vitamin D intake during pregnancy is 50 μg (2,000 IU) (13).

D. **Other nutrient requirements.** The *magnesium* RDA for nonpregnant adult women is in the range of 310 to 320 mg/d (13). This RDA is increased to 350 to 360 mg/d for pregnant women, although no direct experimental data are available to support the increased need (14).

The adult woman's RDA for *vitamin C* is 75 mg/d (14). During pregnancy, this value is increased to 85 mg/d on the basis of declining maternal plasma vitamin C levels and the necessary transfer of vitamin C to the fetus (14). However, no direct experimental data support the need for additional vitamin C during pregnancy. Because of concerns about megadoses of vitamin D for various hypothetical and unproven benefits, and because vitamin C is actively transported from the maternal to the fetal circulation, a tolerable UL for vitamin C intake in pregnancy has been set at 1,800 to 2,000 mg (14) (Appendix B).

With very limited data, and largely on the basis of changes in maternal metabolism during pregnancy and estimations of fetal nutrient accretion, the RDAs for *riboflavin, niacin, vitamin A, vitamin B_6, vitamin B_{12}*, and *zinc* have been modestly increased for pregnant women (4,15) (Table 4-1), as have the RDAs for *copper, iodine,* and *molybdenum* and the AIs for *chromium* and *manganese* (15) (Appendix B1).

IV. **Assessment of nutritional status during pregnancy.** A pregnant woman should be assessed for nutritional risk factors that would jeopardize the outcome of her pregnancy. A history of previous pregnancies should be obtained, with attention to complications, duration of pregnancy, birth weight and length, and development of the child after delivery. A history of eclampsia, abortion, low-birth-weight infant, hyperemesis, or anemia during past pregnancies has implications for the outcome of the present pregnancy. A nutritional assessment also should include the patient's weight, a brief diet history (including alcohol intake and smoking), and a history of the use of medications that might affect nutrient absorption (e.g., folic acid antagonists, anticonvulsants, thyroid medications, vitamins).

A. **Nutritional risk factors at the onset of pregnancy**
   1. **Adolescence.** An adolescent who becomes pregnant within 3 years of menarche is at special risk for a poor outcome of pregnancy. The nutritional demands of pregnancy are added to the needs of a mother who may still be still growing. The demands for calories, protein, and calcium are all increased. Adolescents are more likely than adults to have inadequate diets, and so special attention must be paid to the diet of pregnant adolescents. Pregnant adolescents are also more likely to come from low socioeconomic groups, among which poor nutrition is common.
   2. **Three or more pregnancies within 2 years.** Multiple pregnancies at close intervals deplete stored nutrients, including iron and folate. Iron deficiency is an especially significant problem in this group.
   3. **Poor reproductive performance.** A past history of low-birth-weight infants, abortions, or perinatal loss may reflect nutritional deficiency. The factor most highly correlated with the delivery of a low-birth-weight infant is the past history of a low-birth-weight infant.
   4. **Economic deprivation.** The diets of patients with low incomes are more likely to be deficient in iron, folate, protein, and B vitamins.
   5. **Food faddists.** Women who are on unusual diets deficient in nutrients are at risk.
      a. Those on *weight-loss programs* during pregnancy, especially severely carbohydrate-restricted diets that result in ketosis, are at risk for a poor outcome.
      b. **Strict vegetarians** may be deficient in vitamin B_{12} and riboflavin in addition to iron.
      c. The ingestion of *vitamins* in excessive quantities (megavitamin therapy) may have harmful effects on the fetus. "Rebound" scurvy has been reported in the infants of mothers who have taken massive doses of *vitamin C* (>5g/d). The fetus becomes metabolically dependent on high levels of vitamin C that are provided by the mother *in utero* but not by the infant's diet after birth. Studies in rats have shown unequivocally that high doses of *vitamin A* are teratogenic. Pregnant women are advised not to take more than 800 μg of retinol equivalents per day.

6. **Smoking, drug addiction, and alcoholism**
   a. **Smokers** tend to have low-birth-weight infants. This is thought to be in part a consequence of depressed maternal food intake and inadequate weight gain. The contraindications to smoking are independent of the issues of pregnancy, but pregnancy surely adds one more immediately compelling reason for adult women who smoke to stop.
   b. Heavy *maternal drinking* is associated with prenatal growth retardation. Heavy alcohol consumption is associated with a *diet deficient in B vitamins,* folate, and protein. Maternal alcoholism is associated with fetal toxicity in addition to nutritional deficiencies. Animal studies show that alcohol is a teratogen. Fetal abnormalities associated with heavy maternal alcohol ingestion in humans *(fetal alcohol syndrome)* include microcephaly, cleft palate, and micrognathia. Although it is clear that heavy alcohol consumption is harmful, the *effects of limited or occasional alcohol intake* are undefined. It is not known whether a minimum alcohol intake exists below which risk is not increased. The National Institute of Alcohol Abuse and Alcoholism advises against drinking more than 1 oz of alcohol per day. This is the equivalent of 24 oz of beer, 10 oz of wine, or 2 oz of liquor. In the first trimester, alcohol should be avoided entirely. Because it is possible that the dose–response curve for the effects of alcohol on fetal outcome may extend down into the range of minimal or moderate drinking, the safest course is abstinence from alcohol, as recommended in the *Dietary Guidelines for Americans, 2000* and by the Council on Scientific Affairs of the American Medical Association.
7. **Chronic systemic disease.** Pregnant *diabetic women* must be diligent to avoid both hypoglycemia and hyperglycemia with ketosis. Diabetes in pregnancy is associated with resistance to insulin and an increased insulin requirement. On the other hand, fetal glucose utilization may cause maternal fasting hypoglycemia. Diseases associated with *malabsorption* may cause problems during pregnancy. Primary diseases of the small intestine, such as *Crohn's disease,* may result in malabsorption of many nutrients or malabsorption of selected nutrients, such as vitamin B_{12} or iron. *Chronic pancreatic disease* is associated with malabsorption of fats and, to a lesser extent, fat-soluble vitamins. Usually, malabsorption can be managed either by treating the underlying disease or by appropriate nutritional supplementation.
8. **Prepregnant weight**
   a. **Underweight.** Women who are underweight at the beginning of pregnancy (BMI < 19.8) are at risk for having low-birth-weight babies (5). Underweight mothers also may be at increased risk for toxemia. If a woman who is underweight before pregnancy does not gain enough weight during pregnancy, the risks are increased further.

      Obviously, the optimal time for dealing with the underweight woman is before pregnancy. An underweight woman who is considering pregnancy should be encouraged to gain weight first. When an underweight woman does become pregnant, she should be encouraged to gain more weight than is recommended for the woman who enters pregnancy at a normal weight. Protein–calorie supplements may be necessary to correct previous nutritional deficits and provide for the needs of pregnancy.
   b. **Overweight.** Women whose BMI before pregnancy exceeds 26 are also at risk (5). Obese women are at increased risk for the development of diabetes, hypertension, and thromboembolic events during pregnancy. The appropriate management of pregnancy in obese women to limit these complications is the subject of considerable controversy. Currently, the guidelines for prudent maternal weight gain are within the range of 15 to 25 lb (5) (Table 4-2).

The *reasons to avoid severe calorie restriction* during pregnancy are compelling. When caloric intake is severely restricted, an inadequate intake of calcium, iron, folate, B vitamins, and protein results. If ingested protein is to be used in the synthesis of maternal and fetal proteins, the caloric intake must be adequate. *If caloric intake is inadequate, ingested proteins are catabolized for energy needs.* It has been estimated that 32 kcal/kg of body weight is required for the optimal use of ingested protein (see Chapter 5). Furthermore, severe restriction of total caloric intake, especially when carbohydrate intake is also restricted, results in *ketosis.* Studies of diabetic women indicate that ketosis is poorly tolerated by the fetus. Ketosis may be associated with a reduction in uterine blood flow. Ketone bodies are concentrated in the amniotic fluid and taken up by the fetus. The mental development of the offspring of mothers who have had ketonuria during pregnancy, as a consequence of either diabetes or starvation, may be compromised. Whether this is a direct effect of fetal ketosis or the effect of an associated metabolic problem is not clear.

B. Risk factors developing during pregnancy

1. **Anemia.** Beginning at 3 months' gestation, the maternal blood volume increases markedly. The increase in blood volume precedes the increase in red cell mass, which begins at 6 months, and the increase in blood volume is proportionally greater than the increase in red cell mass. This *dilutional anemia* is characterized by decreased "normal" values for hemoglobin and hematocrit. The decrease begins at 3 to 5 months of gestation. Hemoglobin and hematocrit continue to fall until 5 to 8 months. They begin to rise at term and are normal by 6 weeks after delivery.

   In many pregnant women, a *nutritional anemia* develops along with the normal dilutional anemia. In the vast majority of cases, nutritional anemia is a consequence of *inadequate iron intake.* The hemoglobin levels of up to 40% of women who are not given supplemental iron drop below 11 g/dL. With *iron supplementation,* a hemoglobin level this low is uncommon. Nutritional *megaloblastic anemia secondary to folate deficiency* also occurs, but much less often.

2. **Inadequate weight gain.** The normal pattern of weight gain is a total of about 6 lb during the first trimester, followed by a relatively steady gain of almost a pound per week during the second and third trimesters (3). Inadequate weight gain (<2 lb/mo during the second and third trimesters) is associated with low birth weight, intrauterine growth retardation, and fetal jeopardy. Failure of fetal growth frequently correlates with inadequate weight gain. Negative discrepancy in gestational age versus uterine size or biparietal diameter of the fetal head as measured by sonography are signs of intrauterine growth retardation. Women with inadequate weight gain or actual weight loss should be evaluated. A careful diet history should be taken to determine if protein and calorie intake are adequate, and supplements should be given if needed.

3. **Excessive weight gain.** Rapid weight accumulation (>1.5 to 2 lb/wk) is usually a sign of *fluid retention.* Fluid retention is associated with toxemia, although it does not cause toxemia. Not everyone who retains fluid becomes toxemic, and fluid retention in the absence of hypertension or proteinuria is not an indication for salt restriction or diuretic therapy. Women who retain fluid should be observed for other signs of toxemia.

   Edema in the lower extremities is commonly seen in the later stages of pregnancy; it is caused by the accumulation of interstitial fluid secondary to obstruction of the pelvic veins. The edema can be treated by elevating the legs and wearing support hose.

   Excessive weight gain during pregnancy may be caused by *fat deposition* rather than fluid retention. This should be evaluated by the physician and dietary recommendations offered if weight guidelines exceed those in Table 4-2.

V. Gastrointestinal problems in pregnancy

A. **Nausea and vomiting.** Nausea and vomiting are common in early pregnancy. Eating foods high in carbohydrate, such as crackers, bread, or dry cereal, before rising in the morning may help. Drinking liquids between meals should be encouraged. Fatty foods and caffeine should be avoided.

B. **Constipation.** Constipation is common in pregnancy and is caused by pressure of the enlarging uterus, hormonal changes, and iron supplements. Constipation can be treated with increased exercise, increased fluid intake, and either increased dietary fiber or the use of a supplemental psyllium or polycarbophil preparation (Tables 11-13 and 11-14).

C. **Heartburn.** Reflux esophagitis is common in pregnancy secondary to increased abdominal pressure caused by the enlarging uterus. Hormonal changes may loosen the lower esophageal sphincter. The initial approach is very similar to that used in nonpregnant patients with reflux esophagitis.
   1. Elevate the head of the bed 4 in with bed blocks.
   2. Avoid eating within the 2 to 3 hours before retiring.
   3. Avoid alcohol, especially before retiring.
   4. Eat frequent small meals.
   5. Take antacids as needed. Be alert to their effects on iron absorption.

VI. Nutrition during lactation

A. **Human milk is the optimal food for human infants** (16). It contains a plethora of unique dietary components and host resistance factors that cannot be provided by conventional commercial formulas. Under ordinary circumstances, breast-feeding is recommended for all infants in the United States for at least the first 6 months of life and, preferably, for the first year of life in combination with appropriate supplementation with solid foods. Most women in the United States are capable of breast-feeding their infants adequately (17,18), and nutritional needs during lactation have been extensively reviewed by a panel of the National Academy of Sciences (19).

B. Maternal nutritional status is not related to milk volume in the United States and other industrialized countries. Average milk volumes (750 to 800 mL/d) are comparable in thin, normal-weight, and obese women despite large differences in dietary intakes. Regular exercise also does not appear to affect milk volume.

C. The nutritional quality of human milk is not usually affected adversely by *modest deficiencies in maternal nutrition.* In fact, the mother often loses a small amount of weight gradually during the normal period of lactation.

D. Even milk from malnourished women generally provides an infant with adequate calories, proteins, vitamins, and minerals. The levels of most nutrients in milk, such as calcium and folate, are maintained at the expense of maternal stores. Maternal dietary intake does not affect the macronutrient contents of milk, except that the kinds of fatty acids found in milk are influenced strongly by the maternal diet. Milk calcium, phosphorus, sodium, potassium, and magnesium are not altered by the maternal diet, although the levels of iodine and selenium in milk tend to parallel maternal intake. The concentrations of vitamins in human milk depend on the mother's stores and current intake. However, within usual dietary intake levels, these differences are not practically important. The levels of pyridoxine and vitamins A, D, and B_{12} in milk are the most likely to decline as a result of sustained maternal malnutrition.

E. Increasing maternal nutrient intakes above the RDA level usually does not result in correspondingly high nutrient levels in milk, with the exception of iodine, selenium, vitamin D, and pyridoxine.

F. The *RDAs for most nutrients,* except vitamin D, calcium, magnesium, and iron, are somewhat greater for lactating women than for nonlactating women (Table 4-1). Significant increases are recommended in *calories* (additional 500 kcal/d), *protein* (additional 12 to 15 g/d), vitamin A (additional

70 µg retinol activity equivalents), folate (plus 100 µg dietary folate equivalents), zinc (plus 4 mg), and the B vitamins niacin, riboflavin, B_6, and B_{12} (Table 4-1). Remember, the average 3.5-kg newborn infant doubles his or her weight by 4 months of age. In other words, within 4 months, the mother must supply the infant with the same dietary energy, protein, and other nutrients via the breast that she supplied during a 9-month period *in utero* via the placenta. In general, lactation places a more significant nutritional demand on the mother than pregnancy does (11,13,15,19).

G. The *iron* requirements of the lactating mother are not significantly increased because the amount of iron secreted into milk is less than that normally lost during menstruation. It is common obstetric practice, however, to prescribe an iron supplement.

H. Lactating women should be educated to obtain adequate nutrition from a *well-balanced diet* rather than through the use of nutritional supplements.

I. Women with *specialized dietary habits,* such as vegans, should receive competent nutritional advice from trained professionals to ensure the adequate nutritional health of their infants. There is absolutely no reason to discourage breast-feeding in women with unique dietary patterns. Rather, appropriate educational advice should be provided to ensure adequate dietary nutrients. If necessary, dietary supplements can provide limiting nutrients.

J. As in any human being, *substance abuse* and the *use of illicit drugs* should be actively discouraged in lactating women. Addicted persons should be encouraged to enter appropriate treatment programs. Lactating women should not smoke. Besides the known long-term health risks, smoking reduces milk volume. Modest consumption of coffee and alcohol, less than one to two cups and one to two drinks daily, respectively, is not known to affect lactation or the health of the infant adversely.

K. **Women with HIV/AIDS should not breast-feed their infants.** The main route of transmission of the virus from mother to child is breast-feeding, and transmission can be prevented by not breast-feeding (20,21).

VII. **Overall plan of management**

A. Pregnant women should be evaluated for the presence of *nutritional risk factors,* as already discussed.

B. The most desirable weight gain during pregnancy is determined by the woman's *BMI* before pregnancy (Table 4-2). Almost all the weight gain should occur in the second and third trimesters.

C. **Calorie intake** should be increased during the second and third trimesters to achieve the desired weight gain. The increase is usually an additional 300 kcal/d.

D. **Protein intake** should be increased to about 60g/d during pregnancy.

E. **All women of childbearing age should be sure to consume 400 µg of folic acid daily.**

F. Other *nutritional supplements* recommended routinely for women who begin pregnancy with a normal weight and good dietary habits are iron (15 to 30 mg of elemental ferrous iron per day), 200 µg of food folate equivalents per day, 10 mg of vitamin C, 4 mg of niacin equivalents, 3 mg of zinc, 0.3 mg of riboflavin, 0.6 mg of vitamin B_6, and 0.6 µg of vitamin B_{12}. It is important to realize, however, that the data on which most of these recommendations are based are limited, and the recommendations in fact primarily constitute a judicious form of "nutrition insurance." Additional research is necessary to establish firmly the scientific basis of these recommendations.

G. Modest degrees of *fluid retention* and *ankle edema* are normal during pregnancy, and neither salt restriction nor diuretics are required.

References

1. Osmund C, Barker DJ. Fetal, infant, and childhood growth are predictors of coronary heart disease, diabetes, and hypertension in adult men and women. *Environ Health Perspect* 2000;108[Suppl 3]:545.

2. Phillips DI. Birth weight and the future development of diabetes. A review of the evidence. *Diabetes Care* 1998;21[Suppl 2]:B150.
3. Durnin JVGA. Energy requirements of pregnancy. *Diabetes* 1991;40[Suppl 2]:152.
4. National Research Council. *Recommended dietary allowances,* 10th ed. Washington, DC: National Academy Press, 1989.
5. Institute of Medicine, Food and Nutrition Board, Committee on Nutritional Status during Pregnancy and Lactation. *Nutrition during pregnancy, part I: weight gain; part II: nutrient supplements.* Washington, DC: National Academy Press, 1990.
6. Allen LH, ed. Recent developments in maternal nutrition and their implications for practitioners. *Am J Clin Nutr* 1994;59[Suppl]:437S.
7. Hernandez-Diaz S, Werler MM, Walker M, et al. Folic acid antagonists during pregnancy and the risk of birth defects. *N Engl J Med* 2000;343:1608.
8. Czeizel EA, Dudas I. Prevention of the first occurrence of neural-tube defects by periconceptional vitamin supplementation. *N Engl J Med* 1992;327:1832.
9. Centers for Disease Control and Prevention. Recommendations for the use of folic acid to reduce the number of cases of spina bifida and other neural tube defects. *MMWR Morb Mortal Wkly Rep* 1992;41[RR-14]:1.
10. Food standards: amendment of the standards of identity for enriched grain products to require addition of folic acid. Final rule. (Codified at 21 CFR parts 136, 137, and 139). *Federal Register* 1996;61:8781.
11. Standing Committee on the Scientific Evaluation of Dietary Reference Intakes, Food and Nutrition Board, Institute of Medicine. *Dietary reference intakes for thiamin, niacin, vitamin B_6, folate, vitamin B_{12}, pantothenic acid, biotin, and choline.* Washington, DC: National Academy Press, 1998.
12. Suitor CW, Bailey LB. Dietary folate equivalents: interpretation and application. *J Am Diet Assoc* 2000;100:88.
13. Standing Committee on the Scientific Evaluation of Dietary Reference Intakes, Food and Nutrition Board, Institute of Medicine. *Dietary reference intakes for calcium, phosphorus, magnesium, vitamin D, and fluoride.* Washington, DC: National Academy Press, 1997.
14. Standing Committee on the Scientific Evaluation of Dietary Reference Intakes, Food and Nutrition Board, Institute of Medicine. *Dietary reference intakes for vitamin A, vitamin K, arsenic, boron, chromium, copper, iodine, iron, manganese, molybdenum, nickel, silicon, vanadium, and zinc.* Washington, DC: National Academy Press, 2001.
15. Standing Committee on the Scientific Evaluation of Dietary Reference Intakes, Food and Nutrition Board, Institute of Medicine. *Dietary reference intakes for vitamin C, vitamin E, selenium, and carotenoids.* Washington, DC: National Academy Press, 2000.
16. Lonnerdal B. Breast milk: a truly functional food. *Nutrition* 2000;16:509.
17. Garza C, Hopkinson JM. Physiology of lactation. In: Tsang R, Nichols BL, eds. *Nutrition during infancy.* St. Louis: Mosby, 1986:225.
18. Hopkinson JM, Garza C. Management of breast-feeding. In: Tsang R, Nichols BL, eds. *Nutrition during infancy.* St. Louis: Mosby, 1986:298.
19. Institute of Medicine, Food and Nutrition Board, Committee on Nutritional Status During Pregnancy and Lactation. *Nutrition during lactation.* Washington, DC: National Academy Press, 1993.
20. Mofenson LM and the Committee on Pediatric AIDS. Technical report: perinatal human immunodeficiency virus testing and prevention of transmission. *Pediatrics* 2000;106:e88.
21. Fiore S, Newell ML. Preventing perinatal transmission of HIV-1 infection. *Hosp Med* 2000;61:315.

II. INDIVIDUAL NUTRIENT COMPONENTS

5. PROTEIN AND CALORIES: REQUIREMENTS, INTAKE, AND ASSESSMENT

I. **Estimation of normal daily requirements.** The physician is often faced with patients who are losing weight, are undergoing surgery, or have a disease that increases their usual energy needs. To ensure the proper caloric intake, a reasonable estimate of energy needs must be made. Most of these estimates rely on the carefully measured and standardized determination of the basal metabolic rate and of energy utilization during exercise. The general principles behind the estimation of energy requirements have been reviewed in detail (1,2).

   A. **Energy equation.** It is impossible to predict daily energy use precisely because of the complex factors involved. The methods used to determine energy needs experimentally are flawed, including diet recall and metabolic rates. Current recommendations do not allow for diversity in body composition, dietary intake, or level of activity. Nonetheless, if the principles involved in deriving the recommendations are understood, then one can use the various methods to estimate energy needs. Energy requirements in humans are defined by the following formula:

   $$TDR = BMR\ (60 - 75\%) + EEA\ (15 - 30\%) + TER\ (\sim 10\%)$$

   where TDR = total daily requirement,
   BMR = basal metabolic rate,
   EEA = energy expenditure of activity, and
   TEF = thermal effect of food.

   Basal metabolic rate is a measure of the amount of energy expended to maintain a living state at rest and 12 to 18 hours after a meal; synonyms for this measurement are *basal energy requirement* (BER), *basal energy expenditure* (BEE), *resting metabolic rate* (RMR), and *resting energy expenditure* (REE), except that the REE is not usually measured under basal conditions. REE is the sum of BEE, nonshivering thermogenesis, and stress hypermetabolism. In practice, BMR and REE differ by less than 10%. The BMR or RMR is proportional to the fat-free mass but is influenced by age, sex, body composition, and genetics. It decreases about 2% to 3% per decade and is greater in men than in women of equal weight.

   Energy expenditure of activity, or thermal effect of activity (TEA), is a measure of the energy expended by the body to support a variety of physical activities. This is the most variable item in the energy equation, ranging from about 100 kcal/d in sedentary persons to about 3,000 kcal/d in moderately active persons. The EEA decreases with age and loss of fat-free mass and is greater in men than in women of equal weight.

   Thermal effect of food is an estimate of the number of calories produced as heat during the ingestion and metabolism of food, also called the *specific dynamic action of food* (SDA). The obligatory components of the TEF represent the energy needed for absorption and transport of nutrients plus synthesis and storage. Protein increases heat production by 12%, carbohydrate by 6%, and fat by 2%. A mixed diet yields a 6% increase in heat, but 10% is the usual figure used. The lower the total energy expenditure, the greater the relative importance of the calorigenic effect in determining total energy requirements. The calorigenic effect of food seems to be related closely to the energy required for adenosine triphosphate (ATP) formation and occurs even after food is administered intravenously. The TEF decreases with age and insulin resistance. Excess energy above the TEF is modulated by the sympathetic nervous system.

   In hypermetabolic or infected, febrile patients, the specific dynamic action of food is lower than normal because heat production is already increased.

Thus, the figure used to calculate additional energy requirements for these patients should be 5% rather than 10%. When nutrients are provided continuously, as for hospitalized patients, energy is not needed for storing and recovering nutrients, and the TEF can be ignored for purposes of estimating energy needs.

B. Choice of method. The physician can be confused by the large number of empirically derived methods for estimating the three components of the daily energy requirement. More than 190 methods have been reported to predict energy expenditures (3). The following sections outline a number of the available methods. It is important to use a single method of calculation for each of the three components and to understand the limitations of that method. It is not necessary to learn multiple methods for calculating the BMR or any of the other components because the methods all provide only an estimate and not a precise calculation.

II. Calculation of basal metabolic rate. Energy consumption is assessed by measuring oxygen consumption under carefully controlled conditions. Oxygen uptake is related to carbon dioxide output plus heat. It is translated into calories by assuming the amount of expired carbon dioxide that would yield a nonprotein respiratory quotient of 0.82—that is, a caloric value for oxygen of 4.825 kcal (20.19 kJ)/L. Most of the energy estimates are derived from older measures of BMR. Although measurements of basal metabolism over 1 hour were used to calculate a 24-hour requirement, a more meaningful determination of metabolic rate would reflect the rate at which energy is consumed in a normal life situation while the body is at rest and ingesting food under neutral climatic conditions. This measurement of resting metabolism would include the specific dynamic action of food.

Although the equipment for measuring BMR is not complicated, the actual measurement is time-consuming and considerable variability is involved unless the conditions maintained during measurement are carefully standardized. It has become accepted practice that estimates of BMR are derived from carefully collated data from normal subjects obtained under controlled conditions. Additional energy requirements attributed to the thermal effect of food, growth (in children), and illness are estimated independently and added to the calories required for the BMR. More accurate measurements than are possible with the old, portable BMR apparatus utilize doubly labeled water ($^3H_2^{18}O$). By following the decay in body water for 1 to 2 weeks, one can calculate the rate of carbon dioxide production and estimate total daily energy needs in free-living individuals. This method is technically exacting and not in wide clinical use.

A. Methods for calculating BMR. The BMR can be estimated in a variety of ways by using calculations based on (a) body size (height and weight), (b) weight alone, (c) body size and age, (d) weight and sex, and (e) weight, height, age, and sex. Not surprisingly, the BMR values based on different individual parameters are not identical for each method in the same person. In regard to clinical usefulness, all these methods are satisfactory. The first group of methods presented requires the use of tables to estimate the BMR. Shorter methods not requiring tables are reasonably accurate for estimating the BMR over the entire range of existing body sizes and are currently in widespread use.

1. Physiologic basis for estimate. The cells of the body require oxygen for their integrity; the greater the number of cells, the greater the oxygen consumption. Adipose cells are relatively inert from a metabolic point of view; they constitute about 20% of the body mass but account for only 2% to 4% of the BMR. Thus, in overweight persons, whose adipose cells are increased in number and size, the correlation between weight alone and oxygen consumption is not linear, and oxygen consumption per pound of extra weight is not equivalent to that per pound of lean body weight. Instead of the old, portable BMR apparatus, doubly labeled water ($^3H_2^{18}O$) is used. Body surface area is a more reasonable determinant of lean body mass—that is, metabolically active tissues. Muscle makes up

35% to 40% of body weight but contributes only 20% to the BMR. The brain and liver require high levels of energy but change less with body size than does muscle mass. The increase in BMR per kilogram of body weight or per square meter of surface area depends primarily on the relative proportions of skeletal muscle and adipose tissue and their metabolic activity (different for various states of conditioning). Thus, oxygen consumption increases at the same rate in any person for every unit of increase in body surface area. As body weight increases over normal, when adipose tissue is the major component of body tissue added, the rate of increase in oxygen consumption declines. It is more accurate to have an estimation of BMR that accounts for these changes rather than one based on weight alone.

2. **BMR estimate based on body surface area.** This estimate is made according to the following steps:

   a. Determine body surface area (Fig. 5-1). The BMR is expressed in square meters (m^2).

   b. Identify the metabolic rate for any individual from predicted averages for age and sex (Table 5-1). These rates are given as kilocalories per square meter per day ($kcal/m^2$ per day), an energy equivalent derived from the rate of oxygen consumption. The BMR is highest per square meter in the first few years of life and then steadily declines, although a slight increase occurs at puberty.

   c. The BMR (kcal/d) equals the metabolic rate from Table 5-1 ($kcal/m^2$ per day) times surface area (m^2). Basal metabolism may not be constant throughout the day, and the final calculated estimate does not account for such variations. Nonetheless, it provides a clinically useful guide.

B. **Abbreviated methods for estimating BMR**

   1. **Method based on sex, height, age, and weight (Harris–Benedict equation).** An estimate based on indirect calorimetry was devised by J. A. Harris and F. G. Benedict (4). This method has gained wide acceptance because it requires no tables and is reasonably accurate in comparison with measurements of oxygen consumption (REE prediction is accurate to ± 14%). However, malnutrition is associated with an increase in resting oxygen consumption, apparently only when it is expressed per predicted body mass (5). In malnutrition, a greater preservation of visceral than of skeletal components leads to an increase in REE (BMR) per body cell mass. The apparent hypermetabolism of cancer patients may just be malnutrition, most likely caused by a decrease in food intake (see Chapter 14). The underestimation of BMR by the Harris–Benedict equation in malnourished patients is about 20%, but no constant factor can be applied to all patients. This inaccuracy would be true for all methods of estimating BMR but has been examined most carefully for the Harris–Benedict equation. A similar overestimation occurs in obese patients (6).

      a. **Normally nourished persons.** The BMR can be calculated from the following formulas:

$$BMR \text{ women} = 665 + (9.6 \times W) + (1.8 \times H) - (4.7 \times A)$$

$$BMR \text{ men} = 66 + (13.7 \times W) + (5 \times H) - (6.8 \times A)$$

where W = actual or usual weight (kg),
H = height (cm), and
A = age (years).

The Harris–Benedict data have been reevaluated, and data for a wider age range, but still for normally nourished people, have been added (5).

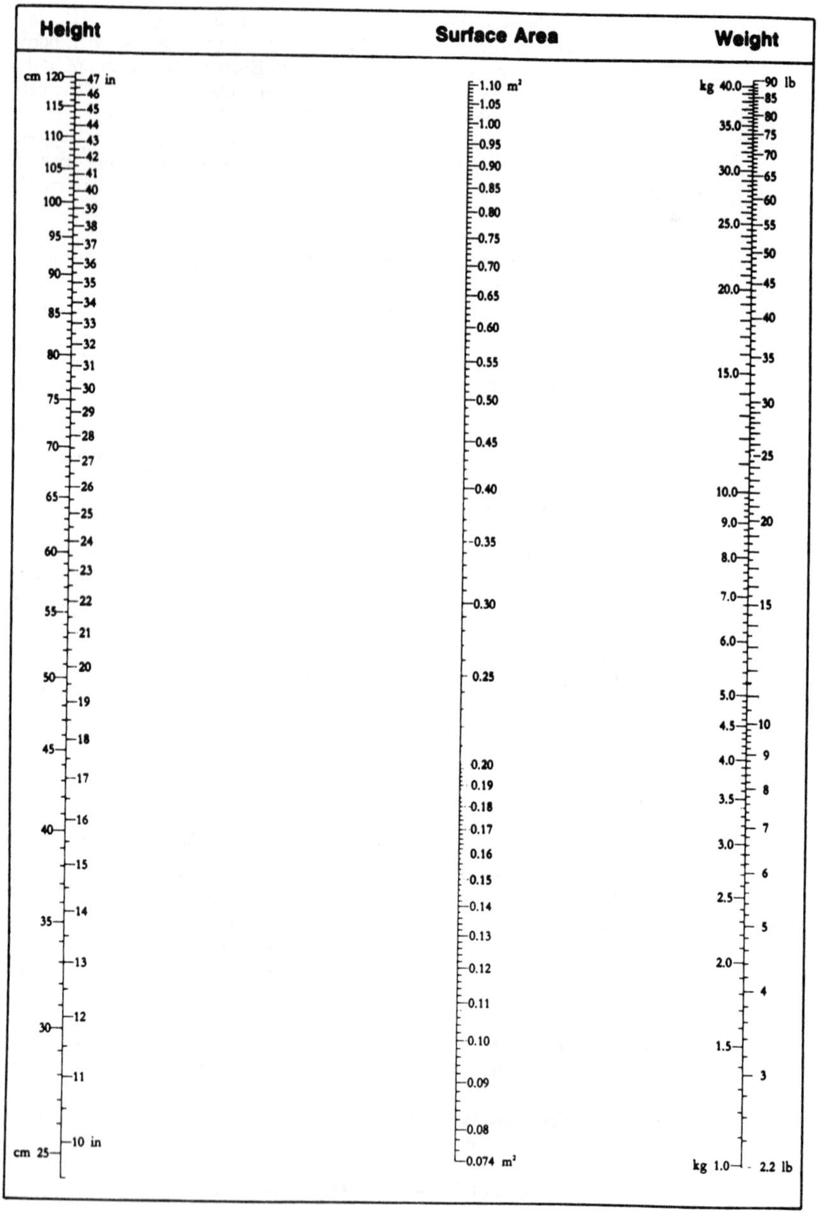

FIG. 5.1. Nomograms for determining body surface area from height and weight.
A: Body surface area of children.

B: Body surface area of adults. (From the formula of DuBois D, DuBois EF. *Arch Intern Med* 1916;17:863. $S = W^{0.425} \times H^{0.725} \times 71.84$, or $\log S = \log W \times 0.425 + \log H \times 0.725 + 1.8564$, where S = body surface area in square centimeters, W = weight in kilograms, and H = height in centimeters. Reproduced from *Scientific Tables, Documenta Geigy*. New York: Geigy Pharmaceuticals, 1962, with permission.)

Table 5-1. Standard basal metabolic rates based on body surface area for age and sex

| Age (y) | Metabolic rate (kcal/m² per day) | |
	Men	Women
1	1,272	1,272
2	1,258	1,258
3	1,231	1,229
4	1,207	1,195
5	1,183	1,162
6	1,160	1,128
7	1,135	1,090
8	1,111	1,051
9	1,085	1,027
10	1,056	1,020
11	1,032	1,008
12	1,020	991
13	1,015	967
14	1,010	941
15	1,003	910
16	994	886
17	979	871
18	960	862
19	941	852
20	926	847
25	900	845
30	883	842
35	876	840
40	871	838
45	869	828
50	859	814
55	850	799
60	838	785
65	826	773
70	811	761
75 and over	797	751

Adapted from Fleish A. Le métabolisme basal standard et sa determination au moyen du "Metabocalculator." *Helv Med Acta* 1951;18:23.

b. Overweight persons. For overweight persons, an adjusted body weight can be used, based on usual body weight (6) (see Table 5-2 or Table 13-2):

$$\text{Adjusted Body Weight} = [(\text{Actual Weight} - \text{Ideal Weight}) \times 0.24] + \text{Ideal Body Weight}$$

Alternatively, ideal body weight may be estimated by using the equations from the Metropolitan Life Insurance Company:

For males, 106 lb for the first 60 in of height plus 6 lb for each additional inch.

For females, 100 lb for the first 60 in of height plus 5 lb for each additional inch.

Add 10% for a large frame size; subtract 10% for a small frame size.

To determine frame size, wrist measurements are used. Small and large frames fall outside the ranges for a medium frame. A medium frame for males taller than 165 cm (65 in) is defined as a wrist cir-

Table 5-2. Average weight for height for ages 25 to 54 from NHANES I and II data sets

Height		Male weight		Female weight	
in	cm	kg	lb	kg	lb
58	147	—	—	63	138.6
59	150	—	—	66	145.2
60	152	—	—	60	132.0
61	155	—	—	61	134.2
62	157	68	149.6	61	134.2
63	160	71	156.2	62	136.4
64	163	71	156.2	62	136.4
65	165	74	162.8	63	138.6
66	168	75	165.0	63	138.6
67	170	77	169.4	65	143.0
68	173	78	171.6	67	147.4
69	175	78	171.6	68	149.6
70	178	81	178.2	70	154.0
71	180	81	178.2	—	—
72	183	84	184.8	—	—
73	185	84	184.8	—	—
74	188	88	193.6	—	—

NHANES, National Health and Nutrition Examination Survey.

cumference of 16.5 to 19 cm. Comparable figures for wrist circumference for females are 14 to 14.5 cm for a height of less than 157 cm (62 in), 15 to 16 cm for a height of 157 to 165 cm, and 16 to 16.5 cm for a height above 165 cm.

2. **World Health Organization/Food and Agriculture Organization (FAO) equations.** These equations for REE (BMR) are simpler than those of Harris and Benedict and are based on more comprehensive data. The sample used includes persons who are thin (body mass index < 20) or overweight (body mass index > 25). People of the same weight but different heights have similar BMRs, but among adults of the same height but different weights, those with lighter weights have higher BMRs per kilogram because of the difference in body composition. For this reason, the simpler formula based only on body weight, age, and sex is reasonable and was used to calculate the data in Table 5-3. The equations to be used are as follows:

Age (y)	Male	Female
0–3	$(60.9 \times W^*) - 54$	$(61.0 \times W) - 51$
3–10	$(22.7 \times W) - 495$	$(22.5 \times W) + 499$
10–18	$(17.5 \times W) + 651$	$(12.2 \times W) + 746$
18–30	$(15.3 \times W) + 679$	$(14.7 \times W) + 996$
30–60	$(11.6 \times W) + 879$	$(8.7 \times W) + 829$
>60	$(13.5 \times W) + 987$	$(10.5 \times W) + 596$

* Weight in kilograms.

With such formulas, one can derive daily REE values for persons of different weights (Table 5-2). The values differ from the 1973 World Health Organization standards mostly for females, in whom an overestimation of weight above 40 kg reached nearly 18% by the end of the scale. For both sexes, the earlier standards underestimated values between 15 and

Table 5-3. Basal metabolic rates according to weight and sex

Body weight (kg)	Metabolic rate (kcal/24 h)	
	Males	Females
3.0	120	144
4.0	191	191
5.0	239	239
6.0	287	311
7.0	357	383
8.0	431	431
9.0	478	502
10.0	550	550
11.0	622	622
12.0	670	670
13.0	718	718
14.0	765	765
15.0	813	813
16.0	861	837
17.0	885	861
18.0	909	885
19.0	933	909
20.0	957	933
22.0	1,005	957
24.0	1,058	981
26.0	1,100	1,005
28.0	1,124	1,055
30.0	1,172	1,076
32.0	1,196	1,100
34.0	1,244	1,124
36.0	1,268	1,148
38.0	1,316	1,172
40.0	1,340	1,172
42.0	1,363	1,196
44.0	1,387	1,220
46.0	1,435	1,220
48.0	1,459	1,244
50.0	1,483	1,268
52.0	1,507	1,268
54.0	1,531	1,292
56.0	1,579	1,316
58.0	1,603	1,316
60.0	1,627	1,340
62.0	1,650	1,363
64.0	1,674	1,387
66.0	1,698	1,411
68.0	1,722	1,435
70.0	1,746	1,459
72.0	1,746	1,459
74.0	1,770	1,483
76.0	1,794	1,507
78.0	1,818	1,507
80.0	1,842	1,532
82.0	1,866	1,555
84.0	1,890	1,579

MJ/24 h have been converted to kcal/24 h as follows: 1,000 kcal = 4.18 MJ (Kleiber M. Joules VS. Calories in nutrition. *J Nutr* 1972;102:307). These figures are not applicable to the elderly. See text for a formula to use for persons older than 60 years.
Modified from James WPT. Basal metabolic rate: comments on the new equations. *Hum Nutr Clin Nutr* 1985;39C[Suppl 1]:5.

20 kg. The overestimation of BMR for healthy women over 40 kg was confirmed in a careful study of 44 women ages 18 to 65 years (7). This study found that other currently available tables and regression equations (including Harris–Benedict) overestimate the BMR of healthy women by 7% to 14%. The authors offered the following equations:

For persons who are not athletes:

$$BMR = 795 + 7.18 \ W \ (\text{kg})$$

For athletes:

$$BMR = 50.4 + 21.1 \ W \ (\text{kg})$$

The World Health Organization/FAO equations offer the most realistic and comprehensive estimates available. One should remember, however, that the predicted BMR in nonathletes may overestimate or underestimate the measured values by 20% to 30% for any individual.

3. **Method based on body size and age.** The resting metabolic rate declines with age by almost 2% per decade in adults 20 to 75 years of age (8). The metabolic rate data compiled by Fleish (Table 5-1) can be converted to Wilmore's equation, which allows the rate to be calculated without consulting the table (9). If one assumes a metabolic rate of 55 kcal/m^2 per hour at birth, then the following equations apply:

From birth to age 19 years:

$$BMR \ (\text{kcal}/\text{m}^2 \text{ per hour}) = 55 - \text{Age (y)}$$

For age 20 years or more:

$$BMR \ (\text{kcal}/\text{m}^2 \text{ per hour}) = 37 - \left[(\text{Age} - 20) \div 10 \right]$$

4. **Estimated BEE for most hospitalized patients.** The goal for caloric intake for most patients is between 25 and 35 kcal/kg per day, or 125% to 175% of the BEE (BMR). The range of total energy expenditure for healthy nonelderly U.S. adults, by comparison, is 167 ± 14% of the BEE (2). To avoid excess provision of glucose, fat, or amino acids, reasonable goals for nonprotein kilocalories per day are as follows: glucose, ≤5 g/kg per day; lipid, ≤1 g/kg per day; and amino acids, 0.75 to 1.5 g/kg per day from a mixed protein diet, depending on the status of protein stores and the need to replace protein losses.

   A simple method for estimating total daily energy requirements in hospitalized patients is based on the body mass index (BMI) (kg/m^2) (Table 5-4). Energy requirements are inversely proportional to the BMI. The lower range in each category should be considered in patients who are insulin-resistant or critically ill, unless they are depleted of body fat, to decrease the risk for hyperglycemia and infection associated with overfeeding.

5. **The total energy requirement in illness** in hospitalized patients on total parenteral nutrition (TPN) rarely exceeds by much the basal rate of the same patient in health. The basal caloric requirement of the usual patient rarely exceeds 2,100 kcal because as a rule such patients do not weigh in excess of 90 kg (200 lb). Thus, the total energy requirement for a patient with severe illness is generally less than 3,000 kcal/d. In fact, the earlier estimates of massively increased caloric requirements in sepsis have not been substantiated by studies of oxygen consumption. Because the energy of activity is quite low in immobilized patients, the total energy requirement in severe illness usually does not exceed the estimated BMR by more than 25% (10). Therefore, although the total energy requirement in patients with illness has been estimated by adding to the REE additional energy requirements for activity, stress, and fever, it is probably most accurate to base the REE on Harris–Benedict or World Health

Table 5-4. Estimate of energy requirements for patients based on body mass index[a]

BMI (kg/m^2)	Energy requirements (kcal/kg per day)	
	Critically ill patients (RMR)	Other patients (RMR + TEF + TEA)
<15	35–40	35–40 + 20%
15–19	30–35	30–35 + 20%
20–29	20–25	20–25 + 20%
≥30	15–20[b]	15–20

[a] Use Harris-Benedict or World Health Organization equations to estimate requirement for patients whose estimate by this method is <1,200 kcal/d.
[b] Do not exceed 2,000 kcal/d.
BMI, body mass index; RMR, resting metabolic rate; TEF, thermal effect of food; TEA, thermal effect of activity.

Organization equations using actual body weight. Equations have been developed for use in estimating the REE of hospitalized patients when indirect calorimetry is not available and when more precision is desired than is provided by the Harris–Benedict equation (11). These equations were developed for both ventilator-dependent and spontaneously breathing patients by correlating indirect calorimetry results and other variables by means of multivariate regression analysis (Table 5-5). Increases above those determined for REE can be estimated, even for medically ill patients. For severely catabolic or malnourished hospitalized patients or for those with high fever or sepsis, an increase of 20% to 25% can be added. Overestimation should be avoided, however, because increased feeding with high-glucose infusions can cause hyperglycemia, hypokalemia, edema, and fatty liver.

III. **The energy expenditure of activity (EEA)** can vary from 1.1 to 10.3 kcal/kg per hour. In fact, a correct calculation of energy requirement over 24 hours would include sleep time (about 90% of BMR) and the metabolic rate per hour of different types of work. In some types of work (e.g., gardening), certain muscle groups become fatigued without a large number of calories being used. Usually, any exercise in which the body leaves the ground (e.g., running) uses a large number of calories. However, one should not overestimate the contribution of sports to overall daily energy use because sports activities generally last for a short time and are followed by a much longer period of inactivity. Table 5-6 provides a more detailed analysis of activity-related energy expenditures. A number of methods are used to estimate or calculate the EEA.

A. **Calculation based on level of activity.** A calculation, albeit imprecise, can be used if the typical activity pattern is known. An average daily activ-

Table 5-5. Estimation of resting energy expenditure in hospitalized patients

For ventilator-dependent patients:
$$REE(s) = 1925 - 10(A) + 5(W) + 281(S) + 292(T) + 851(B)$$
For spontaneously breathing patients:
$$REE(s) = 629 - 11(A) + 25(W) - 609(O)$$

REE, resting energy expenditure (kcal/d); A, age (y); W, body weight (kg); S, sex (male = 1, female = 0); T, diagnosis of trauma (present = 1, absent = 0); B, diagnosis of burn (present = 1, absent = 0); O, obesity (present = 1, absent = 0).
From Breton-Jones CS, Turner WW Jr, Liepa BU, et al. Equations for the estimation of energy expenditures in patients with burns with special reference to ventilatory status. *J Burn Care Rehabil* 1992;13:330.

Table 5-6. Calories used for 10 minutes of activity

Activity	Body weight (lb)				
	125	150	175	200	250
Sedentary					
Sleeping	10	12	14	16	20
Sitting	10–15	12–18	14–21	16–24	18–30
Standing	12	14	16	19	24
Dressing or washing	26	32	37	42	53
Light office work	25	30	34	39	50
Standing (light activity)	20	24	28	32	40
Typing 40 words per minute	25	30	34	39	50
Locomotion					
Walking, downstairs	56	67	78	88	111
Walking, upstairs	146	175	202	229	288
Walking, 2 mph	29	35	40	46	58
Walking, 4 mph	52	62	72	81	102
Running, 5.5 mph	90	108	125	142	178
Running, 7 mph	118	141	164	187	232
Cycling, 5.5 mph	42	50	58	67	83
Cycling, 13 mph	89	107	124	142	178
Light work					
Domestic work	34	41	47	53	68
Weeding garden	49	59	68	78	98
Shoveling snow	65	78	89	100	130
Lawn mowing, power	34	41	47	53	67
Assembly work in factory	20	24	28	34	40
Auto repair	35	46	48	54	69
House painting	29	35	40	46	58
Heavy work					
Chopping wood	60	73	84	96	121
Pick and shovel	56	67	78	88	110
Dragging logs, lifting heavy materials	158	189	220	252	315
Recreation					
Baseball (except pitching)	39	47	54	62	78
Basketball	58	70	82	93	117
Dancing (moderate)	35	42	48	55	69
Football	69	83	96	110	137
Golfing	33	40	48	55	68
Racketball, squash	75	90	104	117	144
Skiing, downhill	80	96	112	128	160
Skiing, cross-country	98	117	138	158	194
Swimming, crawl (20 yd/min)	40	48	56	63	80
Tennis	56	67	80	92	115
Volleyball	43	52	65	75	94

Adapted from Brownell KD. *The partnership diet program.* New York: Rawson-Wade, 1980.

ity factor can be calculated from the estimated level of activity, weighted for the time spent in each activity. Average estimates for different levels of activity are given in Table 5-7. A truly valid estimate would consider activity patterns over days or weeks.

B. Indirect methods for measuring oxygen consumption. An accurate estimation of the BMR, or REE, of patients in intensive care units is important because both overfeeding and underfeeding may produce adverse effects. The calculation made from equations can be inaccurate in critically ill patients (12). Moreover, the effects of stress and infection are difficult to estimate. Therefore, other methods have been used to provide more accurate assessments. It is not yet certain whether this degree of accuracy is required for patients in intensive care units because the World Health Organization and Harris–Benedict equations are useful in determining the REE in many cases. In addition, determinations must be made when the patient's clinical condition is stable. It is unlikely that the risk of providing too much (or too little) energy to critically ill patients will justify the expense of calorimetric measurements. The risks of nutrient provision more often involve fluid and electrolytes when given in excess. If calorimetry is available, it should be used only for selected patients who are very malnourished or who might tolerate the energy provision poorly, such as those in cardiac or respiratory failure.

1. **Indirect calorimetry** involves measuring oxygen uptake ($\dot{V}O_2$) and carbon dioxide output ($\dot{V}CO_2$) at the mouth. Most clinical equipment utilizes the open-circuit method, in which a set of one-way valves directs expired air into a collecting bag. At the end of a timed period, both the volume and composition of expired air are measured and the rates of oxygen consumption and carbon dioxide production are calculated by the difference between the concentrations in the inspired air and the gas collected. The REE is determined from these data by using the respiratory quotient, $\dot{V}CO_2/\dot{V}O_2$. This method requires the use of a metabolic cart and trained personnel but is generally quite accurate. Breath-by-breath systems now allow measurement of the REE even in ventilator patients receiving high levels (>40%) of inspired oxygen (13). If only oxygen consumption data are available, the REE can be estimated by multiplying the oxygen consumption in milliliters per minute by a factor of 7.

Table 5-7. Calculation of energy requirement (kcal/d)

Level of activity	Activity factor ($\times$ REE)	Average energy expenditure (kcal/kg per day)[a]
Very light		
Men	1.3	31
Women	1.3	30
Light		
Men	1.6	38
Women	1.5	35
Moderate		
Men	1.7	41
Women	1.6	37
Heavy		
Men	2.1	50
Women	1.9	44

REE, resting energy expenditure.

[a] Estimated from World Health Organization equations for median weights of persons ages 19 to 74; activity factor 1.0 = 24.0 kcal/kg for men, 23.2 for women.

From National Research Council. *Recommended Daily Allowances,* 10th ed. Washington, DC: National Academy Press, 1989, with permission.

2. **The Fick equation** can be used to calculate energy expenditure in patients who have a pulmonary artery catheter in place (14). The calculation is based on $\dot{V}O_2$ alone, with use of the known caloric value of oxygen (4.86 kcal/L for an estimated respiratory quotient of 0.85). Oxygen consumption is calculated from the Fick equation with measurements of cardiac output (CO), hemoglobin level (Hb), and arterial (SaO_2) and mixed venous ($S\bar{v}O_2$) oxygen saturations.

$$REE \ (\text{kcal/d}) = CO \times \text{Hb} \times (SaO_2 - S\bar{v}O_2) \times 95.18$$

This method appears to be as accurate as indirect calorimetry and uses data available in most intensive care units. In mechanically ventilated nonsurgical patients without sepsis, the Harris–Benedict estimate was comparable (15). In patients with sepsis, an additional requirement of about 20% is appropriate.

IV. **Special energy requirements**
   A. **Additional energy requirements in illness.** Heat production increases with inflammation and infection.
      1. **Infection** increases basal metabolism. The final caloric expenditure depends on the increase in oxygen consumption caused by fever or new cell production and the decrease in oxygen consumption caused by diminished calorie intake and immobility. An estimate for increasing the REE for fever is the following: $(°F - 98.6) \times 0.07$ for Fahrenheit, and $(°C - 37.0) \times 0.13$ for centigrade.
      2. **Fasting and malnutrition** decrease the BMR, or BEE, approximately 25% by day 20. Although the calculations for BEE probably underestimate the REE for malnourished patients, the total REE falls significantly as weight falls.
      3. **Other conditions.** Many conditions associated with weight loss have been thought to be associated with increased energy needs. However, daily energy expenditure is lower than expected in elderly patients with cachexia caused by heart failure and Alzheimer's disease (16). This result is consistent with inadequate intake as the cause of weight loss because in the long term, the balance between daily energy expenditure and food intake must determine body composition.
      4. **Malabsorption.** Malabsorption is a special case of an increased energy requirement in which a loss of nutrients results from incomplete absorption of food. The most accurate way to assess caloric loss would be calorimetry of the feces. However, one can determine daily fat excretion more practically with a 72-hour fecal fat study. Fat accounts for about 40% of caloric intake. If one assumes that protein and carbohydrate are similarly malabsorbed, one then can estimate total calorie malabsorption by multiplying caloric loss from fat by 2.5. Carbohydrate probably is more efficiently absorbed than fat in diseases producing a short-bowel syndrome but not necessarily in diffuse mucosal disease. In practice, no distinction need be made between the proportion of macronutrients as caloric sources in the diet and as caloric losses in the feces.

$$\text{Fat Excretion} \ (\text{g/d}) \times 9 \ \text{kcal/g} = \text{Fecal Kilocalorie Loss from}$$
$$\text{Fat Malabsorption}$$

$$\text{Fecal Kilocalorie Loss from Fat} \times 2.5 = \text{Total Kilocalories}$$
$$\text{Lost from Diet}$$

B. **Pregnancy.** The energy requirement for a full-term pregnancy is estimated at 80,000 kcal. The World Health Organization recommends an increased intake for pregnant women of 150 kcal/d over normal during the first trimester and 350 kcal/d over normal during the rest of the pregnancy. This estimate does not take into account any variation in physical activity or weight gain unrelated to gestation. Because the activity of pregnant women in Western societies is usually decreased, an increase of 300 kcal/d is recommended for the second and third trimesters.

C. **Lactation.** The production of 1 dL of human breast milk requires 67 to 77 kcal. Because the efficiency of converting nutrients to milk energy is 80% to 90%, the total energy requirement is 80 to 95 kcal/dL of milk. If 8.5 dL/d is the average rate of milk production for 3 months, the energy needed will be 750 kcal/d. However, extra fat stores are deposited during pregnancy, and it is estimated that these can provide the mother with 200 to 300 kcal/d for 3 months. Thus, the recommended additional caloric requirement for nursing mothers is 500 kcal/d.

V. Estimation of caloric intake

A. **Total daily caloric intake.** The estimation of a patient's total daily intake of calories requires a careful dietary history. It is most helpful to use a reference in which the caloric contents of foods are listed according to common package limits or portion sizes (i.e., per ounce or per cup). Sources of such data are readily available in the health section of retail book stores, or from the U.S. Department of Agriculture *Food Composition Handbook 8* (*http://www.nal.usda.gov/fmic/foodcomp*). Table 5-8 lists the caloric content of some important common foods.

B. **Calculation of caloric content of foods containing a single macronutrient.** Sometimes, the type of food is known to be homogeneous, and the caloric content can be estimated from the volume ingested.

Nutrient	kcal/g	kJ/g
Carbohydrates		
Monosaccharide	3.75	16
Disaccharide	3.94	16
Starch and glycogen	4.13	17
Total carbohydrate	4	17
Protein	4	17
Long-chain triglyceride	9	37
Medium-chain triglyceride	8.3	34
Alcohol (specific gravity 0.79)	7	29
Intralipid 10% (specific gravity 0.91)	1.1 kcal/mL	4

1. **Caloric content of alcoholic beverages.** The specific gravity of alcohol is 0.79 (rounded off to 0.8). Thus,

(Proof of Alcoholic Beverage $\div$ 2) $\times$ 0.8 $\times$ Deciliters of Beverage = Grams of Alcohol

Grams of Alcohol $\times$ 7 kcal = Kilocalories of Beverage from Alcohol

a. **Example.** Three 2-oz drinks of 86-proof bourbon:

$$(86 \div 2) \times 0.8 \times 1.8 = 62 \text{ g}$$

$$62 \times 7 = 434 \text{ kcal}$$

The alcohol content in grams of some common beverages is listed below:

Beverage	Unit	Alcohol content (g)	kcal/U
Distilled liquor	One jigger		
80 proof		10	70
90 proof		11	80
100 proof		13	90
3.6–4 0% beer	One 12-oz can	12.6–13.5	140–150
12.5–14.5% wine	3½-oz glass	10.0–11.6	70–80

Table 5-8. Caloric content of common foods

Food	Portion size	Kilocalories
Apple	1 ($\frac{3}{4}$ lb)	80
Baby foods		
Vegetables, fruits	$4\frac{3}{4}$ oz	113–207
Meat	$3\frac{1}{2}$-oz jar	99–136
Bacon, cooked	Yield from $\frac{1}{4}$ lb	215
Beans, green, cooked	1 cup	35
Beef		
Sirloin steak, cooked	Yield from $\frac{1}{2}$ lb	596
Ground beef, lean, cooked	Yield from $\frac{1}{2}$ lb	497
Beverages		
Cola	12-oz can	144
Ginger ale, sweet mixers	12-oz can	113
40% Bran flakes	1 cup	106
Bread		
White	1 slice, regular	63–74
Whole wheat	1 slice, regular	56–61
Rye	1 slice, regular	61
Butter or margarine	1 tbs	322
Cake		
Chocolate, no icing	1 piece, $3 \times 3 \times 2$ in	322
White, with chocolate icing	1 piece, $3 \times 3 \times 2$ in	453
Candy		
Chocolate	1 oz	135–144
Chocolate with nuts	1 oz	159
Carrot	1	30
Cheese		
Cheddar	1 slice	96
American	1 oz	113
Cottage (regular)	1 oz	30
Swiss	1 slice	130
Chicken		
Broiled	Yield from 1 lb	273
Fried	Yield from 1 lb	565
	Breast, half	160
	Thigh	122
Cookies		
Brownies	1	97
Chocolate chip	1	52
Sugar	1	46
Corn, cooked	1 ear	70
Crackers		
Saltines	1 cracker	12
Graham	1 cracker	62
Doughnuts		
Raised	1	176
Cake	1	164
Eggs		
Extra large, fried	1	112
Cooking oil	1 tbs	111–120
Grapefruit	1	80–132
Ice cream		
Regular	1 cup	257
Frozen custard	1 cup	334
Rich (16% fat)	1 cup	329

continued

Table 5-8. (*Continued*)

Food	Portion size	Kilocalories
Jam	1 tbs	54
Milk		
Whole	1 cup	159
Skim	1 cup	88
Low fat	1 cup	145
Noodles, egg	Yield from 4 oz	440
Orange		
Navel	1	45–87
Juice	1 cup	112–122
Pastry, Danish	one 4-in-diameter pastry	274
Peanuts, out of shell	1 oz	166
Peanut butter	1 tbs	94
Peas, canned	1 cup	142
Pies		
Fresh, banana	one 3½-in piece (⅛ pie)	253
Fresh, pecan		431
Frozen	one 3½-in piece (⅛ pie)	187–282
Pizza		
Homemade, cheese	⅛ 12-in pie	153
Frozen, cheese	⅛ 12-in pie	139
Ham, roasted or baked	½ lb	848
Pork chops, lean	Yield from ½ lb	442
Potatoes		
Boiled with skin	1	173
Boiled without skin	1	122
French fried	ten 4-in strips	214
Chips	10 chips	114
Rice, white, cooked	¼ cup	56
Salad dressing, Italian	1 tbs	83
Salmon		
Fresh, broiled	½ lb	364
Canned	½ lb	320–477
Sausage		
Bologna	1 slice	67–86
Hot dogs, cooked	1	134–170
Pork, cooked	1 link	62
Salami	1 slice	66–88
Spaghetti, cooked, from 2½ oz dry	¼ lb	168
Sugar, granulated	1 tsp	15
	1 cup	770
Tuna, canned	7 oz	570

b. Abbreviated calculation for caloric content of alcohol:

Kilocalories = $0.8 \times$ Proof of Beverage $\times$ No. Ounces

e.g., 3 drinks (2 oz each) of 86-proof bourbon = $0.8 \times 86 \times 6$, or 413 kcal

2. Caloric content of cooking oil:

Kilocalories = Milliliters $\times$ Specific Gravity of Cooking Oil $(0.91) \times 9$

e.g., 2 tbs of olive oil = $30 \times 0.9 \times 9 = 243$ kcal

3. Caloric content of dextrose infusions:

$$\text{Kilocalories} = \text{Percentage of Nutrient} \times [\text{Volume Infused (mL)} \div 100] \times \text{Kilocalories of Hydrated Dextrose}$$

e.g., 3 L of 5% dextrose in water contains
$$5 \times (3{,}000 \div 100) \times 3.4 \ = 510 \text{ kcal}$$

C. Methods for assessing dietary intake. Even if one allows for the accurate translation of food units into calories, it is difficult to obtain a reliable dietary history with the methods available. The Committee on Food Consumption Patterns, Food and Nutrition Board, of the National Research Council has compiled many data on the methods for assessing food consumption and its relationship to nutritional status (17).

  1. Twenty-four-hour recall. This method is the simplest one available in that it relies on the patient's ability to remember how much food was eaten in a 24- hour period. The 24-hour dietary recall requires a trained interviewer but has been used with success in the National Health and Nutrition Examination Surveys (NHANESs). It takes a minimum amount of time to complete and can provide reproducible data. Although it is notoriously inaccurate in terms of the actual amount of food the patient has ingested (e.g., the intake of alcohol may be neglected), it is often the only technique available for assessing intake. The inaccuracy is compounded by not knowing the nutrient content of the ingested foods, and by the underreporting of intake in women in comparison with men.

  2. Food history. This method is also based on the patient's ability to recall, but the intake of food is averaged over a period of time. For example, the contents of a patient's average breakfast, lunch, or dinner, or all three, are calculated. The food history method is easy to use but suffers from the same inaccuracy of memory as 24-hour recall.

  3. Food records. The patient can keep a written record of the amounts and types of food ingested. This method is accurate if the record is scrupulously maintained, but such thoroughness is rare. Also, people tend to alter their eating behavior during the test period to simplify the record. However, the energy content of foods eaten can be determined accurately, with only moderate overestimates, in a 5-day food record.

  4. Calorie count. This method is useful for the hospitalized patient because it requires the assistance of a dietitian, who understands the need for the calorie count. To ensure the accuracy of the count, no food is ingested by the patient other than what is reported to the dietitian. The dietitian observes the amount of food eaten at each meal and estimates its caloric content. Daily variations in food preparation and serving portions in the central kitchen can produce some inaccuracies. This method is the best of those available for estimating caloric intake. It combines some direct observation of the food actually ingested with a reasonable degree of control over its preparation. The major disadvantage is that it assesses intake of hospital food rather than home-prepared meals.

  5. Weighed diet. This method is very accurate, but it must be carried out on a metabolic ward where the portions of foods are weighed and most of the food is prepared on the floor. In this way, differences in the processing of foods are minimized, and the actual caloric content of foods is best estimated.

VI. Energy balance

  A. Energy balance (kilocalories per day) equals kilocalories obtained minus kilocalories expended (BEE + EEA). *Calories obtained* refers to an estimate of dietary intake or to a calculation of calories fed enterally or parenterally (it can also refer to a combination of estimation and calculation). *Energy expended* includes the energy expended in basal metabolism and through physical activity or disease. When the intake of food exceeds the expenditure of energy, weight is gained. When the expenditure of energy exceeds the intake of food, weight is lost. When the energy balance is zero, weight is stable.

B. Derivation of caloric equivalent to 1 lb of body weight. Although both water and carbohydrate stores are lost in the first few days of fasting, the loss of cell water is proportionally greater than the loss of glycogen. It is generally assumed that a loss of 1 lb of weight (0.45 kg) corresponds to a deficit of about 3,400 kcal. It is instructive to review the data on which this assumption is based (Table 5-9).

The mean composition of tissue lost during the first 11 weeks of semistarvation in otherwise healthy subjects is 40% fat, 12% protein, and 48% water. From weeks 12 to 23, the composition of tissue lost is 54% fat, 9% protein, and 37% water. The BMR per square meter falls an average of 31%, and the physical activity level drops by 55%. Thus, the rate of weight loss decreases with time because expenditure decreases as intake remains constant. The average energy value of weight loss is about 1,900 kcal/lb during the first 11 weeks and about 2,500 kcal/lb during the next 12 weeks of semistarvation.

The mean composition of tissue lost from obese subjects is 78% fat, 5% protein, and 17% water. The energy value of each pound lost is about 3,400 kcal. It appears that obese patients use their adipose tissue reserves more efficiently than persons of normal weight because the percentage of calories available as fat from body stores is higher. In normal persons, weight loss often is associated with a decrease in activity, and total energy expenditure falls. The decrease in physical activity in obese patients during weight loss is less noticeable because they are less active initially. Therefore, weight loss is initially maintained better in very obese than in slightly obese patients because of their more efficient mobilization of fat (high-calorie source) from tissue stores and the fact that they continue to expend energy for a longer period of time at the same rate as before they began to lose weight.

Unfortunately, weight loss during starvation is not the same as controlled weight loss and may approach 50% fat and 50% fat-free mass. Thus, in a starving patient, the decrease in muscle mass and in BMR is larger. This accounts for the lower than expected BMR in severely ill hospitalized patients. It is also misleading to obese patients, who lose less fat while fasting completely than during slower, more controlled weight loss (18).

To calculate an estimated weight loss on a controlled diet, an allowance must be made for the decreased BMR and diminished level of activity noted in nonobese subjects. Because weight loss in normal subjects decreases the BMR by 31% and the energy expenditure of activity decreases by 55%, the average estimated decrease in expenditure is 40%. If this correction is applied to the caloric value per pound of weight loss in nonobese subjects (2,100 kcal/lb ÷ 0.6 = 3,500), the estimated weight loss by nonobese and obese subjects becomes virtually the same. Thus, the figure of 3,400 kcal/lb

Table 5-9. Estimates of energy loss during weight loss

| Subjects | Composition of tissue lost (%) | | | Average proportion of energy deficit provision | |
	Fat	Protein	Water	Fat (%)	Protein (%)
Nonobese	37–54	9–16	37–48	89	11
Obese	76–78	5–6	17–18	97	3

Data derived from Van Itallie TB, Yank MU. *N Engl J Med* 1977;297:1158; Keys A, Brozek J, Henschel A. *The biology of human starvation*. Minneapolis: University of Minnesota Press, 1950; Benedict FC. *A study of prolonged fasting*. Washington, DC: Carnegie Institute, 1915:84, 415; Passmore R, Strong JA, Ritchie FJ. *Br J Nutr* 1958;12:113; Runcie J, Hilditch TE. *Br Med J* 1974;2:352.

lost can be used to calculate weight loss for all subjects without any correction factor. An example of calculating tissue losses during weight loss is summarized below.

	Nonobese subject	Obese subject
Daily caloric intake *(I)*	2,000 kcal	3,000 kcal
Daily expenditure of energy *(E)*	2,800 kcal	3,800 kcal
Weekly caloric deficit *(E − I)* × 7	5,600 kcal	5,600 kcal
Predicted weekly weight change		
Weekly caloric deficit ÷ 3,400 kcal	1.6 lb/wk	1.6 lb/wk

C. **Recommended daily energy intake.** Energy intake must be balanced according to the needs of age, sex, body size, and physical activity if a desirable body weight is to be maintained.

1. **Individual variations.** Despite attempts to estimate energy requirements for groups of adults, a wide range is seen within persons of the same body size and age that reflects differences in activity and individual metabolism. Moreover, it is not possible to establish desirable weights with certainty. For these reasons, the Committee on Dietary Allowances of the Food and Nutrition Board has derived a table of *estimated energy needs* that displays a wide range of values for each group (Table 5-10). The data included are only for persons of average weight and height who perform only light work.

VII. **Estimation of protein requirements.** Normally, nitrogen derived from amino acids, the catabolic product of proteins, is excreted in the urine and feces and lost from the skin. Unlike the energy that is retained and stored in triglyceride and glycogen, proteins and amino acids are not stored in the body. Therefore, protein or nitrogen requirements are often estimated by calculating nitrogen losses on a daily rather than a weekly basis. When excess protein is ingested, the amino acids not needed for protein synthesis are transaminated so that the non-nitrogenous portion of the molecule can be used as a calorie source, as, for example, in pyruvate derived from alanine. The nitrogen that is not needed is converted to urea and excreted in the urine.

A. **Normal losses**

1. **Urinary losses** of nitrogen urea account for more than 80% of urinary nitrogen. Creatinine, porphyrins, and other nitrogen-containing compounds account for the remaining nitrogen.

$$\text{Urinary Nitrogen Loss} = \big[\text{Urine Urea Nitrogen (mg/dL)} \\ \times \text{ Daily Urine Volume (dL)}\big] \div 0.8$$

Urinary nitrogen excretion is related to the BMR. The larger the muscle mass in the body, the greater the number of calories needed to maintain it. Also, the rate of transamination is greater as amino acids and carbohydrates are interconverted to fulfill energy needs in the muscle. Between 1 and 1.3 mg of urinary nitrogen is excreted for each kilocalorie required for basal metabolism. Nitrogen excretion also increases during exercise and heavy work.

2. **Fecal and skin losses** account for a relatively constant proportion of nitrogen loss from the body in normal conditions, but these may vary widely in disease states. Thus, measurement of urinary nitrogen loss alone may not provide a reliable prediction of the daily nitrogen requirement when it is most needed. Fecal losses are a consequence of the inefficient digestion and absorption of protein (93% efficiency). In addition, the intestinal tract secretes proteins into the lumen from saliva, gastric juice, bile, pancreatic enzymes, and enterocyte sloughing. These sources contribute, respectively, about 3, 5, 1, 8, and 50 g of protein daily to the total protein secreted into the intestinal lumen.

Table 5-10. Mean heights and weights and recommended energy intake

Category	Age (y)	Weight kg	Weight lb	Height cm	Height in	REE (kcal/d)	Average energy allowance kcal/kg	Average energy allowance kcal/d
Infants	0.0–0.5	6	13	60	24	320	108	650
	0.5–1.0	9	20	71	28	500	98	850
Children	1–3	13	29	90	35	740	102	1,300
	4–6	20	44	112	44	950	90	1,800
	7–10	28	62	132	52	1,130	70	2,000
Males	11–14	45	99	157	62	1,440	55	2,500
	15–18	66	145	176	69	1,760	45	3,000
	19–22	72	160	177	70	1,780	40	2,900
	23–50	79	174	176	70	1,800	37	2,900
	51	77	170	173	68	1,530	30	2,300
Females	11–14	46	101	157	62	1,310	47	2,200
	15–18	55	120	163	64	1,370	40	2,200
	19–22	58	128	164	65	1,350	38	2,200
	23–50	63	138	163	64	1,380	36	2,200
	51	65	143	160	63	1,280	30	1,900
Pregnancy, second and third trimesters								+300
Lactation								+500

The energy allowances for young adult men and women are derived from the World Health Organization equations for resting energy expenditure (REE) multiplied by an activity factor (see Table 5-7). For men, the activity factor of 1.67 was used for ages 19 to 24, 1.60 for ages 25 to 50; for women, the figures were 1.60 and 1.55, respectively. Beyond age 50, the figure used is 1.50. This allowance accounts for light to moderate activity.
New RDIs for energy will be available in 2001 or 2002.
Reprinted from National Research Council. *Recommended dietary allowances,* 10th ed. Washington, DC: National Academy Press, 1989, with permission.

    3. Total nitrogen losses. Fecal nitrogen averages 1 to 2 g/d in the absence of diarrhea. Skin losses average 0.3 g/d. The total fecal and skin losses can be estimated at about 2 g/d.

$$\text{Total Nitrogen Loss } (g/d) = \text{Urine Nitrogen} + \text{Stool Nitrogen}$$
$$+ \text{Skin Nitrogen} = \text{Urine Nitrogen} + 2$$

    When fecal losses are measured, an estimated nitrogen loss of 1 g/d is used to cover losses in skin and other compartments.

B. Normal daily protein requirement. Obligatory losses of nitrogen are not altered by differences in age or sex, and urinary losses of nitrogen are proportional to body size and weight. The total losses from all sources are approximately 2 mg of nitrogen per basal kilocalorie. Minimal nitrogen loss per day has been estimated for adults. In a series of 11 studies reviewed by the World Health Organization, daily obligatory nitrogen losses averaged 53 mg/kg (range, 46 to 69 mg/kg). On the basis of short- and long-term balance studies, the World Health Organization proposed a mean requirement of 0.6 g/kg per day for reference protein (highly digestible, high-quality protein such as eggs, meat, milk, or fish) (19). If a value of 25% above the average is used to meet the needs of 97% of the population, 0.6 × 1.25, or 0.75 g/kg per day, is the recommended dietary allowance (RDA) for young male and female adults. Although protein turnover in muscle is lower in the elderly (20% vs. 30%), it is not clear how this difference in metabolism affects protein requirements. In the absence of clear data, the RDA for an elderly person is also 0.75 g of protein per kilogram per day. The principles behind protein requirements in the United States have been reviewed (1).

1. **Growth.** Protein requirements are highest during infancy and adolescence. However, total body protein is lowest in infancy, and obligatory losses are greatest, so that protein deficiency is most common in infancy. A modified factorial procedure has been developed to calculate the protein needs of infants and children. Starting with a protein requirement of 1.1 g/kg per day for maintenance, an increment was added for growth and increased by 50% to allow for variability. Efficiency of utilization was assumed to be 70%, and a final calculated growth increment was added to the maintenance figure to recommend daily allowances for average U.S. dietary protein (Table 5-11). Another estimate is needed to convert the figures derived for reference proteins (Table 5-11). The true digestibility of a mixed U.S. diet is estimated at greater than 90%, varying from 95% for milk, meat, eggs, peanut butter, and refined wheat, to 88% for polished rice, to 86% for oatmeal, whole wheat, corn, and soy flour, to 78% for beans (19).

2. **Pregnancy.** About 925 g of protein is synthesized during a pregnancy by the mother for fetal and placental tissues. Protein needs increase as

Table 5-11. Recommended allowances of reference protein and U.S. dietary protein

Category	Age (y) or condition	Weight (kg)	Derived allowance of reference protein[a]		Recommended dietary allowance	
			g/kg	g/d	g/kg[b]	g/d
Both sexes	0.0–0.5	6	2.20[c]	—	2.2	13
	0.5–1	9	1.56	—	1.6	14
	1–3	13	1.14	—	1.2	16
	4–6	20	1.03	—	1.1	24
	7–10	28	1.00	—	1.0	28
Males	11–14	45	0.98	—	1.0	45
	15–18	66	0.86	—	0.9	59
	19–24	72	0.75	—	0.8	58
	25–50	79	0.75	—	0.8	63
	51+	77	0.75	—	0.8	63
Females	11–14	46	0.94	—	1.0	46
	15–18	55	0.81	—	0.8	44
	19–24	58	0.75	—	0.8	46
	25–50	63	0.75	—	0.8	50
	51+	65	0.75	—	0.8	50
Pregnancy	First trimester		—	+1.3	—	+10
	Second trimester		—	+6.1	—	+10
	Third trimester		—	+10.7	—	+10
Lactation	First 6 months		—	+14.7	—	+15
	Second 6 months		—	+11.8	—	+12

[a] Data from World Health Organization, 1985.
[b] Amino acid score of typical U.S. diet is 100 for all age groups, except young infants. Digestibility is equal to reference proteins. Values have been rounded upward to 0.1 g/kg.
[c] For infants 0 to 3 months of age, breast-feeding that meets energy needs also meets protein needs. Formula substitutes should have the same amount and composition of amino acids as human milk, corrected for digestibility, if appropriate.
New RDIs for protein will be available in 2001 or 2002.
From National Research Council. *Recommended daily allowances,* 10th ed. Washington, DC: National Academy Press, 1989, with permission.

the pregnancy progresses. The average additional protein needed per day is estimated at 6.0 g (1.3, 6.1, and 10.7 g for each trimester). This value is increased by 30% to account for variability and by a factor of 70% for efficiency of conversion to tissue protein. Because of uncertainty about the rate of fetal tissue deposition, 10 g of reference protein per day throughout pregnancy is the recommended allowance.

   3. **Lactation.** Milk contains 1.2 g of protein per deciliter, and an average milk output is 750 mL/d. Therefore, the recommended increment is 15 g of protein per day to allow for variation in output and quality of protein ingested for the first 6 months, and 12 g/d for the next 6 months as milk output falls by 20%.

VIII. **Calorie requirement for protein utilization**

   A. **Need for other energy sources.** Nitrogen ingested as amino acids without other sources of energy is not efficiently incorporated into protein because the energy consumed in heat loss during metabolism (thermal effect) is especially high for protein. Moreover, the incorporation of amino acids into peptides requires three high-energy phosphate bonds, so that 10 kcal are used for each molecule derived from the hydrolysis of ATP. Any excess of dietary energy over basic needs improves the efficiency of dietary nitrogen utilization. To achieve a positive nitrogen balance when protein intake is barely adequate, a positive energy balance of about 2 kcal/kg per day is required (20). In other words, when energy intake is limited, protein balance is negative, even when protein intake seems adequate but is not excessive. The exact amount of extra calories required to produce a positive nitrogen balance depends on a large number of factors, including body energy stores, body protein mass, and the ratio of energy to protein sources in the food.

   B. **Nutritional status influences nitrogen utilization.** To ensure positive nitrogen balance in the depleted patient, it is advisable to provide an amount of calories near the estimated energy requirement. Excessive calories may not lead to improvement in meaningful lean body mass.

   C. **Protein–calorie ratios in children.** A safe ratio (protein energy to total energy) that avoids protein–calorie malnutrition in children seems to be 1:20 (21)—that is, for every kilocalorie provided by protein, 19 kcal of nonprotein energy is needed to prevent protein–calorie malnutrition in children. Each gram of protein produces 4 kcal of energy, so 4 × 19 or 76 kcal of nonprotein energy is needed per gram of protein during the period of intense growth in children. When protein is present in excess of needs, even when nonprotein calories are limited, some of the protein is converted to energy that can be metabolized, and the 1:20 ratio is not required.

   D. **Protein–calorie ratios in adults.** Relative requirements also have been estimated for energy and nitrogen in adult patients maintained in nutritional balance (Table 5-12). These estimates are, not surprisingly, somewhat lower than the estimates for children. Estimates of energy–protein require-

Table 5-12. Energy intake required to maintain positive nitrogen balance

Type of patient	Energy (kcal/kg per day)	Nitrogen (mg/kg per day)	kcal/g nitrogen	kcal/g protein
TPN postoperative	46.0	250	184	29
TPN septic	43.3	240	180	29
Ambulatory RDA	38.5	128	308	49

TPN, total parenteral nutrition; RDA, recommended daily allowance.
Data for postoperative patients from Hentley TF, Lee HA. *Nutr Metab* 1975;19:201. Data for patients with septic disorders from Long CL, Crosby F, Geiger JW, Kinney JM. *Am J Clin Nutr* 1976;29:380. Data for ambulatory patients from National Research Council.
Recommended daily allowances, 10th ed. Washington, DC: National Academy Press, 1989, with permission.

ments for normal, ambulatory 70-kg persons call for approximately 50 kcal from nonprotein sources per gram of protein, or about 300 kcal/g of nitrogen. This high ratio cannot usually be achieved with parenteral feeding because caloric intake is limited by the volume that must be infused. Therefore, acceptable figures for parenteral nutrition are about 25 to 30 kcal from nonprotein sources per gram of protein, or 150 to 180 kcal per gram of nitrogen. These figures, however, should not be used as substitutes for independent estimates of energy and protein requirements. Especially in sick patients, energy and protein requirements may be dissociated to some extent. The protein–calorie ratios are important only in so far as they serve as a reminder of the need of calories along with protein replacement.

IX. **Estimation of protein loss in illness.** Obligatory loss of protein from the body (25 to 40 g/d) represents a small fraction of total protein synthesized by the body, which has been estimated to be from 285 to 340 g/d. Thus, the synthesis of protein can be decreased much more severely than is suggested by daily losses alone. Moreover, normal protein losses from the skin and gastrointestinal tract are only a fraction of what can be lost potentially. The average normal gastrointestinal protein loss is 1.7 g of nitrogen times 6.25, or 10.6 g of protein, some of which is recovered in the colon. The value of 6.25 is usually used for conversion of total nitrogen values to grams of protein because this is the factor for the high-quality protein found in meat, fish, and eggs, and also in corn and beans. A lower factor (5.2 to 5.8) is used for other vegetable proteins, and higher values (~6.4) for dairy proteins.

A. **Conditions characterized by excessive protein loss**

1. **Urinary loss.** Loss of protein occurs in nephrosis, chronic renal disease, and states of hypermetabolism with tissue breakdown. The losses from tissue breakdown are accounted for in the usual estimate of urinary nitrogen loss. Estimating urinary urea nitrogen as the sole factor in urinary protein loss is the most logical determination for hypermetabolic conditions in which body proteins are degraded to urea. Protein loss can be estimated by multiplying urinary nonprotein nitrogen loss times 6.25. When protein *per se* is lost into the urine (e.g., in nephrosis or chronic renal disease), the protein itself is often measured.

2. **Loss through other body fluids.** Nasogastric losses or losses through fistulae can be measured and added to the daily protein loss to allow a better estimate of total protein losses, especially if drainage volumes are large.

3. **Loss through gastrointestinal tract, skin, or lungs.** Nitrogen can be lost from organs with a large surface area of epithelial cells. These organs include the intestine, skin, and lungs. A limited number of observations have been made in illnesses involving these organs. Because the losses vary widely, no formula can be devised to estimate them. Intestinal losses are greatest in disorders associated with either decreased digestion or absorption of protein or increased loss of protein into the lumen. Because the small intestine has the largest surface area and the highest normal rate of protein loss of all the enteric organs (about 50 g of protein per day), diseases of the small intestine have the potential to cause the highest rate of protein loss from the body. These *protein-losing enteropathies* may or may not be accompanied by symptoms.

B. **Estimation of protein requirements according to severity of illness.** Nitrogen losses usually cannot be measured in clinical situations. For a hospitalized, adequately nourished adult receiving high-quality protein intravenously, the basal requirements can be estimated to be about 0.4 to 0.6 g/kg. For an ambulatory patient consuming a standard diet of mixed-quality protein, the basal requirements should be estimated at 0.75 g/kg. The estimates in Table 5-13 are used to calculate protein requirements when excessive loss cannot be measured.

X. **Longitudinal measures of growth or body weight.** Assessments are made to describe the nutritional status of populations and individuals. Normal values

Table 5-13. Estimate of recommended daily protein intake

Clinical condition	Protein requirements (g/kg IBW per day)
Normal	0.75
Metabolic "stress/illness/injury"	
Mild/moderate	1.0–1.25
Moderate/severe	1.25–1.5
Severe with extra losses (e.g., skin, urine)	>1.5
Renal failure, acute (undialyzed)	0.8–1.0
Hemodialysis	1.2–1.4
Peritoneal dialysis	1.3–1.5
Hepatic encephalopathy	0.4–0.6

IBW, ideal body weight.

are descriptive of healthy subject groups and may not relate well to the individual patient undergoing evaluation. No single measure in routine use today can accurately reflect the protein–calorie status. Thus, many different anthropometric laboratory tests may be combined to formulate an overall impression. The advantages, disadvantages, and utility of the tests are described, but their routine use in nutritional therapeutics is not necessarily endorsed. Longitudinal measures can be sensitive indicators of malnutrition before static body compartment measurements become abnormal. In the adult, maintenance of the usual body weight is generally expected. Therefore, weight loss with time is a helpful and simple longitudinal measurement in nutritional assessment. In the child, weight gain with growth is expected, and failure to maintain an expected growth rate similarly can be a simple indication of protein and calorie malnutrition. In addition to weight, increases in length and head circumference can be monitored in children because bone is growing.

A. Height should be measured without shoes in adults with the patient erect. Historical data are often erroneous by 1 to 2 in.

B. Weight is a simple measure of nutritional status. It can be compared with ideal weights or with usual weights corrected for height (Table 5-2), derived from representative values of the adult U.S. population sampled in NHANES I and NHANES II.

$$\text{Percentage Reference Body Weight} = (\text{Actual Weight} \div \text{Reference Body Weight}) \times 100$$

To calculate weight change:

$$\text{Percentage Body Change} = [(\text{Usual Weight} - \text{Actual Weight}) \div \text{Usual Weight}] \times 100$$

A loss of 5% of body weight or less is not usually clinically important unless it occurs within a short time. Clearly, the rate of weight loss also must be considered in judging its significance. Weight changes cannot be an assessment of nutritive status in the face of increased extracellular fluid (edema, ascites, congestive failure) or during diuretic therapy. Despite these cautions, body weight is probably the best comprehensive estimate of protein–calorie status.

The definition of healthy weight has traditionally been set at the range of weights associated with the lowest mortality. However, many problems have arisen with this approach (22). A problem with standard weight guidelines is that a person can gain considerable weight (even 15 to 20 kg) and still remain within the recommended range. This has led people to feel that weight gain with age is acceptable. However, it is now clear that smaller gains in weight (e.g., 5 to 10 kg) during adult life are associated with an increased risk for chronic disease, including cancer, diabetes, hypertension, coronary artery disease, and cholelithiasis (22). Thus, it is important for adults to monitor their body weight, best corrected for height as in the BMI, as advocated by both the World Health Organization and the International Obesity Task Force (see also Table 5-15).

C. **BMI.** The BMI is obtained by dividing weight (kg) by the square of the height (m²):

$$BMI = W/H^2 \text{ (Fig. 5-2)}$$

This measure best predicts the percentage of body fat in groups of subjects, but not in individual persons. Because the height is squared, that contributing factor is minimized. A nomogram is useful for quickly determining the BMI. Overweight is now defined as a value greater than 25 (23). This figure is based on excess body weight of 15% or more, according to Metropolitan Life Insurance tables of 1983, which offer ideal weights somewhat lower than those found in the NHANES data for the average U.S. population (Table 5-2). For children, different height–weight data must be used. The BMI may not be representative of some subsets of the population (e.g., elderly, medically ill), and it does not take into account frame size or distribution of fat. The National Institutes of Health Technology Assessment Conference Panel on Methods for Voluntary Weight Loss and Control endorsed use of the BMI to define overweight (24). Its use has been less well documented for identifying conditions associated with weight loss. Simple formulas for calculating the BMI from pounds and inches have been developed:

$$BMI = \left[W \text{ (lb)} \div H \text{ (in)}\right] \div 0.0014192 \text{ (25)}$$

$$BMI = W \text{ (lb)} \div H^2 \text{ (in)} \times 703 \text{ (26)}$$

Tables 5-14 and 13-2 provide a quick conversion of height and weight into BMI for most patients. The advantage of the BMI over linear height and weight is that it provides a simple estimate of disease risk (Table 5-15).

XI. **Measurement of body compartments**

A. **Fat stores.** Adipose tissue comprises about 25% of body weight. This calorie storehouse could theoretically provide more than 150,000 kcal in the average adult. Although reduction of the fat reserves in comparison with those of the normal population is not in itself detrimental, it does suggest inadequate calorie intake for a prolonged period of time and a concomitant protein compartment deficiency. Thus, normal fat reserves in comparison with population standards do not ensure that the protein compartment status is normal. Fat stores can be inferred from the body weight and estimated from subcutaneous fat measurements.

1. **Subcutaneous fat (skinfold) measurement** is a fairly reliable estimate of fat reserves in nutritionally stable persons because about 50% of adipose tissue is subcutaneous; fat losses occur proportionally throughout the body during the utilization of fat reserves. Major problems for measuring this compartment in patients include the lack of complete population standards for comparison and the marked variation in measurements depending on the care and skill with which they are taken. A coefficient of variation of 22.6% has been reported for this procedure when performed by different observers. It is not known whether changes in age or total body water affect the measurement. In addition, skin disease or edema interferes with the accuracy of skinfold measurements. *Triceps skinfold measurements* have been used most frequently in the clinical assessment of fat reserves, but measurement at more than one site appears to provide a better assessment of compart-

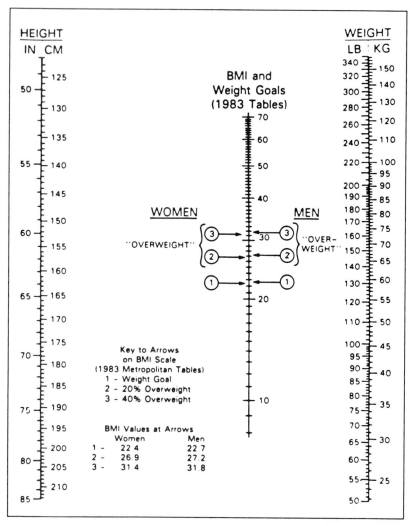

FIG. 5.2. Nomogram for body mass index (kilograms per square meter) and weight goals (1983 tables). The ratio of weight to square of the height (metric units) is read from the central scale after a straight edge ruler is placed between the height and body weight. Weights and heights are without clothing. With clothing, add 5 lb (3.3 kg) for men or 3 lb (1.4 kg) for women, and add 1 in (2.5 cm) in height for shoes. (From Burton BT, Foster WR, Hirsch J, van Itallie TB. Health implications of obesity: NIH consensus development conference. *Int J Obesity* 1985;9:155, with permission.)

ment size. Table 5-16 lists standard values for triceps skinfold thickness for adults of both sexes. Note the considerable variation between males and females.

   a. Technique of triceps skinfold measurement (27)

       (1) Have the patient sit with the right arm hanging freely at the side. (An alternative technique can be followed for bedridden patients. With the patient supine, the right arm is flexed at the shoulder to the vertical position while the forearm crosses the chest.)

(2) Mark the midpoint between the acromion and the olecranon posteriorly over the triceps muscle.

(3) Gently pinch the skin and subcutaneous tissue at the midpoint and apply a pressure-related caliper (Lange, Halipern) for 3 seconds before taking the reading. The caliper should exert 10 g of pressure per square millimeter regardless of the fold thickness for reproducible results and for comparison with normal values. Skinfold thickness can be estimated at the same location by pinching the tissues with the fingers, but variation from careful technique hampers the reproducibility and reliability of skinfold thickness measurements considerably.

(4) Release the caliper and repeat the measurement two additional times.

(5) Record an average of three readings and the percentile of the reference population from Table 5-16.

2. **Interpretation of measurements of fat stores.** Both body weight and skinfold measurements of a patient may be within a low percentile in comparison with measurements from the population in general. These results do not automatically indicate depletion of reserves or malnutrition; they may reflect a slight build of the patient. Therefore, these parameters must be interpreted with caution and in light of other information—for example, the usual body weight. On the other hand, an obese patient can recently have lost a large amount of weight and still have excessive fat reserves. In such situations, fat reserve measurements are not helpful in suggesting concomitant protein compartment depletion. Grading the severity of adipose tissue depletion is arbitrary; a moderate decrease from "normal" may not be unhealthy. Nevertheless, fat reserves below the tenth percentile suggest advanced depletion, and those below the thirtieth percentile suggest mild to moderate depletion.

B. **The "somatic" protein compartment** largely represents muscle mass.

1. **Body weight.** Measurements of body weight also reflect the muscle mass because it constitutes approximately 30% of the total body weight. Protein–calorie malnutrition causes a decrease in the muscle mass as well as in body fat stores, both of which are reflected by a decrease in body weight. Comparison of body weight with values from a reference population can suggest somatic protein depletion, but single measurements can underestimate depletion in large patients and overestimate depletion in patients of small build. Recent weight change or weight as a percentage of usual body weight often better suggests protein depletion, even though these parameters do not measure the compartment directly.

2. **MAMC.** An estimation of muscle mass for comparison with values from a reference population is obtained by measuring the arm at the midpoint between the acromion and the olecranon. From measurements of both the midarm circumference and the triceps skinfold, an estimate of the MAMC can be calculated (Fig. 5-3). This calculation assumes that the compartment is round, that the skinfold measurement is accurate and consistent about the circumference, and that the bone is of constant cross-sectional area. None of these assumptions is completely correct. Considerable variance in reading occurs between observers and even between readings from the same observer. Population percentiles for midarm muscle circumference of adults depending on sex and age are given in Table 5-17. These percentiles are calculated from midarm circumference and triceps skinfold data in the NHANES of 1971–1974. This is largely used for research studies.

Table 5-14. Body mass index for overweight patients

BMI Height (in)	Overweight					Obesity						
	25	26	27	28	29	30	31	32	33	34	35	40
						Weight (lb)						
58	119	124	129	134	138	143	149	153	158	163	167	191
59	124	128	133	138	143	148	154	158	164	169	173	198
60	128	133	138	143	148	153	159	164	169	175	179	204
61	132	137	143	148	153	158	165	169	175	180	185	211
62	136	142	147	153	158	164	170	175	181	186	191	218
63	141	146	152	158	163	169	175	181	187	192	197	225
64	145	151	157	163	169	174	181	187	193	199	204	232
65	150	156	162	168	174	180	187	193	199	205	210	240
66	155	161	167	173	179	186	192	199	205	211	216	247
67	159	166	172	178	185	191	198	205	211	218	223	255
68	164	171	177	184	190	197	204	211	218	224	230	262
69	169	176	182	189	196	203	210	217	224	231	236	270
70	174	181	188	195	202	207	216	223	230	237	243	278
71	179	186	193	200	208	215	222	230	237	244	250	286
72	184	191	199	206	213	221	228	236	244	251	258	294
73	189	197	204	212	219	227	236	243	251	258	265	302
74	194	202	210	218	225	233	241	250	258	265	272	311
75	200	208	216	224	232	240	248	256	264	272	279	319

	Overweight					Obesity						
BMI	25	26	27	28	29	30	31	32	33	34	35	40
Height (cm)						Weight (kg)						
147.3	54.0	56.4	58.6	60.9	62.7	65.0	67.7	69.5	71.8	74.1	75.9	86.8
150	56.4	58.2	60.5	62.7	65.0	67.3	70.0	71.8	74.5	76.8	78.6	90
152.4	58.2	60.5	62.7	65.0	67.3	69.5	72.3	74.5	76.8	79.5	81.4	92.7
155	60.0	62.3	65.0	67.3	69.5	71.8	75.0	76.8	79.5	81.8	84.1	95.9
157.5	61.8	64.5	66.8	69.5	71.8	74.5	77.3	79.5	82.3	84.5	86.8	99.1
160	64.1	66.4	69.1	71.8	74.1	76.8	79.5	82.3	85.0	87.3	89.5	102.3
162.5	65.9	68.6	71.4	74.1	76.8	79.1	82.3	85.0	87.7	90.5	92.7	105.5
165	68.2	70.9	73.6	76.4	79.1	81.8	85.0	87.7	90.5	93.2	95.5	109.1
167.6	70.5	73.2	75.9	78.6	81.4	84.5	87.3	90.5	93.2	95.9	98.2	112.3
170.2	72.3	75.6	78.2	80.9	84.0	86.8	90.0	93.2	95.9	99.1	101.4	115.9
172.7	74.5	77.7	80.4	83.6	86.3	89.5	92.7	95.9	99.1	101.8	104.5	119.1
175.3	76.8	80.0	82.7	85.9	89.0	92.3	95.5	98.6	101.8	105.0	107.3	122.7
177.8	79.0	82.3	85.4	88.6	91.8	94.1	98.2	101.4	104.5	107.7	111.0	126.4
180.3	81.4	84.5	87.7	90.9	94.5	97.7	101.4	104.5	107.7	111.0	113.6	130
182.9	83.6	86.8	90.5	93.6	96.8	100.5	103.6	107.3	111.0	114.1	117.3	133.6
185.4	85.9	88.2	92.7	96.4	99.5	103.2	107.3	110.5	114.0	117.3	120.5	137.3
188	88.2	91.8	95.5	99.1	102.3	106.0	109.5	113.6	117.3	120.5	123.6	141.4
190.5	90.9	94.5	98.2	101.8	105.5	109.0	112.7	116.4	120.0	123.6	126.8	145

Table 5-15. Body mass index as a measure of associated disease risk

Weight category	BMI (kg/m^2)	Risk
Extremely underweight	<14.0	Extremely high
Underweight	14.1–18.4	Increased in smokers, chronic illness
Normal	18.5–24.9	Normal
Overweight	25–29.9	Increased
Obesity		
Class I	30.0–34.9	High
Class II	35.0–39.9	Very high
Class III	≥40.0	Extremely high

Adapted from National Institute of Diabetes and Digestive and Kidney Diseases. Clinical guidelines on the identification, evaluation, and treatment of overweight and obesity in adults—the evidence report. *Obes Res* 1998;6:S53.

a. **Interpretation of percentiles.** A decrease of 15 to 20 percentiles from the expected value suggests a significant reduction of protein mass. As in interpreting fat stores with skinfold thickness or body weight, an absolute measurement that falls below the thirtieth percentile of the population in general suggests a decrease in muscle mass. However, as is also true of the other measurement, this type of interpretation overdiagnoses malnutrition in the patient who has a small build or is lanky and underdiagnoses ongoing malnutrition in the athlete or patient near the other end of the weight spectrum. This explains why the MAMC can be normal even in the presence of protein–calorie malnutrition.

Table 5-16. Percentiles for triceps skinfold thickness of adults in the United States[a]

Age group (y) and sex	Population percentile						
	5	10	25	50	75	90	95
Men							
18–24	4.0	5.0	7.0	9.5	14.0	20.0	21.0
25–34	4.5	5.5	8.0	12.0	16.0	21.5	24.0
35–44	5.0	6.0	8.5	12.0	15.5	20.0	23.0
45–54	5.0	6.0	8.0	11.0	15.0	20.0	25.5
55–64	5.0	6.0	8.0	11.0	14.0	18.0	21.5
65–74	4.5	5.5	8.0	11.0	15.0	19.0	22.0
Women							
18–24	9.4	11.0	14.0	18.0	24.0	30.0	34.0
25–34	10.5	12.0	16.0	21.0	26.5	31.5	37.0
35–44	12.0	14.0	18.0	23.0	29.5	39.5	39.0
45–54	13.0	15.0	20.0	25.0	30.0	36.0	40.0
55–64	11.0	14.0	19.0	25.0	30.5	35.0	39.0
65–74	11.5	14.0	18.0	23.0	28.0	33.0	36.0

[a] Triceps skinfold thickness in millimeters.
Adapted from Bishop CW, Bowen PE, Ritchey SJ. Norms for nutritional assessment of American adults by upper arm anthropometry. *Am J Clin Nutr* 1981;34:2530. Data from Health and Nutrition Examination Survey, 1971–1974.

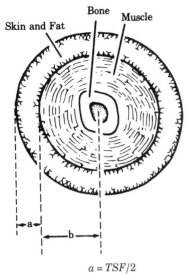

Skin and Fat   Bone   Muscle

FIG. 5.3. Calculation of midarm muscle circumference from midarm circumference and triceps skinfold thickness.

$$a = TSF/2$$

$$MAC \text{ (mm)} = 2\pi\,(a + b)$$

$$MMR = b = (MAC \div 2\pi) - TSF/2$$

$$MAMC \text{ (mm)} = MAC - (TSF)\,\pi$$

where *TSF* is triceps skinfold thickness (mm),
MAC is midarm circumference,
MMR is midarm muscle radius,
and *MAMC* is midarm muscle circumference.

Table 5-17. Percentiles for midarm muscle circumference of adults in the United States[a]

Age group (y) and sex	Population percentile						
	5	10	25	50	75	90	95
Men							
18–24	235	244	258	272	289	308	323
25–34	242	253	265	280	300	317	329
35–44	250	256	271	287	303	321	330
45–54	240	249	265	281	298	315	326
55–64	228	244	262	279	296	310	318
65–74	225	237	253	269	285	299	307
Women							
18–24	177	185	194	206	221	236	249
25–34	183	189	200	214	229	249	266
35–44	185	192	206	220	240	261	274
45–54	188	195	207	222	243	266	278
55–64	186	195	208	226	244	263	281
65–74	186	195	208	225	244	265	281

[a] Midarm muscle circumference in millimeters.
Adapted from Bishop CW, Bowen PE, Ritchey SJ. Norms for nutritional assessment of American adults by upper arm anthropometry. *Am J Clin Nutr* 1981;34:2530. Data from Health and Nutrition Examination Survey, 1971–1974.

b. Technique of MAMC measurement

   (1) Have the patient sit with the right arm hanging freely at the side.
   (2) Mark the midpoint between the acromion and olecranon.
   (3) Measure the circumference at the midpoint with a tape.
   (4) Average the results of three measurements, calculate the MAMC (Fig. 5-3), and record the percentile from the reference population (Table 5-17).

3. **Creatinine–height index (CHI).** Endogenous creatinine production and excretion indirectly reflect the total body muscle mass. Creatinine is a dehydrated end-product of creatine, a complex molecule involved in supplying ATP to muscle cells; it is concentrated in the muscle mass. About 2% of the creatine phosphate in muscle is converted daily into creatinine in an irreversible reaction. Good correlation has been found between lean body mass measured by radioisotope labeling and by 24-hour creatinine excretion. For purposes of clinical assessment, a patient's creatinine excretion is compared with the expected excretion of a person of similar height and ideal weight. Actual population standards for this measurement do not exist. Calculated ideal values are derived from the average 24-hour creatinine excretions of healthy children and adults while on a creatinine- and creatine-free diet; adult values are given in Table 5-18. The CHI compares the actual 24-hour creatinine excretion of a patient with the expected value for a person of the same height:

$$CHI = (\text{Actual 24-Hour Creatinine Excretion} \div \text{Ideal 24-Hour Creatinine Excretion}) \times 100\%$$

Table 5-18. Ideal 24-hour urinary creatinine excretion by adults of various heights (for use in calculation of the creatinine/height index)

Height		Ideal creatinine excretion (mg)	
in	cm	Adult women	Adult men
58	147.3	830	—
59	149.9	851	—
60	152.4	875	—
61	154.9	900	—
62	157.5	925	1,288
63	160.0	949	1,325
64	162.6	977	1,359
65	165.1	1,006	1,386
66	167.6	1,044	1,426
67	170.2	1,076	1,467
68	172.7	1,109	1,513
69	175.3	1,141	1,555
70	177.8	1,174	1,596
71	180.3	1,206	1,642
72	182.9	1,240	1,691
73	185.4	—	1,739
74	188.0	—	1,785
75	190.5	—	1,831
76	193.0	—	1,891

Adapted from Blackburn GL, Bistrian BR, Maini BS, et al. Nutritional and metabolic assessment of the hospitalized patient. *JPEN J Parenter Enteral Nutr* 1977;1:11.

a. **Interpretation of CHI.** The CHI indicates no or mild protein depletion when it is above 80%; moderate protein depletion is indicated at a CHI of 60% to 80%, and severe depletion is indicated by a CHI below 60%. The test is potentially useful when edema or obesity make the measurement of body weight or BMI unreliable as an estimate of malnutrition.

b. **Difficulties with interpretation.** Like other measurements that rely on comparison with reference population standards, the CHI relies on ideal body weight standards for adults and calculated reference standards for children. Estimates of muscle mass may be inaccurate in patients who do not fall into the midrange of ideal body weight for height. The test is not valid in patients whose urine output is impaired or who have undergone amputation. It requires 24-hour urine collection and a constant protein intake. Conditions that alter creatinine excretion include kidney failure, liver failure, sepsis, and trauma. Aging and consumption of a creatinine-free diet also reduce creatinine excretion. Creatinine excretion is increased by vigorous exercise, a diet rich in red meat, corticosteroid and testosterone therapy, and administration of certain antibiotics (some aminoglycosides and cephalosporins). Because so many factors decrease creatinine excretion, the CHI often overestimates muscle mass depletion. For this reason, it is used less frequently than might be expected from its simplicity.

4. **3-Methylhistidine excretion.** 3-Methylhistidine is a biochemical degradation product of myofibrillar muscle protein metabolism. This amino acid is not recycled into protein and is excreted in the urine. However, 3-methylhistidine is not a breakdown product of sarcoplasmic protein, which constitutes about 35% of muscle protein. Like creatinine excretion, 3-methylhistidine excretion is decreased by old age, a decreased protein intake, trauma, or infection, and like the CHI, it overestimates muscle mass depletion.

5. **Muscle strength.** Impairment of muscle function is a detrimental effect of somatic protein compartment depletion. Impaired function may be measurable before anthropometric measurements demonstrate a decrease in muscle mass in comparison with population standards. Measurements of muscle strength are not a routine component of inpatient nutritional assessment but are advocated by some. Measurement of respiratory strength has been suggested as an important determinant of the adequacy of the somatic protein compartment in hospitalized patients. A hand dynamometer also can be used to measure muscle strength (28). Muscle strength can be impaired by sedatives, primary medical disease, depression, and old age.

C. **Circulating proteins.** Serum levels of circulating proteins can be decreased and reflect protein depletion even when other measurements of the protein compartment appear to be normal. Proteins synthesized by the liver have been used as markers for assessing protein status. Presumably, decreased levels of these proteins reflect a decrease in both amino acid precursors and hepatic (and other visceral) mass. Serum levels of some of these protein markers are listed in Table 5-19. The assumption that decreased levels of these proteins are specific for malnutrition is obviously wrong. Levels of liver-dependent circulating proteins reflect not only on adequacy of nutrition but also the synthetic capacity of the liver (not simply in relation to nutrition but also in relation to hepatic disease), rate of metabolic utilization, status of hydration, and excretion. Therefore, no measurable circulating protein is or ever will be specific for assessing visceral protein nutritional status.

1. **Albumin**
   a. **Physiology.** Albumin is a single-chain polypeptide with 575 amino acid residues. The liver is the exclusive site of albumin synthesis, and

Table 5-19. Serum proteins used for nutritional assessment

Protein	Half-life (d)	Reference range	
		Conventional units	SI units
Albumin	18–20	3.3–6.1 g/dL	500–860 µmol/L
Transferrin	8–9	0.26–0.43 g/dL	28.6–47.3 µmol/L
Prealbumin	2–3	0.2–0.4 g/L	3.64–7.27 µmol/L
Retinol-binding protein	0.5	30–60 mg/L	1.43–2.86 µmol/L
Fibronectin, soluble	0.16–1	1.66–1.98 g/L	3.77–4.50 µmol/L

SI, Système International.

the normal adult synthesizes 120 to 200 mg/kg per day (about 12 g/d for the average adult) as part of a total exchangeable pool of 3.5 to 5.0 g/kg of body weight. Only 40% of the pool is located intravascularly. Equilibration is slow between intravascular and extravascular albumin, about 5%/h, so the entire mass of plasma albumin is exchanged daily with the extracellular component. Redistribution of the extravascular pool into the circulating compartment can help maintain normal levels despite protein deprivation.

Albumin represents about half the total exported protein synthesized by the liver. Many factors are involved in regulating albumin synthesis and secretion, and amino acid supply is only one. In short-term exogenous amino acid deprivation, albumin synthesis decreases, serum levels fall, and hepatic albumin degradation decreases such that a new steady state is reached. The total exchangeable albumin pool may decrease to one-third its normal level before a decreased serum albumin concentration is evident. Restoration of amino acid precursors in such cases allows for greater than normal synthesis rates and normalization of serum albumin levels. Long-term protein deprivation results in less rapidly reversible decreases in the translational machinery of the hepatocytes. Providing amino acids only slowly normalizes the albumin-synthesizing capabilities of hepatocytes.

In health, the serum half-life of albumin is 20 days. This long half-life makes albumin a poor marker for rapid changes in metabolic states. Changes in synthesis and degradation rates in addition to body compartment shifts influence the serum level.

b. Interpretation of abnormal values. Because the serum albumin level correlates with morbidity and mortality in hospitalized patients, the concept has developed that such patients need nutritional support. Arbitrary levels of serum albumin have been suggested as indicators of protein malnutrition. A serum albumin level of 2.8 to 3.4 g/dL is associated with a mild degree of protein malnutrition; moderate depletion is suggested by a serum albumin level of 2.1 to 2.7 g/dL, and severe depletion by a level below 2.1 g/dL.

c. Difficulties with interpretation. Albumin levels correlate with disease severity but not necessarily with nutritional status (29). Use of the serum albumin level as an indicator of the protein nutritional state assumes a steady state, which is seldom the case during acute or subacute illness. The long half-life of albumin in serum makes this protein a poor marker of acute changes in nutritional status. Interpretation varies depending on length of protein deprivation. The rapid loss of plasma proteins (e.g., postoperatively, from burns, from the gastrointestinal tract) reduces serum albumin levels but does not necessarily indicate a reduction in protein mass.

Therefore, although the serum albumin level does reflect the size of the intravascular albumin pool, it is simplistic to assume that this measurement, especially during acute illness, always reflects the protein mass. Also, a shift away from the intravascular pool of as much as 16% of the total exchangeable pool can occur with a change in body position from sitting to reclining; this further influences longitudinal measurements. Inflammatory disorders can decrease albumin synthesis and degradation or increase capillary leak. Increased nutrition (e.g., total parenteral nutrition) often does not alter albumin levels (30). Thus, even when protein malnutrition is a component of an illness, restoration of a low serum albumin level to normal with protein or amino acid therapy can be slow, and generally lags considerably behind clinical impressions of successful nutritional therapy.

  d. Reduced serum levels are seen in many conditions, including malnutrition, liver disease, ascites, idiopathic edema, nephrosis, protein-losing enteropathies, thermal burns, severe eczema, hypothyroidism, zinc deficiency, malignant diseases, congestive heart failure, acute stress, and age over 70 years.

2. Transferrin

  a. Physiology. Transferrin is a globulin (molecular weight of approximately 90,000) that binds and transports iron in the plasma. The liver is the principal but not the only site of transferrin synthesis; hepatic synthesis is probably modulated by ferritin within the hepatocytes. Serum levels are similar for men and women and decline only slightly in later life.

  The synthetic rate appears to be the predominant factor in determining serum levels, although in acute illness, enhanced degradation can result in depressed levels. The body pool is only about 5 g, and the serum half-life of the protein is 8 to 10 days. Direct measurement of the protein is not always performed routinely, whereas serum total iron-binding capacity (TIBC) is often obtained when anemia is being investigated. Transferrin concentration can be estimated from the TIBC, but the relationship appears to be less constant at lower concentrations of transferrin, and the constants may vary from institution to institution. The attachment of iron to proteins other than transferrin when the latter is more than half-saturated further contributes to the inaccuracy of this estimate, and the readily measured transferrin is preferred.

  b. Interpretation of abnormal values. Arbitrary levels of serum transferrin have been suggested as indicators of protein depletion. Serum transferrin levels of 150 to 200 mg/dL are associated with a mild degree of protein malnutrition; levels of 100 to 150 mg/dL are associated with moderate depletion, and a level below 100 mg/dL is associated with severe depletion.

  c. Difficulties with interpretation. Like serum albumin levels, serum transferrin levels depend on alterations in synthesis and degradation, both of which are affected by factors other than nutritional status. In particular, the degradation rate increases in acute illness, and synthesis increases in iron deficiency. *Decreased levels* are also seen in pernicious anemia, anemia of chronic disease, liver disease, starvation, burns, iron overload, nephrotic syndrome, and protein-losing enteropathies, and during steroid (glucocorticoid and androgen) therapy. *Increased levels* are observed during hypoxia, pregnancy, and treatment with estrogens or oral contraceptives.

3. Other circulating proteins. Two proteins that are also synthesized by the liver and secreted into the circulation are *retinol-binding protein* (RBP) and *thyroxine-binding prealbumin* (TBPA). Virtually all RBP is bound to TBPA in a 1:1 ratio. Because of their shorter half-lives (10 to 12 hours for RBP, 2 to 3 days for TBPA), and because of the particular amino acid content of TBPA, these two proteins rapidly reflect changes in hepatic protein synthesis.

    a. Interpretation of abnormal values. Any value less than the normal range for these proteins may indicate protein depletion.

    b. Difficulties with interpretation. Unfortunately, levels of both these proteins promptly drop with acute metabolic stress and the accompanying demand for protein synthesis. RBP and TBPA are both metabolized by the kidney, and levels increase in kidney failure. Because of the problems inherent in trying to use the measured level of serum protein to estimate the size and integrity of the organ where it is synthesized, it is unlikely that an ideal circulating protein to assess protein status will be found.

D. Immunocompetence in nutritional assessment

    1. Abnormalities of the immune system. Many aspects of the immune system are frequently abnormal in patients with generalized malnutrition. Decreased numbers of circulating T cells, decreased numbers of total circulating lymphocytes, and an impaired delayed cutaneous hypersensitivity response to skin test antigens in patients with protein depletion or protein–calorie malnutrition indicate concomitant impairment of cell-mediated immunity.

    Depressed levels of various complement components (including C3), reduced amounts of secretory immunoglobulin A in external body secretions, and various abnormalities of the nonspecific cellular mechanisms of host resistance have been observed in malnourished laboratory animals and patients and have been reversed with nutritional repletion. Local nonspecific defenses (e.g., epithelial integrity, mucous production, cilial mobility) are also adversely affected by malnutrition. These adverse effects together make the malnourished patient a likely candidate for infection.

    The precise nutritional deficiency that results in an immunocompromised state in the individual malnourished patient is generally unknown. Although the above-mentioned abnormalities are most frequently associated with protein malnutrition, most protein- and calorie-deficient patients have multiple nutritional deficiencies, not pure protein depletion. Almost any nutritional deficiency, if sufficiently severe, will adversely affect some aspect of the immune system. Therefore, the discovery of immunologic dysfunction does not necessarily imply protein malnutrition. However, if other indicators of macronutrient malnutrition are also present, then correction of protein nutritional status may normalize immune function.

    2. Tests of immune system. Many tests are available to assess immune function (Table 5-20). Two tests of the immune system have been employed most frequently as nonspecific clinical indicators of malnutrition in nutritional assessment: total circulating lymphocyte count and delayed cutaneous hypersensitivity to skin test antigens.

    a. Total lymphocyte count (TLC)

        (1) Physiology. Circulating lymphocytes are mostly T cells. The thymus-dependent immune responses are very sensitive to malnutrition, and involution of tissues that generate T cells occurs early in the course of protein or protein–calorie malnutrition. Reduction in circulating T cells precedes and eventually leads to lymphopenia. The circulating lymphocyte count can be calculated from the peripheral white blood count and the differential:

$$TLC \ (\text{cells/mm}^3) = WBC \ (\text{cells/mm}^3)$$
$$\times (\text{Percentage of Lymphocytes} \div 100)$$

Table 5-20. Methods used to assess nutrient–immune interactions

Tissue tested	Function	Method	Relevance to nutrient status
Mononuclear cells	Disease status	Cell count	Nonspecific
	Proliferation	Cultured blood Culture cells	T-lymphocyte response
	Activation	Isolated cells	T- or B-cell response
	Subtypes	Flow cytometry	T- or B-cell subtypes
	NK cell	Cr release	Subtype of T cell
Cytokine	Serum content	ELISA, RIA	Ability to secrete
	IC content	ELISA, RIA	? Ability to synthesize
Delayed-type hypersensitivity	Cell-mediated	Skin test	Reflect *in vivo* immunity

NK, natural killer; ELISA, enzyme-linked immunosorbent assay; RIA, radioimmunoassay; IC, intracellular; Cr, chromium.

(2) **Interpretation of abnormal values.** Depression of circulating lymphocyte numbers below normal (200 cells/mm^3) is not specific for any particular nutritional deficiency. As a general indicator of malnutrition, the TLC tends to correlate best with other measures of protein status. A TLC of 1,200 to 2,000/mm^3 correlates with mild malnutrition; a count of 800 to 1,200 is associated with moderate depletion, and a count below 800 is associated with severe depletion.

(3) **Difficulties with interpretation.** Infections and immunosuppressant drugs alter the number of circulating lymphocytes. The reason for lymphopenia in chronic or severe disease is generally not specific or identified. The TLC *per se* does not indicate the adequacy of immune function. Its use is complicated in cases of infection, metabolic stress, malignancy, or treatment with corticosteroids or immunosuppressive drugs. In such cases, the TLC may correlate with disease severity but not with nutritional status.

b. **Delayed cutaneous hypersensitivity (DCH) reactions**

(1) **Physiology.** The erythematous, indurated skin response to recall antigens is the standard for studying the cell-mediated immune response *in vivo*. The DCH reaction results from three sequential processes: (a) Processing of antigen by macrophages results in the generation of both effector and memory T cells (the afferent limb); (b) recognition of antigen on rechallenge results in blast transformation, cellular proliferation, and generation of lymphokine-producing effector cells (efferent limb); and (c) local erythema and induration of the skin results from release of lymphokines and chemotactic factors at the antigen site.

A primary DCH response to new antigens requires that both afferent and efferent limbs be intact. Generally, the DCH response is tested by using antigens that the patient has previously encountered. Thus, presumably only the efferent aspects of the system are tested. Such antigens include purified protein derivative (PPD), streptokinase–streptodornase (SKSD), mumps virus, *Candida albicans, Trichophyton,* and coccidioidin.

Failure to react to recall antigens (anergy) has been well described in patients with protein depletion or protein–calorie malnutrition. Unfortunately, many other factors also influence the complex reaction sequence of the normal DCH response. When reactivity to a battery of skin test antigens is examined in relation to circulating liver-dependent proteins and to the TLC, the percentage of patients with anergy increases as protein levels and lymphocyte counts decrease, but anergy cannot be predicted accurately on the basis of any one variable.

The prevalence of nonreactivity to three recall antigens is about 50% in patients with serum albumin levels below 3.0 g/dL but is also reported up to 30% of the time when the serum albumin level is above 3.0 g/dL.

(2) **Normal response** is represented by an induration greater than 5 mm after 24 to 72 hours to at least one of five skin test recall antigens (e.g., mumps virus, PPD, *C. albicans, Trichophyton,* SKSD).

(3) **Interpretation of abnormal response.** Anergy is variably defined but usually implies a failure to respond to any of five skin test antigens (<5 mm of induration). Reactivity is interpreted as a normal DCH response; anergy, or failure of the DCH response, may be the result of protein–calorie malnutrition and reversible with nutritional repletion.

(4) **Difficulties with interpretation.** Recall response depends on prior exposure to the antigen. Because 60% or fewer of subjects respond to many of the antigens used, anergy cannot be assumed on the basis of no response to only one or two antigens. In addition, antigens vary in potency in different lots. A rapid response may occur in subjects tested serially with the same antigen (especially if at the same skin site). The reaction may fade by 48 hours, giving a false-negative test result. Sites should be examined at 24 and 48 hours. The primary illness (e.g., lymphoma, sarcoidosis, cancer, liver or kidney failure, immunosuppressive disease) and medications (e.g., immunosuppressive drugs, chemotherapeutic agents, corticosteroids, warfarin, cimetidine, aspirin) may influence the results. Edema interferes with the local response. Evidence of immune dysfunction on the basis of an impaired DCH response simply cannot be considered to indicate malnutrition.

XII. **Clinical applications of protein and fat nutritional status assessment**
   A. **Indications for assessment of nutritional status**
      1. **Selection of malnourished patients for intensive nutritional therapy.** A comprehensive assessment of protein and fat nutritional status may detect global malnutrition. However, none of the available tests is specific for malnutrition, and results can be abnormal in chronic or acute illness alone. Nutrition provision may be part of the reason for abnormal test results, but it is usually not possible to identify this factor among many others. No "gold standard" exists for determining nutritional status also because no clinical definition of malnutrition is uniformly accepted. Most of the tests discussed below are judged according to their ability to predict clinical outcome. However, this does not necessarily imply that a poor outcome can be reversed by nutrient provision or nutrition support. Deficiencies of individual nutrients are discussed in Chapters 6 and 7.
         a. **Abnormalities in growth and weight maintenance** are the most important clinical indicators of protein–calorie malnutrition in the ambulatory patient population. They are the most frequently used indicators because they are simple and inexpensive. For this reason, growth and weight are routinely monitored by physicians treating children and adults, respectively. Weight loss as a predictor of outcome may be more significant when it is com-

bined with other physiologic measurements in critically ill patients (31).

b. **Subjective global assessment (SGA).** The need for more comprehensive evaluation of protein and fat nutritional status in hospitalized patients is debated. An "eyeball" assessment of nutritional status with the use of routine clinical information from the history and physical examination provides an accurate estimation in more than 70% of patients (32,33). "Subjective" assessments can predict complications in hospitalized patients (34,35), but the findings correlate better with the severity of the underlying disease than with specific nutritional deficiencies of calories or protein. The SGA determines whether the nutrient status has been altered by decreased food intake or poor digestion/malabsorption, notes the effects on organ function and body composition, and evaluates the course of the patient's disease (34,35). The findings of the history and physical examination are then weighted to rank patients as well, moderately, or severely malnourished and predict risk the risk for medical complications (Fig. 5-4). The SGA is not completely subjective because percentage of weight loss and serum albumin levels are taken into account. However, the SGA has been successful in predicting complications of surgery, transplantation, and dialysis (36). The SGA has been found in one study to predict the occurrence of complications during hospitalization in nonsurgical patients (37). This study found similar results when other scales were used, including the nutritional risk index [(1.5 × albumin) + (41.7 × present/usual weight)] and the Maastricht index [(20.68 − (0.24 × albumin) − (19.21 × transthyretin, or prealbumin) − (1.86 × lymphocytes) − (0.04 × ideal weight)].

c. **Prognostic nutritional index.** This technique is designed for use in preoperative patients and is based on objective measurements (38,39) of serum albumin, serum transferrin, triceps skinfold thickness, and reactivity to skin test antigens, calculated in a mathematical relationship. A variant of this technique has been used in a Veterans Administration trial of preoperative total parenteral nutrition (40). Other indices have been proposed, but the prognostic nutritional index was the only one to predict clinical outcome in a prospective study (38). Until the relative importance of the various parameters of protein and fat compartment status are better established, such a stepwise multiple regression analysis may be of no more help to the clinician than determination of a single variable, such as serum albumin, when it can be adequately interpreted.

d. **BMI.** The BMI can help to identify patients at increased risk for medical complications (Table 5-15). Therapy should be provided early for those patients who are extremely underweight (BMI <14 kg/m^2). The upper cutoff of 25 for increased risk for disease is well supported by data, but the much smaller population of underweight persons (BMI <19.0) who do not smoke or who have not lost weight from illness has never been studied. It is possible that such "underweight" persons with stable weight are not at increased risk for illness (22). Of course, a low BMI resulting from unexplained weight loss should signal a search for underlying causes.

2. **Monitoring effects of nutritional therapy.** Assessment of the protein and fat status may be useful in following patients receiving intensive enteral or parenteral support to document improvement in status during therapy. This is particularly true of abnormal protein status. However, most assessment parameters reflect long-term changes in nutritional status and are slow to improve despite successful accomplishment of positive nitrogen and caloric balance. For this reason, evaluation of

A. History
   1. Weight change
      overall loss in past 6 months: _____kg
      change in past week: increase _____kg
                           no change _____
                           decrease _____kg
   2. Dietary intake change compared to normal
      no change _____
      change _____: duration of change _____weeks
      type of change: hypocaloric solid diet _____ full liquid diet _____
            hypocaloric liquids _____ starvation _____
   3. Gastrointestinal symptoms, persisting > 2 weeks
      none_____ anorexia _____ nausea _____ vomiting _____ diarrhea _____
   4. Functional capacity
      no dysfunction _____
      dysfunction _____: duration _____weeks
      type of dysfunction: working suboptimally _____ ambulatory _____
            bedridden _____
   5. Disease and its relation to nutritional requirements
      primary diagnosis (specify) _____
      metabolic demand (stress): none _____ low _____ moderate _____
            high _____

B. Physical exam (for each trait specify: 0 = normal, 1+ = mild, 2+ = moderate,
                  3+ = severe)
   loss of subcutaneous fat (triceps, chest) _____
   muscle wasting (quadriceps, deltoids, temporals) _____
   ankle/sacral edema _____ ascites _____
   tongue or skin lesions suggesting nutrient deficiency _____

C. SGA rating (select one)
   _____A = well nourished (minimal/no restriction of food intake/absorption,
    minimal change in function, weight stable or increasing)
   _____B = moderately malnourished (food restriction, some functional changes,
    little/no change in body mass)
   _____C = severely malnourished (definitely decreased intake, function, and
    body mass)

FIG. 5.4. Subjective global assessment of nutritional status. (From Detsky AS, McLaughlin JR, Baker JP. What is subjective global assessment of nutritional status? *JPEN J Parenter Enteral Nutr* 1987;11:8.)

protein–calorie status has not been widely accepted as necessary in the nutritional management of most patients. As an extreme example, a major weight gain of 25% could increase the total muscle mass by 10%, the midarm muscle area by 8%, and actual midarm muscle circumference by about 5%, changes well within the day-to-day margin of error of this anthropometric measurement.

B. Extent of nutritional assessment. Because the definition of clinically significant malnutrition based on the individual measurements described in this chapter is yet to be determined, a comprehensive evaluation incorporating many parameters often is of little practical clinical value. Weight change remains the most significant parameter and the one best correlated with nutritional status, but it also may reflect chronic illness in its late stages, when nutritional replacement may not be effective. Table 5-21 summarizes the available tests for protein and fat status discussed in this chapter.

Table 5-21. Assessment for the evaluation of protein and fat nutritional status

Measurement	Compartment best reflected by measurement	Normal values	Values suggesting malnutrition or severe disease
Weight (adults)	Fat/protein mass		
% loss in last mo		<5%	>5%
% loss in last 6 mo		<10%	>10%
Weight (children)	Fat/protein mass		
% drop on wt chart		<20th percentile	>20th percentile
Triceps skinfold (mm)	Fat stores	See Table 5-16	Mild = >10th percentile Severe = <10th percentile
Creatinine/height index (%)	Protein mass	>90% (Table 5-18)	Mild = 80–90% Severe = <60%
Midarm muscle circumference (mm)	Protein mass	See Table 5-17	As for triceps skinfold
Serum albumin (g/dL)	Protein mass	3.5–4.5	Mild = 2.8–3.5 Moderate = 2.1–2.8 Severe = <2.1
Serum transferrin (mg/dL)	Protein mass	220–350	Mild = 150–200 Moderate = 100–150 Severe = <100
Total lymphocyte count per cubic millimeter	Nonspecific	>2,000	Mild = 1,200–2,000 Moderate = 800–1,200 Severe = <800
Delayed cutaneous hypersensitivity to skin test antigens	Nonspecific	Reactive to >1/5 antigens	Anergy

C. **Specific indications for nutritional support.** A consensus conference involving the National Institutes of Health, American Society of Parenteral and Enteral Nutrition, and American Society of Clinical Nutrition reviewed the data on nutritional support in gastrointestinal diseases, wasting diseases (especially cancer and AIDS), critical illnesses, and in the perioperative period. The conclusions are summarized in Tables 5-22 and 5-23. It is important to note that these conclusions identify issues for further study but are not recommendations or practice guidelines. In the use of nutritional support therapy, the integration of data from clinical trials, clinical experience in the illnesses being treated, and clinical expertise in nutrition and nutritional therapy will continue to be essential.

D. **Overfeeding and refeeding syndromes.** Although nutritional support is valuable in selected critically ill patients, it is not without risks. Metabolic complications resulting from overfeeding such patients can be serious (41). The clinical characteristics of the syndromes associated with overfeeding are listed in Table 5-24. Most of these are commonly recognized and are detected during the routine follow-up of patients on enteral or parenteral therapy (see Chapters 9 and 10). However, the refeeding syndrome is potentially very serious, can develop rapidly, and, because of its relative rarity, may not be rec-

Table 5-22. Use of nutrition support in gastrointestinal diseases

Condition	Assumptions driving studies	Either (EN or TPN)	TPN alone
IBD	Bowel rest/EN helpful	Steroids > EN[b] EN possibly helpful[b] Mono/oligo/polymeric same outcome[a] Compliance limits use of EN formulations[a] EN/TPN promotes growth in children[b]	Not as primary therapy[a]
Pancreatitis	Support helpful if oral intake limited Jejunal feeding >gastric/duodenal	No effect in mild moderate disease[a] When course is prolonged, timing, route, and formulation unknown[c] EN can be safely given in mild/moderate disease[a]	IV lipid safe if TG <400 mg/dL[a]
Liver disease	Malnutrition can be identified in these patients	EN/TPN improves some parameters in ESLD[a] EN/TPN effect inconclusive in alcoholic ESLD[a]	
	BCAAs improve outcome	BCAA-enriched formulas improve protein intake in intolerant patients[a]	BCAA-rich aid recovery in hepatic encephalitis vs. glutamic acid,[a] untested vs. other amino acids

EN, enteral nutrition; TPN, total parenteral nutrition; IBD, inflammatory bowel disease; BCAA, branched-chain amino acid; ESLD, end-stage liver disease; TG, triglycerides.
[a] Supported by prospective randomized controlled trials of metaanalyses of prospective randomized controlled trial.
[b] Supported by well-designed nonrandomized prospective controlled trials, or by well-designed retrospective or case cohort studies.
[c] Supported by published experience, case reports, or expert opinion.
From Klein S, Kinney J, Jeejeebhoy K, et al. Nutrition support in clinical practice. *JPEN J Parenter Enteral Nutr* 1997;21:133.

ognized early (42). The clinical characteristics of this syndrome are listed in Table 5-25. Cardiovascular and electrolyte abnormalities need to be carefully documented before critically ill patients are refed. Feeding should be restarted slowly, and it should be ascertained that all nutrients, especially nitrogen, phosphorus, potassium, magnesium, and sodium, are adequately provided. The daily intake should be about 20 kcal/kg and should contain about 150 g of carbohydrate and 1.2 to 1.5 g of protein per kilogram. Sodium should be restricted to about 1.5 g/d, but phosphorus, potassium, and magnesium should be liberally provided while weight, electrolytes, and cardiac function are monitored carefully.

Table 5-23. Use of nutrition support in catabolic conditions

Condition	Assumptions driving studies	Either (EN or TPN)	TPN alone
Cancer/AIDS	Reversing weight loss improves	Routine use doesn't ↓ morbidity/morality w/chemo-rad Rx[a] May maintain hydration/ nutrition, ↑ survival in pts who can't eat/drink[b] Restoring body composition/tissue mass probably good[c] Restores cell mass in AIDS pts w/↓d food, no infection[b]	Infections ↑ w/chemo Rx[a] No ↓ morbidity mortality in pts w/BMT[a] Routine use doesn't ↓ mortality or QOL[b]
Critical illness	Hypermetabolic patients should improve w/ support	No good studies to support assumption[c] EN ↓s complications in trauma pts (or ↑d with TPN?)[b]	
	Critical depletion of lean tissue occurs after 14 days	Support should be started in 7–10 days in pts without oral feeding[c] No data available on special additives (e.g., Gln, Arg)	
Perioperative	"Malnourished" pts (weight loss, ↓ plasma protein, SGA) need nutrients for good outcome	EN after hip fracture ↓s morbidity[a] Postop patients who can't eat need calories within 5–10 days[c]	7–10 days of preop Rx↓s complications by 10%[a] Routine postop TPN with no preop Rx ↑s complications 10%[a]

EN, enteral nutrition; TPN, total parenteral nutrition; QOL, quality of life; BMT, bone marrow transplantation; SGA, subjective global assessment.
[a] Supported by prospective randomized controlled trials or metaanalyses of prospective randomized controlled trials.
[b] Supported by well-designed nonrandomized prospective controlled trials, or by well-designed retrospective or case cohort studies.
[c] Supported by published experience, case reports, or expert opinion.
From Klein S, Kinney J, Jeejeebhoy K, et al. Nutrition support in clinical practice. *JPEN J Parenter Enteral Nutr* 1997;21:133.

Table 5-24. Clinical characteristics of overfeeding syndromes

Syndrome	Patients at risk	Management
Azotemia	Age >65, protein intake >2 g/kg, BUN/Cr >15	Provide adequate energy, hydration, protein intake
Fat overload (respiratory distress, bleeding, jaundice)	Lipid intake >3 g/d, onset days to months	Hold lipids for TG >300 mg/dL, monitor PT, PTT, bilirubin
Hepatic steatosis	High CHO, very low fat during parenteral nutrition	Adjust energy and CHO intake, include fat daily
Hypercapnia	Poor ventilatory status	Decrease energy intake, esp. dextrose, add lipid, monitor pCO_2, pH
Hyperglycemia	On steroids, dextrose provision >4 mg/kg/min	Monitor hydration, blood glucose, replace dextrose with lipid
Hyperglycemic, hyperosmolar, nonketotic	High CHO load + diuresis	Monitor CVP, restore intravascular volume, add insulin and K
Hypertonic dehydration	High protein tube feed + fluid loss + old age	↓ Na and protein intake, use isotonic feeding and rehydration
Hypertriglyceridemia	Lipid intake >2g/d, infection	Maintain TG <300 mg/dL, avoid overfeeding
Metabolic acidosis	Formulas with low kcal/g N ratio (<90:1), elderly	Monitor hydration, renal function, pH, ↓ protein intake
Refeeding	Weight <70% of ideal, rapid replacement	Monitor cardiac status, P, Mg, K, ↓ energy load, hydrate

BUN, blood urea nitrogen; Cr, creatinine; TG, triglyceride; PT, prothrombin time; PTT, partial thromboplastin time; CHO, carbohydrate; CVP, central venous pressure.
Modified from Klein CJ, Stanek GS, Wiles CE. Overfeeding macronutrients to critically ill adults: metabolic complications. *J Am Diet Assoc* 1998;98:795.

Table 5-25. Clinical characteristics of the refeeding syndrome

Nutrient/organ system	Clinical findings
Energy balance	Weight <70% of ideal weight
Cardiovascular system	↓ Cardiac mass, stroke volume, end-diastolic volume, heart rate, blood pressure
	↑ Congestive failure, arrhythmias, QT interval
Kidney	↑ Sodium and water retention
Phosphorus	↓ Plasma P, leading to muscle weakness, seizures, acute respiratory failure, tachycardia, death
Potassium/magnesium	↓ Plasma K, Mg because each *g* of N used to form protein leads to retention of 3 mEq of K and 0.5 mEq of Mg
Gastrointestinal tract	Diarrhea with oral feeding secondary to reduced epithelial mass

References

1. Pellett PL. Protein requirements in humans. *Am J Clin Nutr* 1990;51:723.
2. National Research Council. *Recommended daily allowances,* 10th ed. Washington, DC: National Academy Press, 1989.
3. Foster GD, Knox LS, Dempsey DT, et al. Caloric requirements in total parenteral nutrition. *J Am Coll Nutr* 1987;6:231.
4. Harris JA, Benedict FG. *A biometric study of basal metabolism.* Publication No. 279. Washington, DC: Carnegie Institution, 1919.
5. Roza AM, Shizgal HM. The Harris–Benedict equation reevaluated: resting energy requirements and the body cell mass. *Am J Clin Nutr* 1984;40:168.
6. Van Way C. Variability of the Harris–Benedict equation in recently published textbooks. *JPEN J Parenter Enteral Nutr* 1992;16:566.
7. Owen OE, Kayle E, Owen RS, et al. A reappraisal of caloric requirements in healthy women. *Am J Clin Nutr* 1986;44:1.
8. Keys A, Taylor HL, Grande F. Basal metabolism and age of adult men. *Metabolism* 1973;22:579.
9. Wilmore DW. *The metabolic management of the critically ill.* New York: Plenum Press, 1977.
10. Baker JP, Detsky AS, Stewart S, et al. Randomized trial of total parenteral nutrition in critically ill patients: metabolic effects of varying glucose–lipid ratios as the energy source. *Gastroenterology* 1984;87:53.
11. Ireton-Jones CS, Turner WW Jr, Liepa BU, et al. Equations for the estimation of energy expenditures in patients with burns with special reference to ventilatory status. *J Burn Care Rehabil* 1992;13:330.
12. Mann S, Westenskow DR, Houtchens BA. Measured and predicted caloric expenditure in the acutely ill. *Crit Care Med* 1985;13:173.
13. Makk LJ, McClave SA, Creech PW, et al. Clinical application of the metabolic cart to the delivery of total parenteral nutrition. *Crit Care Med* 1990;18:1320.
14. Liggett SB, St John RE, Lefrak SS. Determination of resting energy expenditure utilizing the thermodilution pulmonary artery catheter. *Chest* 1987;91:562.
15. Liggett SB, Renfro AD. Energy expenditures of mechanically ventilated nonsurgical patients. *Chest* 1990;98:682.
16. Toth MJ, Poehlman ET. Energetic adaptation to chronic disease in the elderly. *Nutr Rev* 2000;58:61.
17. National Research Council. *Assessing changing food consumption patterns.* Washington, DC: National Academy Press, 1981.
18. Garrow JS. Energy balance in man—a review. *Am J Clin Nutr* 1987;45[Suppl 5]:1114.
19. WHO/FAO Committee on Nutrition. *WHO energy and protein requirements.* Technical report series 724. Geneva: World Health Organization, 1985.
20. Scrimshaw NS. Shattuck Lecture—strengths and weaknesses of the committee approach. An analysis of past and present recommended dietary allowances for protein in health and disease. *N Engl J Med* 1976;294:198.
21. Waterlow JC, Payne PR. The protein gap. *Nature* 1975;258:113.
22. Willett WC, Dietz WH, Colditz GA. Guidelines for healthy weight. *N Engl J Med* 1999;341:427.
23. Schwartz LM, Woloshin S. Changing disease definitions: implications for disease prevalence. Analysis of the Third National Health and Nutrition Examination Survey, 1988–1994. *Eff Clin Pract* 1999;2:76.
24. NIH Technology Assessment Conference Panel. Methods for voluntary weight loss and control. *Ann Intern Med* 1992;116:942.
25. Frankel HM. Determination of body mass index. *JAMA* 1986;255:1292.
26. Matz R. Calculating body mass index. *Ann Intern Med* 1993;118:232.
27. Jensen TG, Dudrick SJ, Johnston DA. A comparison of triceps skinfold and upper arm circumference measurements taken in standard and supine positions. *JPEN J Parenter Enteral Nutr* 1981;5:519.
28. Windsor JA, Hill GL. Grip strength: a measure of the proportion of protein loss in surgical patients. *Br J Surg* 1988;75:880.
29. Klein S. The myth of serum albumin as a measure of nutritional status. *Gastroenterology* 1990;99:1845.

30. Gray GE, Megried MM. Can total parenteral nutrition reverse hypoalbuminemia in oncology patients? *Nutrition* 1990;6:225.
31. Windsor JA, Hill GL. Weight loss with physiologic impairment: a basic indicator of surgical risk. *Ann Surg* 1988;207:290.
32. Detsky AS, McLaughlin JR, Baker JP. What is subjective global assessment of nutritional status? *JPEN J Parenter Enteral Nutr* 1987;11:8.
33. Windsor JA, Hill GL. Nutritional assessment: a pending renaissance. *Nutrition* 1991;7:377.
34. Baker JP, Detsky AS, Wesson DE, et al. Nutritional assessment: a comparison of clinical judgment and objective measurements. *N Engl J Med* 1982;306:969.
35. Detsky AS. Predicting nutrition-associated complications for patients undergoing gastrointestinal surgery. *JPEN J Parenter Enteral Nutr* 1987;11:440.
36. Klein S, Kinney J, Jeejeebhoy K, et al. Nutrition support in clinical practice: review of published data and recommendations for future research directions. *JPEN J Parenter Enteral Nutr* 1997;21:133.
37. Naber TH, Schermer T, de Bree A, et al. Prevalence of malnutrition in nonsurgical patients and its association with disease complications. *Am J Clin Nutr* 1997;66:1232.
38. Buzby GP, Mullen JP, Matthews DC. Prognostic nutritional index in gastrointestinal surgery. *Am J Surg* 1980;139:160.
39. Harvey KB, Moldawer LL, Bistrian BR. Biological measures for the formulation of a hospital prognostic index. *Am J Clin Nutr* 1981;34:2013.
40. The Veterans Affairs Total Parenteral Nutrition Cooperative Study Group: perioperative total parenteral nutrition in surgical patients. *N Engl J Med* 1991; 325:525.
41. Klein CJ, Stanek GS, Wiles CE. Overfeeding macronutrients to critically ill adults: metabolic complications. *J Am Diet Assoc* 1998;98:795.
42. Alpers DH, Klein S. Refeeding the malnourished patient. *Curr Opin Gastroenterol* 1999;15:151.

6. VITAMINS

I. **Evaluation of vitamin intake and deficiency.** The intake of vitamins (and other nutrients) is calculated in three ways: (a) the amount an individual needs to avoid deficiency (daily requirement), (b) the average daily amount entire population groups should consume in a period of time to prevent deficiency [recommended dietary allowance (RDA) or adequate intake (AI)], and (c) the amount that can be safely ingested when the vitamin is taken to prevent chronic disease [tolerable upper intake level (UL)]. Statistically, the RDA is set 2 standard deviations above the mean requirement, so that it is sufficient for 97% of normal persons. RDAs therefore exceed the needs of many persons and furthermore are established only for healthy persons (1). The RDA takes into account the dietary form of the nutrient, the efficiency of absorption, and other factors, in addition to the estimated daily requirement for the assimilated nutrient. Daily allowances thus may vary depending on whether the vitamin is to be administered parenterally (see Chapter 10) or by mouth. Discussions of controversial recommended dietary intakes of many vitamins and minerals are included in the publications of the Standing Committee on the Scientific Evaluation of Dietary Reference Intakes, Food and Nutrition Board, Institute of Medicine (2–4). RDAs and dietary reference intakes (DRIs) are not designed to provide guidelines for therapy. They should be used only as estimates for normal intake and perhaps as a starting point for therapy in cases of deficiency.

A. **Requirements for vitamin nutrition in selected groups.** These groups include physically active people, the elderly, and persons at increased risk for chronic diseases.

1. **Physically active people.** Only about one-third of people in the United States engage in regular physical exercise—mostly walking, swimming, bicycling, running, and step aerobics. A deficiency of certain vitamins adversely affects physical performance (e.g., by causing anemia, muscle weakness, fatigue, or peripheral neuropathy). These include all the B vitamins. Exercise can increase the need for some nutrients, as in the gastrointestinal blood loss seen during prolonged exercise (5). In addition, some vitamins are considered to be important in reducing the risk for cardiovascular disease. These include vitamin E and the vitamins that lower serum homocysteine levels (vitamin B_6, folate, and vitamin B_{12}). The role of each of these vitamins is discussed later in the chapter.

2. **Elderly people.** The new DRIs include separate recommendations for persons over the age of 70 (6) (see Chapter 3). In the Survey in Europe on Nutrition and the Elderly: a Concerned Action (SENECA) Study, evidence of low vitamin intake/deficiency based on serum levels was found in 47% of European elderly persons for vitamin D, 23% for vitamin B_6, 2.7% for vitamin B_{12}, and 1% for vitamin E (7). Neurocognitive function can be decreased in deficiency states of vitamins B_6 and B_{12} and folate (8), the same vitamins that help to regulate homocysteine levels. The intake of these vitamins is often inadequate in the elderly. Because on average the elderly ingest only about 50% of the RDA for any vitamin, special care must be taken to ensure that the full RDA (or DRI) is taken.

3. **Persons at risk for chronic diseases.** In addition to their potential role in preventing cardiovascular disease, vitamins may play a role in cancer chemoprevention (see Chapter 14) and in preventing cataracts, particularly the vitamins with antioxidant properties (vitamin A, β-carotene, and vitamin E) (4). The data are not yet sufficient to suggest that regular use of these vitamins prevents cancer or nuclear cataracts (9).

B. **Bioavailability of vitamins** differs in various foods. *Bioavailability* refers to the fraction of total dietary vitamin that is absorbed and functions in an organism. The assessment of bioavailability involves assays of tissue content and biologic activity. The accuracy of dietary requirements depends on information about food content and its bioavailability. Nutrient content listed under each vitamin is usually well established. Where data exist concerning bioavailability, they are given.

C. **Vitamin deficiency.** A variety of factors other than dietary intake are related to vitamin deficiency. These are listed in Table 6-1. Dietary deficiency is uncommon in the case of the vitamins that are produced endogenously. Enterohepatic circulation of a vitamin is associated with an increased rate of loss during malabsorption because some portion of the body stores must be reabsorbed each day, along with what is derived from the diet. An enterohepatic circulation of vitamins other than those listed in Table 6-1 is possible, but such data are not available at this time. Hepatic stores of vitamin A and cobalamin are decreased most frequently in cirrhosis. All vitamins may be needed in larger amounts during pregnancy and growth, but folic acid is especially important because body stores are small.

1. **The onset of clinical vitamin deficiency** varies depending on the rate of loss and the size of available body stores. In general, the body stores of water-soluble vitamins are smaller, whereas fat-soluble vitamins are stored in adipose tissue or liver, so that the body stores are larger. Thus, clinical deficiency of fat-soluble vitamins is usually delayed and may take 2 years or more to develop.

2. **Clinical manifestations of deficiency of a given water-soluble vitamin** are relatively late consequences (Table 6-2). Blood levels fall early in the course of deficiency and are thus useful in detecting changes in body stores of the vitamin. This event is followed by altered cell function and finally clinical symptoms. This sequence is not often seen in deficiencies of the fat-soluble vitamins. Vitamin D must be converted to active forms. Thus, even though body stores of the parent vitamin may be normal, activation to the hydroxylated forms may be inadequate. Vitamins A and D are carried in plasma by specific binding proteins. Alterations in the levels of these binding proteins can lead to an erroneous estimate of body stores. The intracellular content of a vitamin sometimes correlates better with body stores than do plasma levels. Thus, the vitamin content of white or red cells is sometimes used to assess body stores.

3. **Therapeutic supplementation.** In many instances, only one or two vitamin deficiencies exist at one time in a patient. However, when generalized malabsorption occurs, extra vitamins are needed each day to prevent deficiencies. This is often best accomplished with one of the mul-

Table 6-1. Pathophysiology of vitamin deficiency

Physiologic factor	Vitamins affected	Comments
Dietary intake	All except K, B_6, biotin	K, B_6, and biotin probably produced by enteric bacteria
Endogenous synthesis	D (skin), K, B_6, biotin	
Enterohepatic circulation	A, polar metabolites of vitamin D, folic acid, cobalamin	
Decreased storage capacity	Cobalamin, A	Stored in liver
Increased utilization	Folic acid	Used in increased amounts during pregnancy, hemolysis
Increased loss from body	All	During malabsorption

tivitamin and mineral preparations. When feeding is only or largely parenteral, multivitamin supplements must be given. (Doses and administration of parenteral therapy are discussed in Chapter 10.) Most of this chapter is devoted to a separate discussion of each vitamin.

    a. Treatment of vitamin deficiency. Most healthy people in the United States do not need vitamin supplements. However, supplements should be given to certain groups of patients at high risk for vitamin deficiency. Details are provided in the sections on the individual vitamins.

        (1) Infancy

            (a) Vitamin K once (0. 5 to 1.0 mg IM or 1 to 2 mg orally) to prevent hemorrhagic disease of the newborn.

            (b) Vitamin E (500 mg/kg daily) to premature infants weighing less than 1.5 kg to prevent hemolytic anemia.

            (c) Vitamin D (400 IU/d) to breast-fed infants if not exposed to sunlight.

            (d) Cobalamin (vitamin B_{12}) to breast-fed infants of strict vegetarian mothers.

        (2) Pregnancy. Folic acid requirements are increased. A dosage of 400 µg/d is recommended for all pregnant women to decrease the incidence of neural tube defects.

        (3) Low-calorie intake/diets. If less than 1,200 kcal is ingested per day, a multivitamin preparation may be used. This is especially true for alcoholics, elderly persons who are poor or homebound, and patients with anorexia nervosa or severe depression.

        (4) Gastrointestinal disorders. Patients with fat malabsorption may require vitamins A and D or, rarely, E. Following ileal resection, vitamin B_{12} is needed (100 µg/mo). Folic acid (1 mg/d) is often required, and all water-soluble vitamins must be administered to patients with short-bowel syndrome.

        (5) Osteodystrophies. Patients in whom activation of vitamin D is defective may require vitamin D, calcifediol (hepatic disease), or calcitriol (renal disease).

    b. Vitamin therapy in conditions other than deficiency. Vitamins are administered in many conditions in which deficiencies are not demonstrated. In most instances, either no effect of the vitamin has been documented, or the data are insufficient to warrant a strong recommendation for their use. Table 6-3 lists some of the clinical areas in which vitamin supplementation has been suggested. Discussions of some of these uses not related to deficiency are included in the sections on the individual vitamins, especially vitamins A and E. Accepted uses of vitamins in states other than deficiency are the administration of pyridoxine to treat pyridoxine-dependent inborn errors of metabolism, and the administration of vitamin A derivatives to treat skin diseases and acute promyelocytic anemia.

  4. Assessment of vitamin status. Guidelines are given for the interpretation of test results (Table 1-19). However, the precise values vary among laboratories. The reader should ascertain the exact normal values of the laboratory providing the information.

II. Water-soluble vitamins. The B-complex vitamins are often considered together because deficiency frequently produces overlapping symptoms. All these vitamins form coenzymes in metabolic processes. Some characteristics of the vitamins are listed in Table 6-2.

  A. Thiamine (vitamin B_1)

    1. Requirements

      a. Relation to energy intake. Thiamine pyrophosphate is important in key reactions in energy metabolism (e.g., the decarboxylation of pyruvic acid). Therefore, the requirement for thiamine is usually

Table 6-2. Summary of vitamin functions and deficiency states

Vitamin	Functions	Results of deficiency	Major food sources
Thiamine B$_1$	Transketolase coenzyme, muscle tone, appetite	Moderate: fatigue, apathy, nausea, irritability, numbness Severe: beriberi with CHF, polyneuritis, edema	Enriched grains, most animal and vegetable products
Riboflavin/B$_2$	Part of FAD, FMN that accept/donate [H$^+$] equivalents	Angular stomatitis, cheilosis, glossitis, seborrheic dermatitis	Organ meats, enriched cereals/flours, cheese, eggs, lean meat
Niacin	Part of NAD, NADP that accept/donate [H$^+$] equivalents	Dermatitis (light-exposed), diarrhea, swollen tongue, delirium, depression	Meat, nuts, dairy products, eggs
Vitamin B$_6$	Coenzyme in transamination, decarboxylation, transsulfuration	Seborrheic dermatitis, red tongue, irritability, weakness, convulsions, neuritis	Grains, seeds, organ meats, lean meats
Pantothenic acid	Part of coenzyme A/acyl carrier protein	Anorexia, nausea, fatigue, numbness, insomnia	Organ meats, cereals/flours, nuts, eggs
Biotin	Coenzyme in decarboxylation, deamination	Scaly dermatitis, anorexia, glossitis, muscle pains	Organ meats, eggs, soy flour
Folate	Formation of purines, pyrimidines, heme, tyrosine, glutamate	Megaloblastic anemia, glossitis, diarrhea	Organ meats, green vegetables, legumes, eggs, fish, nuts, whole wheat products, enriched flour/cereals

Vitamin	Function	Deficiency	Sources
Vitamin B$_{12}$	Transfer of single carbon units, synthesis of CH$_3$–	Sore tongue, weakness, neuropathy, mental changes, pernicious anemia	Organ meats, muscle meats, eggs, dairy products, fish
Vitamin C	Collagen formation, iron absorption, metabolism of folate	Weight loss, fatigue, sore gums/joints, petechiae, bone fractures	Citrus fruits, other fruits, green peppers, leafy vegetables
Vitamin A	Visual adaptation, body/bone growth, gene expression	Night blindness, xerosis, xerophthalmia, follicular dermatitis, abnormal teeth	Organ meats, eggs, dairy (fortified) Carotene: yellow vegetables, fruits
Vitamin D	Calcium/phosphorus absorption, bone mineralization	Rickets, osteomalacia, tetany	Vitamin D-fortified foods (cereals, dairy), fish oils
Vitamin E	Antioxidant against free radicals	Hemolysis, ophthalmoplegia, peripheral neuropathy	Vegetable oils, nuts, seeds, eggs, meats
Vitamin K	Synthesis of clotting factors, glutamate	Delayed blood clotting, hemorrhagic disease of the newborn	Widely distributed (dairy, meat, eggs, fruit, vegetables)

CH$_3$–, methyl groups; CHF, congestive heart failure; FAD, flavin adenine dinucleotide; FMN, flavin mononucleotide; NAD, nicotinamide adenine dinucleotide; NADP, nicotinamide adenine dinucleotide phosphate.

Table 6-3. Proposed uses of vitamins in nondeficiency states

Vitamin	Condition	Dose range per day	Effect	Toxic risk
Riboflavin	Migraine	400 mg	↓ Frequency	None
Nicotinic acid	Hyperlipidemia	3–6 g[a]	↓ TG, cholesterol	Yes
Vitamin B$_6$	Carpal tunnel syndrome	50 mg	Uncertain	None
	Premenstrual syndrome	>500 mg	Uncertain	Yes
	↑ Immune function	50 mg	Uncertain	None
Folate	Depression	15 mg	Uncertain	None
	Prevent dysplasia/cancer	1–10 mg	Uncertain	None
Vitamin A	Acute promyelocytic leukemia	45 mg/d (all-*trans*-retinal) [a]	↑ Survival	Yes
	Pityriasis rubra pilaris	1×10^6 IU (330 mg)	Improvement	Yes
	↓ Measles mortality	0.4×10^6 IU	Uncertain	Yes
	Cancer prevention	unknown	Uncertain	None
Antioxidants (β-carotene, vitamins C, E)	Atherosclerosis and cancer prevention	30–50 mg (β-carotene) 600 IU (vitamin E) 1 g (vitamin C)	Uncertain	None
Vitamin E	Reduce risk for cardiovascular disease	400–1600 mg	Uncertain	None
	Premenstrual syndrome	300 IU	Uncertain	None
	Prevent cataracts	100–300 mg	Uncertain	None
Vitamin C	Common cold	1–2 g	Uncertain	None

TG, triglyceride.
[a] Only these uses have FDA approval.

related to energy intake and more specifically to carbohydrate ingestion. The Food and Nutrition Board recommends 0.5 mg/1,000 kcal
for adults, and the same ratio for infants and children, although fewer
data are available for them. Allowances are based on the effects of
varying dietary thiamine and the relationship of thiamine intake to
signs of clinical deficiency and to urinary excretion of thiamine and
serum erythrocyte transketolase activity. The requirements are listed
in Table 6-4. A minimum of 1.0 mg/d is recommended for all adults,
even those consuming less than 2,000 kcal daily.

   b. Higher requirement in pregnant and lactating women. This
pattern is repeated for all the vitamins for which data are available.
The lactating mother secretes about 0.1 to 0.2 mg/d in milk. This is
available for the suckling child.

2. Food sources. Thiamine is abundant in all foods and is added to many
commercial breads and cereals. Rather small quantities of food provide
the needed daily requirement. Thiamine is easily removed during the
processing of grains or destroyed (10% to 30%) during heating. Because
thiamine is water-soluble, much of the content of the vitamin is extracted in cooking liquid. As much as 80% of the dry food content can be
lost in this way. The method of food preparation must be considered
when lists of food content are consulted. Table 6-5 lists the thiamine content of various foods.

3. Assessment

   a. Intake or absorption. Thiamine in the urine is assayed either
chemically by the thiochrome method or microbiologically with *Lactobacillus viridescens* (10). When thiamine intake equals the requirement of 0.3 to 0.35 mg/1,000 kcal, the urinary excretion is 40 to
290 mg/d. When intake is less than 0.2 mg/1,000 kcal, the urinary
excretion falls below 25 mg/d. To correct for variations in the collection of urine and allow random samples to be utilized, excretion is
usually reported as micrograms of thiamine per gram of creatinine.
When expressed in this way, urinary thiamine is quite sensitive in

Table 6-4. Thiamine dietary reference intakes[a]

Life stage group	Thiamine (mg/d)	Life stage group	Thiamine (mg/d)
Infants		Females	
0–6 mo	0.2[b]	9–13 y	0.9
7–12 mo	0.3[b]	14–18 y	1.0
Children		19–30 y	1.1
1–3 y	0.5	31–50 y	1.1
4–8 y	0.6	51–70 y	1.1
Males		>70 y	1.1
9–13 y	0.9	Pregnancy	
14–18 y	1.2	≤18 y	1.4
19–30 y	1.2	19–30 y	1.4
31–50 y	1.2	31–50 y	1.4
51–70 y	1.2	Lactation	
>70 y	1.2	≤18–50 y	1.4

[a] Estimate based on recommended dietary allowances (RDA).
[b] Recommendation given as adequate intake (AI).
From Standing Committee on the Scientific Evaluation of Dietary Reference Intakes, Food and
Nutrition Board, Institute of Medicine, *Dietary reference intakes for thiamine, riboflavin, niacin,
vitamin B₆, folate, vitamin B₁₂, pantothenic acid, biotin, and choline.* Washington, DC: National
Academy Press, 1998.

Table 6-5. Approximate thiamine content of selected foods

Food	Portion	Thiamine (mg)	Percentage of RDI (1.5 mg)
Grain products			
White bread[a]	Slice	0.131	5–12
Whole wheat bread	Slice	0.1	5–12
Shredded wheat[b]	Biscuit	0.06	
Spaghetti, enriched, cooked	1 cup	0.286	10–24
Rice, white, enriched, cooked	1 cup	0.334	15–30
Meats			
Beef, rib roast, cooked	3 oz	0.056	1–5
Pork center loin chops, cooked	4 oz	0.52	>40
Chicken, roasted			
Breast	4 oz	0.065	1–5
Dark meat, thigh	4 oz	0.042	1–5
Sausage, pork, cooked	2-oz patty	0.2	10–24
Ham, roasted	3 oz	0.551	>40
Vegetables			
Peas, cooked from fresh	½ cup	0.207	10–24
Peanuts or almonds			
Roasted	1 cup	0.364	10–24
Dried	1 cup	0.969	>40
Potato, baked	2 ⅓ in	0.164	10–24
Tomato, raw	2 ⅔ in	0.073	5–12
Milk and eggs			
Whole milk	1 cup	0.093	5–12
Eggs, large	One	0.05	1–5
Beverages			
Beer	12 oz	0.021	1–5

RDI, recommended dietary intake.
[a] Thiamine is added to all-purpose flour.
[b] Ready-to-eat cereals may be fortified with thiamine; check the label.
Derived in part from Hands ES. *Food finder,* 2nd ed. Salem, OR: ESHA Research, 1990.

the detection of low intake. However, this measurement does not assess body stores of the vitamin. Table 6-6 provides some guidelines for interpreting the results of this test.

    b. Body stores. Assessment is either by the direct measurement of thiamine in blood or serum or more commonly by determining the activity ratio of transketolase with and without added thiamine.

        (1) High-pressure liquid chromatography (HPLC) with fluorescent detection is most often used (10). Enzymatic degradation of derivatives produces free B_1, which is converted to a fluorescent form and separated by HPLC. Mean values in normal adults are 11 to 19 nmol/L in serum, 101 to 191 nmol/L in whole blood, and 132 to 284 nmol/L in erythrocytes. Levels of phosphorylated thiamine in whole blood of infants and adults range from a mean of 120 to 177 nmol/L. Erythrocyte thiamine diphosphate levels correlate well with erythrocyte transketolase measurements (Table 6-6).

        (2) Erythrocyte transketolase is a thiamine-requiring enzyme that catalyzes the following reactions in the pentose phosphate pathway:

Table 6-6. Guidelines for the interpretation of thiamine status

| Age of subjects (y) | [RBC thiamine pyrophosphate] (nmol/L) | Thiamine urinary excretion (µg/g creatinine) | |
		Deficient intake (<0.3 mg/1,000 kcal)	Very low intake
1–3	—	<175	<120
4–6	—	<120	<85
7–9	—	<180	<70
10–12	—	<180	<60
13–15	—	<150	<50
15+	>150 (normal) 120–150 (marginal) <120 (deficient)	<65	<27

RBC, red blood cell.
From Sauberlich HE. *Laboratory tests for the assessment of nutritional status,* 2nd ed. Boca Raton, FL: CRC Press, 1999.

$$Xylulose - 5 - PO_4 + Ribose - 5 - PO_4 \rightarrow Sedoheptulose - 7 - PO_4 + Glyceraldehyde - 3 - PO_4$$

$$Xylulose - 5 - PO_4 + Erythrose - 4 - PO_4 \rightarrow Fructose - 6 - PO_4 + Glyceraldehyde - 3 - PO_4$$

When thiamine intake is stable for a period of time, the activity of this enzyme correlates with urinary excretion of thiamine. However, a single determination of urinary excretion detects intake only at one time, whereas transketolase activity (and erythrocyte thiamine diphosphate concentration) assesses cumulative intake and therefore body stores.

The assay is performed on hemolyzed whole blood with ribose-5-phosphate as substrate in the absence and presence of added thiamine. Values obtained without added thiamine reflect the amount of coenzyme present in tissues. The stimulated value gives a measure of the apoenzyme present that lacks coenzyme. Guidelines for interpretation of the test results are as follows (10):

Body stores of thiamine	Thiamine stimulation	Activity coefficient
Normal	0–15%	1.0–1.2
Marginal	16–24%	1.2–1.25
Low	>25%	>1.25

4. Physiology

a. Function. Thiamine pyrophosphate is a coenzyme in the oxidative decarboxylation of α-ketoacids to aldehydes. Lipoic acid, nicotinamide adenine dinucleotide (NAD), and coenzyme A (CoA) are also requirements for the reaction in animals. The reaction yields acetyl CoA and succinyl CoA. Thiamine also catalyzes transketolase activity in the pentose phosphate cycle. This function results in the production of pentose phosphates used for nucleotide synthesis and supplies NAD phosphate (NADP) for synthetic pathways (i.e., fatty acid synthesis). In thiamine deficiency, blood pyruvate levels rise. Because the vitamin plays such an important role in carbohydrate metabolism, the requirement is increased when carbohydrate intake is increased.

   b. **Metabolism.** Thiamine is synthesized by plants. Although intestinal bacteria may make some thiamine, mammals are dependent on dietary intake. The vitamin is rapidly absorbed from the upper small intestine by a specific active transport mechanism (11). Absorption efficiency is greater than 80%, although efficiency decreases at higher doses. Thiamine phosphorylation probably occurs in the intestinal mucosa. Thiamine accumulates in all body tissues, and no storage site is preferred. About 1 mg is degraded in the tissues daily. At low intake (≤1 mg), much of the vitamin is excreted in the urine as pyrimidine metabolites. At high intake, unmetabolized thiamine is excreted.

5. Deficiency
   a. **Mechanisms.** Deficiency may develop from a decrease in intake, an increase in tissue utilization (e.g., pregnancy), or a combination of the two factors. The clinical settings most commonly associated with thiamine deficiency include chronic alcoholism, malabsorption syndromes, and nausea and vomiting of pregnancy. The total amount of thiamine in the human body is about 30 mg, with half this in muscle, largely as thiamine pyrophosphate. With requirements in excess of 1 mg/d, deficiency can develop rapidly within a period of weeks or a few months.

   b. **Anti-thiamine factors** in foods can alter thiamine activity and be a cause of vitamin deficiency. The thermolabile factor found in the viscera of freshwater fish and shellfish and the thermostable factor in tea leaves have both been reported to cause deficiency when coupled with low thiamine intake.

   c. **Signs of deficiency** depend on the duration and severity of the defect, but all degrees of deficiency affect muscle and nerve function. Mild deficiency may result in anorexia, weakness, paresthesias, edema, and lowered blood pressure and body temperature. The infant with acute onset of thiamine deficiency presents with abdominal distension and tenderness, colicky pain and vomiting, and a decreased appetite.

   d. **The usual presentation** of chronic deficiency in the Western world is associated with alcoholism or malabsorption. In these cases, multiple deficiencies may be present that can alter the signs and symptoms of pure thiamine deficiency. The features of thiamine deficiency are cardiac failure, peripheral neuropathy, subacute necrotizing encephalomyelopathy, cerebellar signs, and Wernicke's encephalopathy. Severe deficiency (beriberi) is characterized by neuritis and heart failure (acute mixed type), congestive failure and emaciation (wet type), or polyneuritis and paralysis (dry type). Signs of deficiency may worsen if glucose is administered without thiamine. If lactic acidosis accompanies thiamine deficiency, acute and severe cardiac failure can occur (12). Thiamine deficiency often is neglected as a cause of lactic acidosis. Cardiac failure is suggested by dyspnea, palpitations, cardiomegaly, gallop, increased venous pressure, and a prolonged QT interval. Neuropathy and myelopathy are accompanied by aching and burning and decreased muscle strength, more so in the legs than in the arms. Alcoholic myopathy may complicate the effects of thiamine deficiency.

6. Treatment
   a. **Deficiency.** Thiamine hydrochloride is available in tablets (5 to 1,000 mg), in injectable form (100 or 200 mg/mL), and as an elixir (2.25 mg/5 mL). Mild deficiency may be treated with 15 mg/d parenterally for 1 week, followed by a maintenance oral dose. Severe deficiency may require somewhat larger doses up to 100 mg twice

daily. The amount of thiamine that enters the cerebrospinal fluid is limited; thus, larger doses must be given when the central nervous system is involved.

  b. **Inborn errors.** A few rare and poorly described thiamine-responsive inborn errors of metabolism have been described. These disorders, which require pharmacologic doses for therapy (50 mg/d), include thiamine-responsive megaloblastic anemia, lactic acidosis, branched-chain ketoacidemia, and subacute necrotizing encephalomyopathy.

  c. **Preventive therapy** should be given to patients whose intake is limited, and to those with malabsorption or increased requirements lasting more than 2 weeks. The dose required depends on need but is usually 1 to 2 mg/d.

  d. **Nondeficiency states.** It has been suggested that thiamine improves energy levels during exercise and in the elderly, and increases cognition in patients with Alzheimer's-type dementia, but the small number of studies do not support these uses (13). Low levels of thiamine have been reported in patients with recurrent aphthous mouth ulcers, and in a single trial, replacement therapy with vitamins B_1, B_2, and B_6 led to sustained improvement, but only in those patients with detectable deficiency (14).

7. **Toxicity.** Excess thiamine is rapidly cleared by the kidneys. The UL has not been set because of a lack of suitable data (3). Reported side effects have included headache, irritability, insomnia, tachycardia, and weakness (15). Occasionally, an anaphylactic reaction has been noted after thiamine injection, probably a consequence of hypersensitivity in patients who received the vitamin previously.

B. **Riboflavin (vitamin B_2)**

1. **Requirement.** Riboflavin forms the active portion of the coenzymes involved in biologic oxidation reactions. Therefore, requirements have been linked to protein or energy intake. Requirements have been determined by following the urinary excretion of riboflavin and by monitoring for signs of deficiency. Table 6-7 lists the daily allowances at all ages.

Table 6-7. Recommended riboflavin intakes

Life stage group	Riboflavin (mg/d)
Child	
0–0.5 y	0.3[a]
0.5–1.0 y	0.4[a]
1–3 y	0.5
4–8 y	0.6
Male	
9–13 y	0.9
14–>70 y	1.3
Female	
9–13 y	0.9
14–18 y	1.0
19–>70 y	1.1
Pregnant	1.4
Lactating	1.6

[a] Estimate based on adequate intake (AI). All others based on recommended dietary allowance (RDA). From Standing Committee on the Scientific Evaluation of Dietary Reference Intakes, Food and Nutrition Board, Institute of Medicine. *Dietary reference intakes for thiamine, riboflavin, niacin, vitamin B_6, folate, vitamin B_{12}, pantothenic acid, biotin, and choline.* Washington, DC: National Academy Press, 1998.

In contrast to thiamine requirements, those for riboflavin do not seem to change as energy requirements are increased at any given age. For adults older than 51 years with a low caloric intake, a minimum riboflavin requirement of 1.2 mg/d (women) or 1.4 mg/d (men) is suggested. Otherwise, allowances for all ages have been computed as 0.6 mg/1,000 kcal. For persons engaged in strenuous exercise, the allowance has been estimated as high as 1 to 6 mg/1,000 kcal. The requirement to avoid deficiency symptoms is probably 0.4 to 0.5 mg/1,000 kcal.

2. **Food sources.** Riboflavin is widely distributed, especially in all leafy vegetables and in the flesh of mammals. The best sources are yeast, milk, egg whites, kidney, liver, and leafy vegetables. Fish, meat, and poultry are good sources. Other vegetables and legumes are not as good. Milk, eggs, meat, grains, and green leafy vegetables are the usual dietary sources in Western countries. Table 6-8 lists the riboflavin content of specific foods. Enrichment accounts for much of the riboflavin in dairy products and grains.

   a. **Effects of processing.** Much riboflavin in milk and grains is free, but in other sources, it is conjugated to protein. It is heat-stable but unstable in ultraviolet light. It leaches out into cooking water, with average losses of 15% to 20%. If food is exposed to light during cooking, losses can be as great as 50% of the amount in uncooked food.

Table 6-8. Approximate riboflavin content of selected foods

Food	Portion	Riboflavin[a] (mg)	Percentage of RDI[b]
Grain products			
White bread	Slice	0.087	5–12
Whole wheat bread	Slice	0.059	1–5
Frankfurter rolls	Roll	0.132	5–12
Spaghetti, cooked	1 cup	0.137	5–12
Rice, cooked	1 cup	0.027	1–5
Meats			
Beef, ground, lean	3 oz	0.176	10–24
Beef liver	3 oz	3.52	100
Chicken, light meat, roasted	3 oz	0.098	5–12
Hot dog, beef	One	0.058	1–5
Pork, center loin chop, broiled	4 oz	0.217	10–24
Tuna, canned, water	4-oz can	0.194	10–24
Bacon, cooked	3 pieces	0.054	1–5
Vegetables			
Asparagus, cooked from fresh	½ cup	0.104	5–12
Spinach, cooked from fresh	1 cup	0.425	10–24
Cabbage, raw	1 cup	0.022	1–5
Corn on cob, boiled	1 in	0.08	1–5
Potato, baked	4.75 × 2.3 in	0.067	1–5
Tomatoes	2.4 in	0.059	1–5
Dairy products and eggs			
Milk, whole	1 cup	0.395	10–24
Eggs, large	One	0.265	10–24
Cheese, cheddar	1 oz	0.106	5–12
Cheese, cottage, low fat <2%	1 cup	0.416	10–24
Ice cream	1 cup	0.329	10–24

[a] Data from Hands ES. *Food finder,* 2nd ed. Salem, OR: ESHA Research, 1990.
[b] Recommended dietary intake is 1.7 mg.

However, exposure of processed milk to light does not affect its riboflavin content. Little riboflavin is lost during the pasteurization of milk, but canning of foods can cause up to 30% of the vitamin content to be lost into the water. The riboflavin values listed in Table 6-8 are those of the unprocessed foods in most cases. Riboflavin is lost during the processing of grain and is added back to white flour, corn meal, and rice. The average Western diet contains about 2.7 mg/d, in excess of the RDA.

   b. Colonic bacteria produce riboflavin, but this is not available for absorption in sufficient quantity to fulfill daily need. The bacteria must be lysed or killed for the vitamin to be available.

3. **Assessment**
   a. Intake. Riboflavin is unique among vitamins in that it is minimally metabolized or stored by the body. Thus, urinary excretion correlates well with intake during normal conditions. Urinary levels of riboflavin are measured by means of HPLC with fluorometric detection (10). During fasting or prolonged bed rest, urinary excretion can be falsely elevated. Because urinary levels reflect the recent dietary intake of riboflavin, variations can be considerable. The values are reported as micrograms of riboflavin per gram of creatinine to correct for body size and allow random sampling in 2-hour collections. Samples are usually obtained in the fasting state to avoid the variations caused when the subject consumes a meal near the time of collection. However, a deficient patient retains most of the ingested vitamin, and such variations are minimal in patients whose body stores are depleted. Table 6-9 provides guidelines for the interpretation of this measurement.

   b. Body stores. The riboflavin-dependent enzyme erythrocyte glutathione reductase catalyzes the following reaction:

$$NADPH + H^+ + GSSG \rightarrow NADP^+ + 2GSH$$

where GSSG = oxidized glutathione and
GSH = reduced glutathione.

   This assay is performed on whole blood with and without the addition of flavin adenine dinucleotide. Normally, no stimulation is noted, but when body stores of the vitamin are decreased, activity is markedly stimulated. The activity coefficient value is independent of age and sex. An activity coefficient above 1.40 is diagnostic of severe deficiency. This sensitive assay is the procedure of choice (10).

4. **Physiology**
   a. Coenzyme function. Riboflavin forms a part of the two coenzymes flavin mononucleotide and flavin adenine dinucleotide. The prosthetic group is bound to the enzyme, accepts an H^+ ion, and then is

Table 6-9. Guidelines for interpretation of assessment of riboflavin status

Age (y)	Marginal (moderate risk)	Deficient (high risk)
	Riboflavin excretion (μg/g creatinine)	
All adults	40–119	<40
	Erythrocyte glutathione reductase (activity coefficient)	
All ages	1.2–1.4 (20–40% ↑)	>1.4 (>40% ↑)

From Sauberlich NE. *Laboratory tests for the assessment of nutritional status,* 2nd ed. Boca Raton, FL: CRC Press, 1999.

reoxidized by interacting with another H^+ acceptor, usually a cytochrome of the mitochondrial electron transport chain (16). Flavins participate in both one- and two-electron transfers. Enzymes that require these coenzymes include succinic dehydrogenase; oxidases of fatty acids, glucose, and glycine; and xanthine oxidases. Thus, the richest sources of the vitamin are metabolically active tissues, not storage tissues. The highest concentrations of the vitamin are in the liver, heart, and kidneys. Riboflavin circulates in the blood largely bound to proteins (75%). The mean concentration in blood is 32 µg/L.

   b. **Absorption and excretion.** Riboflavin is absorbed rapidly in the intestine by a site-specific and saturable system that is energy- and sodium-dependent. However, the capacity for absorption is limited. The intestine, along with liver and other tissues, also phosphorylates the vitamin. Urinary excretion is increased by a negative nitrogen balance and by large amounts of thiamine. Excretion is decreased by low-carbohydrate diets, exercise, and pregnancy. Riboflavin is excreted in milk, up to about 10% of the daily intake (i.e., 300 µg/d). Excretion in sweat is much lower.

5. **Deficiency**
   a. **Signs and symptoms.** Early symptoms are related to oral and ocular lesions. Soreness and burning of the lips, mouth, and tongue develop along with photophobia, tearing, burning, and itching of the eyes. Angular stomatitis is characteristic but not specific. This lesion is characterized by maceration and bilateral transverse fissures of the mucocutaneous junction at the angle of the mouth. Lesions of the vermilion of the lips, termed *cheilosis,* frequently occur along the line of closure in riboflavin deficiency. Geographic tongue and denudation of papillae may occur. Desquamation of the skin and seborrheic dermatitis may be seen, especially in the nasolabial fold and scrotum. Corneal vascularization develops around the entire circumference. Hypochromic anemia is associated with erythroid hypoplasia. Growth and appetite are poor. Some of these symptoms also occur in vitamin B_6 deficiency because the oxidase required to produce the functional form of vitamin B_6 is riboflavin-dependent (11). Thus, the symptoms specifically caused by riboflavin deficiency are not known with certainty.
   b. **Associated deficiencies.** Riboflavin-containing foods often contain other B vitamins. Moreover, riboflavin is required for the metabolism of vitamin B_6, folate, niacin, and vitamin K. Thus, multiple other deficiencies often accompany riboflavin deficiency (Table 6-2). The usual settings in which deficiency develops are conditions characterized by poor intake, such as alcoholism or malabsorption. Hemodialysis can lead to losses of water-soluble vitamins, and deficiency can develop if they are not replaced. Drugs can prevent conversion to the active coenzyme; chlorpromazine, imipramine, amitriptyline, and quinacrine have been implicated.
   c. **Differential diagnosis.** The differential diagnosis of lip lesions includes poorly fitting dentures with malocclusion; sensitivity to lipsticks, toothpaste, and similar substances; and iron-deficiency anemia. Similar tongue lesions can be seen with iron deficiency, smoking, pernicious anemia, pellagra, and antibiotic therapy.
6. **Treatment**
   a. **Deficiency states** should be treated with 5 to 10 mg/d by mouth. Often, other B-complex vitamin deficiencies accompany riboflavin deficiency, and some (e.g., niacin deficiency) cannot be distinguished easily on clinical grounds. When malabsorption is present, prophylactic use of the vitamin at a dose of about 3 mg/d is useful. Tablets are available in doses of 5 to 100 mg, and an injectable solution is available at a concentration of 35 mg/mL.

b. Nondeficiency states. Riboflavin is used in rare genetic disorders in which the formation of specific flavoproteins is deficient, and as a supplement during phototherapy for neonatal jaundice. During the photosensitized oxidation of bilirubin to more polar derivatives that can be excreted, riboflavin is destroyed, and additional vitamin needs to be provided. Migraine-like headaches occur in the syndrome of mitochondrial encephalopathy, in which riboflavin therapy appears to be effective. In a randomized, double-blinded, placebo-controlled trial of high-dose (400 mg/d) riboflavin, the frequency of migraine attacks was reduced during a period of 3 months (17). However, the severity of the attacks was not affected, and the benefit of riboflavin was apparent only at the end of the study. More such trials are needed to demonstrate the effectiveness of riboflavin therapy in this condition.

7. Toxicity. Up to 10 mg/kg can be given without any apparent toxic effects. However, insufficient data are available to recommend a UL (3). Riboflavin may cause a yellow-orange discoloration of the urine.

C. Niacin (vitamin B₃)

1. Requirement. The term *niacin* is used for both nicotinic acid and nicotinamide. Estimates of requirement are complicated by the fact that some tryptophan is converted to nicotinic acid in humans. On the basis of three studies in adults, a Food and Nutrition Board task force estimated that 60 mg of ingested tryptophan is equivalent to 1 mg of niacin—that is, when 60 mg tryptophan is ingested, enough is oxidized to provide about 1 mg of niacin. Niacin is required for the function of respiratory enzymes, and therefore allowances are based on energy expenditures. Estimates of the requirement are usually reported in terms of niacin equivalents (NE) (i.e., 1 mg of niacin or 60 mg of tryptophan). The availability of tryptophan for niacin synthesis also depends on the presence of other essential amino acids. Table 6-10 gives the daily requirements and allowances for adults and children.

Most data on deficiency are for adults, but estimates have been made for children. Daily allowances are based on an intake of 6.6 mg NE/1,000 kcal. A minimum for adults over the age of 18 years is 15 (female) or 19 (male) mg NE/d. During lactation, about 1.6 mg of niacin is lost daily in 850 mL of milk.

Table 6-10. Recommended dietary intakes of niacin

Life stage group	Niacin equivalent (mg/d)	Life stage group	Niacin equivalent (mg/d)
Infants		Females	
0–6 mo	2[a]	9–13 y	12
7–12 mo	4[a]	14–>70 y	14
Children		Pregnancy	
1–3 y	6	≤18–>50 y	18
4–8 y	8	Lactation	
Males		≤18–>50 y	17
9–13 y	12		
14–>70 y	16		

[a] Estimate based on adequate intake (AI). All others based on recommended dietary allowance (RDA).
From Standing Committee on the Scientific Evaluation of Dietary Reference Intakes, Food and Nutrition Board, Institute of Medicine. *Dietary reference intakes for thiamine, riboflavin, niacin, vitamin B₆, folate, vitamin B₁₂, pantothenic acid, biotin, and choline.* Washington, DC: National Academy Press, 1998.

2. **Food sources.** Nicotinic acid is present in most foods except fats and oils, mainly as the pyridine nucleotides NAD and NADP. It is removed during grain processing but is added back during enrichment. It is particularly abundant in meat, fish, and grain products. It is sometimes present in a form that is not absorbable (e.g., in corn). It is stable in foods and can survive a reasonable amount of heating, cooking, and storage. Average diets in the United States supply 6 and 24 mg of niacin and 700 and 1,100 mg of tryptophan per day for women and men, respectively. This amounts to a total of 16 to 24 mg NE/d. Animal proteins provide more tryptophan than vegetable proteins (1.4% on average vs. 1.0%). Human milk contains about 0.17 mg of niacin and 22 mg of tryptophan per deciliter and is adequate to supply the needs of an infant. Table 6-11 lists the niacin content of various foods. However, food tables based on niacin content alone are not helpful unless the content is linked to energy, ingested tryptophan, or both.

3. **Assessment**

   a. **Intake or absorption measured by urinary excretion.** Normally, adults excrete 20% to 30% of niacin as N'-methylnicotinamide and 40% to 60% as the 2-pyridone metabolite. Values for these metabolites fall as intake decreases. HPLC procedures provide a

Table 6-11. Approximate niacin content of selected foods

Food	Portion	Niacin content (mg)	Percentage of RDI[a]
Grain products			
White or whole wheat bread	Slice	1.05	5–12
Corn bread	Muffin	0.850	1–5
Frankfurter roll	One	1.58	5–12
40% Bran flakes[b]	½ cup	2.1	5–12
Puffed wheat	1 cup	1.2	5–12
Rice, cooked	1 cup	3.03	10–24
Meats			
Beef, ground, lean	3 oz	4.23	10–24
Pork, center loin chop	4 oz	4.35	>40
Chicken, light meat, roasted	3 oz	10.6	25–39
Fish (e.g., halibut), broiled	3 oz	6.06	>40
Liver, beef	3 oz	12.3	>40
Tuna in water	4-oz can	12.3	10–24
Vegetables and fruits			
Green beans, cooked fresh	1 cup	0.768	1–5
Cauliflower, cooked	½ cup	0.342	1–5
Peas, frozen, cooked	½ cup	1.18	5–12
Potato, baked	4.75 × 2.3 in	3.32	10–24
Tomato, fresh	2.6 in	0.772	1–5
Apple	2.75 in	0.106	<1
Banana	8.75 in	0.616	1–5
Peanuts	1 cup	20.6	100
Peanut butter	2 tbs	4.23	10–24
Milk and eggs			
Milk, whole	1 cup	0.205	1–5
Egg, large	One	0.033	<1

[a] Recommended dietary intake is 20 mg.
[b] Most cold cereals are enriched; check labels.
Data from Hands ES. *Food finder,* 2nd ed. Salem, OR: ESHA Research, 1990.

rapid and sensitive method for determining the levels of both metabolites. The level is usually reported per gram of creatinine to allow for random sampling. However, this method is available only for adults. In children, the level of creatinine excretion is more variable, and good guidelines for the interpretation of excretion have not been worked out. The measurement of the 2-pyridone concentration in plasma may be a more reliable assay than the ratio of the two niacin metabolites in the urine (10). Table 6-12 provides guidelines for interpreting urinary excretion data.

  b. **Body stores.** The levels of 2-pyridone and N'-methylnicotinamide in plasma have been reported in a few small studies to be a more reliable indicator of these metabolites than their urinary concentrations. In addition, the measurement of pyridine metabolites in red cells may be useful and more reliable (Table 6-12). Thus, it is possible that as HPLC methods become more widely available, one of these plasma/red cell measurements may identify patients with low body stores of niacin.

4. **Physiology.** Nicotinic acid is an essential component of the coenzyme nicotinamide adenine dinucleotide and its phosphate (NAD^+ and $NADP^+$). These coenzymes function to carry hydrogen from a substrate through the mitochondrial electron transport system. They are really cosubstrates rather than coenzymes because they join and leave the enzyme along with the substrate. Many dehydrogenases are NAD- and NADP-dependent. Perhaps the most important pathway is that of oxidation of glucose-6-phosphate. The products of oxidation, NADH and NADPH, are then used for other metabolic processes, such as fatty acid synthesis. Nicotinic acid is produced from tryptophan in the liver by a series of enzymes. NAD^+ and $NADP^+$ inhibit the first enzyme of this synthetic pathway, tryptophan oxygenase, thus regulating the production of nicotinic acid. The fourth enzyme in this pathway, kynureninase, requires pyridoxal phosphate, so that deficiencies of these two vitamins are linked.

Table 6-12. Guidelines for interpretation of niacin status

Patient	Acceptable	Deficient intake	Low intake	Deficient intake
	Urinary excretion: ratio of mg N'-methylnicotinamide/g creatinine to 2-pyridone-N'-methylnicotinamide			
Males and nonpregnant, nonlactating females	1.6–4.29	<0.5	0.5–1.50	<1.0
Women, pregnant				
1st trimester	1.6–4.29	<0.5	0.5–1.59	<1.0
2nd trimester	2.0–4.99	<0.6	0.6–1.99	<1.0
3rd trimester	2.5–6.49	<0.8	0.8–2.49	<1.0
	Plasma N'-methylnicotinamide-2-pyridone (μg/dL)			
Young men[a]	16.3 ± 5.9 (28 NE/d)	3.7 ± 0.9 (10 NE/d)	1.2 ± 2.3 (6 NE/d)	
	Erythrocyte NAD/erythrocyte NADP ratio			
Young men[a]	<1.0			

NE, niacin equivalent; NAD, nicotinamide adenine dinucleotide; NADP, nicotinamide adenine dinucleotide phosphate.
[a] Based on a single study of niacin-deficient diets.
From Sauberlich NE. Laboratory tests for nutritional status, 2nd ed. Boca Raton, FL: CRC Press, 1999.

Nicotinic acid, but not nicotinamide, exhibits two pharmacologic properties—peripheral vasodilation and a plasma lipid-lowering effect. The latter effect is more marked when cholesterol levels are high. Nicotinic acid is used to decrease levels of triglycerides and of total and low-density-lipoprotein (LDL) cholesterol, and to increase levels of high-density-lipoprotein (HDL) cholesterol, but the mechanism of action remains unknown.

5. Deficiency

a. Pellagra. The classic deficiency syndrome, pellagra, is associated with skin, gastrointestinal, and central nervous system changes. Dermatitis, which occurs in exposed areas, is symmetric and exacerbated by trauma. Cracking and crusting develop over thickened areas of skin. Soreness is common in the mouth, with a red, swollen, and painful tongue and mucous membranes. Angular stomatitis is often seen but is probably caused by associated riboflavin deficiency. Diarrhea is a common feature of niacin deficiency and may be related to mucosal atrophy. Early neurologic symptoms include headache, sleep disturbances, anxiety, depression, and thought disorders. Psychomotor retardation and stupor may ensue. As the deficiency progresses, confusion, hallucinations, and agitation develop, and finally seizures or catatonia alternating with lucid spells.

b. Associated with vitamin B_6 deficiency. Tryptophan and niacin deficiencies are often compounded by vitamin B_6 deficiency because B_6 is required in the conversion of tryptophan to nicotinic acid. Isoniazid therapy can lead to pellagra because hydrazine drugs form adducts with pyridoxal phosphate. If vitamin B_6 is provided and tryptophan is available, exogenous niacin is not needed. Isoniazid resembles nicotinic acid chemically and acts as an inhibitor. However, other hydrazine drugs that are more potent inhibitors than isoniazid do not cause pellagra. Thus, inhibition of the vitamin alone may not explain the clinical deficiency.

c. Hartnup disease is a rare inherited condition of neutral amino acid malabsorption that produces a clinical syndrome mimicking pellagra. Dermatitis with photosensitivity, ataxia, and psychiatric changes are common. Decreased intestinal and renal tubular absorption of tryptophan may explain in part the relative tryptophan deficiency associated with this condition. Protein synthesis seems adequate, but sufficient extra tryptophan is not available for nicotinic acid synthesis. The fact that the disorder responds to oral niacin confirms the role of tryptophan in daily niacin production.

d. Carcinoid syndrome often presents with low blood levels of tryptophan, probably a result of increased synthesis of serotonin from tryptophan. Rarely, pellagra occurs in the carcinoid syndrome and may be overcome by oral niacin.

6. Treatment

a. Deficiency. Isolated niacin deficiency is uncommon, and usually other B-complex vitamins must also be given. Niacin (nicotinic acid) is available in tablets (20 to 500 mg), as timed-release capsules (100 to 750 mg), and as an injectable solution (10, 50, and 100 mg/mL). Nicotinamide is also available in comparable doses. Nicotinamide does not have hypolipidemic or vasodilating effects. The glossitis, dermatitis, diarrhea, and mental symptoms of pellagra respond to oral doses of 100 to 500 mg/d, depending on the severity of symptoms. The peripheral neuritis seen in pellagra responds to niacin or B_6 replacement, depending on the vitamin deficiency responsible for the syndrome.

b. Pharmacologic effects

(1) Cardiovascular disease. Nicotinic acid (1 to 3 g/d in three or four divided doses), but not nicotinamide, lowers serum levels of triglyceride, total cholesterol, and LDL cholesterol (18). Most randomized, placebo-controlled trials show significant decreases in recurrent myocardial infarction, cerebrovascular events, total mortality, and angiographic progression of atherosclerosis in patients on nicotinic acid monotherapy (3 g/d) (19).

(2) Diabetes mellitus. Despite a protective effect on beta cells in animals and an increase in C-peptide levels as a measure of beta-cell function in humans, no improvement in glycemic control has been found (20).

(3) Osteoarthritis. One preliminary study suggests an effect on joint mobility and the use of antiinflammatory drugs (13).

7. **Toxicity.** The UL for niacin intake has been set at 35 mg/d for subjects over 18 years of age. Large doses of nicotinic acid (>1 g/d) cause flushing secondary to histamine release, with burning of the hands and face. This effect may wear off with time. Taking the drug with meals in divided doses or with aspirin may diminish the flushing (21). At doses of 3 g/d or more, nausea, vomiting, diarrhea, and arrhythmias may occur. Peptic ulcer symptoms may be aggravated by the large acid load. Hyperuricemia secondary to competition for excretion occurs in about 40% of patients. Gout occurs less frequently (7%). Cardiac arrhythmias occur uncommonly. About one-fourth of patients note rash, pruritus, hyperkeratosis (especially at higher doses of >3 g/d), and glucose intolerance. Laboratory evidence of hepatic injury may be found. Elevations of aspartate aminotransferase and bilirubin are common (30% to 50%), even at doses as low as 750 mg/d. Cholestatic jaundice and submassive necrosis have been reported, again at high doses. Rarely, acanthosis nigricans can be seen that is not associated with occult neoplasm. Toxicity is more common with timed-release preparations taken at high doses. A new timed-release preparation may be safer, delivering up to 2,000 mg/d (22).

D. **Pyridoxine (vitamin B₆)**

1. **Requirement.** The term *vitamin B₆* encompasses three naturally occurring pyridines—pyridoxine, pyridoxal, and pyridoxamine. These are all interrelated functionally, and a quantitative requirement would depend on knowledge of the intake and activity of all three. Such data are not readily available in humans. The estimates of requirement are based on production or cure of clinical signs of deficiency or, more often, on production or reversal of abnormal biochemical test results (e.g., excretion of tryptophan metabolites after a tryptophan load). Requirements are increased during intake of large amounts of protein.

The vitamin B₆ allowance has been estimated according to a ratio of 0.016 mg of the vitamin per gram of protein ingested. Thus, the estimates for women and men are based on the lower rates of protein intake in women than in men (Table 6-13). These figures slightly exceed the estimated requirement based on repletion studies. In the elderly, the incidence of biochemical pyridoxine deficiency was nearly 50% (23), but there is little evidence to indicate that this deficiency is based on differences in energy intake (24). Thus, the recommendations are higher in the older aged population. The protein requirements of pregnant and lactating women are increased; in addition, they must supply the fetus with vitamin B₆. The additional allowances suggested for these stresses have been made without much quantitative data to support the recommendations. The vitamin B₆ content of human milk is low in the first few weeks. Oral contraceptive intake for more than 30 months before pregnancy can decrease vitamin B₆ levels.

2. **Food sources.** Vitamin B₆ is produced by intestinal microorganisms, but it is not thought that much of this is absorbed. The three forms of the vitamin are present in low concentrations in all plant and animal tissues. For this reason, dietary deficiency is uncommon. Bound forms of the vitamin are found as β-D-glucosides in plants; about 60% of this is

Table 6-13. Recommended daily dietary intakes of vitamin B_6

Life stage group	Vitamin B_6 (mg/d)	Life stage group	Vitamin B_6 (mg/d)
Infants		Females	
0–6 mo	0.1[a]	9–13 y	1.0
7–12 mo	0.3[a]	14–18 y	1.2
Children		19–50 y	1.3
1–3 y	0.5	50–>70 y	1.5
4–8 y	0.6	Pregnancy	
Males		≤18–50 y	1.9
9–13 y	1.0	Lactation	
14–50 y	1.3	≤18–50 y	2.0
51–>70 y	1.7		

[a] Estimate based on adequate intake (AI). All others based on recommended dietary allowance (RDA).
From Standing Committee on the Scientific Evaluation of Dietary Reference Intakes, Food and Nutrition Board, Institute of Medicine. *Dietary reference intakes for thiamine, riboflavin, niacin, vitamin B_6, folate, vitamin B_{12}, pantothenic acid, biotin, and choline.* Washington, DC: National Academy Press, 1998.

bioavailable. Most vitamin B_6 is associated with glycogen phosphorylase, and this source accounts for much of the storage pool of the vitamin. Table 6-14 lists the content of the vitamin in various foods. Pyridoxal represents 80% of the B_6 vitamins in human milk. This abundance of pyridoxal is needed because the premature infant (<29 weeks) cannot utilize pyridoxine to any extent. Losses of vitamin B_6 have been observed during the heating and storage of some foods as a Schiff base forms between pyridoxal phosphate and the ε-amino lysines in proteins. Bioavailability can be as low as 40% but usually ranges from 60% to 80%. Losses occur during processing, often exceeding 50%. Sometimes, the availability of vitamin B_6 is increased during food processing.

3. Assessment

a. **Intake or absorption.** The vitamin is excreted in the urine mainly as pyridoxal and to a lesser extent as pyridoxamine. About 20% to 50% is excreted as the metabolite *4-pyridoxic acid.* The excretion of free vitamin B_6 correlates closely with intake. Dietary protein does not affect urinary excretion. Urinary excretion reflects recent dietary intake but may not reflect the degree of deficiency. Random samples provide as good data as do 24-hour excretion studies. Chromatographic (HPLC) methods are very reliable for all metabolites, especially 4-pyridoxic acid. Low intake correlates with excretion of less than 5.0 μg of 4-pyridoxic acid per day. Urinary excretion is probably not a reliable measure of pyridoxine status in patients being treated with vitamin B_6 antagonists, such as isoniazid. Table 6-15 provides guidelines for the interpretation of urinary levels.

b. **Body stores**

(1) **Transaminases** are enzymes requiring vitamin B_6. Because the level of transaminase activity is greater in red cells than in serum and less variable, erythrocyte transaminases are used for this determination. The assay is performed with and without the addition of pyridoxal phosphate. However, in contrast to what occurs in the stimulatory tests for thiamine and riboflavin, transaminase activity in normal subjects is increased by the addition of pyridoxal. Activity is reported as a ratio of stimulated to unstimulated activity, termed the *erythrocyte*

Table 6-14. Approximate vitamin B_6 content in selected foods

Food	Portion	Vitamin B_6 content (mg)	Percentage of RDI (2.0 mg)
Grain products[a]			
Bread			
White	1 piece	0.009	<1
Whole wheat	1 piece	0.052	1–5
Rice, cooked	1 cup	0.283	10–24
Spaghetti, enriched	1 cup	0.049	1–5
Corn flakes	3 oz	0.060	1–5
Meats			
Beef, ground, lean	3 oz	0.210	10–24
Pork, center loin chop	4 oz	0.348	10–24
Salmon	3 oz	0.186	5–12
Chicken			
Dark meat, roasted	3 oz	0.304	10–24
White meat, roasted	3 oz	0.510	25–39
Fruits and vegetables			
Banana	8.75 in	0.659	25–39
Apples	2.75 in	0.066	1–5
Grapes	10 each	0.060	1–5
Cauliflower, cooked	½ cup	0.125	5–12
Peas, green, cooked	1 cup	0.250	5–12
Potatoes, baked	1 each	0.701	25–39
Tomatoes, fresh	1 each	0.098	5–12
Peanuts	1 cup	0.367	10–24
Peanut butter	2 tbs	0.124	5–12
Dairy products and eggs			
Milk, whole	1 cup	0.102	5–12
Cheese, cottage, 27% fat	1 cup	0.172	5–12
Egg	One	0.060	1–5

RDI, recommended dietary intake.
[a] Cereals are sometimes fortified with B_6; check label.
Data from Hands ES. *Food finder,* 2nd ed. Salem, OR: ESHA Research, 1990.

Table 6-15. Guidelines for assessment of vitamin B_6 status

Parameter	Acceptable values		
Plasma pyridoxal-5′-phosphate	>30 nmol/L		
Urinary 4-pyridoxic acid	>3.0 µmol/d		
Erythrocyte AST activity coefficient	<1.80		
Erythrocyte ALT activity coefficient	<1.25		
Urinary xanthurenic acid excretion	<65 µmol/d (2 g L-tryptophan load)		
		Plasma [homocysteine][a]	
		<16.3 µmol/L	>16.3 µmol/L
Pyridoxal-5′-phosphate	≥30 nmol/L	83 ± 76	56 ± 50
Plasma folate	≥5 nmol/L	6.7 ± 3.6	5.5 ± 2.9
Plasma cobalamin	±200 pmol/L	275 ± 148	202 ± 61

AST, aspartate aminotransferase; ALT, alanine aminotransferase.
[a] Values from reference 27.
Adapted from Sauberlich HE. *Laboratory tests for the assessment of nutritional status,* 2nd ed. Boca Raton FL: CRC Press, 1999.

transaminase (E-AST or E-ALT) index. Normal subjects have an E-AST index of less than 1.7 and an E-ALT of less than 1.25. Deficiency is correlated with an E-AST index of more than 2.2. Ratios between 1.8 and 2.2 are marginal. This test remains the best readily available functional assessment of vitamin B_6 status.

  (2) Pyridoxal-5′-phosphate (PLP) is also a sensitive measure of vitamin status and correlates with body stores. However, it can be modified by physical exercise, pregnancy, and the level of plasma alkaline phosphatase activity. PLP can be measured in whole blood (50 to 120 nmol/L) and in plasma (17 ± 7 µg/L), with ranges of 30 to 134 nmol/L and 5 to 33 µg/L, respectively (10). If the 95% reference limits for PLP derived from white populations are used, many blacks have low levels of pyridoxine. Thus, low PLP levels in blacks do not necessarily indicate deficiency (25). The assay is currently performed with tyrosine apodecarboxylase as the apoenzyme. HPLC has also been used, but the assay is not so widely available. In some situations, stores are not correctly assessed by PLP measurement. Patients with cirrhosis metabolize PLP more rapidly than normal persons do. However, metabolism is not to pyridoxic acid, so excretion of that metabolite does not assess depletion. PLP is also elevated in hypophosphatasia (26). Thus, its level may vary with alkaline phosphatase activity. The difficulty with assessing body stores is that multiple forms of the vitamin exist and must be measured (10).

  (3) Xanthurenic acid excretion following a 2- or 4-g tryptophan load is also a sensitive functional assay of vitamin B_6 status, perhaps even more sensitive than the transaminase ratio (10). The HPLC assay is reproducible, but because of the convenience of sampling blood or plasma, it has not been used so much as the transaminase ratio and PLP concentrations.

  (4) Homocysteine. Vitamin B_6 is one of three vitamins important in the metabolism of homocysteine, and levels of this metabolite are elevated when the vitamin is deficient. Detection is very accurate by HPLC. Homocysteine is elevated to ≥ 12 µmol/L fasting and ≥ 38 µmol/L after methionine load. When homocysteine is elevated, plasma levels of PLP are significantly lower than in normals. However, elevation of homocysteine is not specific for pyridoxine deficiency (Table 6-15). Folic acid is probably the main determinant of the homocysteine increase associated with coronary artery disease (see sections on folic acid and vitamin B_{12}).

4. Physiology. Very little is known about the factors that influence the absorption of vitamin B_6. It is rapidly absorbed in the upper intestine by passive transport, facilitated diffusion, or both, and is distributed among enzyme proteins as the coenzyme pyridoxal phosphate. Most enzymes use this form, although transaminase can also use pyridoxamine. The ability of the human fetus up to 30 weeks of age to convert pyridoxine phosphate to pyridoxal phosphate via pyridoxine oxidase is limited. Enzymes that require vitamin B_6 are involved in the synthesis and catabolism of all amino acids. Thus, the requirement is linked to protein intake. Most of the transaminases require vitamin B_6, as do many amino acid decarboxylases. Important among this latter group are the enzymes that convert histidine to histamine, ornithine to polyamines, aromatic amino acids to dopamine, and serotonin and glutamate to γ-aminobutyric acid. The enzymes serine deaminase, which produces pyruvic acid, and threonine deaminase, which produces 2-oxybutyrate, require vitamin B_6. The synthesis of coenzyme A, which is the first step in porphyrin (heme) synthesis, the conversion of linoleic to arachidonic acid, and the production of nicotinic acid from tryptophan via kynurenine are all B_6-dependent steps. The vitamin binds to a nuclear steroid hormone receptor and thus acts as a negative control of steroid hormone action.

5. **Deficiency.** Because the vitamin is widely distributed in food and is also made by intestinal bacteria, dietary restriction rarely leads to deficiency. The usual clinical situations in which deficiency arises include malabsorption, old age, alcoholism, and treatment with vitamin B_6 antagonists. The deficiency syndrome is not well defined in humans. The major findings include seborrhea-like lesions about the eyes, nose, and mouth; cheilosis; glossitis; hypochromic anemia; and peripheral neuritis. Nausea, vomiting, dizziness, irritability, insomnia, and convulsions can occur. Vitamin B_6 deficiency can impair interleukin-2 production and lymphocyte proliferation in elderly adults. Most of these symptoms are induced by the use of vitamin B_6 antagonists and may not reflect symptoms of the true deficiency state.

   a. **Hyperhomocysteinuria.** Hyperhomocysteinuria has been identified as an independent risk factor for vascular disease and may be associated with a deficiency of cystathionine synthase, the B_6-dependent enzyme that catalyzes the conversion of homocysteine to cystathionine. Significantly lower levels of PLP, cobalamin, and folic acid were found in patients with moderately elevated levels of homocysteine (≥ 16.3 µmol/L) (27). Supplementation with 10 mg of pyridoxal, 1.0 mg of folic acid, and 0.4 mg of B_{12} normalized serum homocysteine levels. Each of these cofactors may be important in determining homocysteine levels, but it is premature at present to recommend the widespread use of these supplements to alter atherogenesis in this subset of patients with hyperhomocysteinemia.

   b. **Vitamin B_6 antagonists.** The drugs most commonly involved as antagonists are isoniazid, hydralazine and other hydrazines, oral contraceptives, dopamine, and penicillamine. Cycloserine also can act in this way. These compounds increase urinary excretion (e.g., isoniazid) or combine with pyridoxal or pyridoxal phosphate to form inactive drugs (e.g., hydrazones are derived from hydrazines and a thiazolidine derivative from penicillamine). These effects can be reversed with vitamin B_6 supplements, usually in the range of 2 to 5 mg/d. Some experts advocate prophylaxis for all patients on isoniazid; others suggest supplements only for those at risk for neuropathy.

   c. **Pyridoxine-dependent syndromes** have been reported, in which tissue levels of the vitamin are normal but binding of the cofactor to the enzyme is impaired. These inherited disorders respond to larger doses of vitamin B_6 than are required to treat deficiency states. Table 6-16 lists the syndromes.

6. **Therapy**

   a. **Deficiency.** Pyridoxine hydrochloride is available as 5-, 10-, 25-, 50-, 100-, 200-, 250-, and 500-mg tablets and as a solution for injection containing 50 or 100 mg/mL. It is a component of many multivitamin tablets at doses of about 2 mg. In treating deficiencies, it is often advisable also to give other B-complex vitamins because multiple deficiencies frequently occur simultaneously. For *prophylactic* use with isoniazid to prevent peripheral neuropathy, 5 mg/d is probably sufficient, but doses up to 25 mg are used. Treatment of established neuropathy requires 50 to 300 mg/d. Pyridoxine is sometimes given to patients with sideroblastic anemia, dystonia, or Parkinson's disease treated with L-dopa, and to newborns with seizure disorders.

   b. **Pharmacologic doses.** The vitamin has been used to treat a variety of disorders that may or may not be associated with decreased intake, but little evidence of efficacy has been provided by properly conducted trials (28). Pyridoxine has been used in carpal tunnel syndrome,

Table 6-16. Pyridoxine-dependent errors of metabolism

Disorder	Clinical findings	Laboratory findings
Infantile seizures, B₆-dependent	Convulsions	None
Chronic anemia, B₆-dependent	Hypochromic anemia	Increased serum iron
Homocystinuria	Mental retardation, severe collagen disease involving vessels, eye problems, osteoporosis	Homocystinemia, homocystinuria, hypermethioninemia
Cystathioninuria	Mental retardation, blood dyscrasia, heart disease	Cystathionuria
Xanthurenic aciduria	Urticaria	Xanthurenic aciduria

asthma, and autism, with no clear evidence of efficacy from available studies (13). The Atherosclerosis Risk in Communities (ARIC) study was a prospective case–cohort study that found heart disease negatively associated with higher PLP levels (29). A metaanalysis of 10 randomized, controlled trials of premenstrual syndrome found efficacy in doses of 50 mg once or twice a day (30), although the quality of the studies was questioned. Depressive symptoms were helped more than others, and no side effects were noted.

7. **Toxicity.** When pyridoxine is ingested in large amounts (0.5 to 6 g/d), a peripheral sensory neuropathy can occur (10,31) that is completely reversible when treatment is stopped. Possible explanations include neurotoxicity directly caused by pyridoxine, neurotoxicity caused by a minor contaminant, or inhibition of the formation of pyridoxal phosphate by unconverted pyridoxine. The UL for adults has been established at 100 mg/d (3).

E. **Folate (folic acid, folacin, pteroylglutamic acid)**
   1. **Requirement**
      a. **Difficulty of estimation.** Estimating the folate requirement is complex. *Folacin* is a generic term denoting compounds with a structure and function similar to those of folic acid (pteroylglutamic acid), and more than 150 forms are known to exist in foods. However, individual compounds are variably absorbed and retained by the body. Moreover, dietary folates are mostly in the polyglutamate form, which is not quite so available as the unconjugated vitamin. Absorption does not necessarily correlate with retention in the body because more of the monoglutamate form of pteroylglutamic acid is excreted in the urine after ingestion than of other forms.

      Folacin is variably available in foods because of the presence of binders, inhibitors, and other factors. Enterohepatic recirculation of 5-methyltetrahydrofolic acid is important in the retention of body stores, but the relative importance of this factor in individuals can only be guessed at. An exact determination of total body pools of folacin is not available because the data are based on few determinations. The form of folate used commercially, pteroylglutamic acid, is a relatively poor substrate for dihydrofolate reductase; consequently, the rates of tissue utilization and retention for this form are much lower than those for the natural methylated or reduced folates found in food. However, folacin requirements have been assessed by replacement with pteroylglutamic acid.

b. DRIs. The recommendations for folate intake have been modified dramatically (3) since the RDA of 200 μg/d for adults was offered in 1989 in the 10th edition of *Recommended Dietary Allowances*. Subsequently, the need for extra folate to reduce the incidence of neural tube defects was recognized (32), as was the role of folate intake and elevated serum homocysteine concentrations in cardiovascular disease (33). The recent report of the Institute of Medicine expresses dietary folate as folate equivalents, adjusted for the apparently greater bioavailability of synthetic folic acid in comparison with naturally occurring folate, and for the estimated amount of ingested folate needed to maintain folate levels in red blood cells (i.e., body stores) in long-term metabolic studies (3). The resulting recommendations are all higher by 100 to 200 μg/d than previous estimates (Table 6-17). Pregnant and lactating women require extra folate to build red blood cells and produce milk, respectively.

2. Food sources. The folacin content of selected foods is given in Table 6-18. Major sources are orange and other citrus juices, white bread, dried beans, green salads, liver, eggs, and enriched breakfast cereals. However, much dietary folate comes from food sources that are frequently consumed but in which the vitamin is not especially concentrated, and from cereals and grain foods (flour, pasta, rice, cornmeal) that are fortified with folate.

a. Polyglutamate versus monoglutamate forms. Folacins occur in food largely as polyglutamates. The pentaglutamate form predominates, although forms with four and six residues also are common. The assessment of polyglutamate forms in foods is difficult because of rapid breakdown to the monoglutamate form in mammalian tissues. This problem is relevant to estimates of the availability of folacins in foods because they must be deconjugated to the monoglutamate form for absorption. Moreover, the microorganisms used to assay folacin content differ in how they use the monoglutamate and oligoglutamate forms. *In situ* deconjugation in the tissues affects the assessment of nutritional folacin availability. Estimates of folacin available as the monoglutamate form vary from 30% in orange juice to 60% in cow's milk.

Table 6-17. Dietary reference intakes for folate

Life stage group	Folate (μg/d)	Life stage group	Folate (μg/d)
Infants		Females	
0–6 mo	65[a]	9–13 y	300
7–12 mo	80[a]	14–50 y	400 SGA + diet
Children		51->70 y	400
1–3 y	150	Pregnancy	
4–6 y	200	≤18–50 y	600 (400 as SGA)
Males		Lactation	
9–13 y	300	≤18–50 y	500
14->70 y	400		

SGA, synthetic folic acid. Because it is more readily available than dietary folate and is the form shown to prevent some neural tube defects, this form is recommended during the childbearing years and pregnancy.
[a] Estimate based on adequate intake (AI). All others based on recommended dietary allowance (RDA).
From Standing Committee on the Scientific Evaluation of Dietary Reference Intakes, Food and Nutrition Board, Institute of Medicine. *Dietary reference intakes for thiamine, riboflavin, niacin, vitamin B_6, folate, vitamin B_{12}, pantothenic acid, biotin, and choline.* Washington, DC: National Academy Press, 1998.

Table 6-18. Approximate folacin content of selected foods

Food	Portion	Total folacin (µg)	Percentage of RDI (400 µg)
Meat			
Beef or pork, cooked	3 oz	3–4	1–5
Liver, beef, cooked	3 oz	123	25–39
Liver, chicken, cooked	1 each	204	>40
Vegetables			
Asparagus	1 cup	86	10–24
Spinach, cooked	1 cup	164	25–39
Beans, green, cooked	1 cup	41	10–24
Cauliflower	1 cup	42	10–24
Turnip greens	1 cup	52	10–24
Lettuce, head or leaf	1 cup	20	5–12
Lettuce, romaine	1 cup	98	10–24
Nuts			
Walnuts	1 cup	66	10–24
Peanuts	1 cup	153	25–39
Peanut butter	1 tbs	13	1–5
Almonds	1 cup	136	25–39
Breads and cereals			
Bread			
White	1 slice	10	1–5
Whole wheat	1 slice	16	1–5
Rice	1 cup	20	1–5
Eggs			
Egg	1 each	29	5–12
Beverages			
Wine, spirits	8 oz	None	0
Beer	12 oz	21	5–12
Milk, whole	1 cup	12	1–5
Orange juice, fresh or frozen	1 cup	136	25–39

RDI, recommended dietary intake.
Source: An extensive list of folacin content of foods is given by Perloff BP, Britrum RR. Folacin in selected foods. *J Am Diet Assoc* 1977;70:161.

    b. Folacin availability. Most dietary folacins are reduced and methylated forms; 5-methyl pteroylglutamic acid accounts for 60% to 95% of dietary folacin, 10-formyl pteroylglutamic acid for 14% to 40%, and other reduced forms for 10% to 20%. The 5-methyl and N-10-formyl folacins are heat-stable, whereas unsubstituted, reduced pteroylglutamic acids are unstable. Some dietary folates are bound to specific binding proteins (e.g., in milk). In steaming and frying, as much as 90% of the food content can be lost. Boiling for 8 minutes causes a loss of about 80% of folacin activity from most vegetables. Boiling destroys heat-labile folacin in cow's milk; during boiling, the folacin content of milk falls from about 54 µg/L to less than 10 µg/L. Thus, infants fed with boiled milk formulas must receive supplements. Some foods are judged to contain highly bioavailable folacins; examples include bananas, lima beans, liver, and yeast. Foods in which the folacin bioavailability is low include orange juice, lettuce, egg yolk, cabbage, soybean, and wheat germ.

    c. Folacin content of average diets. The new DRIs use the concept of dietary folate equivalents (DFEs) to calculate estimates, and

DFEs are used to estimate dietary content. The DFE converts all forms of dietary folate, including synthetic folate in fortified foods, to an equivalent of food folate (34). The estimated equivalent of food folate for synthetic folate is 50%, and the estimated equivalent for synthetic folate added to food, as opposed to synthetic folate by itself, is 85%. Thus, synthetic folic acid added to food is 85/50 or 1.7 times more available than synthetic folate alone. The diets of adults in the United States and Canada contained 262 to 2,807 µg of DFEs per day, with mean daily intakes of 708 and 718 µg for adult men and women, respectively (in the second National Health and Nutrition Examination Survey, 1988–1994), and of 718 and 644 µg, respectively (in the Continuing Surveys of Food Intakes by Individuals, 1994–1996) (35). With allowances made for the increased availability of foods fortified with folate and the increased use of supplements, it was estimated that 67% to 95% of the U.S. population was meeting the new estimated average requirement (34). However, 68% to 87% of women of childbearing age still had intakes of synthetic folate below the recommended level of 400 µg/d, and about 20% of children under the age of 8 had intakes over the newly established UL of 400 µg/d for that age group (1,000 µg/d for adults).

3. **Assessment**

   a. **Intake or absorption.** Only small amounts of folacin are excreted in the urine (about 1% of dietary intake) (10). Moreover, not all dietary forms are excreted in the same proportions. Thus, urinary excretion is not useful in assessing intake. Oral folic acid tolerance tests have been described, but they do not clearly distinguish between folate and vitamin B_{12} deficiencies because folate utilization is decreased in vitamin B_{12} deficiency. The serum folate level is quite sensitive to changes in dietary folate intake and is a measure of the status at the time of assay (36). A low serum level (2 or 3 to 6 ng/mL) reflects only a recent low dietary intake and may not reflect tissue stores (Table 6-19). Continued low levels (<2 or 3 ng/mL) are usually associated with megaloblastic anemia and decreased tissue reserves. Folate is assayed microbiologically with *Lactobacillus casei*, which uses the 5-methyl vitamers, the only circulating form of folacin. Alternatively, measurements based on binding assays or radioimmunoassay are used. Although the microbiologic assay is the reference method, binding assays are simpler and faster, avoid interference from antibiotics in serum samples, and allow simultaneous measurement of serum B_{12} levels. On the other hand, the results of radioassays are more variable between laboratories, and the radioassays require more expensive reagents and equipment. Single-stage (competitive) and two-stage (noncompetitive) assay kits are available, with the latter providing slightly better sensitivity.

   Most circulating folacin is in the form of 5-methyltetrahydrofolic acid. About 90% is loosely attached to albumin and 10% to specific binding proteins. Therefore, hypoalbuminemia can lead to a low total serum folic acid level, and this result does not necessarily imply a deficiency of the vitamin. Aspirin, at a dose of 650 mg every 9 hours, can produce a reversible decrease in total and bound folate (37). Other albumin-binding drugs produce the same effect. Low values are also associated with decreased intake, malabsorption, or ingestion of drugs that affect folate absorption or utilization. These drugs include folate antagonists, phenytoin, prednisone, alcohol, and oral contraceptive agents. Alcohol lowers serum folate levels by increasing urinary folate excretion (38). Because both red and white cells contain much larger amounts of folacin than serum does, hemolysis or a very high white blood cell count, especially when the white cells

Table 6-19. Guidelines for interpreting folate status

Test	Folate deficiency	Low recent folate intake[a]	Normal	Vitamin B$_{12}$ deficiency
Serum folate (ng/mL)	<2 or 3	3–6	>6	High
Red cell folate (ng/mL)	<140	150–160	>160	<150
Bone marrow	Megaloblasts	Normocytic, normochromic	Normocytic, normochromic	Megaloblasts
Peripheral blood smear	Multilobed polymorphonuclear leukocytes,[b] macrocytosis	Normal	Normal	Multilobed polymorphonuclear leukocytes, macrocytosis
Serum homocysteine (µmol/L)	**Moderate/severe risk** >30	**Low risk** >16	**Normal** <12–15 (40+ y M) <10–12 (40+ y F)	

[a] Low serum levels also may reflect hypoproteinemia or the ingestion of drugs that alter folic acid metabolism or binding, such as folate antagonists, phenytoin, alcohol, and oral contraceptives. Hemolysis may falsely elevate the serum values.
[b] Multilobed: >3.5 lobes per cell on average, or >5% of cells have five lobes, or >1 six-lobed leukocyte per 100 cells.

are abnormal, falsely elevates serum folate levels. One-third of hospitalized patients may have low folate levels, which implies a recent negative folic acid balance. However, few of these patients require long-term supplementation.

b. Tissue stores. Although serum and red cell folate levels decline in parallel, the red cell folate level is a more accurate reflection of tissue stores. It is less variable and reflects the folate status at the time of red cell formation. However, the red cell contains monoglutamate and polyglutamate forms of folic acid, so that the dose–response curves are altered in binding assays. Folate is measured in both serum and whole blood, and the folate level in red cells is calculated based on the hematocrit. In primary vitamin B_{12} deficiency, folate is not well utilized. Thus, in 15% to 25% of cases of vitamin B_{12} deficiency, serum folate levels rise and red cell levels fall. When both the serum and red cell levels are low, folate deficiency is the cause, although the red cell folate level falls after the serum folate level. Table 6-19 outlines the guidelines used for interpreting folate levels.

c. Other assays. The presence of hypersegmented lobes can be helpful, but the determination is somewhat subjective. Macrocytosis (mean corpuscular volume >97) may be present but is not specific. Urinary excretion of formiminoglutamic acid after an oral 20-g load of histidine (normal rate, >50 mg/12 h) is a functional assay, as is the deoxyuridine suppression test. These tests are not routinely available and are not clearly more discriminating than the red cell folate level in detecting deficiency.

d. Serum homocysteine (but not methylmalonic acid) levels are elevated in folate deficiency (see section on vitamin B_{12}). However, they also reflect inadequacies of vitamin B_6 and vitamin B_{12}. Other causes of elevated serum homocysteine concentrations include renal insufficiency, hypovolemia, hypothyroidism, psoriasis, and inherited metabolic defects (39). A common cause of hyperhomocysteinemia is a genetic predisposition secondary to a polymorphic substitution in the methylenetetrahydrofolate reductase gene. In interpreting elevated homocysteine levels, it is best to obtain serum methylmalonic acid levels simultaneously (Table 6-20). Part of the problem in identifying hyperhomocysteinemia is the variability in assay results and normal values. This variability is partly a consequence of the multiple forms of homocysteine in serum (reduced, oxidized, protein-bound), and partly a consequence of the different and noninterchangeable results of HPLC, enzyme immunoassay, and fluorescence polarization immunoassay (40). Reference values for total serum homocysteine increase with age and are higher for men than for women at all ages (41).

Table 6-20. Interpretation of serum methionine metabolite assays

Metabolite(s)	Folate deficiency	Vitamin B_{12} deficiency
	(% in patients with deficiency)	
Methylmalonic acid (MMA) ↑	12	98
Homocysteine (Hcy) ↑	91	96
MMA ↑, Hcy normal	2	4
Hcy ↑, MMA normal	80	1
MMA, Hcy normal	7	0.2

Adapted from Savage DG, Lindenbaum J, Stabler SP, et al. Sensitivity of serum methylmalonic acid and total homocysteine determinations for diagnosing cobalamin and folate deficiencies. *Am J Med* 1994;96:239.

4. Physiology

a. Absorption. Absorption takes place through a pH-dependent active process in the proximal intestine, with maximum transport occurring after deconjugation to the monoglutamate form. Some, but not all, dietary folate is nutritionally available. Polyglutamate forms of folate in food are hydrolyzed by folyl poly-γ-glutamate carboxypeptidase; the products of hydrolysis, which contain decreased numbers of glutamate residues, include the monoglutamate form, found in small amounts in human salivary, gastric, pancreatic, and jejunal juice. The activity of this ubiquitous carboxypeptidase is also increased in intestinal mucosa, liver, pancreas, kidney, and placenta. Both brush border and lysosomal sites of folate conjugase activity have been reported in human jejunum. The brush border enzyme is necessary for the hydrolysis of dietary folates. The intestinal transporter for folate is very similar to the reduced folate carrier found in red cells (42). It is not certain whether a separate mechanism exists for such uptake. Reduced folates are absorbed better than oxidized forms. Pteroylglutamic acid, used in tablets, is not as good a substrate for dihydrofolate reductase and must be reduced before it can be maximally utilized. Methyltetrahydrofolic acid is absorbed rapidly and not changed. Other forms are converted in enterocytes to reduced formylated and methylated derivatives. Some vitamin escapes unreduced and is metabolized in the liver. The reduced methylated form is delivered to all tissues. Folate absorption may be decreased in elderly patients with gastric atrophy, a situation that can be corrected by administering hydrochloric acid to lower the gastric and intestinal pH.

b. Reabsorption. After conversion in the liver to 5-methyltetrahydrofolic acid, the vitamin can enter the plasma as the monoglutamate, be stored in tissue as the polyglutamate, or be reexcreted in bile and reabsorbed. The rate of enterohepatic circulation is estimated to be 100 µg/d. This figure is comparable with the amount of daily tissue folate utilized (50 to 100 µg). Thus, folate deficiency develops more rapidly in malabsorption than in dietary deficiency alone. During deficiency states, the concentration of folate in the bile decreases, so the enterohepatic circulation does not contribute to losses at a constant rate.

c. Intracellular metabolism. Natural forms of folic acid are converted to coenzymes by reduction of the pyrazine ring (two possible sites), elongation of the peptide chain with glutamyl residues (six possible additions), and addition of a one-carbon fragment in position 5 or 10 (six possible fragments). Thus, a large variety of folate coenzymes exist. The tetrahydro form is frequently involved, and it is thought that a polyglutamate form is the active coenzyme. These coenzymes function in many reactions involving one-carbon transfers, including purine and thymidylate synthesis, metabolism of several amino acids (especially serine and homocysteine), methylation of biogenic amines, and initiation of protein synthesis by formylation of methionine. The coenzymes are quite unstable in cells because peptidases degrade the polyglutamyl chain. For mobilization of the storage form in the liver and release into the blood, hydrolysis to the monoglutamate form is required.

d. Protein binding. Two-thirds of plasma folate is protein-bound because it is negatively charged at physiologic pH. This binding, largely to α_2-macroglobulin and albumin, is loose. In addition, folate is tightly bound to a specific binder that recognizes reduced folates. The role of this binder is unclear.

5. Deficiency

a. "Classic" deficiency. Because folate coenzymes are active in RNA, DNA, and protein synthesis, conditions of rapid growth or metabolic utilization (pregnancy, lactation) are associated with a high risk for deficiency. Acute symptoms of folate deficiency have been noted after the administration of antagonists. These include anorexia, nausea, diarrhea, mouth ulcers, and hair loss. Thrombocytopenia occurs frequently. Chronic deficiency is characterized by fatigue, a sore tongue, and anemia, with few neurologic signs. If folate stores are normal at the start, deficiency takes about 4 months to develop. If stores are depleted initially, the symptoms of deficiency can develop in 2 to 3 months. Clinical deficiency cannot be defined by serum folate levels because 10% to 20% of populations in Western nations may have low levels. Some of these are related to low recent intake. If prolonged, a decreased intake leads to deficiency (decreased body stores). Malabsorption of any cause can lead to deficiency. Diseases that are frequent causes of folate deficiency include tropical sprue, gluten- sensitive enteropathy, and alcoholism (43).

b. **Neural tube defects.** The results of randomized trials show that at least half of neural tube defects could be prevented if women consumed adequate amounts of folic acid early in pregnancy (32,44,45). The data have been repeated in areas with a high and low incidence of neural tube defects (3,46). Based on the results of these trials and on uncontrolled observations of the effects of lower doses of folic acid, the U.S. Department of Health and Human Services published *Recommendations for the Use of Folic Acid to Reduce the Number of Cases of Spina Bifida and Other Neural Tube Defects,* with the suggestion that 400 µg of folic acid be ingested daily by all women capable of becoming pregnant. High doses were not recommended because they can mask B_{12} deficiency. These recommendations have been confirmed following extensive review by the Standing Committee on the Scientific Evaluation of Dietary Reference Intakes (3). Not all neural tube defects can be prevented, and folate should be ingested before conception as well as after. Some experts advise women who have had a prior pregnancy in which the fetus had a neural tube defect to take 4.0 mg of folic acid per day. At this dose, folic acid may interfere with anticonvulsant therapy in epilepsy. The synthetic form of folate is recommended. To derive an equivalent intake from the diet, about 10 servings of fruits and vegetables a day would be required, and the folate in foods is less bioavailable.

c. **Bottle-fed infants** are susceptible to folate deficiency because heating can destroy milk folacins.

d. **Pregnancy** is associated with low serum folate levels because of hemodilution and increased requirements. Anemia is often secondary to iron deficiency also. One- third of pregnant women have low serum folate levels at delivery (see Chapter 4).

e. **Anticonvulsant drugs** (especially phenobarbital, phenytoin, and primidone) cause macrocytosis in 40% of patients, but only half of these have low serum and red blood cell levels of folate. Most patients have normal levels of vitamin B_{12}. Thus, the mechanism is not entirely clear. Some alteration in absorption of folates is postulated.

f. **Increased utilization.** Folate deficiency occurs in disorders in which utilization is increased, such as hemolytic anemia, chronic myelofibrosis, leukemia, sideroblastic anemia, and chronic exfoliative dermatitis.

g. **Alcohol ingestion** in excess of 80 g of ethanol per day is associated with macrocytosis (>80%) and low serum levels of folate.

h. **Sulfasalazine** can cause deficiency by decreasing folate absorption. The same effect is not caused by 5-aminosalicylic acid.

i. **Inhibition of dihydrofolate reductase** impairs the conversion of folates to the active coenzyme. Dihydrofolate reductase inhibitors include methotrexate, trimethoprim, pyrimethamine, and triamterene. The frequency of clinical deficiency is greatest with methotrexate.

j. **Smokers with bronchial metaplasia.** Plasma levels of folate are decreased in smokers who have bronchial metaplasia in comparison with smokers who do not have metaplasia. The issue of whether folate deficiency can develop and cause tissue damage is not resolved.

k. **Hyperhomocysteinemia.** Homocysteine levels are consistently higher in patients with atherosclerotic diseases, but the mechanisms for this elevation are multiple (33). It is not clear whether the metabolite itself is sufficient or whether it is a cofactor. However, feeding methionine alone increased the levels of circulating adhesion molecules and altered coagulation parameters; reversal of these findings by the addition of antioxidant vitamins C and E suggests a direct role of homocysteine in vascular damage (47). Hyperhomocysteinemia is considered by many to be an independent risk factor for cardiovascular disease and mortality (48), including the large prospective Women's Health Study (49). However, as of the year 2000, the American Heart Association does not recognize elevated total serum levels of homocysteine as an independent risk factor for cardiovascular disease. Although a low folate status was a strong determinant of elevated total homocysteine levels, it was not associated with an increased risk for coronary atherosclerosis (50). The epidemiologic data linking homocysteine and cardiovascular risk are strong, but data from some prospective studies have been less consistent (51,52).

Other questions have been raised about total serum homocysteine concentrations as a cardiovascular risk factor. Other traditional risk factors are associated with increased homocysteine levels; homocysteine levels rise in renal disease (even in early stages), and the C677T mutation of the methylenetetrahydrofolate reductase gene causes a moderate rise in serum homocysteine concentration, although no significant increase in cardiovascular risk (52). Folate supplementation does decrease homocysteine levels (53,54), but its relationship to lowering cardiovascular risk has not been adequately tested. The role of folate replacement in modifying this increased risk is unclear, and the issue is not likely to be resolved until prospective interventional studies are performed.

l. **Cognitive decline.** Low levels of folate and cobalamin are seen in aged patients with cognitive decline. The low vitamin status is likely secondary to decreased intake. Many poorly controlled trials have suggested a role for folate supplementation in improving cognition, but the severity of cognitive decline is not correlated with the degree of folate deficiency (55). The association of low folate levels with depression is unclear.

m. **Cancer.** The Nurses Health Study found that the risk for the development of colon cancer was lower in women who had used vitamin supplements containing folate for more than 15 years than in women who had used such preparations for shorter periods (56). However, supplemental folate has not yet been shown prospectively to have a protective effect. Data on folate supplementation to treat cervical dysplasia are conflicting (13). Epidemiologic studies also provide some support for a modulating role of folate in breast and pancreatic cancer; however, the findings are only suggestive, despite the prospective nature of some of the studies (57).

6. **Treatment**

a. **Medication.** The form of folacin used therapeutically is the unreduced pteroylglutamic acid. Tablets of 0.1, 0.4, 0.8, and 1 mg are available, and quantities of 0.2 to 1.0 mg are included in some multivitamin preparations; 200 to 500 µg/d is needed to treat most deficiency states. Oral replacement is preferred, except in severe malabsorption, in which parenteral (IM, IV, or SC) folate (5 or 10 mg/mL) can be used. At the concentrations used for total parenteral nutrition, folate is stable if the pH of the solution is above 5.0. Leucovorin calcium (5-CHOH-tetrahydrofolic acid) is available as solutions (3 mg per ampule or 10 mg/mL in 5-mL vials). This compound is used only after methotrexate therapy to avoid toxicity. In the large doses offered, it is not meant as vitamin replacement therapy for deficiency states, especially because the large doses can mask vitamin B$_{12}$ deficiency.

   b. Fortification. The U.S. Food and Drug Administration specified in 1996 that certain grain products (especially most enriched breads, flours, cornmeal, rice, noodles, and macaroni) be fortified with 0.14 mg of folic acid per pound of product. The Food and Drug Administration estimated that this practice would raise the folate intake of women of childbearing age by 100 µg/d yet avoid exceeding the UL of 1,000 µg/d in nontarget populations (58). This UL was selected so as not to mask vitamin B$_{12}$ deficiency and allow neurologic progression. Considerable debate regarding all aspects of the fortification program continues, including the dose added, the effect on nontarget populations, and the risk for masking pernicious anemia. The use of a higher level of cereal-based folate supplementation (499 to 665 µg/d) than that recommended by the Food and Drug Administration (127 µg/d) produced a greater rise in serum folate and a significant fall (11%) in serum homocysteine levels; these findings suggest that more folate should be added to foods (59). However, in a study of a cohort before and after folate fortification was approved, the percentage of subjects with low serum levels of folate fell from 22% to 1.7%, and the percentage of those with high serum homocysteine levels fell from 18.7% to 9.8% (60). The ability of folate to lower serum homocysteine may be related to the intake of other vitamins (e.g., >500 mg of vitamin C per day) that can interfere with vitamin B$_{12}$ metabolism (61). The UL of 1,000 µg/d has been challenged on the grounds that all but eight cases of masked neurologic progression in vitamin B$_{12}$ deficiency occurred in patients taking more than 5 mg of folate per day (35).

7. Toxicity. Folic acid and phenytoin compete for intestinal transport and possibly uptake in the brain. Thus, very large doses of folate (>100 times the RDA) may precipitate convulsions in patients treated with phenytoin (62). A few cases of hypersensitivity have been documented at doses of 1 to 10 mg. Fever, urticaria, pruritus, and respiratory distress have been reported (63).

F. Cobalamin (vitamin B$_{12}$)

   1. Dietary reference intake. The total body content of cobalamin is approximately 2 to 2.5 mg, most of which is in liver. Estimates of half-life vary from 480 to 1,284 days. Thus, daily losses of cobalamin average about 1.3 µg. Because absorption is about 70% efficient at low levels of intake, the RDA for adults of about 2 µg/d was formerly considered sufficient to maintain the body pool. In response to findings that 10% to 30% of people more than 51 years old may have protein-bound vitamin B$_{12}$ malabsorption, the new DRI for this age group has been set at 2.4 µg/d (3). Malabsorption in the elderly is probably a consequence of reduced secretion of pepsin and gastric acid, perhaps related to *Helicobacter pylori* infection. Because intrinsic factor is present, these people can absorb free (synthetic) vitamin B$_{12}$. Thus, it is recommended that the vitamin be ingested mostly in the form of a dietary supplement to ensure that intake is adequate (64). Table 6-21 gives the DRIs for adults and children.

   2. Food sources. The term *cobalamin* refers to cobalt-containing corrinoids with biologic activity in humans. The average diet in the United States provides 5 to 15 µg/d. Cobalamin is produced by bacteria and enters animal tissues during the ingestion of contaminated foods or after

Table 6-21. Dietary reference intakes for cobalamin

Life stage group	Cobalamin (μg/d)	Life stage group	Cobalamin (μg/d)
Infants		Adolescents and	
0–6 mo	0.4[a]	adults (M/F)	
7–12 mo	0.5[a]	14–>70 y	2.4
Children		Pregnancy	
1–3 y	0.9	≤18–50 y	2.6
4–8 y	1.2	Lactation	
9–13 y	1.8	≤18–50 y	2.8

[a] Estimate based on adequate intake (AI). All others based on recommended dietary allowance (RDA).
From Standing Committee on the Scientific Evaluation of Dietary Reference Intakes, Food and Nutrition Board, Institute of Medicine. *Dietary reference intakes for thiamine, riboflavin, niacin, vitamin B₆, folate, vitamin B₁₂, pantothenic acid, biotin, and choline.* Washington, DC: National Academy Press, 1998.

production in the rumen. Microorganisms in the colon synthesize cobalamin, but the vitamin is not absorbed at that site. Thus, cobalamin deficiency develops in strict vegetarians. Most of the cobalamin in normal feces arises from bacterial synthesis in the colon and does not represent unabsorbed vitamin, so that fecal excretion is unrelated to dietary intake. The usual dietary sources are seafood, meat and meat products, fish, eggs, and to a lesser extent milk and milk products. Most cooking methods do not destroy cobalamin. Boiling meat can lead to losses of up to 30% into the water. However, during drying, the cobalamin in some food (e.g.) is converted to inactive analogues (65). Evidence that ingesting megadoses of vitamin C (500 to 1,000 mg) destroys some of the cobalamin in food is conflicting. It is not clear how frequently, if ever, cobalamin deficiency occurs in persons who take megadoses of vitamin C. Table 6-22 lists selected foods containing cobalamin.

3. Assessment

a. Intake or absorption. No reliable method is available to assess intake of cobalamin, but the Schilling test accurately reflects absorption.

(1) Schilling test. This test is based on the fact that free cobalamin does not occur in plasma or elsewhere until all binding proteins are saturated, after which free cobalamin is filtered through the glomerulus. A parenteral injection of 1,000 μg of unlabeled cyanocobalamin is given to saturate binding proteins in tissue and serum. Any serum to be drawn for assessment of body stores must be obtained beforehand. An oral dose of [⁵⁷Co]B₁₂ linked to intrinsic factor is then given. Unfortunately, the dual-isotope Schilling test kit (Dacopac, Nycomed Amersham, Buckinghamshire, U.K.) is no longer available. Excretion of the labeled cobalamin in urine for 24 hours should exceed 8% of the administered dose if absorption is normal. In cases of possible bacterial overgrowth, absorption can be tested after the administration of 1 g of tetracycline per day.

(2) Interpretation. A value above 8% and below 10% is an indeterminate result and accounts for about 25% of test results (66). Problems with the test involve the collection of urine and intertest variability. When urine collection is incomplete or renal disease is present, a low rate of cobalamin excretion is unreliable. Intertest variability can be as much as 30% to 50%. It is a mistake to attach too much importance to an ar-

Table 6-22. Approximate cobalamin content of selected foods

Food	Portion	Cobalamin (µg)	Percentage of RDI (6 µg)
Beef, ground	3 oz	2.4	>40
Liver, beef	3 oz	95	>100
Liver, chicken	1 each	1.87	25–39
Oysters, raw	1 cup	40–48	>100
Crab	1 cup	9.9	>100
Salmon	3 oz	4.93	>40
Egg	1 each	0.59	5–12
Lamb chop	3 oz	1.58	25–39
Pork, center loin chop	4 oz	0.62	5–12
Chicken, light meat, roasted	3 oz	0.291	1–5
Cheese	1 oz	0.2–0.45	5–12
Milk, whole	1 cup	0.871	10–24
Yogurt, low-fat, plain	1 cup	1.28	10–24

RDI, recommended dietary intake.
Data from Hands ES. *Food finder,* 2nd ed. Salem, OR: ESHA Research, 1990.

bitrary normal limit of 10% excretion. Stimulation of urinary excretion by twofold or more with the addition of intrinsic factor is suggestive of intrinsic factor deficiency, even if the excretion without intrinsic factor is in the 8% to 10% range. In 30% to 40% of cases, low serum cobalamin levels cannot be explained by the decreased absorption of free vitamin B_{12}. The multiple causes of a "falsely" normal Schilling test result include the following: (a) erroneous value; (b) dietary insufficiency of cobalamin; (c) metabolic disorder of cobalamin metabolism, such as an inborn error, or inhalation of nitrous oxide; (d) malabsorption of cobalamin that has been corrected by the use of antibiotics; (e) "falsely" low serum cobalamin level, which occurs much less often than formerly assumed (see section on body stores); and (f) malabsorption of food-bound cobalamin. The absorption of cobalamin in food requires the liberation of free cobalamin by gastric proteases. Therefore, the Schilling test result may not always correlate with physiologic alterations in cobalamin absorption, especially when gastric physiology is altered.

When serum levels of cobalamin are low, three patterns of absorption can be seen (67). Decreased dietary intake is associated with low absorption rates of free and protein-bound vitamin B_{12}. In gastric disease, absorption of the free form is normal, but the absorption of bound vitamin B_{12} is decreased. In intestinal disease, absorption of both forms is decreased. If serum gastrin levels are high, absorption of the bound form is frequently decreased, but bound cobalamin is also poorly absorbed in one-fifth of patients with normal gastrin levels. Thus, serum gastrin is not a sensitive test to determine the mechanism of absorption. However, the tests in which food sources of labeled cobalamin are used are neither clinically available nor standardized. No agreement has been reached on the "correct" form of food-bound cobalamin to use. It is unlikely that cobalamin deficiency develops in gastric disease without at least a partial defect in the production of intrinsic factor.

b. Body stores

(1) **Serum vitamin B_{12} (cobalamin).** This parameter usually correlates with body stores. Unlike the folacins, cobalamin is not more concentrated in blood cells than in serum. Thus, hemolysis is not a major factor in producing false results. Transcobalamin II (TCII), the serum carrier protein that delivers cobalamin to tissues, accounts for only 10% to 20% of total serum cobalamin. The rest is bound to haptocorrin. Therefore, in TCII deficiency, serum levels of cobalamin can be normal, but the vitamin is not delivered to tissues and body stores are low. However, it is clear that marginally low levels (140 to 200 or even up to 350 pg/mL) can be associated with neurologic defects.

(a) **Radioisotope dilution assays** are based on the principle that endogenous serum cobalamin competes with radioactive cobalamin for binding to a limited amount of cobalamin-binding protein (10). These assays are now simple and reliable. Some commercial kits make it possible to measure cobalamin and folate simultaneously. Heparinized samples cannot be used because heparin interferes with the assay. A number of studies have found that the results of the radioisotope dilution assay compare well with those of the older microbiologic assay.

(b) **Interpretation of low serum cobalamin levels.** A serum cobalamin level of less than 140 pg/mL is always associated with low body stores if dilution, protein deficiency, folate deficiency, or altered cobalamin binding protein levels are not present (Table 6-23). Cobalamin deficiency should be suspected in patients with levels of 140 to 200 pg/mL. Such patients should undergo further testing (methylmalonic acid, homocysteine levels), or the results should be correlated with abnormal hematologic or neurologic findings. Evidence of cobalamin deficiency will not be found in all patients with marginal serum cobalamin levels. However, in doubtful cases, a therapeutic trial with cobalamin

Table 6-23. Guidelines for interpretation of serum cobalamin levels

Range	WHO	Lindenbaum et al. (68)	Comments
Deficient	<110 pmol/mL <150 pg/mL		
Low	110–147 pmol/mL 150–200 pg/mL		Falsely low: folate deficiency, pregnancy, oral contraceptives, multiple myeloma, haptocorrin deficiency
Acceptable	≥147 pmol/mL ≥201 pg/mL	≥258 pmol/mL ≥350 pg/mL	Falsely normal: myeloproliferative disorders (PV, CML), liver disease, TCII deficiency, intestinal bacterial overgrowth, treatment with cobalamin

PV, polycythemia vera; CML, chronic myelogenous leukemia; TCII, transcobalamin II; WHO, World Health Organization.
From references 10, 35, and 68.

replacement is safe, and reversal of the abnormal findings is diagnostic. Thirty percent of patients with folate deficiency have low serum cobalamin levels, although the reason is not clear. Protein deficiency lowers the amount of total serum cobalamin without having as much effect on delivery of cobalamin to tissues because most of the cobalamin-binding protein in serum is TCI. Up to 75% of strict vegetarians have low serum cobalamin levels without evidence of deficiency. Signs of anemia are likely to develop in patients with continued inadequate dietary intake. In patients with HIV infection, cobalamin deficiency may create cognitive changes when clinical AIDS is not present. Pregnant women have low cobalamin levels secondary to dilution and redistribution of the binding proteins.

For elderly patients, a cutoff of 200 pg/mL may be too low to detect deficiency. A level of 258 pmol/L (350 pg/mL) has been suggested for patients older than 67 years because serum methylmalonic acid was found to be markedly elevated in 11% of patients with cobalamin levels below that threshold (68). Between 8% and 20% of elderly patients and a smaller percentage of others present with a serum cobalamin level below 180 pg/mL, yet they do not exhibit anemia, macrocytosis, clinical deterioration, or a red blood cell response to cobalamin treatment, and their Schilling test result for cobalamin absorption is normal. These patients need to be further evaluated in all cases because subclinical cobalamin deficiency may be present and lead to neurologic damage. Workup should include (a) a careful neurologic examination and (b) measurement of serum metabolites.

(c) **Interpretation of high cobalamin levels.** Concentrations above 1,000 pg/mL are seen in acute liver disease because of release from the hepatocytes and in leukocytosis because white blood cells produce haptocorrin, which increases the total cobalamin-binding capacity. These disorders also can raise the levels of serum cobalamin in patients with cobalamin deficiency to normal values.

(2) **Serum methylmalonic acid and total homocysteine.** Levels of these metabolites increase when the two cobalamin-dependent enzymes, methylmalonyl coenzyme A mutase (methylmalonic acid increased) and methionine synthetase (homocysteine increased), are impaired. Other metabolites that can be assayed include cystathionine (produced from homocysteine by a vitamin B_6-dependent enzyme) and 2-methyl citric acid, a methyl acceptor metabolite derived from methionine via S-adenosyl methionine. These metabolites can be used to differentiate the effects of vitamin B_6 deficiency (increased homocysteine, decreased D-cystathionine) and folate deficiency (increased homocysteine, decreased 2-methyl citric acid) from those of cobalamin deficiency alone (increased homocysteine, increased methylmalonic acid) (Table 6-20). Normal values for methylmalonic acid are less than 376 nmol/L, and for homocysteine they are less than 12 to 15 μmol/L (10). The acceptable level of serum methylmalonic acid was less than 638 nmol/L to correspond with the cutoff of serum cobalamin (258 pmol/mL) that detects nearly all cases of cobalamin deficiency (68). Causes of elevated serum methylmalonic acid besides cobalamin deficiency include renal insufficiency, hypovolemia, and inherited

metabolic defects. Serum homocysteine levels are discussed in this chapter in the section on folate.

   (3) Holo-TCII. The measurement of holo-TCII is the most sensitive method to detect cobalamin deficiency (69) (Table 6-24). It also detects cobalamin deficiency early. The half-life of holo-TCII is only 6 minutes, so levels are low within a week of cessation of oral cobalamin intake. An isotope dilution method is used to measure holo-TCII (i e., cobalamin bound to TCII) by separating TCII from haptocorrin–cobalamin in serum, which is adsorbed onto a microfine precipitate of silica. Because TCII delivers cobalamin to all tissues, a fall in the TCII–cobalamin complex (i.e., holo-TCII) may detect early stages of deficiency, even when serum cobalamin levels are normal. Holo-TCII levels, in parallel with red cell folate and total serum cobalamin levels, are inversely related to serum homocysteine concentrations (69). Values below 30 pmol/L (<40 pg/mL) are considered deficient, with borderline low values ranging from 30 to 44 pmol/mL (40 to 60 pg/mL). Holo-TCII measurements are derived by subtracting a large value (adsorbed haptocorrin–cobalamin) from another large value (total cobalamin) to obtain a small value (holo-TCII). Thus, the reproducibility of holo-TCII measurements in clinical conditions requires careful attention. Plasma cobalamin and holo-TCII levels can both be measured in the same assay (Microparticle Enzyme Intrinsic Factor Assay, Abbott Laboratories, Abbott Park, Illinois).

   (4) Screening. Because abnormal serum parameters of cobalamin metabolism precede manifestations of tissue damage, screening populations at risk for deficiency is recommended. Persons at risk include strict vegetarians; those older than 65 years (especially if institutionalized or with a history of decreased food intake); patients with unexplained neurologic/psychiatric symptoms; those with anemia, *H. pylori* infection (or taking proton pump inhibitors on a long-term basis), thyroid or autoimmune disease, HIV disease, Crohn's disease, chronic pancreatitis, multiple sclerosis, or malabsorption of any cause; and persons who have undergone gastric or small-bowel surgery. If serum holo-TCII measurements are available routinely, they can be used initially or in conjunction with serum cobalamin levels. If serum cobalamin is used alone, values below 350 pg/mL (Lindenbaum criteria, Table 6-23) should be investigated further if cobalamin deficiency is suspected clinically. Tests to confirm deficiency include measurements of serum methylmalonic acid, homocysteine, and serum holo-TCII, depending on availability and cost. When a serum cobalamin level below 350 pg/mL (268 pmol/mL) is used, an elevated methylmalonic acid concentration has a diagnostic sensitivity of 0.4 and a specificity of 0.98, certainly enough to recommend the measurement of methylmalonic acid to detect deficiency (70). If anemia is present, the status of folate, iron, and copper must also be considered.

4. Physiology

   a. Conversion to coenzymes. The stable cyanocobalamin must be converted to active coenzymes in the body. Adenosyl cobalamin is the form of 70% of the vitamin stored in liver, whereas methyl cobalamin is the major form in plasma (60% to 80%). Cobalamin forms the coenzyme for two enzymes, methylmalonyl coenzyme A mutase, and 5-methyltetrahydrofolate-homocysteine methyl-transferase (methionine synthetase). The latter enzyme links cobalamin with folate metabolism by removing the methyl group from methylfolate to re-

Table 6-24. Laboratory tests in sequential stages of cobalamin deficiency

		Stage of cobalamin deficiency			
Parameter	None	I	II	III	IV
CBL balance	None	Negative balance	Depletion of stores (early)	Tissue damage (late)	Tissue damage (late)
Serum holo-TCII	>60 pg/mL	Low	Low	Low	Low
Serum CBL	>201 pg/mL	>201 pg/mL	>201 pg/mL	Low	Low
Serum MMA	<376 nmol/L	<376 nmol/L	<376 nmol/L	High	High
Serum Hcy	<15 µmol/L	<15 µmol/L	<15 µmol/L	High	High
RBC folate	>160 pg/mL	>160 pg/mL	>160 pg/mL	>140 pg/mL	>100 pg/mL
Neurologic symptoms	None	None	None	Sometimes	Frequent
MCV	Normal	Normal	Normal	Normal	High
Hemoglobin	Normal	Normal	Normal	Normal	Low

CBL, cobalamin; TCII, transcobalamin II; MMA, methylmalonic acid; Hcy, homocysteine; RBC, red blood cell; MCV, mean corpuscular volume.
Adapted from Herbert VD. *Round table series 66.* London: Royal Society of Medicine Press, 1999.

generating tetrahydrofolate. Therefore, in cobalamin deficiency, the movement of plasma methyltetrahydrofolate into cells is decreased. Serum folate levels are normal or high, whereas red cell folate levels are low (71).

b. Cobalamin absorption. Cobalamin is bound to enzymes in food and must first be liberated by gastric proteases. The free vitamin is then bound to haptocorrin (non–intrinsic factor-binding protein) in the stomach; haptocorrin has a tenfold greater affinity for cobalamin than does intrinsic factor. In the upper small bowel, pancreatic enzymes hydrolyze haptocorrin to produce free cobalamin (72). Intrinsic factor is not protease-sensitive and now binds cobalamin. The intrinsic factor–cobalamin complex attaches to its specific receptor, cubilin, in the ileal mucosa and is taken up by the cell via receptor-mediated endocytosis (73). In the absence of ileal receptors, only about 1% of the vitamin is absorbed passively. Cathepsin L degrades intrinsic factor within lysosomes, liberating cobalamin to bind to TCII in another compartment of the enterocyte, from which it is released and carried to tissues where it is needed. In the liver, cobalamin is bound again to haptocorrin and excreted in the bile. In the intestine, the biliary haptocorrin–cobalamin complex is digested and absorbed in the same manner as the dietary vitamin. The enterohepatic circulation delivers approximately 5 to 10 µg of cobalamin per day to the intestine, an amount nearly equal to daily dietary intake. Potential daily losses without malabsorption are 1 to 2 µg. With malabsorption, estimated daily losses can approach 10 µg. Therefore, depletion of the 4 to 5 mg of body stores occurs slowly in dietary deficiency but much more rapidly in malabsorption.

5. Deficiency. Deficiency occurs in a variety of clinical situations (Table 6-25). Symptoms are insidious and develop during 2 to 3 years. Weakness,

Table 6-25. Patient populations at increased risk for cobalamin deficiency

Disorder	Prevalence	Pathophysiology
Pernicious anemia	Near 100%	Autoimmune gastritis, lack of IF
Helicobacter pylori gastritis	Variable	Chronic gastritis, some ↓ in IF
Age >65 y	~10%	Atrophic gastritis, malabsorption of food-bound CBL
Crohn's disease	↑ With resection	Ileal disease or resection, loss of IF receptor
HIV disease	~15%	↓ Acid/IF secretion, ↓ ileal absorption
Gastric surgery	High	Loss of parietal cells producing IF
Bacterial overgrowth	Variable	Organisms compete for CBL in bowel
Chronic pancreatitis	Low	Lack of pancreatic enzymes to transfer CBL to IF
Malabsorption	Variable	Loss of IF-CBL receptor, if ileum involved
Zollinger-Ellison syndrome	Moderate	Prolonged inhibition of gastric (and IF) secretion
Hyperhomocystinemia	Moderate	↓ Activity of methionine synthase; r/o folate, B_6 deficiency
Dementia	Moderate	↓ Myelin formation

IF, intrinsic factor; CBL, cobalamin.

fatigue, and dyspnea are related to anemia. However, fatigue is a very nonspecific symptom, and cobalamin supplementation is widely overused for this indication. Sore tongue, paresthesias, anorexia, loss of taste, and dyspepsia are seen, along with diarrhea, hair loss, impotence, irritability, and memory disturbances. Numbness and tingling are noted first in the lower limbs. Some patients present with a psychiatric illness, often depression. Macrocytosis is a feature in many cases. This anemia must be differentiated from the macrocytosis of alcoholism and hypothyroidism.

Dietary deficiency occurs exclusively in persons on a strict vegetarian diet. Cheese, milk, and eggs have low levels of cobalamin but can provide the needed amounts when they are major sources of calories. Increased utilization can occasionally lead to low serum cobalamin levels, as in bone marrow cells in multiple myeloma (74). HIV-infected patients can have low serum levels of vitamin B_{12} without clinical AIDS. The clinical significance is uncertain; not all patients with decreased cobalamin absorption improve when intrinsic factor is replaced. The mechanisms of these changes require clarification. Patients with multiple sclerosis can have low serum cobalamin levels and high homocysteine levels (75). It has been proposed that subclinical cobalamin deficiency aggravates underlying multiple sclerosis, but this association remains to be confirmed. Deficiency can develop during the prolonged use of proton pump inhibitors, but this is usually confined to patients with Zollinger–Ellison syndrome and sustained drug-induced achlorhydria, which does not occur with the usual doses of proton pump inhibitors (76).

   a. **Dementia and neuropsychiatric presentations.** The neurologic manifestations of cobalamin deficiency occur in about 75% of patients (77) (Table 6-26). Moreover, they often develop in the absence of anemia and can be the major presentation in elderly patients. Both folate and cobalamin have been linked to psychiatric disease, especially depression, but direct causal relationships are still uncertain (78). The association of these symptoms in the elderly with cobalamin deficiency is variable, and in one cross-sectional study, no correlation with cognitive impairment or general health was found (79).

   b. **Hyperhomocysteinemia.** This metabolite is regulated by folate, vitamin B_6, and cobalamin. Serum concentrations are also related to age, sex, renal function, drug ingestion, genetic polymorphism, and other factors as yet unknown. The variable rates of prevalence and the still uncertain upper limit of normal values may be associated with the need to use freshly separated plasma so as to avoid homocysteine synthesis by red blood cells *in vitro*. The implications of this finding in regard to cardiovascular disease are still unclear (see section on folate). Even when folate and cobalamin levels are found

Table 6-26. Neuropsychiatric presentations of cobalamin deficiency

Symptoms	Signs	Localization
Paresthesias, numbness, weakness, incontinence	↓ Vibration, touch, position, ↓ reflexes	Peripheral/autonomic nerves
Gait ataxia	Romberg's sign, ↑ reflexes, Babinski's sign, spasticity	Spinal cord
Aphasia, hemiparesis, impaired visual fields	Lateralized signs, optic atrophy	CNS (r/o stroke)
↓ Memory, concentration, depression, confusion, ↓ processing speed	Abnormal symptom scales	CNS (r/o Alzheimer's)

to be below average, it is not clear whether this represents a deficiency state and whether supplemental vitamins will either correct the plasma abnormality or prevent any clinical disorders, particularly cardiovascular disease (48–52,80). The fact that an increase in cardiovascular disease has not been detected in pernicious anemia, the most common cause of cobalamin deficiency, raises a question about the nature of the association with hyperhomocysteinemia.

6. Treatment

a. Dietary deficiency responds to as little as 1 to 3 μg/d taken orally.

b. Malabsorption requires additional supplementation (150 to 300 μg/mo) because the enterohepatic circulation is interrupted. A single injection of 100 μg produces a complete remission of symptoms in most cases. An increased sense of well-being is noted within 24 hours, painful tongue improves in 48 hours, and reticulocytosis begins in 5 to 7 days. Serum folate falls rapidly. Neurologic findings may take 6 months to reverse. Monthly injections of 100 to 200 μg sustain the remission, although 1,000 μg is often used.

c. Patients with rare inborn errors of metabolism, such as vitamin B_{12}-responsive methylmalonic acidemia, require treatment with large amounts of the vitamin because they are resistant to normal levels of cobalamin.

d. Elderly subjects are advised to meet daily needs by taking synthetic cobalamin in enriched foods or supplements (3). The amount of cobalamin found in most multivitamins (≤6 μg) is not sufficient to treat cobalamin deficiency, which is more prevalent in the elderly. Healthy people under age 50 consuming a diet that contains animal products do not require cobalamin supplements. Some healthy people over the age of 50 may require supplements, but it is not clear how many. Thus, it seems reasonable to screen this population, but the best approach to population screening and the best dose to prevent deficiency are still uncertain. If elevated levels of methylmalonic acid are found, treatment with cobalamin in deficiency doses can normalize them (81).

e. Neuropsychiatric presentations. No studies have tested whether Alzheimer's-type dementia responds to cobalamin. Because these patients are elderly, they should be screened and treated if deficiency is present. Some data support the use of cobalamin to treat painful uremic neuropathy (82).

f. Fatigue. Cobalamin injections have been used for years to treat fatigue, but evidence of its efficacy has not been found in controlled trials.

g. Parenteral cobalamin is supplied in solutions of 1,000, 100, and 30 μg/mL.

h. Oral/nasal cobalamin. Oral cobalamin can be used for treatment in most patients with an adequate gastrointestinal tract, although the response is slightly slower than when injectable vitamin is used (83,84). Nasal cobalamin is available (Nascobal, 500 μg/0.1 mL) for maintenance use once a week. It appears to be well tolerated and can even be used more frequently for the initial treatment of mild deficiencies.

7. Toxicity. Cobalamin causes no toxic effects, so no UL has been suggested (3).

G. Vitamin C (ascorbic acid)

1. Requirement. A daily intake of 10 mg of ascorbic acid cures clinical signs of scurvy but does not maintain body stores. When the daily intake is above 200 mg, most of the ingested vitamin is excreted. Between these extremes, body stores vary with intake. Age and sex have only minor effects on the vitamin C requirement. The requirement is compounded by the fact that vitamin C has a chemoprotective effect in many disorders, at doses far in excess of those necessary to prevent scurvy. These include colon cancer, heart disease, and cataracts. A well-designed study has now identified the vitamin C intake and tissue saturation levels that allow maximal protective effects of the vitamin (85). With the ingestion of 60 mg of vitamin C per day (the previous RDA), wide fluctuations in plasma vitamin C were associated with small changes in the amount consumed. The first intake dose at which plasma levels were beyond the first sigmoid part of the saturation curve was 200 mg/d. Saturation did not occur until intake levels were at 1,000 mg/d. These data fit with the estimated vitamin C content of diets (~ 225 mg/d) that appears to be of chemoprotective value (86). The new DRI values represent a compromise between the old RDA value of 60 mg/d and the value needed for chemoprevention (Table 6-27). This compromise also takes into account dietary availability, bioavailability, urinary excretion, potential adverse effects, and biochemical and molecular function in relation to vitamin concentration.

Needs are increased at some life stages. Premature infants have low body pools. Newborn infants ingest about 35 mg from breast milk, and the DRI for them is set to at least equal that source. During pregnancy, about 10 mg of vitamin is added to the fetus each day, which must be added to the DRI for pregnant women. The vitamin C concentration in human milk is about 30 mg/L for a volume of 750 mL (first 6 months), which creates an additional need of 22 mg/d.

2. **Food sources.** Ascorbic acid is widely distributed in foods in high concentrations, especially in green vegetables and citrus fruits. However, the content is quite variable from one food to another and within each type, even for foods from the same region and source, depending on species and degree of ripeness (87). Table 6-28 lists the ascorbic acid content of some common foods. Grain products do not contain ascorbic acid unless they have been enriched. Nuts and sweets contain little or no ascorbic acid. The DRI for adult men (90 mg) can be achieved with 1 ½ glasses of freshly squeezed orange juice, or ¾ cup of raw broccoli. Agencies that suggest vitamin C for chemoprevention of chronic disease (U.S. Department of Agriculture, National Cancer Institute) suggest consumption of five servings of fruits/vegetables each day (200 to 280 mg/d). However, in the third National Health and Nutrition Examination Survey (NHANES III),

Table 6-27. Dietary reference intakes for vitamin C

Life stage group	Vitamin C (mg/d)	Life stage group	Vitamin C (mg/d)
Infants		Females	
0–6 mo	40[a]	9–13 y	45
7–12 mo	50[a]	14–18 y	65
Children		19->70 y	75
1–3 y	15	Pregnancy	
4–9 y	25	≤18 y	80
Males		19–50 y	85
9–13 y	45	Lactation	
14–18 y	75	≤18 y	115
19->70 y	90	19–50 y	120

[a] Evidence sufficient to suggest a DRI based only on adequate intake (AI). All others based on recommended dietary allowance (RDA).
From Standing Committee on the Scientific Evaluation of Dietary Reference Intakes, Food and Nutrition Board, Institute of Medicine. *Dietary reference intakes for vitamin C, vitamin E, selenium, and beta-carotene and other carotenoids.* Washington, DC: National Academy Press, 2000.

Table 6-28. Ascorbic acid content of foods

Food	Serving	Ascorbic acid per portion (mg)	Percentage of RDI (60 mg)
Fruits			
Banana	One (9 in)	10	10–24
Cantaloupe	1 cup	68	>100
Orange	Whole (2½ in)	70	>100
Grapefruit	Half, red	47	>40
Strawberries	1 cup	85	>100
Pear	One Bartlett	7	10–24
Apple	One (2.75 in)	8	10–24
Fruit juices			
Orange, fresh	1 cup	124	>100
Orange, frozen	1 cup	97	>100
Grapefruit, canned	1 cup	72	>100
Pineapple, frozen	1 cup	30	>40
Grape drink[a]	1 cup	250	>100
Vegetables			
Green beans, fresh, uncooked	1 cup	18	25–39
Spinach, cooked from fresh	1 cup	40	>40
Cabbage, cooked	1 cup	36	>40
Broccoli, cooked from fresh	1 cup	116	>100
Peas, frozen	½ cup	8	10–24
fresh, cooked	1 cup	23	25–39
Potato, baked	1 each	26	>40
Lettuce, iceberg	1 cup	2.2	1–5
Tomato, fresh	1 each (2.2 in)	22	25–39
Green pepper, fresh	½ cup	44	>40
cooked	½ cup	50	>40
Dairy products			
Milk, cow's, whole	1 cup	2.3	1–5
Milk, human	1 cup	7–12	10–24
Cheese	1 oz	0	0
Egg	1 each	0	0
Meats			
Beef liver, fried	3 oz	19	25–39
Bacon, lunch meat	2 pieces	10	10–24
Fish	3 oz	4	5–12

RDI, recommended dietary intake.
[a] Vitamin C is fortified in some drinks; check label.
Data from Hands ES. *Food finder,* 2nd ed. Salem, OR: ESHA Research, 1990.

vitamin C intake for adults was only 70 to 80 mg/d (88). Furthermore, ascorbic acid is heat-labile and easily destroyed by oxidation. Prolonged exposure to oxygen, iron, or copper destroys the vitamin. In addition, like other water-soluble vitamins, ascorbic acid can be lost in cooking water. Often, only 50% of the content of the raw food survives processing and cooking.

3. **Assessment**

a. **Intake or absorption.** In general, plasma or serum ascorbate levels reflect intake. Low levels do not necessarily indicate scurvy, but scurvy is invariably associated with low levels. Plasma levels may not always reflect intake. Levels of ascorbate may be reduced in patients with chronic inflammatory diseases, cigarette smokers, persons experiencing acute emotional or environmental stress, and women taking oral contraceptives. The nutritional meaning of these changes is obscure. This test is readily available, and its value is that a normal result rules out scurvy. Vitamin C is stable in plasma when collected in metaphosphoric acid. The method of choice for plasma or blood vitamin C measurement is HPLC, according to the recommendations of the World Health Organization (10). Levels below 23 µmol/L indicate deficient intake or absorption (Table 6-29). Seasonal changes occur, with the highest levels seen in summer, when large amounts of fresh fruits and vegetables are consumed. Levels are very high in the first 3 days of life. When intake is decreased, deficiency develops within 3 to 5 months. Severe infections and acute illness can lower serum levels in the absence of deficiency. Levels should be measured in patients at risk, including those with a poor diet (elderly, alcohol or drug abusers, patients with chronic disease or cancer), patients on dialysis, and smokers.

   b. Body stores. Ascorbate concentrations in leukocytes are more closely related to body stores than concentrations in plasma. Red cell levels of ascorbate do not fall with depleted stores. Separation of cells on a Ficoll density gradient followed by HPLC analysis has made accurate measurement possible in blood samples of 2 mL or less. Both ascorbic acid and the oxidized form, dehydroascorbate, can be measured. Because a fivefold variation in vitamin C content (µg/10^8 cells) is seen between mononuclear cells (higher) and polymorphonuclear cells (lower) (10), vitamin C levels vary with differing degrees of leukocytosis. Because the diagnosis of scurvy must be made quickly, a test must be rapid and readily available to be of any use at all. For these reasons, when an assessment is obtained, plasma ascorbate is preferred, even though it does not measure tissue stores. Guidelines for the interpretation of the results of these tests are listed in Table 6-29.

  4. Physiology

   a. Absorption. The absorption of ascorbic acid is carrier-mediated, active, and sodium-dependent. Two sodium-dependent vitamin C cotransporters have been cloned, SVCT1 and SVCT2 (89). SVCT1 is found in kidney, intestine, and liver; SVCT2 is in choroid plexus and retinal pigmented epithelium. Efflux across the basolateral membrane is mediated by an unknown sodium-independent mechanism. Neither cotransporter recognizes oxidized ascorbic acid (dehydroascorbate). This metabolite crosses the blood–brain barrier via the GLUT1 glucose transporter, and ascorbic acid is regenerated in the brain and thus trapped in that tissue.

    The efficiency of ascorbic acid absorption decreases with a daily intake above 180 mg. In such cases, 55% to 90% of the ingested vitamin appears in the urine. The stool contains the rest, with the proportion increasing as the oral dose increases. When excessive ascorbate is

Table 6-29. Guidelines for interpreting vitamin C status

Test	Deficient (high risk)	Low (moderate risk)	Acceptable (low risk)
Serum ascorbic acid (µmol/L)	<11	11–23	>23
Leukocyte ascorbate (µmol/L)	<150	<200	300–600

From second National Health and Nutrition Examination Survey, Canada Nutrition Survey, and reference 10.

ingested, osmotic diarrhea ensues. Ascorbic acid is catabolized to oxalate and accounts for 20% to 30% of urinary oxalate under normal conditions. Ingestion of more than 4 g/d increases urine oxalate excretion. Large doses of vitamin C increase oxalate excretion to 60 to 100 mg/d. The range of molar conversion varies from 2.5% to 3.0%. Average stores are about 900 mg, and the mean daily excretion of dietary vitamin C is 2.7%. At higher doses, the vitamin is uricosuric.

    b. Metabolic functions of ascorbic acid are not completely understood (90). It is important in the hydroxylation of proline and lysine and affects collagen formation. It enhances the hydroxylation of lysine to hydroxylysine, and of proline to hydroxyproline. The collagen matrix produced under stimulation by ascorbic acid may potentiate differentiation. Ascorbic acid influences tyrosine metabolism when large amounts of tyrosine are ingested. It is involved in the formation of norepinephrine from dopamine and in converting tryptophan to 5-hydrotryptophan and subsequently to serotonin. Vitamin C also aids in the synthesis of carnitine and adrenal hormones, and enhances microsomal drug metabolism, wound healing, and leukocyte functions. Ascorbic acid is an excellent antioxidant, scavenging free radicals. The half-life in the body is 10 to 20 days. By its reducing power, the vitamin enhances the absorption of inorganic iron and the transfer of iron from transferrin to ferritin, and it may function as an antioxidant for vitamins A and E. The formylation of tetrahydrofolinic acid is enhanced by vitamin C.

5. Deficiency. Scurvy is manifested by weakness, irritability, bleeding gums, gingivitis, joint pains, and loosening of teeth. Interference with neurotransmitter synthesis may explain the fatigue, weakness, and vasomotor instability associated with scurvy. Hemorrhaging occurs in the skin, especially the perifollicular regions, conjunctivae, nose, and gastrointestinal and genitourinary tracts. Anemia and hyperkeratosis of hair follicles are common. Infants are subject to weight loss and subperiosteal hemorrhage. Cessation of the growth of long bones is a prominent feature of infantile scurvy. Scurvy is a rare disorder in the United States because of the wide availability of fresh fruits and vegetables and the common supplementation of packaged foods with vitamin C. When scurvy occurs, it is usually in alcoholics. Because the assessment of vitamin C stores is difficult, information is lacking about other possible deficiency syndromes. Despite many claims to the contrary, no deficiency state for vitamin C other than scurvy has been documented.

6. Therapy

    a. Scurvy responds to as little as 10 mg of vitamin C per day. A dose of 60 to 100 mg/d is recommended for replenishing body stores. Tablets are available in doses of 25, 50, 100, 250, 500, and 1,000 mg. As a syrup, it is available at a dose of 500 mg/5 mL. Parenteral preparations offer 100, 250, and 500 mg/mL.

    b. Low serum levels of vitamin C. Persons at risk include the elderly (older than 65 years), smokers (especially men), diabetics, and oral contraceptive users. They should be encouraged to increase their vitamin C intake, most likely via a supplement, because five to 10 servings of fruits/vegetables are needed to fulfill their increased requirement.

    c. Prevention of chronic disease. In addition to its antiscorbutic role, many potential benefits of vitamin C have been suggested, so that vitamin C supplements are now more widely used than any others in the United States. Evidence exists for a role of vitamin C in the prevention of cataracts, diabetes, hypertension, coronary heart disease, cancer, asthma, and the common cold (13,90). The data on the prevention of rhinovirus infection are still equivocal (13), but a metaanalysis of the six largest supplementation trials found no benefit for vitamin C (91). Similarly, the evidence for a role in relieving asthma or allergy is equivocal (92). Evidence in small numbers of subjects suggests a possible role for vitamin C in enhancing immune function, but none in exercise-induced oxidative stress (13). Many epidemiologic studies show an inverse correlation between vitamin C levels and coronary artery disease and also between vitamin C levels and hypertension (93,94), but prospective trials have not been performed. The same correlations and lack of prospective interventional studies have been noted for cataracts (13) and gastric, esophageal, oral, and pharyngeal cancers (95). It is reasonable to suggest an increased dietary vitamin C intake for these patients, but it is premature to recommend supplements.

  d. **Iron absorption.** The addition of ascorbate to inorganic iron preparations enhances absorption. The uptake of iron in food is not affected.

  e. **Industrial uses** of ascorbic acid include prevention of food spoilage, maintenance of the red color of canned meat, prevention of rancidity of fats, and stabilization of milk.

7. **Toxicity.** Earlier reports of adverse effects with supplemental vitamin C have largely not been substantiated in normal healthy populations (96). However, a UL for adults has been set at 2,000 mg/d (3) (Appendix B). Although the urinary excretion of oxalate increases with high doses of the vitamin, no relationship with kidney stones has been found in normal persons. Likewise, the inorganic iron-enhancing feature of the vitamin does not affect serum ferritin. High doses of vitamin C do not appear to destroy cobalamin. Nonetheless, it would be well to remember that this lack of toxicity applies only to normal populations, and that high doses of supplemental vitamin C have not been shown to be beneficial. Moderation of intake can be suggested for any patients considered at risk for iron overload or renal oxalate stones.

  The pH of chewable vitamin C tablets (500 mg) is less than 2.0. Because vitamin C acidifies the urine, it can decrease the excretion of acidic drugs such as aspirin and increase the excretion of basic drugs such as tricyclic antidepressants. Large doses (>500 mg) also can interfere with the laboratory measurement of levels of serum bilirubin, glucose, lactic dehydrogenase, and transaminases, and with tests to detect fecal occult blood. Such doses can cause false-negative determinations of urine glucose with glucose oxidase and false-positive determinations with copper reduction or Benedict's solution.

H. Biotin

1. **Requirement.** Biotin is synthesized by many microorganisms, and it is felt that colonic flora contribute to the available biotin in humans. Thus, estimation of the requirement is difficult. It has been suggested that a biotin intake of 60 µg/1,000 kcal prevents deficiency. The estimated safe dietary intake ranges from 30 to 100 µg/d in adults because data on the availability in foods and the intestinal contribution are incomplete. The DRIs for biotin are 5 to 12 µg/d in infants and children, 20 to 25 µg/d in adolescents, and 30 µg/d in adults.

2. **Food sources.** The average diet in the United States contains 100 to 300 µg of biotin. It is present in free and bound forms. In egg yolks, biotin is bound by the protein avidin. Biotin is liberated in the intestine by enzymatic hydrolysis. The vitamin is heat labile, but much of it is retained in processed foods. Rich sources (600 to 2,000 µg/100 g) include yeast extracts, liver and other organ meats, soybeans, and egg yolks. Poor sources (<10 µg/100 g) include muscle meats, dairy products, grains, fruits, and vegetables.

3. **Assessment.** Biotin is measured with *Lactobacillus plantarium* as the assay organism. Values for plasma and whole blood in the literature are variable (10). Normal whole blood levels are 244 ± 61 pmol/L. Mean

urinary excretion is 35 ± 14 nmol/24 h (10). Values well below these have been reported in biotin deficiency. Recent data suggest that decreased urinary excretion of biotin and its metabolite bisnorbiotin, increased urinary excretion of 3-hydroxyisovaleric acid, and decreased activity of propionyl coenzyme A and β-methylcotonyl carboxylases in lymphocytes are good indicators of marginal biotin deficiency (97).

4. **Physiology.** Biotin is a cofactor for carboxylating enzymes. Biotin accepts carbon dioxide to form an intermediate compound and then transfers carbon dioxide to the substrate. It is thus essential as an intermediary in the metabolism of carbohydrate, protein, and fat. Biotin is absorbed by the small intestine and by the colon in the process of facilitated diffusion. An electrogenic sodium–biotin cotransport system has been identified. Colonic and small-bowel absorption explains the rarity of human deficiency states. Fecal synthesis by bacteria is prominent but can be inhibited by broad-spectrum antibiotics.

5. **Deficiency**

   a. **Dietary biotin deficiency** is rare in humans (98). High levels of phenylpyruvate, seen in phenylketonuria, inhibit pyruvate carboxylase and lead to a functional biotin deficiency. In experimental deficiency, a maculopapular dermatitis (along with lingual atrophy) and pallor are noted after many weeks. Lassitude, muscle pain, paresthesias, and anorexia with nausea occur. In some children with seborrheic dermatitis, biotin levels are low. Ingestion of large amounts of raw egg has produced a deficiency as a result of an excess of avidin, which binds biotin. Biotin deficiency as a complication of long-term total parenteral nutrition can produce alopecia and dermatitis (99). Dermatitis and alopecia are also seen in deficiencies of essential fatty acids and zinc. Biotin deficiency produces a scaly dermatitis, whereas in zinc deficiency, the dermatitis is more moist. A correlation between marginal biotin status and teratogenicity has been reported during pregnancy (100).

   b. **Biotin-responsive carboxylase deficiencies** have been rarely reported. The affected children present with an erythematous rash, alopecia, and keratoconjunctivitis. It is not clear that the syndrome is caused by biotin deficiency, but at least one case has responded to biotin supplements of 10 mg/d (101).

   c. **Biotinidase deficiency** is an autosomal recessive disorder in which biotin cannot be cleaved from peptides and recycled. Patients may become biotin-deficient during early childhood, with seizures, rash, alopecia, ataxia, hearing loss, delayed development, coma, and death. A simple screening test is available for blood in neonates, and the symptoms are reversed by pharmacologic doses (10 mg) of biotin provided they are given early in the course (102).

6. **Therapy.** The addition of 200 to 1,000 μg of biotin daily reverses the symptoms of deficiency. The vitamin is available in multivitamin preparations and as 1-, 5-, and 10-mg tablets.

7. **Toxicity.** No toxic effects have been reported, and no UL has been established.

I. **Pantothenic acid (vitamin B₅)**

   1. **Requirement.** When they consume 5 to 7 mg of pantothenic acid daily, normal subjects excrete 2 to 7 mg/d in the urine and 1 to 2 mg/d in the stool. The data are insufficient to base the DRIs for pantothenic acid on RDAs. The AI-based recommendations are 4 mg for adolescents 9 to 13 years old and 5 mg/d for older adolescents and adults (3). The AI for children is 1.7 to 3 mg/d. During pregnancy and lactation, deficiency has not been reported, but increments of 1 and 2 mg/d are suggested, respectively.

   2. **Food sources.** Pantothenic acid is widely distributed in foods, especially in animal tissues, whole-grain cereals, and legumes. Cow's milk

contains 3.5 mg/L. An egg contains 1 mg, and liver contains about 8 mg/100 g. Beef and pork contain about 0.3 to 0.6 mg/100 g. Vegetables and fruits contain less vitamin. Microflora may produce some vitamin, although this has not been clearly demonstrated in humans. Some vitamin is lost during the heating and processing of foods.

3. **Assessment.** Urinary excretion correlates with intake, and excretion of more than 1.0 mg/d is probably normal. No good method exists to determine body stores of pantothenic acid.

4. **Physiology.** Pantothenic acid is the "backbone" of coenzyme A, which is needed to activate acetate for its many functions in the synthesis of fatty acids, cholesterol, and sterols and in acetylation reactions. In addition, it is a key participant in the formation of citric acid, which enters the Krebs cycle.

5. **Deficiency.** A syndrome of spontaneous human deficiency is not clearly recognized. Experimental deficiency induced by an antagonist, ω-methylpantothenic acid, leads to tenderness of the heels and feet, fatigue, paresthesias, weakness, sleep disturbances, irascibility, and leg cramps. The "burning feet" syndrome seen in malnourished persons responds to pantothenic acid and may represent a specific deficiency.

6. **Treatment**
   a. **Deficiency.** If deficiency is suspected, it is treated by the oral administration of 10 mg/d. The vitamin has been used to treat paralytic ileus, with 50 to 100 mg/d given parenterally. No evidence for its effectiveness has been noted. Tablets of 25 and 500 mg are available as calcium pantothenate.
   b. **Conditions other than deficiency.** Pantothenic acid has been studied for its effects on hypercholesterolemia, exercise performance, and arthritis, but data are too fragmentary for any conclusions to be made (13). The vitamin is marketed as an "antistress" treatment, but no evidence supports this claim.

7. **Toxicity.** Daily administration of as little as 10 to 20 mg of the calcium salt has been reported to produce diarrhea. Ordinarily, larger doses are required before this complication is seen. As a result, no UL has been established.

III. **Fat-soluble vitamins.** The functions, symptoms of deficiency, and common food sources of the fat-soluble vitamins are summarized in Table 6-2.
   A. **Vitamin A**
      1. **Requirement**
         a. **RDAs.** The estimated average requirement on which the current RDAs are based is intended to ensure adequate stores of vitamin A (103). The term *vitamin A* refers to retinoids with the biologic activity of retinol, and also includes retinal, the aldehyde, and retinoic acid. The infant AI is derived from the average retinol content of human milk (485 µg/L). If 780 mL of milk is ingested, breast-feeding supplies about 385 µg of retinol. Because of the large body stores in the liver and the lack of functional criteria for vitamin A status in infants, a precise daily requirement for infants is not known. The allowance for adults is based on many experimental nutritional studies and amounts to 900 µg of retinol per day for men and 700 µg for women. The allowance for children and adolescents is extrapolated to fall between the values for infants and those for adults. The allowance is increased only slightly in pregnancy, based on the small fetal hepatic content. The increase during lactation is based on the vitamin A content of milk.

         The determination of dietary vitamin A is complex, and the determination of β-carotene is even more so. Dietary provitamins (of which carotene is the major one) are used much less efficiently than retinol or its esters. No reproducible biologic activities in humans are available to use in establishing the AI. Epidemiologic studies show a correlation between low (but within normal range) serum levels and a variety of chronic diseases, but intervention trials have not produced positive results (104). In addition, some carotenoids (e.g, lutein and zeaxanthin) are preferentially accumulated in the retina and other ocular tissues (105), whereas others lack provitamin A activity but exhibit other biologic activities (e.g., lycopene) (106). Although many observational studies suggest that higher blood levels of β-carotenes and other active carotenoids are associated with a lower risk for several chronic diseases, evidence is not currently convincing that a certain percentage of dietary vitamin A must be derived from provitamin A carotenoids as part of the RDA for vitamin A. However, recommendations to increase the consumption of fruits and vegetables rich in carotenoids for their health-promoting benefits are supported strongly by the Standing Committee on the Scientific Evaluation of Dietary Reference Intakes (4). The RDAs for vitamin A are included in Table 6-30.

   b. Retinol equivalents. Most often, vitamin A activity in foods is expressed in international units; 1 IU is the equivalent of 0.3 μg of all-*trans*-retinol or of 0.6 μg of β-carotene. Since 1969, the RDAs have been expressed as retinol equivalents (REs). This change was considered desirable because of the poorer utilization of dietary provitamins in comparison with retinol. The Committee currently uses retinol activity equivalents (RAEs) to measure dietary provitamin A carotenoids, mainly β-carotene, α-carotene, and β-cryptoxanthin (103). The RAE values of these nutrients have been set at 12, 24, and 24 μg, respectively. The RAE has been estimated as one-half the vitamin A activity in comparison with the RE. This change in equivalence was made because of the observation that β-carotene activity in oil is twice that of dietary β-carotene. As a result of the change, more darkly colored, carotene-rich fruits and vegetables are needed to meet the vitamin A requirement; the change also means that vitamin A intake was overestimated in the past. When the RAE is used, approximately 26% and 34% of vitamin A consumed by men and women, respectively, is derived from provitamin A carotenoids. Ripe or cooked colored fruits and yellow tubers contain more read-

Table 6-30. Recommended daily dietary intakes of vitamin A

Life stage group	Vitamin A (μg/d)	Life stage group	Vitamin A (μg/d)
Infants[a]		Females	
0–6 mo	400	9–13 y	600
7–12 mo	500	14–18 y	700
Children		19–>70 y	700
1–3 y	300	Pregnancy	
4–8 y	400	14–18 y	750
Males		19–50 y	770
9–13 y	600	Lactation	
14–18 y	900	14–18 y	1200
19–>70 y	900	19–50 y	1300

[a] Estimate based on adequate intake (AI). All others based on recommended daily allowance (RDA). From Standing Committee on the Scientific Evaluation of Dietary Reference Intakes, Food and Nutrition Board, Institute of Medicine. Dietary reference intakes for vitamin A, vitamin K, arsenic, boron, chromium, copper, iodine, iron, manganese, molybdenum, nickel, silicon, vanadium, and zinc. Washington, DC: National Academy Press, 2001. Available on line at *http://www.nap.edu/books, Crawler list 0309072794.* Accessed May 30, 2001.

ily converted carotenoids than do equal weights of dark green, leafy vegetables. By the 2001 definition,

1 REA = 1 μg of all-*trans*-retinol
       = 12 μg of all-*trans*-β-carotene
       = 24 μg of other provitamin A carotenoids
       = 3.3 IU of activity from retinol
       = 10.8 IU of activity from β-carotene

The previously accepted 6:1 equivalence of β-carotene to vitamin A has been questioned, also because of the inefficient bioconversion of plant carotenoids (107). Until 10 years ago, the provitamin A content of foods was measured by extinction at 450 nm of a nonpolar organic extract. However, this measurement included carotenoids with no vitamin A activity. Food content is now measured with HPLC, which correctly identifies the provitamin A content. The equivalence from the older measurements may vary from 1:2 in orange fruits to 1:26 in green plants. β-Carotene in red palm oil has an equivalence of 1:2 to 1:3. Thus, with vegetarian diets and in areas where intake from animal sources is poor, a conversion of 21 μg of β-carotene per microgram of retinol has been proposed, which reduces retinol intake to well below the RDA (107). In many regions in Africa, South America, and Asia, supplementation with preformed vitamin A should be considered.

2. Food sources

a. Median daily intake in the United States is about 624 RE. Vitamin A as retinyl esters is found only in animal foods, whereas provitamin or vitamin A precursors are found in the vegetable kingdom. Unfortunately, our knowledge of the content of retinol or β-carotene in many foods is incomplete. Grains and flours are not sources of vitamin A unless egg, milk, or fruit is added to baked goods. More than 600 carotenoids are found in food among the five to 10,000 bioactive plant compounds, only about 50 of which have provitamin A activity and 40 of which are part of the usual diet in the United States. Only about 20 carotenoids are found in human blood and tissues, the most abundant of which (in the United States) are β-carotene, lycopene, α-carotene, lutein, and zeaxanthin. Table 6-31 lists the vitamin A content and RE values of selected foods. Losses of vitamin A during cooking are small. Many food lists are still given in IUs. When IUs are given for vegetable sources, the total must be divided by 6 to estimate the REs because of poor absorption and conversion to retinol. The Committee on Dietary Allowances of the Food and Nutrition Board recommends that food tables list retinol and provitamin carotenoids separately so that the total REs (μg) can be calculated.

b. Bioavailability. In many countries, including the United States, dairy products and margarines are supplemented with retinyl esters, which are the main dietary source (108). Factors that affect bioavailability include fiber intake (109), cholesterol-lowering drugs (110), and fat-free foods. Human milk contains 400 to 600 RE/L. A linear decline in levels is seen during the first 6 weeks after childbirth. Esters (85% of the total) are split by milk lipase, which is activated by bile salts (111). Richer sources among animal foods are liver and enriched dairy products.

Many factors affect the absorption of vitamin A and carotenoids, and therefore their bioavailability. These factors are generally more significant for carotenoids. In general, pigmented vegetables and fruits, especially the yellow ones, contain large amounts of β-carotene. Dried fruits are concentrated sources. Table 6-32 provides an estimate of carotenoid sources in foods.

Table 6-31. Approximate vitamin A content of selected foods

Food	Portion	RE As retinol	RE As pro-vitamins	Percentage of RDI (1,000 RE)
Grains				
Corn bread	1 muffin	16	16	1–5
Wheat bread	1 slice	0	0	0
Meats				
Salmon	3 oz	43		1–5
Liver, beef	3 oz	9,119		>100
Chicken, roasted	1 cup	22		1–5
Shrimp	1 oz	6		>1
Tuna, fresh broiled	3 oz	642		>40
Tuna, canned, water	4 oz	62		5–12
Fruits and vegetables				
Apple	2.75 in		7	1–5
Orange	2.6 in		27	<1
Strawberries	1 cup		5	>40
Cantaloupe	1 cup		516	>40
Watermelon	1 cup		59	5–12
Green beans, fresh	1 cup		83	5–12
Spinach, cooked, fresh	1 cup		1,750	>100
Corn, cooked, fresh	½ cup		18	1–5
Potatoes, white	8.75 in		0	0
Potatoes, sweet	1 each		2,450	>100
Carrots, cooked	½ cup		1,292	>100
Tomatoes	1 each		139	10–24
Dried apricots	16 halves		676	>40
Dried prunes	7 halves		187	10–24
Dairy				
Milk				
Whole	1 cup	76		5–12
Skim, enriched	1 cup	149		10–24
Eggs, large	1 each	97		5–12
Butter	1 tbs	106		5–12
Ice cream	1 cup	133		10–24

RE, retinol equivalents; RDI, recommended dietary intake.
Data from Hands ES. *Food finder,* 2nd ed. Salem, OR: ESHA Research, 1990.

3. Assessment

a. Intake or absorption. Carotene is not stored in the body. Thus, persons with only preformed vitamin A in their diet will have vitamin A in their serum without carotene. The intake of both carotene and vitamin A is reflected in the serum levels. Total and individual carotenoids are easily determined by HPLC methods; when this test is performed, it is important to determine whether carotene has been ingested recently.

When intake is persistently low, the serum vitamin A level falls, reflecting the low intake and marginal body stores. With continued low intake, serum levels fall further and reflect decreased body stores. Low carotene levels are meaningful only if carotene is being ingested in the diet. Furthermore, low levels do not distinguish low intake from

Table 6-32. Relative content of carotenoids in food sources

Food	β-Carotene	α-Carotene	Lutein/ zeaxanthin	Lycopene
Apricots	4+	—	—	1+
Beet greens	1+	tr	—	—
Broccoli, cooked	1+	—	1+	—
Carrot, cooked	3+	2+	—	—
Corn	tr	—	—	1+
Mango	1+	tr	—	—
Spinach, raw	2+	—	3+	—
Tomato juice, canned	1+	—	—	1+

1+, 8–25 mg/3.5 oz; 2+, 25–60 mg/3.5 oz; 3+, 60–110 mg/3.5 oz; 4+, >110 mg/3.5 oz.
From Sauberlich HE. *Laboratory tests for the assessment of nutritional status,* 2nd ed. Boca Raton, FL: CRC Press, 1999.

poor absorption. Therefore, spot vitamin A and carotene levels by themselves are poor screening tests for malabsorption.

b. Body stores. The stellate (Ito) cells contain stores of vitamin A as esters, which are hydrolyzed and taken up by hepatocytes or parenchymal cells when needed. These stores turn over at a rate of 0.5%/d in adults. The storage efficiency of dietary vitamin A is about 50% in the repleted state. The liver produces retinol-binding protein, which is secreted into the serum and metabolized by the kidney. Vitamin A nutritional status is tested by serum/plasma retinol concentrations, serum retinol-binding protein levels, and relative dose–response assay (10).

   (1) Retinol can be measured by fluorometric, spectrophotometric, or HPLC methods, and retinol measurement is the most commonly used method to determine vitamin A status. The World Health Organization recommends HPLC methods for population surveys. The vitamin is stable in serum or plasma for up to 2 years. Serum vitamin A levels reflect body stores, but only when the level is very low is the interpretation clear (Table 6-33).

Table 6-33. Guidelines in interpreting serum vitamin A and carotene levels

Interpretation	Vitamin A (µg/dL)	Vitamin A (µmol/L)	Carotene (µg/dL)	Carotene (µmol/L)
Normal	>20	>0.7	>40	>1.4
Normal, not ingesting vegetables	>20	>0.7	<40	<1.4
Low intake, marginal stores	10–19	0.35–0.66	20–39	0.7–1.34
Deficient stores	<10	<0.35	Variable	
Severe liver disease	<20	<0.7	>40	>1.4
Excess vitamin A ingestion	>65	>2.28	>40	>1.4
Excess carotene ingestion (also, hypothyroidism, hyperlipidemia, anorexia nervosa, hypercholesterolemia of diabetes)	>20	>0.7	>300	>10.5

From Sauberlich HE. *Laboratory tests for the assessment of nutritional status,* 2nd ed. Boca Raton, FL: CRC Press, 1999.

Serum vitamin A levels increase somewhat with age but usually do not exceed 65 μg/dL. Samples should be obtained in the fasting state to avoid the fluctuations that follow meals. Retinol levels can decline with fever, physical exercise, and prolonged exposure to the sun. Occasionally, the serum level of vitamin A may be normal in the face of depleted hepatic stores. This situation may be seen in alcoholic liver disease—either fatty liver or alcoholic hepatitis. The therapeutic implications of such a discrepancy are not clear because an adequate serum level would imply adequate tissue delivery.

Low levels of vitamin A can be unrelated to decreased intake or absorption, as in chronic infection and liver disease. In severe liver disease, the vitamin A level falls because retinol-binding protein is not produced. However, carotene is not converted to vitamin A, and carotene levels tend to rise. The serum retinol concentration usually decreases transiently because of a diminished release of retinol-binding protein during an acute-phase response to trauma or inflammation (112).

This finding complicates the use of serum retinol as an indicator of vitamin A stores. It is unclear whether the fall in serum retinol occurs only in patients who have a marginally sufficient vitamin A status and whether they require therapy. Levels of vitamin A can be elevated (>100 μg/dL) in patients on hemodialysis because of impaired conversion of retinol to retinoic acid in the kidney. Elevated carotene levels with low vitamin A levels are sometimes seen in anorexia nervosa. Pregnancy and the use of oral contraceptives raise vitamin A levels by increasing serum retinol-binding protein. Because retinol-binding protein is catabolized in kidney, vitamin A levels rise in renal disease.

(2) **Retinol-binding protein and transthyretin (prealbumin).** Retinol-binding protein circulates as a 1:1 molar complex; filtration and loss from the kidney are prevented by prealbumin. The normal concentrations in plasma are 40 to 50 μg/mL (1.9 to 2.4 μmol/L) for retinol-binding protein and 200 to 300 μg/mL for prealbumin. Radial immunodiffusion assay kits are commercially available. Retinol and retinol-binding protein levels are lowered in diabetes, zinc deficiency, and protein–calorie malnutrition, and in response to trauma and infection. Levels of both parameters are elevated in women taking oral contraceptive pills. Liver disease lowers the levels of retinol-binding protein and transthyretin, whereas renal disease raises them. In these situations, the serum levels of vitamin A do not correlate with body stores.

(3) **Relative dose–response assay.** This test is based on the fact that when vitamin A stores are low, aporetinol-binding protein accumulates in the liver. Thus, the test measures the changes in retinol concentration in serum following the administration of a small oral dose (450 to 1,000 μg) of retinol. An increase of more than 20% implies low hepatic stores of retinol. Because the test depends on hepatic synthesis of the binding protein, a false-negative result can be obtained in the presence of liver disease, protein malnutrition, infection, inflammation, or trauma.

(4) **Functional assays.** The conjunctival impression cytology assay provides an early measure of histologic ocular changes. Examination for night blindness also can be sensitive in establishing vitamin A deficiency (113). The clinical demonstration of night blindness also provides evidence of inadequate body stores. Impaired dark adaptation is an early sign of vita-

min A deficiency in patients with cirrhosis. However, this finding is not specific, resulting also from zinc and protein deficiency.

4. **Physiology** (103)

   a. **Absorption.** Vitamin A is usually ingested as the ester or as
carotene and is hydrolyzed by pancreatic and brush border enzymes
before absorption. Carotenes in food are bound to macromolecules
and are more poorly absorbed than either dietary or synthetic vitamin A. Factors that influence vitamin A or carotenoid release from
food and its inclusion in lipid droplets in the intestinal lumen include heating (increased), ingestion of lipid-rich foods (increased),
and lipid malabsorption or ingestion of lipid drugs or additives (decreased). Such compounds include mineral oil, cholestyramine (which
causes fat malabsorption), and olestra. In addition, some carotenoids
are more lipophilic (carotenes, lycopene) than others (lutein, zeaxanthin), which affects their relative rates of absorption (106). Lycopene
is absorbed more slowly in cigarette smokers.

   b. **Metabolism of retinol and carotene.** Inside the enterocyte, retinol
is converted back to a retinyl ester by the action of acyl coenzyme A:
retinol acyltransferase or lecithin coenzyme A: retinol acyltransferase
and is incorporated into chylomicrons (114). Carotene is either hydrolyzed in the enterocyte to two retinol molecules or absorbed intact. In
the former case, it is handled like dietary retinol; in the latter, it is
transported intact in the lymphatics. About 10% of the carotene
cleaved in the gut is converted to retinoic acid, a metabolite that supports cell growth but does not function in the visual cycle or in reproduction. Most absorbed retinol arrives at the liver in chylomicron
remnants, and uptake is mediated by LDL receptors on hepatocytes.
Retinol is released bound to retinol-binding protein and taken up by
stellate (Ito) cells. The retinyl esters are stored in lipid droplets in Ito
cells in the liver or are converted to retinol for transport to the tissues.
Absorbed carotene is also converted to retinol in the liver. A small percentage ($\sim 10\%$) of hepatic retinol is converted to retinoic acid via the
aldehyde retinal.

   c. **Enterohepatic circulation of retinoic acid.** Retinoic acid is conjugated with glucuronide and excreted in the bile to be reabsorbed
by the intestine via the portal vein. This enterohepatic circulation
retains retinoic acid, which is not helpful for visual functions. The
concentration of vitamin A metabolites in bile is low when liver
stores are low, but the excretion rate increases proportionally as hepatic reserves enlarge (115). However, in malabsorptive states,
those metabolites are lost from the body. Because body stores of
retinol are converted in part to retinoic acid, this loss can lead to a
further depletion of the body pool of retinol, but the significance of
the loss is unknown. In vitamin A deficiency, little of the incoming
vitamin is deposited in the liver but is delivered to depleted tissues.

   d. **Function of retinol.** Retinol maintains normal epithelia by aid-
ing in glycoprotein synthesis. It (but not retinoic acid) also forms an
essential part of the visual cycle and is required for normal reproductive function. Vitamin A is felt to play a role in cell growth. It
suppresses malignant transformation of cell lines, prevents chemical induction of some animal tumors *in vivo,* and has been reported
to induce regression of basal cell carcinomas. Vitamin A plays a
major role in cell differentiation and morphogenesis. Thus, it is important in reproduction, bone development, skin integrity, and immunity. Retinoic acid, transported to the nucleus, interacts with one
or more retinoic acid receptors, which are members of the super-
family of secosteroid receptors. The effect of retinoic acid is not limited to embryonic tissues, but the precise mechanism by which it
mediates differentiation is not known.

e. **Function of carotenoids.** Carotenoids mediate many functions, including antioxidation, intercellular communication, immune response, neoplastic transformation, and modification of detoxifying enzymes (116). These effects can be mediated by the parent carotenoid or by retinoid metabolites and are influenced by other carotenoids and metabolic products. Thus, it is not possible to estimate the overall effect of carotenoids in humans, and no reproducible effect has been identified other than their provitamin A activity.

The evidence that carotenes are antioxidants is crucial to their use in nondeficiency states, but in fact, it is not clear that they are general antioxidants. They are good scavengers of singlet oxygen, but they are neither generalized reducing agents (like vitamin C) nor universal antioxidants (like vitamin E). β-Carotene differs greatly in potency from system to system in comparison with vitamin E (116). Moreover, its antioxidant properties are unpredictable in humans. Although β-carotene has been approved as an antioxidant in foods and supplements, the Food and Drug Administration has noted that no direct scientific evidence exists for such activity in humans and has based its decision to allow the antioxidant label on the antioxidant properties of β-carotene demonstrated *in vitro*.

5. **Deficiency.** The only unequivocal clinical signs of deficiency in humans occur in the eye. These changes have been classified in five stages, listed in order of increasing severity:

X0—Effect on the retina: poor dark adaptation.
X1—Effect on the conjunctiva: xerosis (dryness) detected by dullness of the conjunctiva in bright light; frequent presence of Bitot's spots, an accumulation of foamy white debris and fatty material near the limits of the eye, especially laterally.
X2—Effect on the cornea: xerosis along with superficial erosion.
X3—Effect on the cornea: irreversible corneal ulceration.
X4—Effect on the cornea: scarring and softening.

In the United States, only night blindness is usually encountered, most frequently in chronic alcoholics. Persons with malabsorptive states are the other major group at risk for vitamin A deficiency. When zinc deficiency is also present, the effect on visual adaptation may be magnified.

6. **Therapy.** When vitamin A is used for therapy, it is provided entirely in the form of retinol, and its biologic potency is expressed in IUs. In this use, therefore, 1 IU and 1 RE are identical. Because of continued frequent use, the doses are listed here in IUs.

a. **Deficiency.** Deficiency states respond to daily doses of vitamin A from 5,000 to 30,000 IU. The higher doses should be used when severe malabsorption is the cause of the deficiency. A dose of 5,000 IU three times weekly has been effective in treating vitamin A deficiency in low-birth-weight infants, and in slightly decreasing the risk for lung disease (117). Vitamin A is available in liquid form (5,000 IU/0.1 mL); an emulsifier solubilizes the vitamin but probably does not enhance absorption when bile acids are deficient in the intestinal lumen. The vitamin is also available as capsules of 5,000 to 50,000 IU and in injectable forms (50,000 IU/mL).

Therapeutic doses of vitamin A are available as retinol, whereas the RDA of 5,000 IU (1,000 μg RE) per day assumes an intake that is half retinol and half β-carotene. Thus, 5,000 IU of retinol, the "standard" replacement dose, is in fact excessive. This is one of the reasons why vitamin A toxicity develops in some persons when it is taken in large doses.

b. **Vitamin A derivatives.** 13-*cis*-Retinoic acid and eretrinate, an aromatic analogue, have been used to treat severe acne, rosacea, fulminant psoriasis, and Darier's disease. Eretrinate has been reported to decrease bronchial metaplasia in heavy smokers, but serum levels of vitamin A are normal in patients with cancer. All-*trans*-retinoic acid is effective in the treatment of acute promyelocytic leukemia by causing blast cells to differentiate (118). However, no other differentiating agents have been useful in other forms of leukemias.

  c. **Prevention of chronic disease.** Because of their antioxidant properties *in vitro,* carotenoids have been implicated in many chronic diseases often linked with vitamins E and C, the other vitamin antioxidants (13,104,116). Several epidemiologic cohort and case–control studies have shown that the ingestion of foods containing carotenoids (but not preformed vitamin A) is associated with a lower risk for breast cancer. In the Alpha-Tocopherol Beta-Carotene (ATBC) Cancer Prevention Study, male smokers were given either 20 mg of β-carotene and 50 mg of α-tocopherol versus placebo, or 30 mg of β-carotene with 25,000 IU of retinyl palmitate for 5 to 8 years (119,120). Neither study showed a reduction in lung cancer incidence or mortality. The effect of 20 mg of β-carotene and 50 mg of α-tocopherol on the incidence of major coronary events in male smokers was also examined, but no effect was found (121). More deaths occurred in a subgroup with previous myocardial infarction, so that it was recommended that such supplements not be used by male smokers with heart disease (122). In another large study, in which male physicians took 50 mg of β-carotene every other day for a period of 12 years, no benefit or harm was noted, even among the smokers (123). Only limited evidence in small studies suggests a role for β-carotene in improving immune function (13). Intake of lutein and zeaxanthin has been inversely correlated with the risk of cataract extraction (104,124), but in another report of the ATBC Study, taking supplements had no effect on either the prevalence of cataracts or age-related maculopathy (13).

  d. **Prevention of infection.** Vitamin A has been used to treat children severely ill with measles (125) and at doses of 8,333 IU/d to prevent mortality from infection in children less than 3 years old in areas where deficiency is endemic (126).

7. **Toxicity**
  a. **Amount of intake.** Because vitamin A is readily stored in the body, toxic levels can accumulate if intake is excessive. At levels of daily intake above 4,000 IU/kg (especially >500,000 IU/d), toxic symptoms can develop (127). These levels can easily be achieved by the use of supplements that offer the vitamin in capsules of 50,000 IU. Unfortunately, these higher doses of vitamin A can be obtained without a prescription. Toxicity is correlated with serum levels above 1,000 µg/dL, with intake of 18,000 IU/d for 1 to 3 months in infants less than 6 months old, and with intake of 1 million IU for 3 days, 50,000 IU/d for more than 18 months, or 500,000 IU/d for 2 months in adults. UL values have been set for adults at 3,000 µg of retinol per day (~ 10,000 IU) (103) (Appendix B).
  b. **Manifestations.** In children with acute hypervitaminosis A (>10 times the RDA), vomiting and bulging fontanelles are noted. In older children, growth failure, pseudotumor cerebri, sixth nerve paresis, and optic atrophy develop. At all ages, nonspecific findings such as irritability, skin dryness, desquamation of the skin over the palms and soles, myalgia, arthralgia, abdominal pain, and hypoplastic anemia may be present. Hepatosplenomegaly also occurs. In chronic hypervitaminosis, cortical thickening of bones of the hands and feet develops, with tenderness and weakness. Premature closure of the epiphyses has been observed.

In adults, early symptoms of overdose include nausea, vomiting, anorexia, malaise, cracking of skin and lips, headache, and irritability. Long-term use of vitamin A by the elderly can lead to increased plasma levels of retinol and biochemical evidence of liver damage (10). Hepatic fibrosis has been associated with excessive ingestion of vitamin A in a few cases. In adults receiving 50,000 to 100,000 IU/d, nausea, vomiting, skin desquamation, fatigue, hair loss, bone pain, and hepatomegaly can occur (128). One case–control study has shown that a high intake of dietary retinol is associated with an increased risk for osteoporosis (129).

c. **Teratogenicity.** Doses of 15,000 IU/d ingested between days 14 and 40 of gestation can cause microcephaly, dilated ventricles, and aqueduct stenosis. Spontaneous abortions have been reported with isotretinoin. Microphthalmos and atresia of the external auditory meatus have been reported. The risk of a malformation in the newborn was 1 in 57 for mothers who ingested more than 10,000 IU of preformed vitamin A as a supplement during pregnancy (130). However, mothers ingesting supplemental vitamin A in current multivitamin preparations (up to 6,000 IU/d) were not found to be at increased risk for delivering infants with birth defects. Thus, it is probably safe for mothers to ingest an amount of vitamin A not in excess of the RDA (800 RE, or 2,640 IU of vitamin A as retinol). Because folate supplementation, needed to prevent neural tube defects, is most readily available in multivitamin preparations, it is important that mothers not shun both supplements for fear of excessive vitamin A ingestion.

d. **Retinoic acid syndrome.** Retinoic acid syndrome is the main adverse event resulting from tretinoin therapy for promyelocytic leukemia. It is characterized by elevated and rising leukocyte counts, weight gain, respiratory distress, serous effusions, and cardiac and renal failure (131). The average time of onset is 7 to 12 days, but it can begin after 1 day of treatment. It can be reversed or controlled with dexamethasone.

B. Vitamin D

1. Requirement

a. **Types of vitamin D.** Vitamin D_2 is produced during ultraviolet irradiation of ergosterol, a plant sterol. Vitamin D_3, cholecalciferol, is formed from 7-dehydrocholesterol in the skin by the action of ultraviolet light. About 100 IU is produced per day from endogenous sources in persons living in temperate zones. The maximum amount of previtamin converted to vitamin D_3 is increased by an elevated skin temperature and is limited to 15% to 20% daily regardless of the amount of light. This limitation is a consequence of photoisomerization to other compounds. Because more than 90% of circulating 25-hydroxycholecalciferol (25-hydroxyvitamin D_3) in the plasma is derived from vitamin D_3 and thus is endogenously produced, the daily requirement has not been established. Moreover, intake becomes important in persons with normal absorption only when exposure to sunlight is limited. Estimated allowances were previously given in IUs but now are usually expressed as micrograms of cholecalciferol (10 µg of cholecalciferol = 400 IU of vitamin D).

b. **DRI.** Vitamin D in a dose of 2.5 µg (100 IU) prevents rickets, but 10 µg (400 IU) was recommended previously as the RDA for growing children. This recommendation represented in part the underdeveloped 25-hydroxylase activity in the liver of newborns. After the age of 24 years, 5 µg (200 IU) was considered adequate. After a careful review of the literature in 1997, the Institute of Medicine concluded that it is not possible to determine an RDA for vitamin D, but suggested an AI of 5 µg for infants, older children, and young adults

(Table 6-34). This AI recommendation was based on the literature and assumed some exposure to sunlight. In some elderly patients (>70 years), calcium intake and exposure to the sun may be decreased, and they may convert less of the dietary previtamin to the active form and produce less active metabolites of vitamin D in response to calcium depletion. Vitamin D deficiency is more prevalent in persons over the age of 50 than in younger adults. Thus, the recommended AI of vitamin D for adults older than 50 years is now set at twice that of younger adults, and for adults older than 70 years, it is three times greater (15 µg or 600 IU/d). A UL for infants 0 to 12 months of age has been set at 25 µg/d (1,000 IU), and for older children and adults it has been set at 50 µg/d (2,000 IU).

Some estimates of vitamin D requirements in the absence of the skin supply exceed 15 µg/d, so that concern has been expressed that the current recommendation is not high enough for patients not exposed to sunlight (132). Moreover, oral vitamin D is inactivated by the liver, unlike that supplied by skin, which makes vitamin D supplements more problematic in patients with chronic liver disease. The DRI of 5 µg is considered adequate for all healthy children and adults exposed to some sunlight, but at least 15 µg should be supplied daily to people not exposed to sunlight.

2. **Food sources.** Endogenous production is the most important source. The usual dietary intake in the United States is 1.25 to 1.75 µg/d (U.S. Department of Agriculture, *National Food Consumption Survey, 1977–1978*). The major natural food sources are fatty fish (e.g., mackerel, salmon), fish liver and oils, egg yolk, and beef liver. Fortified foods now provide the major dietary source. The reason for the high vitamin D content of fish liver is not apparent. It has been speculated that fish liver contains a nonphotochemical system for making vitamin D, but no real evidence for such a system has been found. Table 6-35 lists the major dietary sources of vitamin D. The content in cow's milk varies with the seasons from 4 IU/qt in winter to 40 IU/qt in summer, unless supplements are added. The mean concentration of vitamin D in human milk is 0.5 µg/L and is proportional to maternal intake. This is well below the level needed to prevent rickets, yet rickets occurs only when milk is not given and sunshine is not provided. Thus, vitamin D in milk may be more biologically available than that from other dietary sources.

In NHANES III (1988–1994), 5% to 7% of men more than 20 years of age had 25-hydroxyvitamin D serum concentrations of 15 ng/mL or less, whereas 12% to 15% of women had these levels (133). However, almost no adults had a vitamin level above 50 ng/mL. Thus, relatively more

Table 6-34. Dietary reference intakes of vitamin D[a]

Life stage group	Vitamin D (µg/d)	Life stage group	Vitamin D (µg/d)
Infants/children		Females	
0–8 y	5	9–50 y	5
Males		51–70 y	10
9–50 y	5	>70 y	15
51–70 y	10	Pregnancy/lactation	
>70 y	15	≤18–50 y	5

[a] All values based on adequate intake (AI).
From Standing Committee on the Scientific Evaluation of Dietary Reference Intakes, Food and Nutrition Board, Institute of Medicine. *Dietary reference intakes for calcium, phosphorus, magnesium, vitamin D, and fluoride.* Washington, DC: National Academy Press, 1997.

Table 6-35. Foods sources of vitamin D

Food	Portion	Vitamin D content (IU)
Milk, whole	1 cup	100
Butter	1 tsp	1.4
Cheese, cottage	1 cup	5
Egg yolk	1 each	23
Egg white	1 each	0
Beef liver	3 oz	11.9
Oysters, raw	4 each	2.9
Canned sardines	1 oz	85
Canned salmon	1 oz	142
Lunch meats	1 piece	8–12
Margarine	1 tsp	15
Cod liver	1 tsp	400

Data from Hands ES. *Food finder,* 2nd ed. Salem, OR: ESHA Research, 1990.

older persons in the United States have a marginal vitamin D status and are at risk for complications related to vitamin D deficiency. In fact, postmenopausal women presenting with hip fractures have evidence of vitamin D insufficiency (lower 25-hydroxyvitamin D levels) in comparison with women undergoing elective hip replacement (134).

3. **Assessment.** Assessment of vitamin D status may include measurement of serum 25-hydroxyvitamin D (body stores), serum 1,25-dihydroxyvitamin D (renal metabolism), or serum levels of total and ionized calcium, inorganic phosphate, and alkaline phosphatase (late-stage tissue damage) (10).

   a. **25-Hydroxyvitamin D_3.** The 25-hydroxyvitamin D_3 level is low when body stores, intake, or endogenous production is low, and measurement of this level is a satisfactory (but not sensitive) method for assessing deficiency of the vitamin D body pool. The available methods include HPLC, competitive protein binding, and radioimmunoassay. HPLC methods are good for determining both vitamin D metabolites in a single serum sample. Commercial radioimmunoassay kits are also available that are equally sensitive and practical, but they measure only one metabolite at a time. The cutoff values for vitamin D deficiency are below 30 nmol/L (Table 6-36).

Table 6-36. Suggested guidelines for evaluating vitamin D status

Test	Deficient	Low	Acceptable	High
25-Hydroxyvitamin D				
(nmol/L)	≤12	<25	≥30	>200
(ng/mL)	≤4.8	<10	≥12	>80
1,25-Dihydroxyvitamin D				
(pmolL)			48–100	
(pg/mL)			20–42	
24 Hour urinary calcium (mg/kg)	<2		>2	
Bone density (SD from mean)	>2.5	>2	1–1.5	

Data derived in part from Sauberlich HE. *Laboratory tests for the assessment of nutritional status,* 2nd ed. Boca Raton, FL: CRC Press, 1999.

(1) Regulation. More than 90% of plasma 25-hydroxyvitamin D is derived from cholecalciferol produced by the skin. However, the production of this vitamin is not closely regulated—that is, levels rise or fall as its precursor is made available. The mitochondrial 25-hydroxylase is not regulated by vitamin D, unlike the microsomal enzyme, which is regulated by its substrate. Concentration in plasma is five to 10 times greater than in other tissues, except for adipose tissue. The 25-hydroxyvitamin D_3 in plasma is bound to a protein that binds all metabolites and is less than 5% saturated. Finally, the plasma half-life of 25-hydroxyvitamin D_3 is long (24 hours). Thus, the level reflects recent intake or exposure to sunlight, so that the sensitivity of this measurement in the assessment of vitamin D deficiency is limited.

(2) Interpretation. The binding capacity of the plasma for excess 25-hydroxyvitamin D_3 is very great, and levels rise as intake increases. Moreover, levels remain elevated for some time. Therefore, the 25-hydroxyvitamin D_3 level reflects vitamin D intake or production only in a general way but does correlate with body stores until they become depleted. Levels of 25-hydroxyvitamin D_3 are low in states of dietary deficiency, decreased absorption, deficiency of ultraviolet light, prematurity, and severe liver disease, and when drugs are ingested that alter its metabolism (e.g., anticonvulsants). Levels are low when plasma binding capacity is decreased. Levels are high in growing children, conditions associated with hyperparathyroidism, sarcoidosis, and certain forms of idiopathic hypercalciuria (135). Factors other than intake affect plasma levels of 25-hydroxyvitamin D_3. The amount of ultraviolet irradiation reaching production sites in the skin is affected by the intensity of sunlight, thickness of the ozone layer, and pigmentation of the skin. Thus, the 25-hydroxyvitamin D_3 level rises in summer and falls in winter. Pregnancy, ovulation, and the use of oral contraceptives increase the plasma level of vitamin D-binding protein. Because this protein is normally unsaturated, usually only the capacity of the plasma to retain vitamin D metabolites is increased, not the steady-state levels of the metabolites. Despite these confounding factors, the 25-hydroxyvitamin D_3 level is the best available test for determining vitamin D status. The level is almost always low when deficiency is present.

(3) Intoxication. The 25-hydroxyvitamin D_3 level is an accurate parameter of vitamin D intoxication because the level rises progressively as intake is increased. Intoxication is indicated by levels above 150 ng/mL (375 nmol/L).

b. 1,25-Dihydroxyvitamin D_3

(1) Regulation. The production of this vitamin is regulated, but not by vitamin D stores unless they are extremely low. The metabolite is assayed by HPLC or by radioimmunoassay with use of a nuclear receptor. The normal concentration of 20 to 42 pg/mL (48 to 100 pmol/L) cannot be increased by feeding 1,25-dihydroxyvitamin D_3. Normal ranges differ with the age and calcium intake of the population studied. Fluctuations occur during the ovulation cycle and also diurnally. Levels are higher during periods of growth and decline during growth retardation. The serum concentration responds to calcium and phosphate levels and is part of the endocrine system of vitamin D metabolism. The production rate and concentration of this vitamin are altered rapidly and inversely by high (3 g/d) and low (0.5 g/d) intakes of phosphorus (136). The plasma half-life is 4 to 6 hours, hence the rapid functional changes. The level of this form of vitamin D correlates with certain functions of vitamin D but not with intake, absorption, or body stores until deficiency is apparent. Values of 25-hydroxyvitamin D_3 fall in the winter and are lower in patients over 60 years of age.

    (2) **Interpretation.** Various conditions are associated with abnormal values. 1,25-Dihydroxyvitamin D_3 levels are low in profound vitamin D deficiency, chronic renal disease (if serum phosphorus levels are high and renal enzyme activity is decreased despite elevated parathyroid hormone levels), hypoparathyroidism, vitamin D-resistant rickets type I, and osteolytic states not related to parathyroid hormone (cancer, hyperthyroidism, and possibly osteoporosis of the elderly). However, 1,25-dihydroxyvitamin D_3 levels do not always reflect total body stores. In primary biliary cirrhosis, this metabolite is not excreted in bile, so that synthesis is decreased and plasma levels are normal, yet malabsorption of vitamin D and osteopenia develop (137). Primary hyperparathyroidism, vitamin D-resistant rickets type II, and pregnancy are conditions in which 1,25-dihydroxyvitamin D_3 levels are elevated. In hypervitaminosis D, the 25-hydroxyvitamin D_3 level is markedly elevated, but the 1,25-dihydroxyvitamin D_3 level is altered only slightly.

  c. Twenty-four–hour urinary calcium excretion. Because of problems with the interpretation or availability of vitamin D metabolite levels, the state of vitamin D repletion is often assessed by functional measurements. This is best accomplished in patients with a normal intestine by measuring the 24-hour urinary calcium excretion as an estimate of calcium absorption. At steady state, urinary calcium excretion equals net intestinal absorption. If no intestinal disease is present and the serum parathyroid hormone level is normal, calcium absorption depends in large part on the active vitamin D metabolites. Patients should be kept on a constant calcium intake of 800 to 1,200 mg/d for 4 to 5 days before a 24-hour urine sample is collected. Normal urinary calcium levels range from 100 to 300 mg (about 2 to 4 mg/kg of body weight).

  d. Serum alkaline phosphatase levels become elevated in osteomalacia secondary to vitamin D deficiency. However, the increase develops late in deficiency states, and elevations of phosphatase occur for a large number of other reasons. Thus, the usefulness of this test is limited.

  e. Bone densitometry. Single-photon absorptiometry of the forearm and os calcis is rapid (15 minutes) and relatively inexpensive. However, in patients under the age of 60 years, it does not assess risk for vertebral fracture. Computed tomography and dual-photon absorptiometry of the spine are better predictors of vertebral fracture (see section on assessment of calcium deficiency in Chapter 7). For patients at risk for vitamin D deficiency, these screening tests are very useful. Their role in screening postmenopausal women for osteoporosis is much less clear. 25-Hydroxyvitamin D_3 levels vary directly with vertebral bone density in some studies of postmenopausal women (138). Thus, vitamin D deficiency may be more common than appreciated in this group of patients.

4. Physiology

  a. Calcium and phosphate absorption is increased by vitamin D to maintain blood levels of calcium and phosphorus (139). Because the plasma is supersaturated with both minerals, bone mineralization results. In addition, the vitamin mobilizes calcium (and phosphate) from bone and increases the renal reabsorption of calcium. All these effects result in increased serum levels of calcium and phosphate and normal mineralization. Evidence for an independent effect of the vitamin (especially 25-hydroxyvitamin D) on bone mineralization is limited. 1,25-Dihydroxyvitamin D plays an important role in mobilizing calcium from bone to maintain serum calcium and phosphorus levels within a normal range.

   b. Other functions. Vitamin D improves muscle function and corrects decreased phosphate concentrations in muscle in deficiency states. Some vitamin D metabolites, especially 25-hydroxyvitamin D, may have a direct effect on bone to improve calcium deposition. Insertion of a 24-hydroxyl group into 1,25-dihydroxyvitamin D reduces the affinity of the vitamin for the nuclear vitamin D receptor and thus its classic activity. Other hydroxylations (C23 and C26) may lead to various selective activities on growth and differentiation via effects on the nuclear receptor.

   c. Metabolism. Vitamin D from the skin is bound to a plasma-binding protein, so that its uptake by the liver is limited. Dietary vitamin D is absorbed by incorporation into mixed micelles and enters very-low-density lipoproteins or chylomicrons, which are taken up by the liver. Thus, hepatic uptake is not limited by the plasma-binding protein, and toxic levels of metabolites can be reached after oral ingestion. The liver adds a 25-hydroxyl group, whereas the kidney adds hydroxyl groups at positions 1 and 24. Adipose tissue is the major storage site of vitamin D metabolites. Both 1,25-dihydroxyvitamin D_3 and other polar metabolites of vitamin D are excreted in bile and participate in an enterohepatic circulation, although the quantitative importance of this in humans is not clear. In deficiency of either calcium or phosphorus, the formation of 1,25-dihydroxyvitamin D_3 is increased. Parathyroid hormone, calcitonin, estrogens, prolactin, and growth hormone enhance the formation of active dihydroxyvitamin D. Many of these factors also regulate (reciprocally) the formation of 1,25-dihydroxyvitamin D_3, but some other metabolites are also functional. The production of 24,25-dihydroxyvitamin D_3 in the kidney is not closely regulated. The biologic importance of this metabolite is not established, but it may alleviate bone disease in uremic patients.

5. Deficiency. Several syndromes result from vitamin D deficiency, all related to decreased body stores of calcium or phosphorus.

   a. Rickets, the major deficiency syndrome, is caused by poor bone mineralization. The newborn infant is at high risk because the vitamin D content of unfortified milk (<1 µg/L) is low and 25-hydroxylase activity in the liver is not fully developed. The incidence seems to be increasing in children, most of whom do not ingest the recommended intake of vitamin D. In rickets, or childhood osteomalacia, the calcification of newly formed bone and epiphyseal cartilage is decreased. Decreased amounts of calcium are deposited in the collagen elaborated by cartilage cells. Wide osteoid seams are found most often in the long bones because they grow the fastest. Craniotabes, chest deformity, bending of long bones, enlarged epiphyses of long bones, greenstick fractures, swollen wrists, muscle weakness, seizures, tetany, inability to initiate walking, and decreased growth are all noted. Serum calcium levels may be normal or low. The tetany associated with vitamin D deficiency results from hypocalcemia. Muscle weakness is probably caused by a decrease in muscle phosphate.

   b. Adult osteomalacia. In adults, the endochondral growth of long bones has ceased; consequently, decreased calcification of cartilage is not a factor. Osteoblast-mediated mineralization is affected by vitamin D deficiency, but changes occur over a longer period of time, and the clinical presentation is not so fulminant as in children. Subclinical bone disease occurs with normal blood calcium levels. By the time bone disease has become severe, hypocalcemia and hypophosphatemia are often present. Skeletal pain and muscle weakness occur anywhere in the body, but the long bones are less affected than are bones in the shoulders, hips, and spine. Adult osteomalacia is associated with aging, renal disease (lack of 1-α-hydroxylase), severe hepatic disease (decreased 25-hydroxylase activity), and intestinal resection (decreased absorption); it is also seen after gastric surgery (possibly because of decreased uptake) and after use of anticonvulsant medication (which may cause inactive metabolites to form). Vitamin D-resistant rickets is the cause of osteomalacia in a few patients. The contribution of an interrupted enterohepatic circulation to vitamin D deficiency in malabsorption is probably small. Fewer than one-third of highly polar metabolites are excreted in bile, and virtually no 25-hydroxyvitamin D_3. It has been suggested that a loss of bile salts alters the hepatic metabolism of vitamin D and leads to the rapid half-life of the vitamin in malabsorption.

   c. **Involutional osteoporosis.** This disorder is defined by a low bone mass. Although vitamin D and calcium are the primary nutrients involved, other vitamins (K, C, and B_6) also play a role in bone formation (140). Three etiologic categories of osteoporosis are recognized: early postmenopausal, late postmenopausal (after 70 years of age), and drug-induced. A decline in renal 1-α-hydroxylase activity with age may result in decreased calcium absorption and increased secretion of parathyroid hormone. Chronic vitamin D deficiency may be a factor in osteoporosis in elderly patients in nursing homes. In about 15% of elderly people, dietary intake is poor or outdoor activity is decreased. Vitamin D deficiency develops because of decreased skin production, decreased metabolism of vitamin D to the 1,25-dihydroxylated form, and decreased oral intake (141). Chronic abuse of alcohol is a frequently overlooked cause of osteoporosis in men (142). The cause(s) are probably multifactorial and include vitamin D deficiency. Chronic pancreatitis and small-bowel injury resulting from alcohol abuse may impair calcium and amino acid absorption. Elevated blood levels of cortisol and parathyroid hormone may contribute to bone destruction. Decreased intake of vitamin D, lack of sunlight, and altered vitamin D metabolism (in cirrhotics) are probably important. The hypomagnesemia seen in many alcoholics may play a role. Reversal of important factors in individual patients may retard the otherwise progressive bone loss. Although some evidence has been found that short-term therapy with low-dose 1,25-dihydroxyvitamin D_3 relieves osteoporosis, improvement is not maintained. This result is consistent with the transient improvement seen in patients with osteoporosis after various forms of therapy.

6. **Therapy**
   a. **Deficiency.** Oral vitamin D maintains vitamin D status less effectively than skin-derived vitamin D; with the latter, release is more constant and the rate of hepatic metabolism to less active isomers slower. Nevertheless, oral supplements are sometimes needed. Dietary deficiency still occurs, especially in hospitalized patients (143). Indications for supplementation include breast-feeding in infancy, fat malabsorption, advanced age, institutionalization (especially if the patient is not exposed to the sun), uremia, and long-term use of corticosteroids. Many forms of vitamin D are available. Some vitamin D products contain tartrazine, which may cause allergic reactions in susceptible persons.

b. **Bone health.** When taken with calcium, vitamin D increases serum 25-hydroxyvitamin D levels, minimizes bone loss observed on bone density testing, and may reduce the incidence of fractures (13). Calcium absorption is only about one-third of normal (10% vs. 33%) when vitamin D is deficient (144). When both nutrients are taken together [20 µg of vitamin D with 1.2 g of calcium (145) or 17.5 µg of vitamin D with 500 mg of calcium (146)], the incidence of hip fractures can be decreased. Calcium (1 g/d) and vitamin D (12.5 µg/d) have prevented loss of bone mass in patients with rheumatoid arthritis and corticosteroid-induced osteoporosis (147). Vitamin D may also be effective when given in combination with other drugs that diminish bone loss (148).

c. **Cancer.** Epidemiologic studies are not consistent in finding an association between vitamin D and colon cancer risk (13). This may be because both calcium and the vitamin are needed, or because other vitamins and foods differ among the cohort groups.

d. **Vitamin D preparations**

   (1) **Vitamin D$_2$ (ergosterol)** is available in large doses of 600 or 1,200 µg (25,000 or 50,000 IU per capsule) for daily replacement. These large doses are used for patients with refractory rickets or malabsorption. Although an injectable form in sesame oil contains 500,000 IU/mL, its bioavailability is still questionable. In liquid form, ergosterol is available solubilized with polysorbate 80 or polyethylene glycol at a concentration of 200 µg (8,000 IU) per milliliter (Drisdol, Sanof; Winthrop Pharmaceuticals, New York, NY). These preparations contain 200 IU (5 µg) per drop, if it is assumed that a milliliter contains 40 drops. The liquid form, which is adequate for most needs, provides the greatest flexibility. Cholecalciferol (vitamin D$_3$) is provided in tablets of 400 or 1,000 IU (10 or 25 µg). For breast-fed children, a safe and inexpensive preparation containing vitamin D is Tri-Vi-Sol.

   (2) **Dihydrotachysterol,** a vitamin D$_2$ derivative that is active without 1-α-hydroxylation, is available in tablets of 0.125, 0.2, or 0.4 mg and in oral solution (0.2 mg/5 mL). It is used to treat postoperative tetany; 1 mg is equivalent to 3 mg of vitamin D$_2$.

   (3) **1,25-Dihydroxyvitamin D$_3$ (calcitriol)** is marketed as 0.25- and 0.5-µg tablets and in injectable form (1 or 2 µg/mL). 1,25-Dihydroxyvitamin D$_3$ is available for IV use in concentrations of 1 or 2 µg/mL. The usual dosage is 0.01 to 0.05 µg/kg three times per week. It is most often given to patients undergoing renal dialysis, in whom such frequent IV dosing is possible. This form of vitamin D does not alter serum levels of 25-hydroxyvitamin D or 1,25-dihydroxyvitamin D, so repletion should be monitored by measurement of serum or 24-hour urinary calcium. Daily requirements are met by 0.5 to 1.0 µg/d. No good information exists to estimate dose when malabsorption is present. To avoid toxicity, serum and urinary calcium levels should be followed, although toxicity is unlikely in the presence of malabsorption. Although 1,25-dihydroxyvitamin D$_3$ is more water-soluble than the parent compound and does not require incorporation into bile acid micelles for solubility, its advantages in the treatment of malabsorption have yet to be demonstrated, and it is more expensive. Its use should be confined mostly to patients who cannot form 1,25-dihydroxyvitamin D$_3$ (e.g., those with renal failure) when the aim is rapid reversal of hypocalcemia. It is often use to induce the mild hypercalcemia required to offset excess calcium secretion in renal failure. 1,25-Dihydroxyvitamin D$_3$ is degraded in the gut (149). Thus, the oral drug is not

delivered to tissues as efficiently as the IV drug. Parenteral use suppresses parathyroid hormone levels more effectively.

(4) **25-Hydroxyvitamin D₃ (calcifediol, Calderol)** is also available in 20- and 50-μg tablets. At doses from 50 to 150 μg/d, it is useful in treating osteomalacia, especially as this vitamin may have a direct effect on bone. Whereas 25-hydroxyvitamin D₃ appears to have a direct effect on bone by increasing its calcium content, 1,25-dihydroxyvitamin D₃ seems to have an osteolytic effect. Thus, the 25-hydroxylated form may be useful in some cases of renal disease, even though it lacks the 1-hydroxyl group. Although 25-hydroxyvitamin D₃ is slightly more water-soluble than the parent compound, some bile acid micelles are still required for absorption. However, 25-hydroxyvitamin D₃ is absorbed better than vitamin D in patients with steatorrhea (150).

7. **Toxicity.** Hypervitaminosis D occurs because the plasma binding capacity for 25-hydroxyvitamin D₃ is relatively unlimited. Although serum 1,25-dihydroxyvitamin D concentrations are regulated by calcium levels, 25-hydroxyvitamin D levels are not. Because 25-hydroxyvitamin D₃ itself has physiologic effects, albeit less potent than those of 1,25-dihydroxyvitamin D, hypercalcemia and hypercalciuria can ensue. Toxicity is caused by excessive oral ingestion rather than ultraviolet irradiation because skin production of the active vitamin is limited to 15% to 20% of the provitamin content per day. Total body sun exposure potentially provides up to the equivalent of 250 μg (10,000 IU) of vitamin D per day (151). A UL of 50 μg/d has been recommended for adults (3) (Appendix B).

Acute hypercalcemia causes nausea, anorexia, itching, polyuria, abdominal pain, constipation, bone pain, metallic taste, and dehydration. In chronic cases, nephrocalcinosis, metastatic calcification, renal failure, and kidney stones may develop. Weight loss, irritability, psychosis, pancreatitis, photophobia, hypertension, cardiac arrhythmias, and elevated levels of blood urea nitrogen, cholesterol, aspartate aminotransferase, and alanine aminotransferase have been reported. For treatment, prednisone, diuresis, and a low-calcium diet may be required, along with withdrawal of vitamin D. Periodic measurement of 25-hydroxyvitamin D is essential, as levels below 140 nmol/L are not associated with adverse effects (150). The 24-hour urine calcium excretion provides a functional assay because it reflects excessive absorption of calcium. If this method is used to assess vitamin D toxicity, measurement should be frequent, perhaps monthly, during the initiation of therapy if malabsorption is not the cause of deficiency and should be repeated every 3 to 6 months for patients on long-term replacement. The product of serum calcium times phosphate (Ca × P) should not exceed 70 to prevent precipitation of calcium phosphate.

C. Vitamin E
1. Requirement
a. **Chemical forms.** It is not possible to determine vitamin E requirements accurately for several reasons: (a) the vitamin is heterogeneous chemically; (b) the requirements depend on the intake of natural oxidants, such as polyunsaturated fatty acids (PUFAs) and selenium; and (c) evidence of vitamin E deficiency develops uncommonly (152). The term *vitamin E* refers to all tocopherols showing biologic activity of D-α-tocopherol. In mixed diets, the non–α-tocopherols account for about 20% of the total activity, although they are less potent than α-tocopherol. One international unit of vitamin E equals 1 mg of DL-α-tocopherol acetate. The natural form of the vitamin, D-α-tocopherol, has a biopotency of 1.36 IU (acetate) and 1.21 IU (succinate). Commercial vitamin E is made from a mixture of many stereoisomeric synthetic forms of α-tocopherol acetate or succinate. The synthetic DL-α-tocopherol succinate has a potency of 1.49 IU.

The requirement for vitamin E increases as PUFA intake increases, but dietary fats also contain vitamin E, so that dietary deficiency is unlikely. About 0.4 to 0.8 mg of vitamin is needed for each gram of PUFA, and possibly more than 1.5 mg/g in diets containing high numbers of long-chain PUFAs. Variability in requirement can be related both to dietary PUFA intake and to tissue composition depending on prior dietary habits.

b. DRIs. The RDA was based previously on assumptions of a diet containing no more than 0.1 part per million of selenium, average amounts of sulfur amino acids, 0.4 mg of vitamin E for each gram of PUFA, and less than 1.5% linoleic acid in 1,800 to 3,000 kcal. Current recommendations take into consideration the possible role of vitamin E as an antioxidant in preventing chronic disease and the increased intake of PUFAs in the U.S. diet, in addition to serum vitamin E concentrations from NHANES III. However, these levels were not corrected for serum lipid or cholesterol, which might exaggerate the prevalence of low vitamin E body stores. The new DRIs are set at levels about 50% higher than the RDAs of 1989 (Table 6-37).

2. Food sources. Vitamin E is found in lipids of green leafy plants and in oils or seeds. Animal sources derive most of the vitamin from alfalfa, corn, and soybean foods. The richest sources for humans are salad oils, shortenings, and margarines, especially those derived from soybean, cottonseed, peanut, corn, and safflower oils, and wheat germ and nuts. Some of these oils contain more γ-tocopherol than α-tocopherol. Animal sources containing the highest amounts include eggs, liver, and muscle meats.

a. Vitamin E content in foods (Table 6-38) is greatly affected by processing, storage, and preparation, especially if cooking in oil is followed by storage. Freezing does not prevent peroxide formation and the destruction of biologic activity. Many foods (e.g., milk) show a seasonal variation in vitamin E content, which is highest in summer. A 2,000- to 3,000-kcal diet in the United States contains 8 to 11 mg equivalents of tocopherol, just barely sufficient for the average adult. An extensive summary of the food content of vitamin E has been published (153).

b. The ratio of vitamin E to PUFAs is lower in vegetable oils than in animal products, and the proportion of non–α-tocopherols is often

Table 6-37. Dietary reference intakes for vitamin E[a]

Life stage group	Vitamin E (mg/d)	Life stage group	Vitamin E (mg/d)
Infants[b]		Adults (M/F)	
0–6 mo	4	9–13 y	11
7–12 mo	6	14–>70 y	15
Children		Pregnancy	
1–3 y	6	≤18–50 y	15
4–8 y	7	Lactation	
		≤18–50 y	19

[a] Values refer to α-tocopherol forms occurring naturally, and to the synthetic isomers with comparable biologic activity that occur in fortified foods and supplements.
[b] Estimate based on adequate intake (AI). Other values based on recommended dietary allowance (RDA).
From Standing Committee on the Scientific Evaluation of Dietary Reference Intakes, Food and Nutrition Board, Institute of Medicine. *Dietary reference intakes for vitamin C, vitamin E, selenium, and beta-carotene and other carotenoids.* Washington, DC: National Academy Press, 2000.

Table 6-38. Approximate vitamin E content of selected foods

Food	α-Tocopherol (mg/100 g)	Non-α-tocopherol (mg/100 g)
Grains		
Bread		
White	0.1	0.13
Whole wheat	0.45	1.75
Oatmeal	2.27	1.7
Meat		
Bacon	0.53	0.06
Beef	0.3	0.3
Beef liver	0.6	1.0
Chicken	0.4	1
Pork chops, fried	0.16	0.44
Salmon	1.35	0.46
Shrimp	0.6	6
Vegetables		
Carrots	0.11	0.1
Celery	0.38	0.19
Onion	0.22	0.12
Peas		
Fresh	0.55	1.2
Frozen	0.23	0.4
Canned	0.02	0.02
Peanuts	7	5
Potatoes, French fried	0.3	1
Fruits		
Apple	0.31	0.2
Banana	0.22	0.2
Orange juice	0.04	0.16
Dairy		
Milk, whole	0.036	0.057
Butter	1	0
Margarine	13	48
Eggs	0.46	1
Fats		
Corn oil	12	53
Olive oil	4	—
Peanut oil	19	14
Safflower oil	34	7
Sesame oil	—	53
Soybean oil	10	85

much greater. Olive oil, however, contains much less vitamin E than other vegetable oils (154). Its ability to retard LDL oxidation is attributed to polyphenol compounds. Fish oils are higher in PUFAs but lower in vitamin E. Fortunately, the vitamin is ubiquitous. The tocopherol–linoleic acid ratio in milk is 0.79 mg/g, more than the 0.5 mg/g recommended for newborns. Tocopherol levels are higher in colostrum than in milk.

c. **Intake.** Median intake in the United States is less than the RDA, 7.3 and 5.4 mg/d in men and women, respectively (NHANES II), and only about half of the current DRI for adults over the age of 19 years. NHANES III data show that serum concentrations of vitamin E are below 20 µmol/L (low normal) in 20% of whites and 41% of African-

Americans (155). The vitamin E– PUFA ratio is more than 0.4 mg/g, which is acceptable. About 20% of intake is derived from fruits and vegetables and 20% from fats and oils. Fortunately, most foods high in vitamin E are also high in PUFAs.

3. **Assessment.** No measures are available that reflect recent intake because absorption is poor and the tocopherols are carried as part of the lipoprotein complex. Thus, all available assays correlate with body stores (Table 6-39).

   a. **Erythrocyte hemolysis.** Serum tocopherol levels and the erythrocyte hemolysis test correlate well, but the latter is a functional assay. It is based on the ability of hydrogen peroxide to liberate hemoglobin from red cells. In the absence of the natural antioxidant, vitamin E, the reaction proceeds more rapidly. Erythrocyte hemolysis above 10% or a serum α-tocopherol level below 0.5 mg/dL is often associated with vitamin E deficiency. The test result is affected by circulating PUFA levels and is positive only at very low serum levels of vitamin E. Unfortunately, it is not clear that this assay (or serum tocopherol itself) indicates α-tocopherol status in body tissues other than blood, especially the major storage pool in adipose tissue. Thus, the exact usefulness of this test has not yet been determined.

   b. **Serum vitamin E.** The vitamin E levels of infants and children are lower than those of adults, in fact below 0.5 μg/mL. Therefore, both serum α-tocopherol levels and the erythrocyte hemolysis test should be performed to see whether both suggest a deficiency state. Earlier methods for assessing vitamin E levels have been largely replaced by HPLC procedures (10). The levels are highly correlated with total lipid, and the ratio of vitamin E to total lipid is considered a better indicator of vitamin E stores. This is because vitamin E is carried in plasma exclusively on lipoproteins. Thus, in hypolipidemic states (e.g., malabsorption), vitamin E levels are characteristically low. Premature infants are at special risk for vitamin E deficiency because their levels fall after birth. The ratio of α-tocopherol to cholesterol is the one most conveniently obtained (156). All the samples must be taken in a fasting state, and total lipids can be the sum of triglyceride and cholesterol because the phospholipid concentrations are much lower.

   c. **Tissue damage in vitamin E deficiency.** End-organ damage is more common than once thought, but detection requires sophisticated techniques in some instances. Neurologic examination may

Table 6-39. Guidelines for interpreting vitamin E status

Test	Vitamin E status category		
	Deficient	Low	Acceptable
Plasma α-tocopherol			
μmol/L	<11.6	11.6–16.2	≥16.2
μg/ml	<5.0	5.0–7.0	≥7.0
Erythrocyte hemolysis (%)	>20	10–20	≤10
α-Tocopherol/lipid ratios			
Plasma α-tocopherol/total lipid (μg/mg)			>8
Plasma α-tocopherol/cholesterol (μg/mg)			>2.22
Serum/plasma α-tocopherol (μmol/L)			≥11.6

From Sauberlich NE. *Laboratory tests for the assessment of nutritional status,* 2nd ed. Boca Raton, FL: CRC Press, 1999.

disclose ataxia or peripheral neuropathy. Examination of the fundus may reveal retinal pigment degeneration, and examination of the visual fields can disclose central scotomata. The electroretinogram shows delayed and reduced potentials. Sensory evoked potentials are delayed in the lower limb.

d. Breath ethane and pentane. Ethane and pentane are generated though peroxidation of n-3 and n-6 fatty acids, respectively. Breath ethane has been used to evaluate vitamin E status in children, in whom it correlates negatively with vitamin E serum levels. This test may be useful to screen children and assess response to therapy (157). High doses of vitamin E decrease breath pentane in heavy smokers. Breath pentane and ethane levels are also elevated in vitamin C deficiency, β-carotene deficiency, and low glutathione levels.

4. Physiology

a. Function. Vitamin E is localized in membranes and provides a defense against lipid peroxidation of PUFAs. Selenium in glutathione peroxidase is located in the cytosol and provides another defense system. Other antioxidant defense mechanisms include the enzymes catalase, glucose-6-phosphate dehydrogenase, and glutathione reductase; the plasma proteins ceruloplasmin and transferrin; sulfhydryl-containing amino acids; and zinc, copper, and riboflavin. Vitamin E protects the membranes of intracellular organelles from damage. If all the peroxide formed by superoxide dismutase is not destroyed, then singlet oxygen is formed in the presence of ferric ions. Vitamin E acts to destroy these peroxides, which promote peroxidation of LDL in the subendothelial space. Oxidized LDL in turn can induce cytokine production in endothelial cells, which leads to recruitment of macrophages, proliferation of smooth muscle, vasoconstriction, and platelet aggregation. Vitamin E delays these effects and so plays a role in preventing cardiovascular disease (158).

Platelet adhesion is impaired by an antioxidant-independent action of vitamin E, although a daily dose of 400 IU is required to show an effect *in vivo*. Fewer platelet pseudopods are produced during vitamin E-induced inhibition of protein kinase C (159), which is likely to be the basis of the effect of the vitamin in ischemic damage and the rationale for conjoint therapy with inhibitors of platelet aggregation.

b. Absorption. Absorption requires biliary (bile salt micelles) and pancreatic (esterase) secretions. Less than 40% of an oral dose is absorbed, and this amount is decreased by excess unsaturated fatty acids in the lumen. The natural form ingested is D-α-tocopherol acetate, which must be hydrolyzed in the intestine by a bile salt-dependent pancreatic esterase. Only free α-tocopherol is found in the intestinal lymph. In serum, two-thirds of the vitamin is bound to LDL, with the rest in other lipoproteins; 70% absorption requires 6 to 7 hours. No carrier is specific for vitamin E; therefore, its serum level is proportional to the total lipid level. The percentage of vitamin E that is absorbed decreases at doses above 30 mg because the vitamin is passively absorbed. Most is deposited initially in liver as lipoprotein lipase acts on lipoproteins, and vitamin E is then distributed to adipose tissue. Specific binding proteins have been found in hepatic and cardiac cytosol that transfer the vitamin to mitochondria. Plasma and tissue α-tocopherol are exchanged rapidly. The vitamin is excreted largely in feces, where it is mostly degraded (160). It is not known whether an enterohepatic circulation exists or whether all fecal vitamin derives from oral sources. Less than 1% is excreted in urine.

5. Deficiency

a. Persons at risk include newborns and premature infants, food faddists, and patients with fat malabsorption or biliary obstruction.

Vitamin E crosses the placenta poorly, and adipose tissue stores are small in the fetus *in utero*. The antioxidant properties of the vitamin cannot explain all manifestations of the uncommon deficiency state. Moreover, in most cases, no symptoms have been noted that respond to vitamin E when serum α-tocopherol levels are low. Low serum concentrations of vitamin E, ranging from 0.5% to 24%, were found in a variety of populations, but these were not correlated with serum lipid content, and the significance in regard to risk for disease is uncertain (161).

b. **Deficiency as part of medical conditions.** In some muscular dystrophies, the pathologic features are similar to those of experimental vitamin E deficiency in animals, but no relationship of human dystrophies to the vitamins is known. Hemolytic anemia can occur in the premature infant with low body stores, especially if supplementation with linoleic acid and iron is given. Edema, tachypnea, and restlessness are noted. In adult malabsorption syndromes, especially in association with biliary obstruction, α-tocopherol levels decline, and red cell hemolysis and creatinuria have been reported. When serum levels are very low, a ceroid pigment has been found in smooth and skeletal muscle. In short-bowel syndrome and abetalipoproteinemia, unsteady gait, tremor, weakness, ophthalmoplegia, pigmentary retinopathy, and proprioceptive impairment have been noted. Patients with hereditary abetalipoproteinemia also can present with myopathy and cerebellar dysfunction. In cystic fibrosis, changes in posterior column axons and nuclei and sensory nuclei of the fifth cranial nerve in the medulla have been observed, but without clinical neurologic defects. A progressive neurologic syndrome associated with low serum vitamin E concentrations has been described in children with cholestatic liver disease. The syndrome includes areflexia, gait disturbance, decreased proprioceptive and vibratory sensation, and paresis of gaze (162). Lipofuscin pigment accumulates in neurons but has no obvious harmful effect.

c. **Isolated vitamin E deficiency.** A genetic abnormality in which defective hepatic α-tocopherol transfer protein prevents vitamin E from reaching tissues results in ataxia and peripheral neuropathy (163).

d. **Cardiovascular disease and cancer.** Patients with these conditions have been noted to have serum levels of vitamin E lower than those of control groups. In nearly all such studies, the serum tocopherol levels were not corrected for lipid content. There are theoretical reasons for a response to antioxidants, and many studies have examined the effect of supplemental vitamin E (sometimes given together with β-carotene). Table 6-40 lists some of the prospective, double-blinded, randomized studies that have been performed. The results are promising (but inconclusive) for heart disease, although not for cancer. The American Heart Association consensus statement on vitamin E does not consider that vitamin E can yet be recommended for routine use (164). The Health Professionals Follow-up Study of Males showed no correlations between vitamin E, vitamin C, or β-carotene intake and the risk for stroke (165).

e. **Other conditions.** Because of its antioxidant properties, supplements or intake of vitamin E have been examined in a variety of other conditions (13) (Table 6-40). Preliminary evidence in small numbers of patients suggests that vitamin E may play a role in immune function, Alzheimer's disease, tardive dyskinesia, lung function, diabetes, and exercise performance in highly trained athletes. Serum vitamin E levels (corrected for cholesterol), but not for vitamin C and β-carotene levels, did correlate with short-term recall (memory) in an elderly population (166).

Table 6-40. Randomized double-blinded controlled studies of vitamin E to prevent chronic disease

Condition and study	Patients		Intervention	Outcome
	Characteristics	No.		
CV disease				
ATBC[1]	Finnish M smokers, no MI, 50–69 y	27,271	E 50 mg, β-car 20 mg or both, 5–8 y	No Δ fatal, nonfatal MI
ATBC[2]	M smokers, Hx of MI	1,862	"	↑ Deaths on β-car
ATBC[3]	M smokers, angina	1,795	"	No benefit
CHAOS[4]	Angiogram-positive atherosclerosis	2,002	E 528/264 mg, ~2 y	72% ↓ Nonfatal MI, no Δ death
Hodis[5]	CABG, cholestipol/niacin	156	E 100 mg, 2 y	↓ Progression on angiogram
Tardif[6]	Probucol, undergoing angioplasty	317	E 700 mg, C 500 mg, β-car 30,000 IU	No Δ in restenosis
HOPES[7]	>55 y with CV risk factors	1,509	E 400 mg, 4.5 y	No Δ in CV outcomes
Cancer				
ATBC[8] gastric	M smokers	20,113	E 50 mg, β-car 20 mg or both, 5–8 y	No Δ colorectal
ATBC[9] gastric	M smokers with atrophic gastritis	2,132	"	No Δ prevalence
ATBC[10]	M smokers	409	"	No Δ in oral lesions
Immunity				
Meydani[11]	Healthy >65 y	88	E 60 or 200 or 800 mg, 0.5 y	↑ DTH, HBV/tetanus titers
DeWaart[12]	Healthy >65 y	83	E 100 mg, 3 mo	No Δ IgG, cell immunity
Neuropsychiatric				
Alzheimer Coop Study[13]	Alzheimer's disease	341	E 1,320 mg, selegiline 10 mg or both	20% ↓ Time to death, loss of function
Lohr[14]	Tardive dyskinesia	35	E 1,056 mg, 2 mo	24% ↓ Dyskinesia
Adler[15]	Tardive dyskinesia	40	E 1056 mg, 9 mo	↓ Dyskinesia

		n	Dose, duration	Outcome
Lung function				
Grievink[16]	Dutch cyclists	38	E 100 mg, C 500 mg, 15 wk	↑ FEV_1, ↓ ozone effects
Cataracts				
ATBC[17]	M smokers, 50–69 y	1,828	E 50 mg, 5–8 y	No Δ prevalence
Diabetes				
Tutuncu[18]	T2 DM, peripheral neuropathy	21	E 900 mg, 6 mo	↑ Nerve conduction velocity
Paolisso[19]	Elderly, nonobese, normal GTT	20	E 900 mg, 4 mo	↑ Body glucose disposal
Paolisso[20]	T2 DM	25	E 900 mg, 3 mo	↓ [Glucose], [HbA_{1c}]
Exercise performance				
Meydani[21]	Adults 22–29 y	9	E 528 mg, 7 wk	↓ Peroxide formation
	Adults 55–74 y	12	"	
Simon-Schnass[22]	Mountaineers	13	E 400 mg, 4 wk	↑ Hct
Simon-Schnass[23]	"	12	E 400 mg, 10 wk	↑ Anaerobic threshold

ATBC, Alpha Tocopherol Beta Carotene cancer prevention study; CHAGS, Cambridge Heart Antioxidant Study; HOPES, Heart Outcomes Prevention Evaluation Study. [1]Arch Intern Med 1998;158:668; [2]Lancet 1997;349:1715; [3]Heart 1998;79:454; [4]Lancet 1996;347:781; [5]JAMA 1995;273:1849; [6]N Engl J Med 1997;337:365; [7]N Engl J Med 2000;342:154; [8]Cancer Epidemiol Biomarkers Prev 1998;7:335; [9]Scand J Gastroenterol 1998;33:294; [10]Oral Dis 1998;4:78; [11]JAMA 1997;277:1380; [12]Br J Nutr 1997;78:761; [13]N Engl J Med 1997;336:1216; [14]J Clin Psychiatry 1996;57:167; [15]Biol Psychiatry 1998;43:868; [16]Am J Epidemiol 1999;149:306; [17]Acta Ophthalmol Scand 1997;75:634; [18]Diabetes Care 1998;21:1915; [19]Am J Clin Nutr 1994;59:1291; [20]Diabetes Care 1993;16:1433; [21]Am J Physiol 1993;264:R992; [22]Int J Vitam Nutr Res 1990;60:26; [23]Int J Vitam Nutr Res 1988;58:49.

6. **Therapy.** The premature infant absorbs vitamin E poorly, and large doses are required orally (30 to 60 mg or 45 to 90 IU). Larger doses may be needed for malabsorption syndromes. Vitamin E is available in tablets of 200, 400, 500, 600, and 1000 IU and in aqueous suspension at 50 mg/mL. The therapeutic use of vitamin E falls into three categories (167).

   a. **Correction of deficiency states.** Examples include the hemolytic anemia of premature infants and the malabsorption syndromes of patients with cystic fibrosis, cholestatic liver disease, and hereditary abetalipoproteinemia. Large doses may be needed for a response. Up to 100 to 200 IU/kg per day can be given as a liquid emulsion with breakfast or 2 hours after medication that can interfere with absorption (e.g., cholestyramine, vitamin A, antacids). Parenteral (IM) vitamin E has been used as an investigational drug (Ephynal, Hoffman-LaRoche, Nutley, New Jersey) at a dose of 1 to 2 IU/kg (168). A truly water-soluble form, such as D-α-tocopheryl polyethylene glycol 1000 succinate (169), is available over the counter as Liqui-E (Twin Lab, Hauppauge, NY). This compound forms micelles when given at doses of 25 mg/kg per day. Blood levels of vitamin E may rise with replacement in 2 to 3 weeks unless hypolipidemia persists, as in abetalipoproteinemia. It is not clear what this means in terms of transfer of vitamin E to peripheral tissues. Oral vitamin E emulsion (1,000 to 2,000 IU/d) was reported to reverse a deficiency state when given orally three times a week with 0.7 to 3.0 mmol of desiccated ox bile (170).

   b. **Countering effects of prooxidants.** Large doses have been used in conditions in which no deficiency exists but large amounts of oxygen or other oxidants are administered. Examples of such use include the prevention or partial relief of retrolental fibroplasia in premature infants, to whom 100 mg of vitamin has been given per kilogram of body weight per day (171). Large doses of the vitamin have been given to lessen the severity of pulmonary dysplasia in infants exposed to prolonged oxygen treatment for respiratory distress syndrome and also to prevent the cardiotoxic effects of the chemotherapeutic drug doxorubicin.

   c. **Compensation for preexisting defects in the antioxidant systems of the body.** Large doses of vitamin E have been used in the absence of defined vitamin E deficiency to treat hemolytic anemia secondary to deficiencies in glutathione synthetase and in glucose-6-phosphate dehydrogenase (172). A decrease in the percentage of sickled cells in sickle cell anemia has been reported with 450 IU/d for 6 to 35 weeks (173). Of all the conditions associated with vitamin E listed in Table 6-40, cardiovascular disease is the most prevalent, and prevention of cardiovascular disease has the most support. Although no routine recommendations can be made for this use of vitamin E, doses between 100 and 400 IU/d might be considered for patients with or at high risk for cardiovascular disease, with the higher doses given to patients with documented disease (174). If vitamin E is used, it must be understood that the optimal dosage, duration of use, and appropriate source of the vitamin (diet or supplements) are not known.

7. **Toxicity.** No consistent ill effects are noted after ingestion of up to 2,112 mg (3,200 IU) per day in healthy volunteers or in patients with a variety of disorders (175). Occasionally, muscle weakness, fatigue, headaches, and nausea have been reported with these doses. High doses may impair the absorption of other fat-soluble vitamins by displacing them from the mixed bile acid–fatty acid micelle. At doses of 100 to 1,100 mg/d, vitamin E can block the oxidation of vitamin K to its active form, mimicking the action of warfarin, and therefore high-dose vitamin E may be contraindicated in patients with disorders of bleeding. However, no changes in prothrombin time have been noted in patients taking 800 to

1,200 IU/d while on coumadin therapy (13). Thus, the UL for adults has been set at 1,000 mg/d (3) (Appendix B). Multiple organ toxicity has been reported in premature infants receiving IV vitamin E with polysorbate 80 as an emulsifier.

D. Vitamin K

1. **Requirement.** Two forms of vitamin K occur naturally—K_1 (phylloquinones) in green plants and K_2 (menaquinones) in bacteria and animals. Colonic bacterial synthesis provides an unknown amount of vitamin K that has been estimated to be about 2 μg/kg of body weight. Because of the bacterial synthesis, dietary requirements are uncertain. The role of intestinal bacteria in providing any vitamin K in humans has been questioned (176). When antibiotics are given to alter intestinal flora, a vitamin K intake of 1 μg/kg per day prevents deficiency and is presumably adequate. The RDAs of 1989 were based on the function of the vitamin for the coagulation proteins, but the requirement may be greater for the nonhepatic vitamin K-dependent proteins, including those in bone (177). Because of the lack of data to estimate an average requirement, an AI is based on representative dietary intake data from healthy persons (103). The lower limit of the AI for vitamin K is set at 120 μg for adult men and 90 μg for adult women (Table 6-41). The RDA for other age groups is based on the need for 1 μg/kg of body weight in infants and children. Because human milk contains low levels of vitamin K (2 μg/L) and intestinal flora are underdeveloped, breast-fed infants receiving no other food source are at risk for deficiency and intracranial hemorrhage.

2. **Food sources.** Phylloquinone concentrations of plant leaves are proportional to their chlorophyll content. Thus, the best dietary sources are green leafy vegetables and broccoli. Although the food content varies widely, the vitamin is associated with chloroplasts, and bioavailability is also variable. Other primary dietary sources are certain plant oils, namely soybean, canola, cottonseed, and olive (177). However, other commonly used oils (peanut, corn, safflower, and sesame) have a very low content. Fruits, cereals, dairy products, and meat contain less vitamin K. The average diet in the United States contains 60 to 200 μg/d (177). Some vitamin K in the body is derived from bacteria, but this is poorly absorbed, and diet is the major source. The content of representative foods is listed in Table 6-42. Only a small number of vegetables

Table 6-41. Recommended dietary allowances for vitamin K

Life stage group	Vitamin K (μg/d)	Life stage group	Vitamin K (μg/d)
Infants		Females	
0–6 mo	2	9–13 y	60
7–12 mo	2.5	14–18 y	75
Children		19–>70 y	90
1–3 y	30	Pregnancy, lactation	
4–8 y	55	14–18 y	75
Males		19–50 y	90
9–13 y	60		
14–18 y	75		
19–>70 y	120		

All estimates are based on adequate intake (AI).
From Standing Committee on the Scientific Evaluation of Dietary Reference Intakes, Food and Nutrition Board, Institute of Medicine. Dietary reference intakes for vitamin A, vitamin K, arsenic, boron, chromium, copper, iodine, iron, manganese, molybdenum, nickel, silicon, vanadium, and zinc. Washington, DC: National Academy Press, 2001. Available on line at *http://www.nap.edu/ books, Crawler list 0309072794*. Accessed January 12, 2001.

Table 6-42. Vitamin K content of selected foods

Food	Portion	Vitamin K content (µg per serving)
Vegetables		
Broccoli	½ cup	88
Brussels sprouts	½ cup	225
Cabbage	½ cup	73
Collard greens	½ cup	374
Nuts, mixed (no peanuts)	1 oz	3.2
Potato, baked with skin	1 medium	1.5
Spinach	½ cup	324
Dairy		
Milk, 2%	8 oz	0.5
Meat		
Beef, ground	3 oz	2.0
Chicken breast, roasted	3 oz	<0.01
Chicken breast, home fried	3 oz	3.8
Oils		
Cottonseed, olive	1 oz	15
Corn	1 oz	1.5

From Booth SL, Suttie JW. Dietary intake and adequacy of vitamin K. *J Nutr* 1998;128:785.

contribute substantially to dietary phylloquinones. Oral phylloquinone at a dose of 500 µg can overcome therapeutic doses of warfarin, but some reports have suggested that a much lower content in enteral products can cause dietary resistance to warfarin (178). If the dietary intake of green vegetables or high-content oils is reasonably constant, there is no need to be concerned with a dietary cause of unstable warfarin effect. However, it is not known how much dietary vitamin K patients on warfarin therapy require if function of their extrahepatic vitamin K-dependent proteins is to be maintained.

3. **Assessment**

   a. **Intake: plasma phylloquinone.** HPLC methods have made this a straightforward measurement. Normal plasma concentrations range from 1.04 nmol/L ± 0.13 in younger adults to 1.45 nmol/L ± 0.22 in older (70 years) adults (10). The dietary intake of vitamin K correlates best with the plasma level.

   b. **Body stores**

      (1) **Prothrombin time.** Because vitamin K stimulates the production of clotting factors II, VII, IX, and X in the liver, the one-stage prothrombin time is used to assess its presence indirectly. For this test, sources of tissue factor (thromboplastin) and calcium are added in excess. Under these conditions, all the clotting factors tested (II, V, VII, X) are responsive to vitamin K except for factor V. The rate of formation of clot is an indirect measure of factors II, VII, and X. In practice, factor VII is the usual rate-limiting factor. Factor V has a longer half-life than the vitamin K-dependent proteins and is not rate-limiting in the reaction. Normally, the test sample clots within 1.5 seconds of the control (international normalized ratio of 1.0 to 1.1). The prothrombin time does not test vitamin K stores and is abnormal only when deficiency is present, synthesis of clotting factors is impaired by hepatic disease, or clotting fac-

tors are consumed in intravascular coagulation. Therefore, the test is nonspecific. It is most helpful when acute serious illness or liver disease is not present. In these situations, the interpretation regarding vitamin K is simple. If parenteral administration of vitamin K (5 to 10 mg) restores the prothrombin time to normal, deficiency in vitamin K becomes evident.

(2) **γ-Carboxyglutamic acid (Gla)-modified proteins.** Because vitamin K mediates the addition of Gla to proteins, detection of these proteins has been examined to evaluate vitamin K status. These assays are still not widely available, and more studies are needed before they can become clinically valuable. The assays used, and their "normal" values in adults, include plasma undercarboxylated prothrombin, protein induced by vitamin K absence (PIVKA)-II (1.58 μg/L), plasma undercarboxylated osteocalcin (2 to 3.3 μg/L), plasma carboxylated osteocalcin (7 to 10 μg/L), and urine Gla–creatinine ratio (3.16 in women, 3.83 in men) (10).

4. **Physiology**
   a. **Absorption and metabolism.** Vitamin K absorption requires bile acids and is passive, occurring largely in the small bowel. Other fat-soluble vitamins in very large amounts can displace vitamin K from the bile acid micelle and limit absorption. After absorption in the lymphatics, vitamins K_1 and K_2 are metabolized in the liver and retained there. The vitamin is reduced and converted to the epoxide before the original vitamin is re-formed, all by microsomal enzymes.
   b. **Tissue stores.** Unlike other fat-soluble vitamins, vitamin K is not stored in large quantities in adipose tissue, and the total body pool is small. The amount in tissue is low, but the vitamin is found in adrenals, lungs, marrow, kidney, and lymph nodes after it leaves the liver. The storage form differs from the plasma form, which is carried in lipoproteins. Long-chain menaquinones are the predominant hepatic form. Phylloquinones account for only 10% of liver reserves, do not cross the placenta, and are depleted first in cases of deficiency.
   c. **Function.** Vitamin K acts by carboxylating selected glutamic acid residues of proteins (α-Gla) so that they bind calcium. The Gla reaction is catalyzed by a microsomal enzyme, vitamin K-dependent carboxylase, and requires four substrates: reduced vitamin K, oxygen, carbon dioxide, and the Gla-containing peptide. A microsomal electron transport system is coupled with carbon dioxide fixation during the reaction. This vitamin K cycle oxidizes vitamin K hydroquinone to vitamin K-2,3-epoxide in a process that provides the energy for carboxylation of glutamic acid residues (179). Warfarin blocks the reduction of the epoxide to the quinone and the subsequent hydroxylation to the hydroquinone. The coagulation function of hepatic proteins is proportional to the degree of carboxylation. Vitamin K-dependent procoagulants include prothrombin and factors VII, IX, and X. Vitamin K-dependent anticoagulants include proteins C and S. Osteocalcin (bone Gla protein) is important in the extracellular matrix of bone, and matrix Gla proteins in the extracellular matrix of other tissues. Other vitamin K-dependent proteins of unknown function include protein Z, nephrocalcin, plaque Gla protein, Gas-6, PRGP-1, and PRGP-2 (179).

5. **Deficiency.** To avoid deficiency, a person must have adequate intraluminal vitamin K, a normal concentration of bile acids, and a normal small bowel, colon, and liver. Deficiency is manifested by easy bruising and clotting abnormalities. Subjects at risk for deficiency include newborn infants, whose intestinal flora is not established; others are patients with malabsorption resulting from loss of intestine or bile acid

insufficiency, patients with liver disease, and persons receiving no oral intake while on broad-spectrum antibiotics.

a. Hemorrhagic disease of the newborn occurs because the placenta transports lipids poorly, the intestine is sterile in the first days of life, and human milk is a poor source of vitamin K. Premature infants are at highest risk.

b. Drugs interfere with vitamin K metabolism as well as with production in the intestine. Warfarin inhibits vitamin K epoxide formation, hydantoins antagonize vitamin K in some way, certain antibiotics (e.g., moxalactam, cefamandole) decrease peptide carboxylation, salicylates inhibit vitamin K reductase, and the diuretic ticrynafen inhibits part of the microsomal electron transport system.

Table 6-43. Drugs that affect vitamin utilization and plasma concentrations

Drug class	Drug	Vitamin affected	Mechanism
Antibacterial	Isoniazid	Niacin, B_6	Competition with active coenzyme
	PAS	B_{12}	↓ Absorption
	Neomycin	B_{12}, K	↓ Absorption (bile salt sequestration)
	Pyrimethamine	Folate	Inhibits folate reductase
	Tetracycline	C	↑ Excretion
	Trimethoprim	Folate	Inhibits folate reductase
	Broad-spectrum	K	↓ Endogenous production
Anticoagulant	Warfarin	K	Blocks Gla formation
Anticonvulsant	Phenytoin	Folate	↓ Absorption
		D	↓ Hepatic metabolism to 1,25-$(OH)_2$ D
		K	Induction of hepatic inactivating enzyme
Antihypertensive	Hydralazine	B_6	Competition with active coenzyme
Antiinflammatory	Aspirin	C	↑ Excretion (competes with binding)
	Sulfasalazine	Folate	↓ Absorption
	Colchicine	B_{12}	↓ Absorption (intestinal damage)
	Phenylbutazone	Niacin, K	Displacement from albumin binding
Antineoplastic	Methotrexate	Folate	Inhibits folate reductase
Bile salt sequestrants	Cholestyramine	A, B_{12}, folate	↓ Absorption (binding of water-soluble, luminal sequestration of fat-soluble)
	Cholestipol	A, D, K	
Chelating	Penicillamine	B_6	↑ Urinary excretion (adduct formed)
Hormones	Birth control pills	B_1, B_2	↑ Function
		B_6	↓ Plasma binding
		Folate	↓ Absorption, ↑ plasma binding
		B_{12}	↓ Plasma binding

Gla, Carboxy-glutamic acid; PAS, *para*-aminosalicylate.

     c. **Postmenopausal osteoporosis.** Although vitamin K is essential for the biosynthesis of some bone proteins, it is not clear whether some patients with osteoporosis are also vitamin K-deficient (180). High doses of vitamin K administered to postmenopausal women for 24 to 48 weeks increase bone mass (181), but the link between vitamin K deficiency, if it occurs, and hip fracture in elderly women is not clear (182). Two studies of warfarin use and the risk for fractures reached opposite conclusions, one showing no increase (183) and one showing no overall increase but more rib and vertebral fractures (184).

    6. **Therapy.** Vitamin K is available in solutions of 2 or 10 mg/mL for parenteral use. Injection should be SC or IM when possible. For anticoagulant-induced or other deficiency of prothrombin in adults, use 2.5 to 10 mg initially or up to 25 mg. If the prothrombin time has not shortened satisfactorily within 6 to 8 hours, repeat the dose. When necessary hemodynamically, use blood replacement. For hemorrhagic disease of the newborn, prophylactic therapy consists of a single IM dose of 0.5 to 1 mg within 1 hour of birth or 1 to 5 mg to the mother 12 to 24 hours before delivery. Hemolytic anemia and hepatotoxicity have been reported with high doses. Long-term use should be limited to patients with malabsorption. Vitamin K_1 is not a component of any multivitamin preparation and must be prescribed individually as 5 mg tablets of phytonadione (Mephyton).

    7. **Toxicity.** More than 500 times the RDA can be given without toxicity. Thus, no UL has been recommended (103). Large amounts of vitamin K given during pregnancy or to the newborn (>10 mg) can produce jaundice in the newborn infant. It has been suggested that phylloquinone in infant formulas not exceed 20 µg/100 kcal (10). Hydantoin antagonizes vitamin K and can produce hemorrhagic disease in the newborn when taken by the mother during pregnancy.

IV. Effect of drugs on assessment of vitamin status. Many drugs can alter the results of tests used to assess vitamin status. These are listed in Table 6-43. Many of the drugs listed alter only the laboratory assessment of nutrient status, and a clear clinical deficiency state is not always described. Therefore, unless treatment is prolonged, replacement therapy is usually not required.

References

1. National Research Council. *Recommended dietary allowances,* 10th ed. Washington, DC: National Academy Press, 1989.
2. Standing Committee on the Scientific Evaluation of Dietary Reference Intakes, Food and Nutrition Board, Institute of Medicine. *Dietary reference intakes for calcium, phosphorus, magnesium, vitamin d, and fluoride.* Washington DC: National Academy Press, 1997.
3. Standing Committee on the Scientific Evaluation of Dietary Reference Intakes, Food and Nutrition Board, Institute of Medicine. *Dietary reference intakes for thiamine, riboflavin, niacin, vitamin B_6, folate, vitamin B_{12}, pantothenic acid, biotin, and choline.* Washington, DC: National Academy Press, 1998.
4. Standing Committee on the Scientific Evaluation of Dietary Reference Intakes, Food and Nutrition Board, Institute of Medicine. *Dietary reference intakes for vitamin C, vitamin E, selenium, and beta-carotene and other carotenoids.* Washington, DC: National Academy Press, 2000.
5. Haymes EM. Trace minerals and exercise. In: Wolinsky I, Hickson JF Jr, eds. *Nutrition in exercise and sport,* 2nd ed. Boca Raton, FL: CRC Press, 1994:224.
6. Russell RM. New views on the RDAs for older adults. *J Am Diet Assoc* 1997;97:515.
7. Haller J. The vitamin status and its adequacy in the elderly: an international overview. *Int J Vitam Nutr Res* 1999;69:160.
8. Selhub J, Bagley LC, Miller C, et al. B vitamins, homocysteine, and neurocognitive function in the elderly. *Am J Clin Nutr* 2000;71:614S.
9. Lyle BJ, Mares-Perlman JA, Klein BEK, et al. Serum carotenoids and tocopherols and incidence of age-related nuclear cataracts. *Am J Clin Nutr* 1999;69:272.

10. Sauberlich HE. *Laboratory tests for the assessment of nutritional status,* 2nd ed. Boca Raton, FL: CRC Press, 1999.
11. Laforenza U, Patrini C, Alvisi C, et al. Thiamine uptake in human intestinal biopsy specimens, including observations from a patient with acute thiamine deficiency. *Am J Clin Nutr* 1997;66:320.
12. Oriot D, Wood C, Gottesman R, et al. Severe lactic acidosis related to acute thiamine deficiency. *JPEN J Parenter Enteral Nutr* 1991;15:105.
13. Sarubin A. *The professional's guide to popular dietary supplements.* Chicago: American Dietetic Association, 1999.
14. Snodgrass SR. Vitamin neurotoxicity. *Mol Neurobiol* 1992;6:41.
15. Alhadeff L, Gueltieri CT, Lipton M. Toxic effects of water-soluble vitamins. *Nutr Rev* 1984;42:33.
16. McCormick D. Riboflavin. In: Shils ME, Olson JA, Shike M, et al., eds. *Modern nutrition in health and disease,* 9th ed. Baltimore: Williams & Wilkins, 1998:391.
17. Schoenen J, Jacquy J, Lenaerts M. Effectiveness of high-dose riboflavin in migraine prophylaxis. A randomized controlled trial. *Neurology* 1998;50:466.
18. Cervantes-Laurean D, McElvaney NG, Moss J. Niacin. In: Shils ME, Olson JA, Shike M, et al., eds. *Modern nutrition in health and disease,* 9th ed. Baltimore: Williams & Wilkins,1999:401.
19. Guyton JR. Effect of niacin on atherosclerotic cardiovascular disease. *Am J Cardiol* 1998;82:18U.
20. Pozzilli P, Browne PD, Kolb H. Meta-analysis of nicotinamide treatment in patients with recent-onset IDDM. The Nicotinamide Trialists. *Diabetes Care* 1996; 19:1357.
21. Jungnickel PW, Maloney PA, van der Tuin EL, et al. Effect of two aspirin pretreatment regimens on niacin-induced cutaneous reactions. *J Gen Intern Med* 1997;12:591.
22. Capuzzi DM, Guyton JR, Morgan JM, et al. Efficacy and safety of an extended-release niacin (Niaspan): a long-term study. *Am J Cardiol* 1998;82:74U.
23. Bailey AL, Maisey S, Southon S, et al. Relationships between micronutrient intake and biochemical indicators of nutrient adequacy in a "free-living" elderly U.K. population. *Br J Nutr* 1997;77:225.
24. de Groot CP, van den Broek T, van Staveren W. Energy intake and micronutrient intake in elderly Europeans: seeking the minimum requirement in the SENECA study. *Age Ageing* 1999;28:469.
25. Stabler SP, Allen RH, Fried LP, et al. Racial differences in prevalence of cobalamin and folate deficiency in disabled elderly women. *Am J Clin Nutr* 1999;70:911.
26. Whyte M, Mahuren JD, Vrabel LA, et al. Markedly increased circulating pyridoxal-5′-phosphate levels in hypophosphatasia. Alkaline phosphatase acts in vitamin B_6 metabolism. *J Clin Invest* 1985;76:752.
27. Ubbink JB, Vermaak WJ, van de Merse A, et al. Vitamin B-12, vitamin B-6, and folate nutritional status in men with hyperhomocystinemia. *Am J Clin Nutr* 1993; 57:47.
28. Bender DA. Non-nutritional uses of vitamin B_6. *Br J Nutr* 1999;81:7.
29. Folsom AR, Nieto FJ, McGovern PG, et al. Prospective study of coronary artery disease incidence in relation to fasting homocysteine, related genetic polymorphisms, and B vitamins. The Atherosclerosis Risk in Communities (ARIC) Study. *Circulation* 1998;98:204.
30. Schaumberg H, Kaplan J, Windebank A, et al. Sensory neuropathy from pyridoxine abuse. a new megavitamin syndrome. *N Engl J Med* 1983;309:445.
31. Wyatt KM, Dimmock PW, Jones PW, et al. Efficacy of vitamin B-6 in the treatment of premenstrual syndrome: systematic review. *BMJ* 1999;318:1375.
32. Botto LD, Moore CA, Khoury MJ, et al. Neural-tube defects. *N Engl J Med* 1999; 341:1509.
33. Welch GN, Loscalzo J. Homocysteine and atherosclerosis. *N Engl J Med* 1998; 338:1042.
34. Bailey LB. Dietary reference intakes for folate: the debut of dietary folate equivalents. *Nutr Rev* 1998;56:294.

35. Lewis CJ, Crane NT, Wilson DB, et al. Estimated folate intakes: data updated to reflect food fortification, increased bioavailability, and dietary supplement use. *Am J Clin Nutr* 1999;70:198.
36. Bailey LB. Folate status assessment. *Br J Nutr* 1990;120[Suppl 11]:1508.
37. Laurence VA, Loewenstein JE, Eichner ER. Aspirin and folate binding: *in vivo* and *in vitro* studies of serum binding and urinary excretion of endogenous folate. *J Lab Clin Med* 1984;103:944.
38. Weir DG, McGing PG, Scott JM. Folate metabolism, the enterohepatic circulation and alcohol. *Biochem Pharmacol* 1985;34:1.
39. Miner SES, Evrovski J, Cole DEC. Clinical chemistry and molecular biology of homocysteine metabolism: an update. *Clin Biochem* 1997;30:189.
40. Ubbink JB, Delport R, Riezler R, et al. Comparison of three different plasma homocysteine assays with gas chromatography-mass spectrometry. *Clin Chem* 1999;45:670.
41. Selhub J, Jacques PF, Rosenberg IH, et al. Serum total homocysteine concentrations in the Third National Health and Nutrition Examination Survey (1991–1994): population reference ranges and contribution of vitamin status to high serum concentrations. *Ann Intern Med* 1999;131:331.
42. Said HM, Kumar C. Intestinal absorption of vitamins. *Curr Opin Gastroenterol* 1999;15:172.
43. Davis RE. Clinical chemistry of folic acid. *Adv Clin Chem* 1986;25:233.
44. MRC Vitamin Study Research Group. Prevention of neural tube defects: results of the Medical Research Council Vitamin Study. *Lancet* 1991;338:131.
45. Czeizel AE, Dudas I. Prevention of the first occurrence of neural-tube defects by periconceptional vitamin supplementation. *N Engl J Med* 1992;327:1832.
46. Berry RJ, Li Z, Erickson JD, et al. Prevention of neural-tube defects with folic acid in China. *N Engl J Med* 1999;341:1485.
47. Nappo F, De Rosa N, Marfella R, et al. Impairment of endothelial functions by acute hyperhomocysteinemia and reversal by antioxidant vitamins. *JAMA* 1999;281:2113.
48. Bostom AG, Silbershatz H, Rosenberg IH, et al. Nonfasting plasma total homocysteine levels and all-cause and cardiovascular mortality in elderly Framingham men and women. *Arch Intern Med* 1999;159:1077.
49. Ridker PM, Manson JE, Buring JE, et al. Homocysteine and risk of cardiovascular disease among postmenopausal women. *JAMA* 1999;281:1817.
50. Siri PW, Verhoef P, Kok FJ. Vitamins B-6, B-12, and folate—association with plasma total homocysteine and risk of coronary atherosclerosis. *J Am Coll Nutr* 1998;17:435.
51. Eikelboom JW, Lonn E, Genest J Jr, et al. Homocysteine and cardiovascular disease: a critical review of the epidemiologic evidence. *Ann Intern Med* 1999;131:363.
52. Ueland PM, Refsum H, Beresford SAA, et al. The controversy over homocysteine and cardiovascular risk. *Am J Clin Nutr* 2000;72:324.
53. Collaboration HRT. Lowering blood homocysteine with folic acid-based supplements: meta-analysis of randomized trials. *BMJ* 1998;316:894.
54. Boushey CJ, Beresford SA, Omenn GS, et al. A quantitative assessment of plasma homocysteine as a risk factor for vascular disease. Probable benefits of increasing folic acid intakes. *JAMA* 1995;274:1049.
55. Fioravanti M, Ferrario E, Massaia M, et al. Low folate levels in the cognitive decline of elderly patients and the efficacy of folate as a treatment for improving memory deficits. *Arch Gerontol Geriatr* 1997;26:1.
56. Giovannucci E, Stampfer MJ, Colditz GA, et al. Multivitamin use, folate, and colon cancer in women in the Nurse's Health Study. *Ann Intern Med* 1998;129:517.
57. Kim Y-I. Folate and cancer prevention: a new medical application of folate beyond hyperhomocysteinemia and neural tube defects. *Nutr Rev* 1999;57:314.
58. Mills JL. Fortification of foods with folic acid—how much is enough? *N Engl J Med* 2000;342:1442.
59. Malinow MR, Duell PB, Hess DL, et al. Reduction of plasma homocysteine levels by breakfast cereal fortified with folic acid in patients with coronary artery disease. *N Engl J Med* 1998;338:1009.

60. Jacques PF, Selhub J, Bostom AG, et al. The effect of folic acid fortification on plasma folate and total homocysteine concentrations. *N Engl J Med* 1999; 340:1449.
61. Mix JA. Do megadoses of vitamin C compromise folic acid's role in the metabolism of plasma homocysteine? *Nutr Res* 1999;19:161.
62. Herbert V. Recommended dietary intakes (RDI) of folate in humans. *Am J Clin Nutr* 1987;45:661.
63. Sesin GP, Kirschenbaum H. Folic acid hypersensitivity and fever: a case report. *Am J Hosp Pharm* 1979;36:1565.
64. Ho C, Kauwell GPA, Bailey LB. Practitioners' guide to meeting the vitamin B-12 recommended dietary allowance for people aged 61 years and older. *J Am Diet Assoc* 1999;99:725.
65. Yamada K, Yamada Y, Fukuda M, et al. Bioavailability of dried asakusanori *(Porphyra tenera)* as a source of cobalamin (vitamin B-12). *Int J Vitam Nutr Res* 1999;69:412.
66. Fairbanks VF, Wahner HW, Phyliky RL. Tests for pernicious anemia: the "Schilling test." *Mayo Clin Proc* 1983;58:541.
67. Miller A, Furlong D, Burrows BA, et al. Bound vitamin B_{12} absorption in patients with low serum B_{12} levels. *Am J Hematol* 1992;40:163.
68. Lindenbaum J, Rosenberg IH, Wilson PW, et al. Prevalence of cobalamin deficiency in the Framingham elderly population. *Am J Clin Nutr* 1994;60:2.
69. Flynn MA, Herbert V, Nolph GB, et al. Atherogenesis and the homocysteine–folate–cobalamin triad: do we need standardized analyses? *J Am Coll Nutr* 1997;16:258.
70. Holleland G, Schneede J, Ueland PM, et al. Cobalamin deficiency in general practice. Assessment of the diagnostic utility and cost–benefit analysis of methylmalonic acid determination in relation to current diagnostic strategies. *Clin Chem* 1999;45:189.
71. Shane B, Stokstad EL. Vitamin B_{12}–folate interrelationship. *Annu Rev Nutr* 1985;5:115.
72. Seetharam B, Alpers DH. Cobalamin absorption. In: Field M, Frizzell RA, eds. *Handbook of physiology: the gastrointestinal system, section 6,* vol. IV. Bethesda, MD: American Physiological Society, 1991:437.
73. Christensen EI, Birn H, et al. Synergistic endocytic receptors in renal proximal tubules. *Am J Physiol Renal Physiol* 2001;280:F562.
74. Ermens AA, Sonneveld P, Michiels JJ, et al. Increased uptake and accumulation of cobalamin by multiple myeloma bone marrow cells as a possible cause of low serum cobalamin. *Eur J Haematol* 1993;50:57.
75. Reynold EH. Multiple sclerosis and vitamin B_{12} metabolism. *J Neuroimmunol* 1992;40:225.
76. Howden CW. Vitamin B-12 levels during prolonged treatment with proton pump inhibitors. *J Clin Gastroenterol* 2000;30:29.
77. Healton EB, Savage DG, Grust JC, et al. Neurologic aspects of cobalamin deficiency. *Medicine (Baltimore)* 1991;70:220.
78. Hutto BR. Folate and cobalamin in psychiatric illness. *Compr Psychiatry* 1997;38:305.
79. Bernard MA, Nakonezny PA, Kashner TM. The effect of vitamin B-12 deficiency on older veterans and its relationship to health. *J Am Geriatr Soc* 1998;46:1199.
80. Langman LJ, Cole DEC. Homocysteine: cholesterol of the 90s? *Clin Chim Acta* 1999;286:63.
81. Bjorkegren K, Svardsudd K. Turn of tide for oral vitamin B_{12} treatment. *J Intern Med* 1999;246:237.
82. Kuwabara S, Nakazawa R, Azuma N, et al. Intravenous methylcobalamin treatment for uremic and diabetic neuropathy in chronic hemodialysis patients. *Intern Med* 1999;38:472.
83. Lederle FA. Oral cobalamin for pernicious anemia. Medicine's best kept secret? *JAMA* 1991;265:94.
84. Kuzminski AM, Giacco EJD, Allen RH, et al. Effective treatment of cobalamin deficiency with oral cobalamin. *Blood* 1998;92:1191.

85. Levine M, Conry-Cantilena C, Wang Y, et al. Vitamin C pharmacokinetics in healthy volunteers: evidence for a recommended dietary allowance. *Proc Natl Acad Sci U S A* 1996;93:3704.
86. Lachance P, Langseth L. The RDA concept: time for a change? *Nutr Rev* 1994;52:266.
87. Vanderslice JT, Higgs DJ. Vitamin C content of foods: ample variability. *Am J Clin Nutr* 1991;54:1323S.
88. Ausman LM. Criteria and recommendations for vitamin C intake. *Nutr Rev* 1999;57:222.
89. Friedman PA, Zeidel ML. Victory at C. *Nat Med* 1999;5:620.
90. Packer L, Fuchs J, eds. *Vitamin C in health and disease.* New York: Marcel Dekker Inc, 1997.
91. Hemila H. Vitamin C intake and susceptibility to the common cold. *Br J Nutr* 1997;77:59.
92. Bielory L, Gandhi R. Asthma and vitamin C. *Ann Allergy* 1994;73:89.
93. Ness AR, Powles JW, Khaw KT. Vitamin C and cardiovascular disease: a systematic review. *J Cardiovasc Risk* 1996;3:513.
94. Ness AR, Chee D, Elliott P. Vitamin C and blood pressure—an overview. *J Hum Hypertens* 1997;11:343.
95. Weber P, Bendich A, Shcalch W. Vitamin C and human health—a review of recent data relevant to human requirements. *Int J Vitam Nutr Res* 1996;66:19.
96. Johnston CS. Biomarkers for establishing a tolerable upper intake level for vitamin C. *Nutr Rev* 1999;57:71.
97. Zempleni J, Mock DM. Biotin biochemistry and human requirements. *J Nutr Biochem* 1999;10:128.
98. Roth KS. Biotin in clinical medicine—a review. *Am J Clin Nutr* 1981;34:1967.
99. Mock DM, de Lorimer AA, Liebman WM, et al. Biotin deficiency: an unusual complication of parenteral alimentation. *N Engl J Med* 1981;304:820.
100. Zempleni J, Mock DM. Marginal biotin deficiency is teratogenic. *Proc Soc Exp Biol Med* 2000;223:14.
101. Thoene J, Baker H, Yoshino M, et al. Biotin-responsive carboxylase deficiency associated with subnormal plasma and urinary biotin. *N Engl J Med* 1981;304:817.
102. Wolf B, Heard G , Jefferson LG, et al. Clinical finding in four children with biotinidase deficiency detected through a statewide neonatal screening program. *N Engl J Med* 1985;313:16.
103. Standing Committee on the Scientific Evaluation of Dietary Reference Intakes, Food and Nutrition Board, Institute of Medicine. *Dietary reference intakes for vitamin A, vitamin K, arsenic, boron, chromium, copper, iodine, iron, manganese, molybdenum, nickel, silicon, vanadium, and zinc.* Washington, DC: National Academy Press, 2001. Available on line at *http://www.nap.edu/books, Crawler list 0309072794.* Accessed May 30, 2001.
104. Cooper DA, Eldridge AL, Peters JC. Dietary carotenoids and certain cancers, heart disease, and age-related macular degeneration: a review of recent research. *Nutr Rev* 1999;57:201.
105. Brown L, Rimm EB, Seddon JM, et al. A prospective study of carotenoid intake and risk of cataract extraction in U.S. men. *Am J Clin Nutr* 1999;70:517.
106. Clinton SK. Lycopene: chemistry, biology, and implications for human health and disease. *Nutr Rev* 1998;56:35.
107. West CE. Meeting requirements for vitamin A. *Nutr Rev* 2000;58:341.
108. Dimitrov NV, Meyer C, Ullrey DE, et al. Bioavailability of beta-carotene in humans. *Am J Clin Nutr* 1988;48:298.
109. Rock CL, Swendseid ME. Plasma β-carotene response in humans after meals supplemented with dietary pectin. *Am J Clin Nutr* 1992;55:96.
110. Elinder L, Hadell K, Johansson J, et al. Probucol treatment decreases serum concentrations of diet-derived antioxidants. *Arterioscler Thromb Vasc Biol* 1995; 15:1057.
111. Fredrikzon B, Hernell O, Blackberg L, et al. Bile salt-stimulated lipase in human milk: evidence of activity *in vivo* and of a role in the digestion of milk retinol esters. *Pediatr Res* 1978;12:1048.

112. Stephenson CB. When does hyporetinolemia mean vitamin A deficiency? *Am J Clin Nutr* 2000;72:1.
113. Underwood BA. Method for assessment of vitamin A status. *J Nutr* 1990;120 [Suppl 11]:1459.
114. Blomhoff R, Green MH, Norum KR. Vitamin A: physiological and biochemical processing. *Annu Rev Nutr* 1992;12:37.
115. Hicks VA, Gunning DB, Olson JA. Metabolism, plasma transport and biliary excretion of radioactive vitamin A and its metabolites as a function of liver reserves of vitamin A in the rat. *J Nutr* 1984;114:1327.
116. Pryor WA, Stahl W, Rock CL. Beta carotene: from biochemistry to clinical trials. *Nutr Rev* 2000;58:39.
117. Tyson JE, Wright LL, Oh W, et al. Vitamin A supplementation for extremely low-birth-weight infants. *N Engl J Med* 1999;340:1962.
118. Fenaux P, Degos L. Differentiation therapy for acute promyelocytic leukemia. *N Engl J Med* 1997;337:1076.
119. Albanes D, Heinomen OP, Huttunen JK, et al. Effects of alpha-tocopherol and beta-carotene supplements on cancer incidence in the Alpha-Tocopherol Beta-Carotene Cancer Prevention Study. *Am J Clin Nutr* 1995;62:1427S.
120. Albanes D, Heinonen OP, Taylor PR, et al. Alpha-tocopherol and beta-carotene supplements and lung cancer incidence in the Alpha-Tocopherol Beta-Carotene cancer prevention study: effects of base-line characteristics and study compliance. *J Natl Cancer Inst* 1996;88:1560.
121. Virtamo J, Rapola JM, Ripatti S, et al. Effect of vitamin E and beta-carotene on the incidence of primary nonfatal myocardial infarction and fatal coronary heart disease. *Arch Intern Med* 1998;158:668.
122. Rapola JM, Virtamo J, Ripatti S, et al. Randomized trial of alpha-tocopherol and beta-carotene supplements on incidence of major coronary events in men with previous myocardial infarction. *Lancet* 1997;349:1715.
123. Hennekens CH, Buring JE, Manson JE, et al. Lack of effect of long-term supplementation with beta-carotene on the incidence of malignant neoplasms and cardiovascular disease. *N Engl J Med* 1996;334:1145.
124. Chasan-Taber L, Willett WC, Seddon JM, et al. A prospective study of carotenoid and vitamin A intakes and risk of cataract extraction in U.S. women. *Am J Clin Nutr* 1999;70:509.
125. Hussey GD, Klein M. A randomized, controlled trial of vitamin A in children with severe measles. *N Engl J Med* 1990;323:160.
126. Rahmathullah L, Underwood BA, Thulasiraj R, et al. Reduced mortality among children in Southern India receiving a small weekly dose of vitamin A. *N Engl J Med* 1990;323:929.
127. Bendich A, Langseth L. Safety of vitamin A. *Am J Clin Nutr* 1989;49:358.
128. Ovesen L. Vitamin therapy in the absence of obvious deficiency. What is the evidence? *Drugs* 1984;27:148.
129. Melhus H, Michaelsson K, Kindmark A, et al. Excessive dietary intake of vitamin A is associated with reduced bone mineral density and increased risk for hip fracture. *Ann Intern Med* 1998;129:770.
130. Oakley GP, Erickson JD. Vitamin A and birth defects: continuing caution is needed. *N Engl J Med* 1995;333:1414.
131. Fenaux P, DeBooton S. Retinoic acid syndrome. recognition, prevention and management. *Drug Saf* 1998;18:273.
132. Glerup H, Mikkelsen K, Pousen L, et al. Commonly recommended daily intake of vitamin D is not sufficient if sunlight exposure is limited. *J Intern Med* 2000;247:260.
133. Looker AC, Gunter EW. Hypovitaminosis D in medical inpatients. *N Engl J Med* 1998;339:344.
134. LeBoff MS, Kohlmeier L, Hurwitz S, et al. Occult vitamin D deficiency in postmenopausal U.S. women with acute hip fracture. *JAMA* 1999;281:1505.
135. Avioli L, Haddad JG. The vitamin D family revisited. *N Engl J Med* 1984;311:47.
136. Portale AA, Halloran BP, Murphy MM, et al. Oral intake of phosphorus can determine the serum concentration of 1,25-dihydroxyvitamin D by determining its production rate in humans. *J Clin Invest* 1986;77:7.

137. Kumar R. Hepatic and intestinal osteodystrophy and the hepatobiliary metabolism of vitamin D. *Ann Intern Med* 1983;98:662.
138. Sahota O, Masud T, San P, et al. Vitamin D insufficiency increases bone turnover markers and enhances bone loss at the hip in patients with established vertebral osteoporosis. *Clin Endocrinol* 1999;51:217.
139. Jones G, Strugnell SA, DeLuca HF. Current understanding of the molecular actions of vitamin D. *Physiol Rev* 1998;78:1193.
140. Weber P. The role of vitamins in the prevention of osteoporosis—a brief status report. *Int J Vitam Nutr Res* 1999;69:194.
141. MacLaughlin J, Holick MF. Aging decreases the capacity of human skin to produce vitamin D_3. *J Clin Invest* 1985;76:1536.
142. Spencer H, Rubio N, Rubio E, et al. Chronic alcoholism. Frequently overlooked cause of osteoporosis in men. *Am J Med* 1986;80:393.
143. Thomas MK, Lloyd-Jones DM, Thadhani RJ, et al. Hypovitaminosis D in medical inpatients. *N Engl J Med* 1998;338:777.
144. NIH Consens Statement. Optimal calcium intake. 1994;12:1.
145. Chapuy MC, Arlot ME, Duboeuf F, et al. Vitamin D_3 and calcium to prevent hip fractures in elderly women. *N Engl J Med* 1992;327:1637.
146. Dawson-Hughes B, Harris SS, Krall EA, et al. Effect of calcium supplementation on bone density in men and women 65 years of age or older. *N Engl J Med* 1997;337:670.
147. Buckley LM, Leib ES, Cartularo KS, et al. Calcium and vitamin D_3 supplementation prevents bone loss in the spine secondary to low-dose corticosteroids in patients with rheumatoid arthritis. *Ann Intern Med* 1996;125:961.
148. Nuti R, Martinin G, Giovani S, et al. Effect of treatment with calcitriol combined with low-dosage alendronate in involutional osteoporosis. *Clin Drug Invest* 2000;19:55.
149. Slatopolsky E, Weerts C, Thielan J, et al. Marked suppression of secondary hyperparathyroidism by intravenous administration of 1,25-dihyroxy-cholecalciferol in uremic patients. *J Clin Invest* 1984;74:2136.
150. Leichtman GA, Bengoa JM, Bolt MJ, et al. Intestinal absorption of cholecalciferol and 25-hydroxycholecalciferol in patients with both Crohn's disease and intestinal resection. *Am J Clin Nutr* 1991;54:548.
151. Vieth R. Vitamin D supplementation, 25-hydroxyvitamin D concentrations, and safety. *Am J Clin Nutr* 1999;69:842.
152. Weber P, Bendich A, Machlin LJ. Vitamin E and human health: rationale for determining recommended intake levels. *Nutrition* 1997;13:450.
153. Bauernfeind JC. The tocopherol content of food and influencing factors. *Crit Rev Food Sci Nutr* 1977;8:337.
154. McLaughlin PJ, Weihrauch JL. Vitamin E content of foods. *J Am Diet Assoc* 1979;75:647.
155. Ford ES, Sowell A. Serum alpha-tocopherol status in the United States population: findings from the Third National Health and Nutrition Examination Survey. *Am J Epidemiol* 1999;150:290.
156. Thurnham DI, Davies JA, Crump BJ, et al. The use of different lipids to express serum tocopherol:lipid ratios for the measurement of vitamin E status. *Ann Clin Biochem* 1986;23:514.
157. Refat M, Moore TJ, Kazui M, et al. Utility of breath ethane as a noninvasive biomarker of vitamin E status in children. *Pediatr Res* 1991;30:396.
158. Chan AC. Vitamin E and atherosclerosis. *J Nutr* 1998;128:1593.
159. Steiner M. Vitamin E, a modifier of platelet function: rationale and use in cardiovascular and cerebrovascular disease. *Nutr Rev* 1999;57:306.
160. Berdanier CD. *Advanced nutrition: micronutrients*. Boca Raton, FL: CRC Press, 1998.
161. Euronut SENECA study. Nutritional status: blood vitamins A, E, B_6, B_{12}, folic acid, and carotene. *Eur J Clin Nutr* 1991;45:63.
162. Rosenblum JL, Keating JP, Prensky AL, et al. A progressive neurologic syndrome in children with chronic liver disease. *N Engl J Med* 1981;304:503.
163. Kayden HJ. The neurologic syndrome of vitamin E deficiency: a significant cause of ataxia. *Neurology* 1993;43:2167.

164. Tribble DL. Antioxidant consumption and risk of coronary heart disease: emphasis on vitamin C, vitamin E, and β-carotene: a statement for healthcare professionals from the American Heart Association. *Circulation* 1999;99:591.
165. Ascherio A, Rimm EB, Hernan MA, et al. Relation of consumption of vitamin E, vitamin C, and carotenoids to risk for stroke among men in the United States. *Ann Intern Med* 1999;130:963.
166. Perkins AJ, Hendrie HC, Callahan CM, et al. Association of antioxidants with memory in a multiethnic elderly sample using the Third National Health and Nutrition Examination Survey. *Am J Epidemiol* 1999;150:37.
167. Horwitt MK. Therapeutic uses of vitamin E in medicine. *Nutr Rev* 1980;38:105.
168. Sokol RJ, Guggenheim MA, Iannaccone ST, et al. Improved neurologic function after long-term correction of vitamin E deficiency in children with chronic cholestasis. *N Engl J Med* 1985;313:1580.
169. Sokol RJ, Butler-Simon N, Conner C, et al. Multicenter trial of d-alpha-tocopheryl polyethylene glycol 1000 succinate for treatment of vitamin E deficiency in children with chronic cholestasis. *Gastroenterology* 1993;104:1727.
170. Sitrin MD, Lieberman F, Jensen WE, et al. Vitamin E deficiency and neurologic disease in adults with cystic fibrosis. *Ann Intern Med* 1987;107:51.
171. Hittner HM, Godio LB, Rudolph AJ, et al. Retrolental fibroplasia: efficacy of vitamin E in a double-blind clinical study of preterm infants. *N Engl J Med* 1981;305:1365.
172. Corash L, Spielberg S, Bartsocass C, et al. Reduced chronic hemolysis during high-dose vitamin E administration in Mediterranean-type glucose-6-phosphate dehydrogenase deficiency. *N Engl J Med* 1980;303:416.
173. Natta CL, Machlin LJ, Brin M. A decrease in irreversibly sickled erythrocytes in sickle cell anemia patients given vitamin E. *Am J Clin Nutr* 1980;33:968.
174. Spencer AP, Carson DS, Crouch MA. Vitamin E and coronary artery disease. *Arch Intern Med* 1999;159:1313.
175. Bendich A. Safety issues regarding the use of vitamin supplements. *Ann N Y Acad Sci* 1992;669:300.
176. Lipsky JJ. Nutritional sources of vitamin K. *Mayo Clin Proc* 1994;69:462.
177. Booth SL, Suttie JW. Dietary intake and adequacy of vitamin K. *J Nutr* 1998;128:785.
178. Booth SL, Centurelli MA. Vitamin K: a practical guide to the dietary management of patients on warfarin. *Nutr Rev* 1999;57:288.
179. Ferland G. The vitamin K-dependent proteins: an update. *Nutr Rev* 1998;56:223.
180. Vermeer G, Knapen MHJ, Schurgers LJ. Vitamin K and metabolic bone disease. *J Clin Pathol* 1998;51:424.
181. Szulc P, Chapuy MC, Meunier PJ, et al. Serum undercarboxylated osteocalcin is a marker of the risk of hip fracture in elderly women. *J Clin Invest* 1993;91:1769.
182. Feskanich D, Willett WW, Rockett H, et al. Vitamin K intake and hip fractures in women: a prospective study. *Am J Clin Nutr* 1999;69:74.
183. Jamal SA, Browner WS, Bauer DC, et al. Warfarin use and risk for osteoporosis in elderly women. *Ann Intern Med* 1998;128:829.
184. Caraballo PJ, Heit JA, Atkinson EJ, et al. Long-term use of oral anticoagulants and the risk of fracture. *Arch Intern Med* 1999;159;1750.

7. MINERALS

I. **Evaluation of mineral intake and deficiency.** The minerals important in human nutrition can be classified into three groups: those stored in the body in large quantities (Na, K, Ca, Mg, P); those present in trace amounts whose role in human nutrition has been determined (Fe, Zn, Cu, I, F, Se, Cr); and those present in trace amounts (Co, Mo, Mn, Cd, As, Si, V, Ni) that are clearly important in laboratory animals but whose role in human nutrition is uncertain. Of this last group, only manganese is discussed in this chapter because some deficiency of that element has been demonstrated in humans.

   A. **Intestinal absorption and secretion**

      1. **Divalent cations.** The major divalent cations (Ca, Mg, Zn, Cu) are not absorbed efficiently. They are ingested in forms that are poorly soluble and must be converted to more soluble salts, and transport across the apical membrane is relatively slow. Moreover, significant amounts of these ions are secreted into the intestinal lumen each day via intestinal, pancreatic, and biliary juices. Thus, deficiency develops in the setting of either diarrhea or malabsorption. Iron is absorbed best in its divalent form and is lost mainly through bleeding into the gastrointestinal tract or from the uterus.

      2. **Monovalent cations.** The major monovalent cations (Na, K) are also secreted in digestive juices, but they are very efficiently reabsorbed. Nonetheless, their concentrations are so high that deficiency can develop when large amounts of body fluids are lost. Therefore, intestinal diseases often lead to decreases in the body stores of many minerals. Many minerals are reabsorbed by renal (Na, K, Ca, Mg, P) as well as intestinal cells. Thus, the potential for loss is great when these organs are diseased.

   B. **Evaluation of deficiency.** Only in the case of iron do blood levels correlate with body stores. Bone is the major storage site of several minerals (Ca, P, Mg, F), and levels of these minerals in bone do not equilibrate rapidly with blood levels. In the case of some minerals (Na, K, Ca), many compensatory mechanisms exist to maintain blood levels within the normal range. These mechanisms are designed to regulate extracellular fluid concentrations rather than body stores. Because blood levels do not usually correlate well with body stores, deficiencies of many minerals are difficult to assess from a practical point of view. The diagnosis of mineral deficiency should be suspected first by the presence of appropriate symptoms or signs in a high-risk setting. Table 7-1 outlines these general features. The details of each deficiency state are described in the sections on each mineral.

   C. **Mineral overload.** Many minerals are widely available in foods; moreover, they are easily provided as supplements. For these reasons, and because it is difficult to assess body stores, it is not surprising that overload syndromes occur more frequently in the case of minerals than of vitamins. Sodium, potassium, calcium, iron, and fluoride are the minerals most commonly involved in overload syndromes. Table 7-1 outlines the general features of overload syndromes.

   D. **Treatment of mineral deficiency.** Oral therapy is discussed in detail in this chapter. Parenteral therapy with major minerals (Na, K, Ca, Mg, P) is discussed in Chapter 10. Most healthy people do not require mineral supplements. However, certain groups of patients at high risk for deficiency of individual minerals should receive supplements.

      1. **Infancy.** Iron may be needed at 6 to 8 weeks of life, especially if the mother has been deficient. Low-birth-weight infants require zinc.

      2. **Menstruation.** Iron supplements are often required.

      3. **Pregnancy.** Iron and calcium are needed because requirements are increased (see also Chapter 4).

Table 7-1. Clinical manifestations of mineral deficiency and toxicity states

Mineral	Major functions	Major causes of deficiency	Clinical signs	
			Deficiency	Toxicity
Na	ECF volume, muscle and nerve function, nutrient absorption	GI, renal, and skin losses	Hypovolemia, weakness, nausea	Confusion, stupor
K	Acid/base balance, membrane transport, muscle contraction, protein synthesis	GI (nausea, diarrhea) renal (diuretics) losses	Arrhythmias, muscle weakness, nausea, irritability	Paresthesias, confusion, cardiac depression
Cl	Acid–base balance, osmotic pressure, HCl in stomach	GI (vomiting, diarrhea), renal (diuretics) losses	Alkalosis, muscle cramps, anorexia	Acidosis with renal failure
Ca	Bone/tooth formation, blood clotting, nerve transmission, muscle contraction, secretion	↓ Intake, malabsorption, ↑ PTH	Tetany, arrhythmia, osteomalacia	Anorexia, constipation, vomiting, coma
Mg	Cell metabolism, enzyme activation, nerve/muscle action	Malabsorption, renal tubular leak, EtOH	Muscle twitching, arrhythmia, nausea, weakness, confusion	Nausea, ↓ BP, confusion, ↓ reflexes
P	Bone/tooth formation, metabolic functions, nucleic acid formation	↑ renal excretion, wasting diseases	Weakness, bone pain, rhabdomyolysis,	Secondary ↑ parathyroidism

	Heme formation, enzyme cofactor	Blood loss (GI, gynecologic) ↑ needs (pregnancy), ↓ intake (infants)	Anemia	Cirrhosis, heart failure, skin pigmentation
Fe	Heme formation, enzyme cofactor	Blood loss (GI, gynecologic) ↑ needs (pregnancy), ↓ intake (infants)	Anemia	Cirrhosis, heart failure, skin pigmentation
Zn	Enzyme cofactor, CO_2 transfer, DNA function, wound healing	Diarrhea, malabsorption	Stunted growth, skin changes, anorexia, lethargy, alopecia	Cu deficiency, ↓ immunity
Cu	Enzyme cofactor function of nerves, vascular/bone structure	Malnutrition, prematurity	Anemia, neutropenia, skeletal defects, nerve degeneration	Vomiting
I	Thyroxine synthesis	↓ Intake	Goiter, hypothyroidism	Hyperthyroidism
Mn	Enzyme cofactor	One case reported	↑ Cholesterol, weight loss	Neural damage
Cr	Insulin cofactor	TPN	Glucose intolerance	None
F	Bone/tooth formation	↓ Intake	Dental caries	Brittle bones
Se	GSH peroxidase cofactor	↓ Intake, TPN	Cardiomyopathy	Hair loss, fatigue

ECF, extracellular fluid; GI, gastrointestinal; PTH, parathyroid hormone; EtOH, ethyl alcohol; BP, blood pressure; TPN, total parenteral nutrition; GSH, reduced glutathione.

4. **Restricted diets.** Persons who consume little or no milk require calcium; those on vegetable diets require iron.
5. **Gastrointestinal disorders.** Patients with malabsorption may require calcium, magnesium, and zinc. In acute disorders characterized by severe vomiting or diarrhea, sodium and potassium must be replaced. Patients with chronic gastrointestinal bleeding may require iron replacement.
6. **Osteodystrophies.** Elderly patients whose calcium intake is decreased or who have osteopenia may require calcium supplements. The sections on the individual minerals should be consulted for details.

II. Major minerals
A. Sodium

1. **Requirements.** Total body sodium levels range from 52 to 60 mEq/kg in male adults and from 48 to 55 mEq/kg in female adults. The body of a 70-kg man may contain between 3,600 and 4,200 mEq of sodium (83 and 97 g). About one-fourth of this, largely in the skeleton, is not exchangeable. Exchangeable sodium averages 40 mEq/kg in males and 37 mEq/kg in females. Changes in sodium concentration are corrected even at the expense of volume distribution. The kidney regulates sodium excretion by producing aldosterone. When intake falls, aldosterone levels increase and urinary excretion of sodium falls. When sodium intake is high, urinary excretion rises. Thus, obligatory sodium losses are small in comparison with body stores. Minimal urinary and fecal losses are each about 23 mg (1 mEq) daily. Total body water losses contain from 46 to 92 mg of sodium (2 to 4 mEq) daily.

   a. **Minimal sodium needs** in normal persons, therefore, can be met by an intake of 4 to 8 mEq (92 to 184 mg) daily. The requirement increases when the production of sweat (containing 25 mEq of sodium per liter) increases or losses in the urine or stool increase in disease states. Because of wide variations in physical activity and ambient temperatures, the safe minimum intake is set at 500 mg for adults (1). The sodium requirement in children is set somewhat below that for adults: 120 mg for infants ages 0 to 5 months, 200 mg for infants ages 6 to 11 months, 225 mg for children 1 year old, 300 mg for children 2 to 5 years old, and 300 mg for children 6 to 9 years old. The requirement in infants is largely provided by human milk (7 mEq/L) or cow's milk (21 mEq/L). In pregnancy, another 11 kg is added to the mother's body weight, of which 35% to 40% is extracellular fluid. This amounts to an additional 700 mEq of sodium, or 3 mEq (69 mg) per day, throughout the pregnancy. When sweating is increased, the additional amount required varies from 2 to 7 g of sodium chloride per liter of water lost.

   b. **U.S. dietary guidelines.** The Intersalt study (2) examined blood pressure measurements versus 24-hour urine sodium excretion in more than10,000 persons and found a positive and linear relationship between these parameters across all the populations. This result was confirmed in a more recent analysis (3). However, within a single population, the relationships were modest if present at all. Metaanalyses of randomized trials of the effect of reducing sodium on blood pressure demonstrated a direct relationship (4), but not for normotensive persons (5). Because of these data, the American Heart Association suggests limiting sodium intake to 3 g/d, and the World Health Organization and National Academy of Science recommend 2.4 g/d (6 g of NaCl per day) (6). Data from the first National Health and Nutrition Examination Survey (NHANES I) showed an inverse relationship between sodium intake and all-cause and cardiovascular mortality (7), but confounding factors such as smoking and calorie intake were not accounted for. Because the data are so difficult to obtain and interpret, debate continues regarding the need for limiting sodium intake.

One view states that sodium is only one of many factors in hypertension, and that even randomized interventions (30% to 50% decrease in sodium intake) produce very modest changes (decrease of ~ 1 mm Hg in systolic pressure) (8). The Dietary Approaches to Stop Hypertension (DASH) study compared a typical American diet (high in fat, low in fiber, low in potassium and calcium) with a diet rich in fruits and vegetables, both without and with low-fat dairy products (DASH diet); sodium intake and weight were kept stable throughout the 8-week trial in patients with systolic pressures below 160 mm Hg and diastolic pressures between 80 and 95 mm Hg (9). The DASH diet lowered systolic blood pressure by 11.4 mm Hg and diastolic blood pressure by 5.5 mm, much better results than those obtained with low-sodium diets. The National Heart, Lung, and Blood Institute 1999 Workshop on Sodium and Blood Pressure agreed that sodium restriction is most beneficial for older persons with established hypertension, but that only a small percentage of the U.S. population is sensitive to the hypertensive effect of sodium (8). Moreover, much of the effect may represent a lower intake of potassium, calcium, and other minerals, rather than an excessive intake of sodium. Thus, the argument is made for revising the safe sodium intake.

Proponents of the other point of view discount the small effects of randomized low-sodium trials because of their short time frame and cite data suggesting a high prevalence of sodium sensitivity (10). For these reason and because most people do not reach the currently recommended level of sodium intake, the argument for keeping the presently "restricted" figure seems reasonable to some. The issue is still unresolved, but both groups agree that sodium restriction for elderly hypertensives is a reasonable approach.

2. **Food sources.** In Western societies, an adult with free access to salt consumes from 2.3 to 6.9 g (100 to 300 mEq) of sodium per day, or from 8 to 12 g (140 to 250 mEq) of sodium chloride. Most of the sodium is added to foods as salt (NaCl). Of total dietary sodium, about one-third comes from the shaker, one-third from processing, and one-third from the food itself. Cheese, milk, and shellfish, in addition to meat, fish, and eggs, are good natural sources of sodium. Cereals, fruits, and vegetables are low in salt unless it is added during processing. The amount of salt added in processing can be considerable. Table 7-2 lists the sodium content of some foods at different stages of preparation.

Normally, sodium must be added to some cereals, such as those containing bran or fiber, to increase palatability. In other cereals (e.g., wheat cereals), the range of sodium content is very wide. The sodium content of some natural foods is listed in Table 7-3.

Table 7-2. Effect of food processing on sodium content

Food	State	Portion	Na content (mg)[a]
Corn	Fresh kernels	½ cup	12
	Canned kernels	½ cup	190
	Canned, creamed	½ cup	365
Potato	Baked	1 each	16
	Mashed, instant	1 cup	733
	Chips	14 chips	133
Tomato	Fresh chopped	1 cup	11
	Canned whole	1 cup	390
	Juice	1 cup	881

[a] These are representative figures, not brand-specific.

Table 7-3. Approximate sodium content of natural foods

Negligible	2–5 mg	5–9 mg	25 mg	120 mg
Butter, unsalted	Fruits (½ cup)	Bread without salt (slice)	Muscle or organ meat (1 oz)	Milk (1 cup)
Cream (tbs)	Corn, potato, peas, beans (½ cup)	Selected dry cereals (puffed rice, puffed wheat, shredded wheat (1 cup)	1 egg Fish (1 oz)	
Cooking fat (tsp)		Most vegetables (½ cup)		

Much sodium can be added to foods in the form of condiments, fats, and salad dressings. Some of the most commonly used products are listed in Table 7-4.

A full list of the sodium content of foods is presented in the U.S. Department of Agriculture booklet entitled *The Sodium Content of Your Food* (Home and Garden Bulletin No. 233, U.S. Government Printing Office, Washington, D.C.). Some labels express sodium content in grams or milligrams. Some diets list salt content or milliequivalents of sodium. To convert salt to sodium content, multiply milligrams of salt by 0.4, the fraction of sodium chloride weight that represents sodium. To convert sodium in milligrams to milliequivalents, divide milligrams by 23, the atomic weight of sodium.

Table 7-4. Representative sodium content of condiments

Product	Portion	Na content (mg)	Na content (mEq)
Baking powder	1 tsp	339	15
Baking soda	1 tsp	821	36
Catsup	1 tbs	202	9
Garlic salt	1 tsp	1,620	70
Meat tenderizer	1 tsp	1,750	76
Monosodium glutamate	1 tsp	492	21
Mustard, prepared	1 tsp	65	3
Onion salt	1 tsp	1,650	72
Olives, green	10 ea	936	41
Pickle, dill	1 medium	928	41
Pickle, sweet	1 tbs	107	40
Table salt	1 tsp	1,938	84
A-1 sauce	1 tbs	275	12
Barbecue sauce	1 tbs	130	6
Soy sauce, regular	1 tbs	1,029	45
Soy sauce, low-sodium	1 tbs	300	13
Worcestershire sauce	1 tbs	206	9
Butter, regular	1 tbs	116	5
Margarine	1 tbs	140	6
Salad dressing, bottled	1 tbs	109–224	5–10

a. **Sodium in prepared foods.** In food preparation, a number of compounds are added besides sodium chloride to increase the sodium content. These are listed below as they appear on labels:

Monosodium glutamate (MSG)—in packaged and frozen foods
Baking powder—in breads and cakes
Baking soda (sodium bicarbonate)—in breads and cakes
Brine—in processed foods (e.g., pickles)
Disodium phosphate—in cereals and cheeses
Sodium alginate or caseinate—as thickener and binder
Sodium benzoate or nitrite—as preservative
Sodium hydroxide—to soften skins of fruits and olives
Sodium propionate—to inhibit mold in cheeses
Sodium sulfate—as preservative in dried fruit
Sodium citrate—as buffer for canned and bottled citrus drinks

b. **Sodium in water and medications.** In addition to food, sodium is present in drinking water and in medications. Water may contain very little sodium or as much as 1500 mg/L, depending on the degree of softening, a process that raises the sodium content of water. The various departments of public health can usually supply information on the sodium content of local water supplies.

Most medications do not contain enough sodium to present a problem, but a few are very high in sodium. Table 7-5 lists some of these. In general, liquid formulas contain more sodium than do capsules or tablets.

3. **Assessment**

a. **Clinical.** The signs of total body sodium excess are weight gain and edema. The signs of total body sodium deficiency are manifestations of hypovolemia and can include decreased skin turgor, hypotension, tachycardia, dry tongue or axillae, sunken eyes, and weight loss. In older adults, other explanations are often present for all these signs (11). Orthostatic hypotension is often used, defined in the American Academy of Neurology consensus statement as a decrease in systolic blood pressure of 20 mm Hg or in diastolic blood pressure of 10 mm Hg within 3 minutes of standing (12). Some clinicians prefer an increase in the pulse rate of 5 to 12 beats/min (13). However, postprandial hypotension resulting from splanchnic blood pooling is common in older patients, and blood loss is a common cause of postural hypotension. Usually, the decision to proceed with hydration therapy depends on a consideration of all the findings of the clinical and laboratory evaluation.

b. **Serum sodium.** Sodium is measured by ion-selective electrodes in either clotted blood or anticoagulated blood (not ethylenediaminetetraacetic acid, or EDTA). The serum sodium level (normal, 135 to 145 mEq/L) does not reflect the total body sodium but rather the relationship between total body sodium and extracellular fluid (ECF) volume. A patient with excess total body sodium, manifested by edema, may have a low, normal, or high serum level of sodium depending on whether ECF volume is increased to a level in excess of, even with, or less than that of the total body sodium. Thus, a patient with edema and a serum sodium level of 125 mEq/L has a total body excess of sodium, but the serum sodium level is low because of retained water in excess of sodium. The serum sodium level can be high in hyperadrenalism, severe dehydration, diabetic coma, or treatment with sodium salts. Serum values above 160 mEq/L or below 120 mEq/L are usually associated with symptoms and must be verified and corrected.

c. **Other laboratory evaluation.** Laboratory findings associated with hypovolemia include a high urine specific gravity, elevated

Table 7-5. Sodium content in selected medications (sodium per therapeutic unit[a])

<5 mg	5–25 mg	25–100 mg	>100 mg
Penicillin, potassium	Phenytoin	Penicillin, sodium	Alka-Seltzer (521 per tablet)
Analgesics (most)	Maalox liquid	Synthetic penicillins, sodium	Bromo-Seltzer (717 per tablet)
Nonpenicillin antibiotic tablets	Amphojel suspension	Dramamine	Sal Hepatica (1,000 per tsp)
Vitamin tablets	Titralac liquid[a]	Antibiotic suspensions	
Metamucil	Kaopectate	Colace	
Diuretics	Milk of magnesia		
Antihypertensives	Metamucil instant mix		
Antihistamines	Endocrine agents		
Mg/Al(OH)$_3$ antacid tablets (many)	Cold syrups		
Mylanta liquid	Sedative elixirs		
Riopan liquid	Liquid vitamins		
Laxatives (many)	Di-Gel liquid		
Psychoactive drugs			
Sedative capsules			

[a] The therapeutic unit of antacids is considered to be 30 mL of liquid or two tablets. The therapeutic dose of Titralac is 5 mL.

hematocrit, and a blood urea nitrogen (BUN) elevated in excess of the serum creatinine level. The urinary sodium level does not correlate with intake or body stores except in the normal condition when excess sodium is excreted. The normal range is 27 to 287 mmol/24 hours. In sodium retention syndromes, the urinary sodium level can be low when stores are high; in renal salt wasting, the urinary sodium level can be elevated when body stores are low. For acute assessment, the body weight provides a better measure of extracellular volume. When the glomerular filtration rate (GFR) per nephron ratio is decreased, as in prerenal azotemia, the urinary–plasma (U/P) creatinine ratio is greater than 20 (range, 20 to 50) and the urine sodium concentration is greater than 20 mEq/L. The fractional excretion of sodium is defined as $100 \times (U/P_{sodium} \div U/P_{creatinine})$ and is less than 1% in prerenal azotemia or total body sodium deficiency. In acute renal failure, the fractional excretion of sodium is more than 4%, the U/P creatinine ratio is less than 10, and the urinary sodium level is more than 40 mEq/L.

4. Physiology

    a. Excretion. Sodium is present in most body secretions. Excessive loss of sodium can occur when any of these secretions is lost in large amounts from the body. The secretions and their ion contents are listed in Table 7-6. Only the kidney (and the colon and terminal ileum to a limited extent) is able to restrict or increase its loss of sodium. Because the urinary sodium level is so variable, it is not included in the list. Renal conservation involves a balance between filtration and reabsorption. The urinary sodium level reflects the sodium that escapes reabsorption in the nephron; therefore,

Table 7-6. Electrolyte concentrations in gastrointestinal fluids

Fluid source	Na (mEq/L)	Na (mEq/d)	K (mEq/L)	K (mEq/d)	Cl (mEq/L)	Cl (mEq/d)	HCO₃ (mEq/L)	HCO₃ (mEq/d)
Stomach[a]	65	40–100	10	10–15	100	140–200	—	—
Bile	150	100	4	5	100	40	35	40
Pancreas[b]	150	130	7	6	80	70	75	65
Duodenum	90	180	15	30	90	180	90	180
Mid-small bowel	140	280	6	12	100	200	20	40
Terminal ileum	140	70	8	4	60	30	70	35
Rectum/stool	40	10	90	23	15	4	30	8
Diarrhea, moderate	50–100		20–30		50–100		<20	
Diarrhea, severe	100–140		20–40		80–100		30–50	

[a] Na and Cl vary inversely according to the rate of H⁺ secretion.
[b] Cl and HCO₃ vary inversely, according to the rate of secretion.

sodium excretion depends on the GFR. Thus, renal regulation is well adapted to conserving the major extracellular cation.

   b. **Intestinal reabsorption.** The small bowel reabsorbs most of the electrolytes and water from luminal secretions under normal circumstances. Most of the sodium is absorbed from the jejunum and ileum by solute-dependent sodium cotransport along with sugars and amino acids. Non–nutrient-dependent sodium absorption in the proximal small intestine occurs mainly by Na/H exchange. The ileum and colon absorb sodium actively by a coupled Na/Cl cotransport and also secrete bicarbonate in exchange for chloride. The colon retains sodium most avidly and secretes potassium into the lumen. In small-bowel malabsorption, the colon is presented with an increased sodium load, which it reabsorbs at least partially. The colon and terminal ileum can respond to aldosterone but are not able to retain sodium as efficiently as the kidney. Sodium absorption in the rectum occurs mainly through apically located sodium channels.

   (1) **Potential losses of sodium.** When diarrhea is mild or moderate and the colon is intact, sodium losses are moderate and proportional to the stool volume (Table 7-7). Potassium losses are also proportional to the stool volume when it is not excessive (<3 L/d). Chloride is lost as the predominant anion, and systemic alkalosis develops, so that the potassium loss is exacerbated through increased urinary excretion. In secretory diarrheas, stool sodium is less than 70 mEq/L; in osmotic diarrhea, sodium is usually less than 70 mEq/L.

   When diarrhea is severe, the colon is maximally stimulated to conserve sodium chloride. In the process, it secretes more potassium and bicarbonate. The result is greater loss of sodium (because the colonic capacity is exceeded) and greater loss of

Table 7-7. Common metabolic consequences of electrolyte depletion syndromes

Syndrome	Major ions lost	Acid–base status	ECF volume	Renal response	[K]
Vomiting	H, Cl, K >Na	Alkalosis	↓	Na, HCO$_3$ Retained K lost	↓
Pancreatic fistula	Na, HCO$_3$	Acidosis	↓↓	Na, Cl retained	NL
Malabsorption	Na, Cl, K All > HCO$_3$	NL, alkalosis	↓	Na, Cl retained, K lost	↓
Ileostomy	Na, Cl > HCO$_3$	Alkalosis	↓	Na, HCO$_3$ retained, K lost	NL, ↓
Diarrhea, moderate	Na, K	NL	NL	K retained	NL, ↓
Diarrhea, severe	Na, HCO$_3$, K, Cl	Acidosis	↓↓	Na, Cl retained	↓
Salt wasting	Na, Cl	Alkalosis	↓	None	NL, ↑
↑ Sweating	Na, Cl	Alkalosis	↓	Na, Cl retained,	NL, ↓
↑ Diuretics	Na, K, Cl	Alkalosis	↓	None	↓

ECF, extracellular fluid; NL, normal.

potassium. Sodium loss can increase without limit, depending on fecal volume. Large amounts of sodium can be lost in a short time whenever intestinal secretions are lost in large quantities. Sodium is the major extracellular cation and is involved in the maintenance of electrogenic potentials across the cell membrane. Because the body preserves serum sodium concentration at the expense of extravascular volume, early sodium deficiency is accompanied by signs of volume depletion rather than by hyponatremia.

(2) **Potential losses of other electrolytes.** Potassium loss is limited somewhat by the degree of sodium exchange, and the potassium concentration tends to plateau when fecal volumes are above 3 L/d. Bicarbonate losses can be large in severe diarrhea, and metabolic acidosis may result.

5. **Deficiency.** Sodium deficiency is nearly always the result of excessive losses and results in hypovolemia and dehydration (see Section 3, Assessment). Hyponatremia may accompany signs of dehydration. The differential diagnosis of hyponatremia with contracted ECF volumes is aided by determining the urinary sodium levels. When the urinary sodium concentration is less than 10 mmol/L, sodium intake may be inadequate, but hypovolemia resulting from excessive sodium loss (sweating, diarrhea) is a more likely cause. When the urinary sodium concentration is more than 10 mmol/L, vomiting or excessive urinary loss of sodium may be the likely cause. When the cause of hyponatremia is not clear, the serum osmolality should be measured. Normal osmolality can be associated with hyperlipidemia or markedly elevated glucose or urea levels (*pseudohyponatremia*). To ascertain whether the serum sodium concentration is normal in the presence of hyperglycemia or an elevated BUN value, the serum osmolarity can be estimated (normal, 275 to 295 mOsmol/kg):

$$\text{Estimated Serum Osmolality} = 2 \times [\text{Na}] + ([\text{Glucose}] \div 18) + ([\text{BUN}] \div 2.8)$$

where [Na] is expressed in mEq/L and [glucose] and [BUN] are expressed in mg/dL.

Dilutional (hypotonic) hyponatremia occurs when water is retained in excess of existing sodium stores. Although sodium depletion is a major cause of this syndrome, any water-retaining disorder may present with a similar serum sodium profile, although signs of dehydration are not present. Both sodium depletion and retention syndromes are characterized by low urinary sodium levels and an impaired capacity for renal water excretion.

The serum sodium level is not a guide for volume loss, but symptoms (confusion, anorexia, lethargy, vomiting, seizures) can develop when the serum sodium level falls below 120 to 125 mEq/L. Other metabolic consequences accompany clinical situations in which sodium depletion develops (Table 7-8). These situations largely involve losses from the gastrointestinal tract. Losses of sodium from the gastrointestinal tract are proportional to the volume lost. The other ions lost (K, Cl, HCO_3) are determined by the source of the fluid. The serum sodium level is normal or low in these syndromes depending on how rapidly the losses occur. With large losses of gastric secretions, hypochloremia and alkalosis ensue. With severe losses from diarrhea, metabolic acidosis can develop when the colon is intact to generate bicarbonate. In mild to moderate cases of diarrhea, chloride is lost in proportion to or in excess of bicarbonate, and alkalosis is present if any acid–base disturbance is noted.

6. **Therapy.** In sodium replacement, the amount given depends on the salt administered. Because 1 g of sodium equals 43 mEq of sodium and 1 g of

Table 7-8. Causes of dilutional hyponatremia

Pathophysiology	ECF volume	Causes
Renal sodium loss	↓	Diuretic drugs, adrenal insufficiency, nephropathy, osmotic diuresis
Intestinal sodium loss	↓	Diarrhea, vomiting, blood loss
Skin sodium loss	↓	Excessive sweating/climatic heat
Fluid sequestration	↓	Burns, pancreatitis, bowel obstruction
Renal sodium retention	↑	CHF, cirrhosis, renal failure, pregnancy
Inappropriate antidiuretic	NL	Cancer, CNS lesions and disorders, medications, pulmonary conditions, postoperative, HIV hormone
↓ Solute intake	NL	Beer potomania, tea-and-toast diet
Excessive water intake	NL	Primary polydipsia, dilute infant formula

ECF, extracellular fluid; NL, normal; CHF, congestive heart failure; CNS, central nervous system.

sodium chloride equals 17 mEq of sodium, a 4-g sodium diet is roughly equivalent to a 10-g salt (NaCl) diet. Each gram of sodium bicarbonate represents 12 mEq of sodium. Sodium preparations are listed in Table 7-9.

  a. **Parenteral replacement.** When hyponatremia causes symptoms (lethargy, seizures), IV treatment is needed with normal or hypertonic saline solution. Replacement should raise the serum concentration to above 120 mEq/L but should not increase it by more than 24 mEq/L in the first 24 hours. Permanent neurologic damage has been attributed to excessively rapid sodium replacement when deficiency is severe. When IV fluid is needed, the choice of additive or solution used (Table 7-9) sometimes depends on the source of lost fluid (Tables 7-6 and 7-8). When signs of volume depletion are obvi-

Table 7-9. Sodium supplements

Product	Anion	Na per dose (mEq)	Na per dose (mg)	ECF distribution (%)
Oral supplements				
NaCl	Cl	17/1-g tablet	391	100
NaHCO₃	HCO₃	7.8/0.650-g tablet	138	?
Parenteral fluids				
Normal saline	Cl	154/L	3541	100
3% Saline	Cl	517/L	11,891	100
NaHCO₃	HCO₃	44.6/50 mL or 50/50 mL		?
Lactated Ringer's solution	Lactate	130/L	2990	97
0.45% Saline in water	Cl	77/L	1771	73

ECF, extracellular fluid.

ously present, at least a 10% reduction in the ECF volume has occurred. In a normal person, the ECF volume is about 20% of body weight. Because the sodium concentration is 135 to 146 mEq/L of ECF fluid, the milliequivalents of sodium required can be estimated to replace 10% of the ECF volume or 20% if the signs of volume depletion are severe. The sodium deficit can be estimated as follows:

$$Na_{deficit} \, (mEq) = ([Na]_{desired} - [Na]_{observed}) \times 0.6 \times Weight \, (kg)$$

Alternatively, one can estimate the effect on the serum sodium concentration of adding 1 L of infusate:

$$Change \, in \, [Na]_{serum} = [Na]_{infusate} - [Na]_{serum} \div (Total \, Body \, Water + 1)$$

where total body water is estimated in liters as a fraction of body weight (0.6 for children; 0.6 and 0.5 for nonelderly men and women, respectively; 0.5 and 0.45 for elderly men and women, respectively) (14).

b. Oral replacement

    (1) Oral replacement solutions. In general, oral therapy is effective, less costly, and as effective as parenteral therapy for dehydration. Many oral rehydration solutions are available, but they are often underutilized in young children and infants because of concern that they are not as efficient as IV solutions (15), and in adults because of the general availability of IV solutions in hospitals (16) (Table 7-10). The mechanism of oral substitution is to restore fluid and electrolyte content by driving water across intestinal mucosa following sodium-coupled glucose uptake via the sodium–glucose cotransporter, SGLT1. The exact composition of the oral replacement solution for infants is still being debated because diarrheal stool sodium concentration is lower in children than in adults. Thus, when dehydration is severe, too much sodium (90 mEq/L) in a short time can occasionally cause hypernatremia. In this situation, solutions with 40 to 60 mEq/L are recommended (17). However, for children with mild to moderate dehydration and for adults with normal intestine, the World Health Organization solution containing 90 mEq/L is probably just as good. The use of rice-based and other cereal-based oral rehydration solutions (as a substitute for glucose) is thought to reduce diarrhea by providing glucose slowly in the gut lumen without increasing osmolarity. In fact, fecal losses have been reduced by adding resistant starch to the oral rehydration solution in the form of high-amylose maize starch, which allows colonic fermentation to short-chain fatty acid and sodium and fluid absorption in the colon (18).

    Solutions with higher sodium and glucose concentrations are used for rehydration, although whether 75 or 90 mEq of sodium per liter is better is unclear. The Washington University formula has been developed for patients with short-bowel syndrome who require IV rehydration. The higher sodium concentration has been shown to convert such patients from fluid secretors to fluid absorbers (16). The oral rehydration solutions with lower sodium and glucose contents are used for maintenance. The World Health Organization oral rehydration solution can be bought in many countries in dried packets to be rehydrated at home, or can be made from ingredients readily available at home. Recent modifications of the World Health Organization solution contain less glucose to avoid osmotic diarrhea, and less sodium (50 mEq/L) to avoid hypernatremia and convulsions. The

Table 7-10. Composition of selected oral rehydration solutions

Solution	Sodium	Potassium	Chloride	Base	Glucose	Osmolality (mOsm/kg)
			(mEq/L)			
Rehydration						
WHO	90	20	80	30	111[a] (2.0%)	310
Rehydrylyte	75	20	65	30	139 (2.5%)	310
CeraLyte 70	70	20	60	30	[b]	230
EquaLyte	78	22	68	32	139 (2.5%)[d]	305
Washington U*	105	0	100	10	111 (2.0%)	250
Maintenance						
Pedialyte	45	20	35	30	139 (2.5%)	269
Resol	50	20	50	34	111 (2.0%)	265
Ricelyte	50	20	50	34	[b]	?
Infalyte	50	20	40	30	111 (2.0%)	270
Lytren	50	25	45	30	111 (2.0%)	?
Naturalyte	45	20	35	48	139 (2.5%)	?
Diocalm Junior[c]	60	20	50	10	111 (2.0%)	251
Dioralyte[c]	60	20	60	10	90 (1.6%)	240
Electrolade[c]	50	20	40	30	111 (2.0%)	251
Rapolyte[c]	60	20	50	10	111 (2.0%)	251
Unsuitable						
Gatorade	20	3	27	3	278 (4.5%)[c]	330
Colas	1.6	<1	—	13.4	(5–15%)	550–750
Orange juice	<1	50	—	50	(12%)	High
Chicken broth	250	8	—	0	0	500

* Washington University formula: Mix ¾ tsp NaCl, ½ tsp sodium citrate, and 3 tbs + 1 tsp Polycose powder in 1 L (4¼ cups) of distilled water. Potassium may need to be added.
[a] May contain glucose or sucrose.
[b] Rice-based carbohydrate.
[c] Available in the U.K.
[d] Also contains fructooligosaccharides.

standard recipe involves ¾ tsp of salt, ½ tsp of baking soda (or 1 tsp of baking powder), 4 tbs of table sugar, and 8 oz of orange juice diluted in 1 L (4¼ cups) of water. A Crystalite packet (or other product without sugar or electrolytes) can be added for flavor if needed.

The daily dose for adults is 2 to 3 L, for children 1 L plus food, and for infants 0.5 L plus food. The more substrate present, the better the cotransport of sodium. For this reason and to replace deficits resulting from malnutrition, infants and children should also be fed the regular diets appropriate for their age.

(2) **Food-based solutions.** Food-based solutions may be less practical because the sodium and fluid may not be so readily available for rapid absorption. Most sodas contain 1 to 4 mEq of sodium per liter and 0.1 to 0.6 mEq of potassium per liter along with about 10% carbohydrate. Thus, they are inadequate for the treatment of dehydration. Fluid replacement drinks are available in grocery stores. The characteristics of some of these preparations are listed in Table 7-10. Gatorade was designed to provide energy and replace electrolytes lost in sweat, and consequently the sodium concentration is too low to treat significant dehydration. However, it is isotonic, and all therapeutic oral replacement solutions are isotonic or mildly hypotonic.

When fluid loss from vomiting or diarrhea is not severe in adults, Gatorade or similar beverages may be well tolerated because of their near-isotonicity. These products are helpful in maintaining fluid volume but not in treating volume depletion because the sodium concentration is too low. If fluid loss is moderate to severe, one of the other solutions is indicated.

   7. **Toxicity.** Sodium toxicity occurs in only two situations.

   a. **Hypernatremia.** Sodium may be ingested or provided in excess of water to cause hypernatremia. Hypertonic sodium gain can be caused by the use of hypertonic IV or feeding solutions, ingestion of sodium chloride tablets, or the administration of hypertonic dialysis or saline enemas (19). Hypernatremia also develops during net water loss (usually renal) in diabetes insipidus, the use of loop diuretics, osmotic diuresis, postobstructive diuresis, the polyuric phase of acute tubular necrosis, and intrinsic renal disease. The loss of hyponatremic gastrointestinal fluids (e.g., in vomiting) can also cause hypernatremia. The major signs of hypernatremia are evidenced in the central nervous system by confusion, obtundation, stupor, and even coma. These signs are similar to those of other hyperosmolar syndromes (e.g., hyperglycemia). The effect of 1 L of any infusion can be estimated by using the formula presented in the section on sodium deficiency. The rapid correction or overcorrection of hypernatremia should be avoided because shifts in cerebral edema can have major clinical consequences (19).

   b. **Abnormal sodium retention,** as in conditions associated with edema, is the more common cause of toxicity. Signs and symptoms are related to fluid overload. Treatment involves decreasing dietary or infused sodium and the use of diuretics. Booklets with low-sodium diets are available from the dietary divisions of most hospitals. The principles involved in dietary management are discussed in Chapter 11 in the section on low-sodium diets. Seasoning food can be a problem. Salt substitutes can be used, and other spices can be very helpful in making food more palatable. Table 7-11 outlines alternative seasonings and their suggested uses. Many commercial products are available offering various combinations of these spices.

B. Potassium

   1. **Requirements.** The requirements for potassium are not as clearly defined as those for sodium because of adjustments in urinary excretion that follow changes in intake. The minimum requirement for healthy adults has been set at 2,000 mg/d (1). All but a small amount of potas-

Table 7-11. Natural low-sodium seasonings that can be substituted for salt

Uses	Alternate seasonings
General cooking	Lemon juice, garlic, onion and sour cream the most useful; pepper and chili powder good if tolerated
Meat	Lemon, garlic, onion, pepper, oregano, curry powder, rosemary, thyme, paprika, ginger, sour cream
Fish and poultry	Lemon, garlic, onion, pepper, ginger, oregano, paprika, parsley, sesame seed, savory, tarragon, thyme
Egg dishes	Pepper (red or black), basil, marjoram, onion, oregano, tarragon, thyme
Vegetables	Pepper, basil (especially for tomatoes), dill, thyme, oregano, chervil, rosemary, sour cream (potatoes especially)
Soups	Garlic, onion, pepper, bay leaf, basil, thyme

sium is normally absorbed by the gastrointestinal tract. The kidney is the major excretory organ for potassium and regulates output. The normal kidney can adjust the amount of potassium excretion from 5 to 1,000 mEq/d. Moreover, sodium intake determines, in part, the amount of potassium excreted, as both are affected by the action of aldosterone. Thus, the sodium–potassium ratio in the diet is a factor in defining the daily excretion rate and requirement (1).

   a. Dietary effects. Potassium excretion is also affected by changes in recent dietary intake. Maximal values for potassium excretion occur early after a few days of adaptation to a high intake of potassium. On the other hand, sodium excretion increases within hours of a sodium load. With potassium restriction, maximal renal preservation occurs after 1 to 2 weeks, whereas sodium adaptation is more rapid. These considerations further confuse the determination of minimal daily requirements based on urinary excretion. With all factors considered, the estimated minimal potassium intake for adults more than 18 years of age on a high-salt, Western-style diet has been estimated at 2,000 mg (62.5 mEq) per day. This is below the usual dietary intake. Probably an intake as low as 800 mg (20 mEq) per day is adequate to prevent deficiency. However, moderate obligatory losses of potassium do occur, whereas obligatory losses of sodium do not.

   b. Potassium needs of infants. During infancy, growth (increase in lean body mass) and fecal losses determine the potassium requirements more than urinary excretion does. The intestine during infancy does not absorb electrolytes and water as efficiently as it does after age 2. Obligatory losses plus growth requirements for children of all ages should be met by 78 mg (2 mEq) per 100 kcal daily. Minimum requirements for children ages 0 to 5 months are 500 mg; ages 6 to 11 months, 700 mg; 1 year old, 1,000 mg; 2 to 5 years old, 1,400 mg; 6 to 9 years old, 1,600 mg; and 10 to 18 years, 2,000 mg (1). The average intake of infants from milk and other foods ranges from 780 to 1,600 mg/d (20 to 80 mEq/d) (1).

2. Food sources

   a. Average intake of potassium in adults varies from 2,000 to 6,000 mg/d (50 to 150 mEq/d). Hospitalized patients generally receive adequate dietary sources of potassium. The average hospital diet provides about 4,000 to 4,800 mg. Low-sodium diets provide 3,800 to 4,000 mg, and full-liquid diets supply the same amount. Because potassium is an intracellular ion, meat is a rich source. Therefore, low-protein and low-calorie diets provide somewhat less potassium (2,000 to 3,000 mg). A clear liquid diet is low in potassium (~ 750 mg) and in other essential nutrients. Table 7-12 lists some major good sources of potassium. Meat, fluid milk, and fruits are good sources. In general, fruits and meats provide 200 to 400 mg of potassium per serving, vegetables slightly more, milk 370 mg per glass, and dried fruits, nuts, and juices somewhat more. Foods high in sodium, processed foods, and diets low in fruits, vegetables, dairy, and whole grains may not provide enough potassium to meet minimum requirements. Because many potassium-rich foods also contain fiber and other vitamins and minerals, the consumption of dietary fruits, vegetables, and dairy products should be encouraged, rather than the use of potassium supplements.

   b. The effect of food processing on potassium content can be significant, as it is on sodium. Potassium content can increase or decrease with processing, but not so much as sodium content (Table 7-2). Water itself contains very little potassium and does not affect food content after cooking. Table 7-13 lists some examples of the effects of processing on potassium content.

3. Assessment. Ionic potassium is measured in serum or plasma with the use of ion-selective electrodes. Hemolysis elevates values through

Table 7-12. Food sources of potassium

Food	Portion	Potassium content (mg)
Grains		
White bread	1 slice	28
Whole wheat bread	1 slice	62
Rice, cooked	1 cup	80
Spaghetti noodles, cooked	1 cup	43
Meats		
Muscle red meats, broiled	3 oz	250
Organ meats	3 oz	250–300
Bacon, cooked	3 slices	92
Fish, broiled	3 oz	340–400
Chicken, white meat roasted	3 oz	209
Vegetables		
Asparagus, fresh, cooked	½ cup	279
Avocado	½ medium	530
Broccoli, cooked	1 cup	456
Potato, baked	1 each	844
Green beans, cooked	1 cup	373
Kidney beans	1 cup	713
Tomato	1 each	273
Tomato juice	1 cup	537
Peanuts, almonds	1 cup	960
Carrot, raw	1 each	233
Fruits		
Applesauce, canned	1 cup	295
Cantaloupe	1 cup	494
Banana	1 medium	451
Dried apricots	10 each	482
Orange	1 medium	273
Grapefruit, white	½ grapefruit	175
Grapefruit juice, canned	1 cup	378
Orange juice, frozen	1 cup	474
Watermelon slice	1 cup	186
Dairy Products		
Milk	1 cup	350–370
Cheese	1 oz	25–40
Egg	1 each	63
Other		
Coffee, brewed	4 oz	80
Tea, brewed	4 oz	16

the release of intracellular potassium. Of all the potassium in the body (~ 54 mEq/kg of body weight), only about 10% is extracellular. Moreover, only about 0.4% (0.2 mEq/kg) is found in the plasma or serum. The distribution of potassium depends on an energy-consuming process in which sodium is extruded from cells and potassium enters. At normal rates of dietary intake, the transfer of ingested potassium into cells occurs so rapidly that extracellular concentrations do not change noticeably.

    a. Body stores. The serum potassium concentration (normal, 3.5 to 4.5 mEq/L) reflects both total body stores and availability of energy (glucose). Values from 3.0 to 3.5 mEq/L correspond to mild hypokalemia, and values below 2.5 mEq/L define severe hypokalemia. The serum potassium level does reflect body stores in the absence

Table 7-13. Effect of processing on potassium content of food

Food	Portion	Potassium content (mg)
Potato		
Fresh baked	1 each	844
Instant mashed	1 cup	428
Canned	2 each	160
Chips	14 (1 oz)	369
Tomato		
Sliced	1 cup	400
Canned	1 cup	529
Catsup	1 tbs	82
Peas, green		
Fresh cooked	1 cup	434
Frozen, cooked	1 cup	268
Canned, without liquid	1 cup	194

of impaired energy utilization, (e.g., diabetes mellitus). It does not reflect changes in recent or chronic intake because the plasma level is adjusted fairly rapidly. However, the serum potassium level, at best, provides only an approximation of total body stores. A serum level not below 3.3 mEq/L often corresponds to a loss of 10% of body potassium; a level below 3.0 mEq/L suggests a loss greater than 20%. Small shifts in the transport of potassium can rapidly shift the equilibrium between intracellular and extracellular compartments. Hypokalemia also may occur during acute alkalosis or acute attacks of familial periodic paralysis. Conversely, the serum potassium level may be normal when body stores are low (or high) as measured by isotope studies.

   b. Losses from the body. Urinary potassium levels reflect excretion on any given day. However, the ability of the kidney to alter potassium excretion is great, and adults on an average diet excrete 25 to 125 mEq/d (20). Therefore, the urinary potassium level may be useful in assessing losses from the body when potassium depletion is present. When the kidney is normal, potassium excretion should be low but still significant (10 to 20 mEq/d). When losses from the gastrointestinal tract occur, the measurement of potassium in the appropriate fluid provides an additional assessment of the requirement for that patient (see Table 7-6 for the average daily potassium content of gastrointestinal fluids). Once hypokalemia is detected, measurement of the urinary potassium level may be helpful in determining the source of loss. A low urinary potassium level (<15 mEq/L) implies near-maximal renal conservation and suggests an extrarenal source of depletion. This interpretation is correct only if the patient has not been treated recently with diuretics. After diuretics are discontinued, the kidney responds to induced hypokalemia with maximal potassium conservation. However, if the urinary potassium level is high (>30 mEq/L), then renal conservation is inadequate, and this result suggests that the kidney is the source of potassium loss.

4. Physiology. Potassium is the major intracellular cation. Along with sodium and calcium, it is responsible for the maintenance of normal electric potentials across cell membranes. The membrane depolarization needed for muscle contraction depends on an influx of sodium into the cell coupled with an efflux of potassium. Membrane repolarization involves the reverse process. Thus, potassium helps to regulate neuromuscular contraction in addition to glycogen formation, protein synthesis, and acid–base balance.

   a. Absorption. Potassium is absorbed by bulk fluid movement after sodium/solute absorption in the intestine. It is also present in gastrointestinal secretions, from which it must be reabsorbed (Table 7-6).

   b. Excretion. The kidney is the major regulatory site of potassium excretion, through the action of aldosterone. Potassium excretion by the kidney is regulated by a secretory process, largely independent of the GFR and the amount of filtered potassium. All filtered potassium is reabsorbed in the proximal nephron. The amount in the urine is regulated by the potassium ion concentration in the cells of the distal tubule and is high when the intracellular concentration is high. Thus, excretion is regulated in part by the intracellular content of renal cells. The kidney responds rapidly to alterations in potassium intake. The colon, the other aldosterone-sensitive organ, also secretes potassium. In the colon, potassium secretion is aided by the electronegativity of the intestinal lumen. Ordinarily, stool volumes are low, so the relatively high potassium concentrations in stool are not the cause of serious losses. In diarrhea, large potassium losses may occur. Changes in colonic secretion do not alter the overall potassium balance unless the colon is removed, when losses through the ileostomy can be significant.

5. Deficiency. If one assumes that no metabolic factors are altering the serum potassium level, each decrease of 1 mEq/L corresponds to a loss of body potassium of 200 to 300 mEq. The major causes of deficiency include increased renal excretion and extrarenal losses, largely intestinal. Because of the widespread presence of potassium in foods, decreased intake is an uncommon cause of deficiency. However, clear liquid diets are low in potassium and may lead to deficiency after prolonged use.

   a. Causes. Increased renal excretion, one cause of deficiency, may be secondary to the use of potent diuretics, chronic metabolic alkalosis (e.g., chronic obstructive pulmonary disease), diabetic ketoacidosis (with osmotic diuresis), and states associated with the development of edema. Distal renal tubular acidosis also can lead to large losses of potassium. Potassium can be lost at the rate of 150 to 300 mEq/d in these situations. Major causes of extrarenal losses include gastric or biliary drainage and chronic diarrhea. Because potassium is secreted by the colon, moderate diarrhea can lead to hypokalemia before sodium or volume depletion is clinically evident. The concentration of potassium in sweat is low (5 to 10 mEq/L), so large losses are not common with increased sweating. Nondiuretic medications, such as steroids, digoxin, and excess natural licorice, may cause an increase in potassium excretion (21).

   b. Symptoms and signs. The loss of 5% to 10% of body stores (200 to 300 mEq) is tolerated without many symptoms. Manifestations of hypokalemia usually appear at serum levels below 2.5 to 3.0 mEq/L. If the loss of potassium is rapid, symptoms may develop at a higher serum level. Prominent symptoms include weakness, paresthesias, orthostatic hypotension, and cardiovascular abnormalities. With depletion, the membrane electrical potential gradient increases, and muscle contraction is impaired. Muscle weakness and delayed cardiac repolarization are early effects. Electrocardiographic abnormalities include depressed ST segments, low T waves, and the presence of U waves. However, these findings are neither constant nor specific and cannot be relied on for diagnosis. The effects of digitalis are exaggerated by potassium deficiency. If depletion is chronic, the concentrating ability of the kidneys is impaired and polyuria results. Glucose intolerance, polydipsia, constipation, ileus, and metabolic alkalosis can occur. Common causes of depletion are gastrointestinal (vomiting and diarrhea) and urinary (diuretics) losses, glucocorticoid excess, and inadequate intake in the face of obligatory urinary excretion.

c. **Hypertension.** Potassium supplementation is associated with a significant but small reduction in systolic (3 mm Hg) and diastolic (2 mm Hg) pressures (22,23). This effect is noted most in patients with a high intake of sodium. However, in the DASH study, in which the diet of participants was rich in fruits and vegetables (average potassium intake of 4,100 mg/d), blood pressures fell (9). This diet also included low-fat dairy foods and reduced amounts of saturated and unsaturated fat, so the role of potassium alone is not clear. It is usually not necessary to prescribe potassium supplements for hypertensive patients except when hypokalemia is present.

6. **Treatment.** Hypokalemia is treated by oral replacement if possible. The reason for choosing this route is to allow the serum potassium level to rise slowly in equilibrium with the intracellular component. For mild deficiency, table foods may be adequate (Table 7-12). Foods high in potassium are those with more than 300 mg per portion.

a. **Supplements.** The Food and Drug Administration now allows manufacturers to claim on the labels of certain foods that "diets containing foods that are good sources of potassium and low in sodium may reduce the risk of high blood pressure and stroke." To qualify, the food must contain more than 10% of the recommended dietary value of potassium (or 350 mg), be low in sodium (<140 mg), and also be low in fat, saturated fat, and cholesterol, as defined by the Food and Drug Administration.

Potassium salts (gluconate, aspartate, citrate, chloride) are available as liquid, tablets, and capsules. Individual doses of nonprescription preparations are limited by the Food and Drug Administration to less than 99 mg (~ 2.5 mEq) because of the dangers associated with self-dosing. The salt most often used to treat moderate deficiency is potassium chloride. However, it has a bitter taste, and if it is not well tolerated, other salts are available. If the source of the potassium loss is in the intestine, fixed base will also be lost, so that a basic salt of potassium (e.g., potassium gluconate) may be more appropriate as replacement therapy. Although the risk for mucosal damage in the gastrointestinal tract caused by potassium chloride, a sclerotic agent, is smaller with currently available slow-release, wax matrix, and microencapsulated forms than with liquid potassium chloride, esophageal and small-bowel damage does still occur when slow-release tablets containing high doses of potassium chloride are ingested. Such preparations should not be used by patients with any condition that may delay transit through the gastrointestinal tract. For such patients, the gluconate or citrate salt is more appropriate. Liquid or effervescent preparations are preferable if they are well tolerated and should be mixed in 3 to 8 oz of water or juice and drunk slowly. Potassium chloride can be given IV to severely depleted patients if the salt is diluted to 20 to 40 mEq/L of fluid, no more than 40 mEq is administered per hour, and electrocardiographic monitoring is provided. Without such monitoring, replacement should not exceed 20 mEq/h. A partial list of oral potassium preparations available by prescription is given in Table 7-14.

b. **Salt substitutes.** Many patients who require potassium supplements are also on a low-sodium diet. As part of this diet, they may be using a salt substitute. The potassium content of salt substitutes is considerable. If significant amounts of these salts are used, they may contribute a major supplementary source of potassium and should be considered in the overall oral intake. In addition, potassium chloride in the form of commercial salt substitutes is 10 times less expensive than potassium chloride solutions and powders.

Table 7-14. Potassium supplement preparations[a]

Usual preparation[b]	Anion	K+ content/unit dose (mEq/15 mL or per tablet)
Liquids		
Kaochlor 10%	Cl	20
Kaon Cl 20%	Cl	40
Kay Ciel	Cl	20
Klorvess 10%	Cl	20
Klor-Con 10%		20
Rum-K	Cl	20
Potassium chloride solution 5%, 10%, or 20%	Cl	20
Kaon Elixir	Gluconate	20
Kolyum	Gluconate/Cl	20
Potassium triplex (Tri-K)	Acetate, HCO₃, citrate	45
Twin-K	Gluconate, citrate	20
Polycitra-K	Citrate, citric acid	30
Tablets[c]		
Effer K	HCO₃, citrate	25
K+ Care	HCO₃	20, 25
Slow-K	Cl	8
Klotrix	Cl	10 in wax matrix
Klor-Con/EF	HCO₃, citrate	25
Klor-Con 10	Cl	10 in wax matrix
Micro-K Extencaps	Cl	8, 10 controlled-release
K-tab	Cl	10
Kaon	Gluconate	5
K-lyte effervescent	HCO₃, citrate	25 (DS = 50)
Klorvess Effervescent	HCO₃, Cl	20
K-Dur	Cl	10, 20 microencapsulated
Potassium chloride	Cl	10 in wax matrix, controlled-release, or microencapsulated
Powder		
Effervescent Kaon-Cl	Cl	6, 7, 10
K+ Care	Cl	15, 20, 25
K-Lor	Cl	15, 20
Klor-Con	Cl	20, 25
K-Lyte/Cl	Cl	25 (DS = 50)
Kay Ciel	Cl	20
Kolyum	Gluconate/Cl	20
Klorvess Effervescent	HCO₃, Cl	20
Micro-K LS	Cl	20 (extended-release)
Potassium chloride	Cl	20

DS = double strength.
All liquid preparations should be diluted in juice or water (4 oz for each 20-mEq dose). All packets or effervescent tablets should be dissolved in the same amount of liquid. Tablets (slow release in wax matrix or microencapsulated) should be swallowed whole with 4 oz of liquid.
[a] The K content (mEq/g) of potassium salts is K gluconate, 4.3; K citrate, 9.8; K bicarbonate, 10; K acetate, 10.2; K chloride, 13.4.
[b] Many preparations are available in liquid, tablet, and powder forms.
[c] Most tablets are either covered by wax matrix, microencapsulated, or in controlled-release forms.

Characteristics of the salt substitutes are listed in Table 7-15. "No salt" products are the only ones with a nutritionally significant potassium content and an acceptably low sodium content but are poorly accepted by patients who find them unpalatable.

7. **Toxicity.** Toxicity occurs when hyperkalemia develops (serum level >5.0 to 5.5 mEq/L). Because of the largely intracellular distribution of potassium, toxicity can be manifested without significant changes in total body levels of potassium.

  a. Causes

    (1) **Impaired renal excretion** is the major cause of hyperkalemia because this mechanism is so important for normal function. When diuretics are used, potassium often must be replaced. Potassium-sparing diuretics increase potassium retention and can cause hyperkalemia. The concurrent use of angiotensin-converting enzyme (ACE) inhibitors may lead to hyperkalemia in certain patients.

    (2) **Increased potassium intake** may also produce hyperkalemia, especially the use of prescription supplements. An increase in oral intake of 50 to 100 mEq within a short period can raise the serum potassium level by 0.5 to 1 mEq/L, but the abnormality is transient once cellular redistribution occurs. The use of salt substitutes along with other potassium supplements can result in excessive intake.

    (3) **Other causes.** Potassium penicillin contains 1.7 mEq per million units and can provide a large dose of potassium. The sudden breakdown of cells with disruption of the transcellular gradients can acutely raise the serum potassium level and produce toxic effects in the absence of changes in total body potassium.

  b. Na content and Na:K ratio are provided for the class of "no salt" subsitutes.

Table 7-15. Characteristics of salt substitutes[a]

Product	Na content (mEq/g)	K content (mEq/g)	Na:K ratio
Table salt	16.6	0.004	4150
Flavored salt	11.9	0.049	243
Monosodium glutamate	5.3	0.004	1325
Seasonings and marinades	7.0	0.087	80
Lemon pepper	4.4	—	—
Marinades	1.4	—	—
Meat tenderizer	12.0	—	—
"Low salt" substitutes	9.45	5.29	1.8
"No salt" substitutes[b]	0.014	12.8	<0.01
Adolph's salt substitute	—	12.8	—
Adolph's seasoned salt substitute	—	7	—
Morton's salt substitute	—	12.8	—
Morton's seasoned salt substitute	—	11.2	—
Nosalt	—	12.8	—
Neocurtasal	—	12	—
Nu-salt	—	13.6	—
Lawry's seasoned salt-free	—	6	—

[a] Mean values for classes of products are listed.
Adapted from Greefield H, et al., *Med J Aust* 1984;140:460 and from Hands ES. *Food finder,* 2nd ed. Salem, Or.: ESHA Research, 1990. Data for salt substitutes adapted from Cannon-Babb MT, Schwartz AB, *Hosp Pract* 1986;21:99, and from *Drugs: facts and comparisons.* C.V. Mosby: St Louis: 1998.

b. **Signs and symptoms** of hyperkalemia include those associated with decreased membrane potential, rapid repolarization, and slowed conduction velocity. Neuromuscular effects include paresthesias, weakness, mental confusion, and paralysis. The cardiovascular effects are a decrease in blood pressure and direct cardiac effects. The electrocardiogram shows peaked T waves, loss of P waves, a depressed ST segment, widened QRS complex, and prolongation of the PR interval. If severe, these features lead to heart block, atrial arrest, and asystole. The rate of onset of hyperkalemia, accompanying acid–base disturbances, and use of other drugs modify the degree of cardiac toxicity. In general, cardiac toxicity is rare when the serum potassium level is below 6.5 mEq/L, and common when it is above 8.0 mEq/L.

c. **Treatment.** Treatment should be started immediately. For mild hyperkalemia, cessation of potassium intake may be enough if renal function is normal. With more severe toxicity, active intervention should be used.

   (1) **Calcium gluconate.** Ten to thirty milliliters of 10% calcium gluconate be given IV over a few minutes, but the effect is transient (1 to 2 hours).

   (2) **Glucose and insulin** can be used to drive the potassium intracellularly. A dose of 10 to 20 U of insulin per 100 g of glucose can be given after the glucose is started, and the effect lasts 6 to 12 hours.

   (3) **Sodium bicarbonate** is used when systemic acidosis is present. Two ampules (90 to 100 mEq) can be given IV over 5 to 10 minutes.

   (4) **Potassium exchange.** Oral exchange can be accomplished by giving the resin sodium polystyrene sulfonate (Kayexalate) orally (20 to 30 g) or by enema (50 to 100 g in 200 mL), as indicated by the serum potassium level. In severe toxicity or renal failure, hemodialysis is used.

C. Calcium

1. **Requirement.** Calcium is the major cation of bone. Three factors define the requirements for calcium and explain the discrepancy between the actual requirement and the larger dietary reference intake (DRI): (a) Calcium is needed in increased amounts during periods of growth or new bone formation. (b) Because absorption is not efficient (~ 30%), the amount ingested must exceed the actual requirement. (c) There is an obligatory daily loss of calcium in the stool and urine. Thus, the requirement is greatest during childhood, adolescence, pregnancy, and lactation.

   a. **Effect of luminal contents**

      (1) **High intake of phytate and fiber** may decrease calcium absorption.

      (2) **Phosphorus.** Animal data suggest that the optimal dietary calcium–phosphorus ratio is from 2:1 to 1:2. The ratio of the average U.S. diet is 1:1.5. Although phosphate is an additive in many processed foods, especially canned foods and soft drinks, the effect of the added phosphorus on calcium absorption is unclear. At a luminal pH above 6, calcium forms complexes with phosphorus and with other anions. Thus, fecal calcium and phosphorus are usually correlated. Because calcium absorption is inefficient in adults, changes in the phosphorus intake increase the fecal output relatively little.

      (3) **Protein.** As protein intake increases, so does urinary calcium excretion, but the effect is not always proportional to the protein intake. In balance studies, when phosphorus intake was stable, 1 g of dietary protein increased urinary calcium excretion by

1 to 1.5 mg (24). Thus, diets high in protein but with limited calcium intake (e.g., high in meat, low in dairy products) may increase urinary calcium loss and alter daily requirements. The practical significance of this effect in making diet recommendations is not clear because diets with low intakes of calcium should be avoided.

(4) **Sodium.** Sodium and calcium excretion are linked in the proximal tubule of the kidney. Each gram of sodium leads to the urinary excretion of about 15 mg of calcium when calcium intake is high or moderate (24).

b. **Effects of physiologic conditions**

(1) **Infants and children.** Until puberty, calcium absorption is increased up to twofold (60%) in comparison with absorption in adults.

(2) **Pregnancy.** Absorption and retention of calcium are increased.

(3) **Old age.** After the age of 60, calcium absorption decreases, and the ability of the intestine to respond to a low-calcium diet by increasing the rate of absorption is impaired.

c. **Obligatory/insensible calcium losses.** The bowel and kidney excrete about 160 mg of calcium daily even when calcium intake is low. In addition, about 40 mg is lost per day through the skin (25). Thus, an intake of 200 mg/d is needed to offset these obligatory losses.

d. **DRIs.** Bone density increases during the first 25 to 30 years of life and decreases thereafter. The Food and Drug Administration has approved the claim that the use of calcium supplements reduces the risk for osteoporosis (26). The revised dietary recommendations for calcium intake (24) are close to those formulated by the National Institutes of Health consensus development conference on optimal calcium intake (27).

The recommendations in Table 7-16 are meant to be reflections of national policy. They are not intended to be nutrient requirements for individuals. This issue is particularly troublesome for calcium because a long time may elapse before the effects of calcium deficiency are noted. Thus, an optimal intake is better stated for populations than for individuals. The debate over calcium guidelines continues to stress the need for calcium intake versus the complex relationship between calcium intake and bone health (28). The increased recommendation for adolescents is based on their rapid growth of bone. The increased recommendation for older persons is based on data showing that their rate of calcium absorption is decreased.

Table 7-16. Dietary reference intakes for calcium

Age group	DRI (mg/day)
0–6 mo	210
7–12 mo	270
1–3 yrs	500
4–8 yrs	800
9–18 yrs	1,300
19–50 yrs[a]	1,000
51+ yrs	1,200

[a] No alterations for pregnancy or lactation are recommended

From Standing Committee on the Scientific Evaluation of Dietary Reference Intakes, Food and Nutrition Board, Institute of Medicine. *Dietary reference intakes: calcium, phosphorus, magnesium, vitamin D, and fluoride.* Washington, DC: National Academy Press, 1997.

The current recommendations imply that a single universal requirement exists for calcium, regardless of the intake of protein, sodium, and fiber/phytate. This view has been challenged because of the fact that calcium intake is low in parts of the world where fracture rates are low, and high where fracture rates are high (25). It has been estimated that a diet low in sodium and protein can reduce the calcium requirement by as much as 200 to 300 mg/d. These considerations have not been included in the DRI calculations of the U.S./Canadian Committee (24).

2. **Food sources.** Primitive diets containing vegetables, bones of small animals or fish, and possibly insects have a high calcium density that approaches 80 to 100 mg/100 kcal (27). In contrast, the median calcium density of the diet of women in NHANES III was only about 36 mg/100 kcal, and the new DRIs suggest about 50 mg of calcium per 100 kcal (25). Milk contains 350 mg of calcium per 100 kcal (~ 300 mg/cup), and so dairy products are the most calcium-dense foods in the diets of most countries. Three hundred milligrams of calcium can be found in 1½ oz of cheese, 1¾ cup of ice cream, 6 oz of low-fat yogurt, 1½ cup of cooked greens (e.g., kale, spinach, bok choy), and 5 oz of canned salmon. Other foods that contribute to daily calcium intake include dried beans, broccoli, and tofu (chemically set with calcium). In animal products, calcium is bound largely to protein, which must first be digested before calcium can be absorbed. Organic anions, such as phytates, are found in many green leafy vegetables and inhibit calcium absorption, so bioavailability is variable. Calcium-fortified foods (e.g., fortified orange juice) contain up to 350 mg of calcium per 8 oz and may constitute a major source of dietary calcium for persons who do not use dairy products. Table 7-17 lists the calcium content of selected foods.

Table 7-17. Calcium content of selected foods

Food	Serving size	Calcium content (mg)
Calcium-fortified orange juice	1 cup	up to 350
Milk, all types (liquid)	1 cup	280–300
Yogurt, plain	1 cup	274–315
Hard cheeses	1 oz	213–287
Soft cheeses	1 oz	159–219
Figs, dried	10	269
Tofu, raw, firm	½ cup	258
Calcium-fortified cereals	¾ cup	250
Spinach, cooked	1 cup	244
Collards, cooked	½ cup	179
Cottage cheese	1 cup	126–180
Ice cream	1 cup	176
Peanuts, roasted	1 cup	126
Beans (navy, pinto)	1 cup	80–120
Salmon, canned with bones	1 oz	110
Sardines, in oil	Two	92
Vegetables (carrots, kale, broccoli)	½ cup	36–52
Fruits	1 cup/piece	18–25
Pasta, rice	1 cup	10–23
Bread, white	Slice	35
Meat, fish	3 oz	3–10

From Hands ES, Food Finder, 2nd ed. Salem, Or.: ESHA Research, 1990; Pennington JAT. Bowes and Church's food values of portions commonly used, 17th ed. Philadelphia: Lippincott-Raven, 1998.

3. Assessment

    a. Intake/absorption is best measured by 24-hour urinary calcium excretion. This varies from 100 to 240 mg/d, with much individual variation noted. In adults, the amount excreted correlates with calcium absorption above 2 mg/kg per day (i.e., intake >6 mg/kg per day) because only about 30% is absorbed. When calcium intake or absorption is low, urinary calcium does not decline proportionally. The range of values for urinary calcium found with an inadequate calcium intake of less than 200 mg/d (30 to 160 mg of urinary calcium per day) overlaps with the range of values found with a normal calcium intake (100 to 240 mg/d). Thus, the values for urinary calcium excretion should not be interpreted too rigorously. Even when net calcium absorption is zero, the obligatory loss of urinary calcium continues. This situation is in contrast to what is observed with other minerals, such as sodium, potassium, magnesium and phosphorus, the urinary excretion of which is regulated at low levels of intake/absorption. Thus, urinary excretion is not a good test for calcium deficiency; it is better used to monitor the adequacy of calcium intake when supplemental calcium is prescribed. It should be measured only after 3 to 4 days on a constant calcium intake and when drugs that alter urinary calcium (e.g., thiazide diuretics, tetracycline, glucocorticoids) are not being taken. A high intake of protein or renal leak may increase calcium excretion. Treatment with 1,25-dihydroxyvitamin D_3 can cause bone resorption and an increase urinary calcium that is unrelated to calcium absorption. In patients with bone disease, urinary calcium excretion may be constant and independent of calcium absorption.

    b. Calcium determination. Serum calcium and alkaline phosphatase measurement is the conventionally used test of calcium status but is inadequate for this purpose. Ionized calcium is maintained within a very narrow range as calcium is mobilized from the bones. The non-ionized calcium is protein-bound and pH-dependent, increasing with alkalosis and decreasing with acidosis. Thus, alkalosis or hyperproteinemia can cause a false-positive result for hypercalcemia, and acidosis or hypoproteinemia a false-positive result for hypocalcemia.

    Calcium is measured by rapid automated procedures; the o-cresolphthalein complex method is used most often, and sometimes flame photometry or atomic absorption spectroscopy (20). Normal values for serum calcium are given in Table 7-18. Because of the tight metabolic regulation of serum calcium, values outside this range cannot be interpreted according to nutritional status; rather, they usually suggest a pathologic mechanism. Ionized calcium levels reflect calcium metabolism better than total calcium does. Serum levels of ionized calcium can be low when calcium (or vitamin D) deficiency is severe and skeletal pools of calcium are

Table 7-18. Serum calcium biochemical parameters

Parameter	Young men	Young women	Adults	Elderly
Total calcium (mmol/L)	2.41 ± 0.2	2.40 ± 0.2	2.43 ± 0.02	2.28 ± 0.12
Ionized calcium (mmol/L)	1.48	1.21	1.25 ± 0.04	1.24 ± 0.07
Alkaline phosphatase (IU/L)	63 (21–155)		80 (43–110)	

From Sauberlich HE. *Laboratory tests for the assessment of nutritional status*, 2nd ed. Boca Raton, FL: CRC Press, 1990.

low, but this is a late finding. Hypocalcemia is defined as less than 2.18 mmol/L (<85 mg/L), and hypercalcemia as more than 2.6 mmol/L (>105 mg/L).

c. **Alkaline phosphatase.** Activity in serum represents the sum of liver and bone isozyme activity. During active bone resorption, alkaline phosphatase activity in serum increases, but this result is neither sensitive nor specific. Origin of the enzyme in bone can be suggested by heat inactivation at 56° (<15% remaining indicates origin in bone), or by determination of γ-glutamyl transpeptidase, a bile canalicular enzyme present in liver and biliary tissue but not in bone. When calcium deficiency is advanced and osteomalacic bone disease is present, alkaline phosphatase is elevated. The enzyme level is high in any condition in which bone remodeling is taking place, so that it is elevated in children and adolescents and in patients with metastatic bone disease or Paget's disease.

d. **Bone density measurements.** Changes in bone density are measured for several years to follow the effects of dietary calcium supplements and other interventions on bone density, especially in the prevention and treatment of postmenopausal osteoporosis in women. The measure is not recommended for routine screening but may be useful in guiding treatment decisions for selected postmenopausal women (29,30). The World Health Organization study group has emphasized the differences that may occur depending on the site tested for bone density and warns against using density to assess fracture risk, although a low bone density is one of the strongest risk factors for fracture. The World Health Organization has suggested that intervention be recommended for persons with a T-score value less than 2.5 SD below the age-adjusted mean, but the U.S. Department of Agriculture has accepted a score less than 2.0 SD below the mean.

(1) **Guidelines for the use of bone density measurement.** In 1996, the American Association of Clinical Endocrinologists (AACE) developed guidelines for the treatment of osteoporosis that included bone density measurement (31). They recommended bone density measurement to assess risk in perimenopausal or postmenopausal women concerned about osteoporosis. They also recommended testing for women with radiographic evidence of the diagnosis, undergoing treatment for osteoporosis, with asymptomatic primary hyperparathyroidism, or receiving long-term glucocorticoid therapy, situations in which evidence of skeletal loss might alter clinical strategy. In 1996, the European Foundation for Osteoporosis and Bone Disease (EFFO) also published practical guidelines for the use of bone density measurement (32). These guidelines were similar but did not include a recommendation to perform a baseline hip measurement. All these guidelines recommend the use of multiple skeletal sites, with the caveat that each site (e.g., spine, hip) best predicts fractures at that site but not at others (33). The U.S. Department of Agriculture recommends bone density measurement if "it is reasonable and necessary for diagnosing, treating, or monitoring the condition of a beneficiary" as indicated in "estrogen deficiency . . . vertebral abnormalities . . . glucocorticoid (steroid) therapy . . . hyperparathyroidism" (34). Potentially modifiable features in postmenopausal women (and others) that might encourage testing include current cigarette smoking, low body weight, estrogen deficiency, low calcium intake (lifelong), alcoholism, recurrent falls, inadequate physical activity, and glucocorticoid therapy (35).

(2) **Method.** Most centers now use dual-energy absorptiometry (DEXA) to assess trabecular bone in the vertebrae and hips. The x-ray source in DEXA, which replaced the isotopic source of the original dual-photon absorptiometry, is preferable because of its wider range and shorter scanning speed. Quantitative computed tomography (QCT) is also useful for the spine and wrist. Bone mass values from DEXA or QCT are difficult to interpret if metal in the spine, contrast material in the gastrointestinal tract or spinal canal, or focal bone lesions are present. Aortic calcification and prior spinal bone surgery can affect the measurement, although QCT is more useful with aortic calcification. Accuracy is only about 90% because of variation in marrow fat content. More radiation is delivered by QCT than by DEXA, about 250 mrad.

e. **Bone biopsy.** Calcium (or vitamin D) deficiency can sometimes be diagnosed by bone biopsy, which can demonstrate increased osteoid seams. Tetracycline labeling allows a distinction to be made between delayed mineralization (osteomalacia) and increased osteoid synthesis (bone remodeling states) by revealing the calcification front. This technique is not often needed to make clinical decisions.

4. **Physiology.** Calcium provides part of the matrix structure of bone. It is necessary for blood coagulation and for controlling membrane potential and the excitability of nerves and muscles. Through the protein calmodulin, it helps to control myocardial function and contractility. It supports membrane integrity and is a second messenger for many secretory processes. It helps to maintain intracellular integrity and intercellular tight junctions (35). Because of the importance of all these functions, serum levels are maintained with precision at the expense of bone matrix if exogenous calcium is not available. The calcium content of the human adult body is about 1,000 mg. More than 99% of this is in the skeleton. Young adults typically retain about 68 mg of calcium per day, with average retention efficiency of about 7.6% (35). About half of circulating calcium is turning over in the bone.

a. **Absorption.** When calcium intake is adequate, differences in calcium bioavailability probably play little role (36). When dietary calcium is low, however, or ingested in poorly soluble forms (e.g., green vegetables), then availability may be a problem. Absorption of vegetable calcium has proved to be quite variable because effective digestion is difficult to predict and assess (35). The high solubility of dairy calcium has been attributed to its presence as the citrate salt, and also to the presence of peptides, amino acids, and lactose. Milk substitutes lack many of these features and are not as good a source of available calcium and phosphorus as milk or milk products. Synthetic triglycerides improve calcium absorption (35). Gastric acid does not have much effect on the absorption of dietary calcium when the calcium is ingested with a meal (37). However, when calcium enters the relatively alkaline lumen of the duodenum, less calcium is solubilized, and calcium carbonate, when taken alone, is poorly absorbed.

Active calcium absorption (entry and secretion) depends on vitamin D intake and the presence of calbindin in duodenal enterocytes (35). Most calcium is absorbed passively in the jejunum and ileum because transit time through the duodenum is so short. The degree of passive ileal absorption depends on many factors, including luminal solubility, residence time in the lumen, and the rate of paracellular diffusion. Only a small amount (<10%) of calcium is absorbed in the human colon, all of it passively; active transport of larger amounts occurs in rat and sheep.

b. **Enteroenteric circulation.** About 300 to 400 mg of calcium is absorbed each day in a normal adult, but 200 to 300 mg is reexcreted into the lumen via pancreatic, biliary, and intestinal secretions. The newly absorbed calcium in the blood mixes with an exchangeable pool of about 1 g. The calcium pool is filtered through the kidney many times, so that 10 g is filtered each day, of which 99% is absorbed secondary to the action of parathyroid hormone and 100 mg is excreted in urine. When intestinal or urinary losses are excessive, the rate of bone resorption increases until it cannot compensate for the losses and hypocalcemia develops.

5. **Deficiency**

a. **Incidence.** Dietary deficiency of calcium is more common than magnesium or phosphorus deficiency; dietary sources of calcium are more limited than those of magnesium and phosphorus, absorption is not as good as that of phosphorus, and the obligatory daily excretion (300 mg in stool, 100 mg in urine) is large in comparison with the exchangeable pool size (1 g) and the daily flux from bone (200–300 mg). Dietary deficiency is most likely to develop during infancy, adolescence, and pregnancy (when requirements are large) and during old age (when absorption is decreased and bone mass is lower).

b. **Hypocalcemia.** The usual causes of hypocalcemia are not related to deficiency but to metabolism. Hypocalcemia leads to enhanced neuromuscular transmission, tetany, altered myocardial function and arrhythmias (prolonged QT interval), and altered nerve conduction. Severe weight loss (e.g., anorexia nervosa) can lead to a prolonged QT interval and arrhythmia by a mechanism that is not explained by hypocalcemia (38).

c. **Chronic deficiency.** The body contains about 1,000 g of calcium. A net loss of 100 mg/d would lead to a 20% (detectable) loss of bone calcium in about 2,000 days, or 6 years. Because bone loss is a slow process, the state of calcium nutrition at the time of clinical presentation, such as fracture, may bear little relationship to an earlier cause of bone loss. Thus, calcium intake should aim to achieve a peak bone density at ages 25 to 30 as well as to alter the rate of bone loss with aging (39). The expected rate of bone loss with aging is 0.5% yearly after age 40, except for the 5 years after menopause, when it increases to 2% annually.

Osteopenia can occur unevenly in different bones, so the bone density analysis must be performed on those most at risk in a given patient. As a person ages, however, the bone loss from various sites tends to equalize. Thus, measurements of density in the spine, proximal femur, middle portion of the radius, and os calcis all reflect similar degrees of bone loss in the elderly. In women 20 to 45 years old, the site of measurement may be critical (33). The spine is most often followed in postmenopausal osteoporosis; the rate of bone turnover in trabecular bone, such as that of the spine, is high, and measurement with DEXA is most precise in the spine.

d. **Causes.** Malabsorption of calcium usually occurs in short-bowel syndrome and untreated celiac disease, but malabsorption may be of many causes. Renal failure and vitamin D deficiency lead to hypocalcemia and bone disease. The factors most often associated with low bone mass (not necessarily calcium deficiency) are postmenopausal osteoporosis (especially if the patient or a first-degree has a history of fracture), Caucasian race, female sex, advanced age, dementia, low body weight, current cigarette smoking, low calcium intake (lifelong), alcoholism, and poor general health.

6. **Treatment.** Any patient with calcium deficiency should also be evaluated for vitamin D deficiency (see Chapter 6), and if this is present, it should be treated.

a. Hypocalcemia. Acute symptomatic hypocalcemia is a medical emergency. It should be treated with 10 to 20 mL of a 10% solution of calcium gluconate (90 to 180 mg of elemental calcium) administered IV over 10 to 15 minutes. This initial therapy should be followed by more prolonged IV infusion (e.g., six to eight 10-mL ampules of 10% calcium gluconate per liter in D5W) until serum calcium levels can be maintained with oral supplements.

b. Nutritional deficiency. Nutritional rickets still occurs in Third World nations. When rickets was caused by a low intake of calcium (200 mg/d), it responded better to treatment with calcium alone (1,000 mg/d) or in combination with vitamin D than to vitamin D alone (40). When calcium intake was below recommended levels but not very low (e.g., 800 mg/d) in mothers who were lactating or post weaning, supplementation with calcium (1,000 mg/d) enhanced bone density only modestly (~ 5%) in 6 months (41).

c. Osteoporosis in medical disorders. In certain intestinal diseases, fecal calcium loss is increased by diarrhea or malabsorption; patients with such diseases should undergo bone density screening, and any osteoporosis should be treated. Clinical risk factors are not good predictors of bone mass in these patients, and the threshold for measuring bone density should be low. Patients with celiac disease and inflammatory bowel disease should be given adequate dietary calcium and supplementation to 1,500 mg/d in the form of tablets if necessary (42). Vitamin D deficiency should be sought and treated (see Chapter 6). If patients are on glucocorticoids, the dose taken should be the lowest required to obtain benefit, and it should be taken for the shortest possible time. Physical activity and adequate nutrition should be promoted, and cigarette smoking should be discouraged (43). Early studies suggest that supplementation with calcium, vitamin D, or both prevents bone loss in patients with Crohn's disease (44). If low bone density persists, drug therapy for osteoporosis should be provided, with the addition of hormone replacement therapy for postmenopausal women, testosterone for men with low testosterone levels, and biphosphonates or calcitonin for others as indicated.

d. Osteoporosis. Good evidence is available to support the role of calcium supplementation in improving bone density in elderly and adolescent populations (23). This relationship has been supported by the Food and Drug Administration, the National Institutes of Health, and the National Academy of Sciences. The beneficial effect of 1,000 mg of supplemental calcium, with or without vitamin D, has been seen in early postmenopausal women, even those with good initial calcium and vitamin D status. Some studies also show a decrease in the fracture rate with calcium alone (1,200 mg/d for 4 years) (45). Studies assessing the efficacy of estrogen therapy in postmenopausal women showed improved bone density in those whose dietary calcium exceeded 1,000 mg/d, but not in those whose dietary calcium was only half that amount (46). When adequate calcium (>1,000 mg/d) and vitamin D (to maintain 25-hydroxyvitamin D levels ≥ 75 nmol/L) were taken, bone sparing with low-dose hormone replacement therapy was as good as that achieved with high-dose hormone replacement therapy (47).

e. Hypertension. A small decrease in systolic, but not diastolic, pressure was observed with calcium supplementation between 500 and 2,000 mg/d (48,49). However, use of the DASH diet, low in fat and rich in fruits, vegetables, whole grains, and low-fat dairy products that provide 1,265 mg of calcium per day, produced a greater fall in pressure (9). Thus, calcium supplements are not often indicated for the treatment of hypertension.

    f. Colon cancer. Controlled studies measuring the effect of calcium on colonic proliferative rates have provided mixed answers (50). One large study showed a modest effect of calcium supplementation (1,200 mg/d) for 4 years in preventing colorectal polyps (51).

    g. Premenstrual syndrome. The use of 1,200 mg of calcium per day for three cycles led to fewer symptoms in women ages 18 to 45 years (52). The use of calcium for this condition should still be considered uncertain until more studies have been reported.

    h. Oral preparations. Calcium carbonate is given to most patients because it contains the largest amount of elemental calcium per unit weight. However, it is less soluble than some other salts (glubionate, gluconate, citrate), which may be useful in selected cases because they are better absorbed (53). Calcium carbonate contains 40% elemental calcium. Tricalcium phosphate contains 33% elemental calcium, acetate 25%, dibasic phosphate 23%, citrate 21%, lactate 13%, gluconate 9%, and glubionate 6.5%. Table 7-19 lists some of the available preparations.

   7. Toxicity. The tolerable upper intake level (UL) for calcium has been set for adults at 1,200 mg/d (24) (Appendix B). When intake exceeds 4,000 mg/d, hypercalcemia develops, along with renal damage and metastatic calcification.

Table 7-19. Selected calcium-containing products for oral use

Calcium supplement	Elemental calcium (mg per tablet)	Vitamin D (IU per tablet)
Calcium carbonate		
Alka 2	200	—
Alka-Mints	340	—
Biocal	250, 500	—
Calburst	500	200
Calciday	667	—
Calsup	300, 600	200
Caltrate + D	600	200
Os-Cal + D	250, 500	200
Oystercal	250, 375, 500	—
Titralac	200 (405/5 mL)	—
Tums	200, 500	—
Viactiv	500	100
Calcium citrate		
Citracal	200 (500 per effervescent tablet)	—
Citracal + D	315	200
Calcium citrate + D	315	200
Calcium complex/components		
Calcium acetate	167–668 mg	—
Calcet (carbonate, lactate, gluconate)	150	100
Calcium gluconate	45/500 mg	—
Calcium lactate	42/325 mg	—
Ca Plus (protein)	280	—
Calcium glubionate		
Neo-Calglucon	115/5 ml)	—
Calcium phosphate		
Dical-D	350	400
Posture-D	600	125

   a. Populations at risk. In patients on thiazide diuretics or with renal disease, urinary calcium excretion may be decreased. Patients with absorptive or renal hypercalciuria are at an increased risk for kidney stones, although normal persons are not (54). Patients with primary hyperthyroidism and sarcoidosis are at risk for hypercalcemia and should avoid calcium supplements. Patients with calcium oxalate stones, especially if they are secondary to malabsorption of fat, should be treated with oral calcium to precipitate the soluble sodium oxalate in the intestinal lumen.

   b. Interference with absorption. Oral calcium may interfere with the absorption of many drugs (e.g., salicylates, bisphosphonates, fluoride, tetracyclines, atenolol, iron). Calcium supplements should not be taken at the same time as iron and other medications. Calcium supplements do not interfere with magnesium absorption in normal persons but may do so in cases of magnesium depletion, as in patients with diabetes, malabsorption, or acute alcoholic intake. In such cases, 100 mg of magnesium should be provided for every 500 mg of supplemental calcium used (54).

   c. Hypercalcemia. Serum calcium levels above 11 mg/dL can be associated with symptoms related to decreased neuromuscular transmission and muscle contraction. These include weakness, ileus, altered cardiac conductivity, anorexia, nausea, vomiting, constipation, dry mouth, polyuria, and thirst. Serum calcium levels above 12 mg/dL can produce confusion, delirium, stupor, and coma, especially in the elderly. Changes on the electrocardiogram include short PR, ST, and QT intervals, with a prolonged QRS complex. Arrhythmias can occur, especially at levels above 13 mg/dL. The treatment of severe exogenous hypercalcemia should begin with IV normal saline solution (500 to 750 mL/h or as tolerated) and furosemide (80 to 120 mg/h) if renal function is adequate. These measures are usually rapidly effective. Long-term management consists of adjusting the doses of exogenous calcium, vitamin D, or both.

D. Magnesium

1. **Requirement.** Magnesium requirements have been determined by balance studies and urinary measurements because the kidney is the main excretory organ. With an average U.S. dietary intake of 120 mg/1,000 kcal per day and maintenance of the serum concentration at 2 mg/dL ($\sim$ 1.7 mEq/L), the mean urinary excretion is about 72 mg/d. Because average absorption is 30% to 40%, the daily requirement should be about 200 mg for an adult. However, the requirements for infants and children have not been accurately assessed. Human milk contains 40 mg of magnesium per liter, and the average infant ingests about 850 mL/d. The 1997 DRIs are noted in Table 7-20.

2. **Food sources.** Magnesium is bound to protein and phosphate ions, and to porphyrin in green leafy plants and vegetables. Hard water and mineral waters can contain as much as 120 mg/L. The sources of magnesium are widespread. Good dietary sources include whole grains, legumes, dark green leafy vegetables, nuts, fish, whole grains, and cocoa. Table 7-21 lists the magnesium content of selected foods.

3. **Assessment**

   a. Intake and absorption. When dietary information is available, urinary magnesium can be helpful because dietary intake and urinary excretion are strongly correlated (20). The kidney avidly retains magnesium when dietary intake is low, and urinary levels fall. However, dietary deficiency of magnesium is uncommon because the mineral is widely distributed among foods. Thus, low urinary levels of magnesium usually reflects disease (e.g., prolonged diarrhea).

Table 7-20. Dietary reference intakes of magnesium

Life stage group	Magnesium (mg/d)	Life stage group	Magnesium (mg/d)
Infants		Females	
0–6 mo	30[a]	9–13 y	240
7–12 mo	75[a]	14–18 y	360
Children		19–30 y	310
1–3 y	80	31–>70	320
4–8 y	130	Pregnancy	
Males		≤18 y	400
9–13 y	240	19–30 y	350
14–18 y	410	31–50 y	360
19–30 y	400	Lactation	
31–>70 y	420	≤18 y	360
		19–30 y	310
		31–50 y	320

[a] Adequate intake (AI) is estimated from ingestion of human milk content. Other values reflect recommended dietary allowance (RDA).
From Standing Committee on the Scientific Evaluation of Dietary Reference Intakes, Food and Nutrition Board, Institute of Medicine. *Dietary reference intakes: calcium, phosphorus, magnesium, vitamin D, and fluoride.* Washington, DC: National Academy Press, 1997.

Elevated urinary levels of magnesium often reflects diuretic therapy, not high dietary intake.
  b. **Body stores.** Serum magnesium is measured by colorimetric or fluorometric methods, although atomic absorption spectroscopy is more reliable. Hemolysis falsely elevates serum magnesium levels because the mineral is an intracellular cation. Extracellular ionized magnesium (filterable magnesium) is the biologically active fraction, so that the total serum magnesium level does not reflect total stores in a reliable fashion. Magnesium-selective electrodes are now available and have been incorporated into commercially available instruments (20). About 70% of the total magnesium in plasma is ionized, but the usefulness of measuring ionized magnesium in disease states is not well studied. Hypomagnesemia, defined as levels below 1.25 to 1.50 mEq/L (Table 7-22), is often accompanied

Table 7-21. Magnesium content of selected foods

Food	Serving size	Magnesium content (mg)
Cereals	3 oz	90–120
Legumes	1 cup	80–120
Nuts	½ cup	130–210
Fish, cooked	3 oz	20–60
Baked potato with skin	One	55
Spinach, cooked	½ cup	80
Vegetables, cooked	1 cup	5–30
Fruit	1 cup	20–30
Meat, cooked	3 oz	10–20
Milk	1 cup	28–33
Yogurt	1 cup	27–40
Beer	12 oz	23

Table 7-22. Reference values for magnesium assessment

Parameter	Magnesium levels	
	(mmol/L)	(mEq/L)
Serum magnesium (adult)	0.75–1.25	1.5–2.5
NHANES I (18–74 y)	0.75–0.96	1.5–1.92
Hypomagnesemia	<0.62–0.75	<1.25–1.5
Hypermagnesemia	>1.25	>1.5
Serum ionized magnesium	0.58 ± 0.006	
Erythrocyte magnesium (adult)	1.88 ± 0.12	
	Magnesium urinary excretion per day	
Magnesium load test	94–95% (normal)	33–69% (deficient)

NHANHES, National Health and Nutrition Examination Survey.
From Sauberlich HE. *Laboratory tests for the assessment of nutritional status.* 2nd ed. Boca Raton, FL: CRC Press, 1990.

by hypokalemia and hypocalcemia. Low levels can occur with pregnancy, malabsorption, reduced intake, diabetes mellitus, severe illness, acute alcoholism, or renal leak (or diuretic use). A normal level does not rule out deficient stores because the serum level is corrected by the action of parathyroid hormone and calcitonin. Hypermagnesemia is found in renal failure and with the use of magnesium-containing antacids or laxatives.

Tissue magnesium levels should be the best measure of body stores of this intracellular cation, but practical methods are not available. Red and white cells have been isolated for this purpose, but the results are not sufficiently consistent for general use. The magnesium loading test has been used to assess deficiency (20). Thirty millimoles of magnesium chloride is infused over 12 hours, and urine is collected for 24 hours. Magnesium status is based on the amount of magnesium retained in the body. Normally, only 5% to 6% is retained. However, the care required to perform the test has limited its clinical usefulness.

4. **Physiology.** Magnesium is the fourth most abundant cation in the body, after sodium, potassium, and calcium. The 70-kg adult body contains about 2,000 mEq of magnesium, or 21 to 28 g. About 60% is in the bone, with the rest distributed equally between muscle and other soft tissues. Less than 5% is in the extracellular fluid. The exchangeable magnesium pool is about 5 g, but extracellular magnesium is only about 250 mg. Magnesium flux from bone replenishes the exchangeable pool, but the daily rate of this flux is not precisely known.

   a. **Function.** More than 300 enzymatic reactions require magnesium. These involve transfer of phosphate groups, acylation of coenzyme A, hydrolysis of phosphates and pyrophosphates, and nucleic acid synthesis. All enzymatic reactions in which adenosine triphosphate is involved require magnesium. In addition, the cation is necessary for ribosomal RNA and DNA stability, activation of amino acids, degradation of DNA, neurotransmission, and immune function. Magnesium is a calcium antagonist in some reactions, and interacts with potassium, pyridoxine, and boron.

   b. **Absorption.** Magnesium is absorbed by both passive diffusion and active transport. Absorption varies from 30% to 70% of ingested magnesium, depending on how much magnesium is presented to the gut. At the usual intake levels of 300 mg/d, absorption is about 33%.

Active magnesium absorption is more readily detected in magnesium-deficient states, such as idiopathic hypomagnesemia (55). At physiologic concentrations, the effect of 1,25-dihydroxyvitamin D_3 on magnesium absorption is very small and is probably related to changes in calcium or phosphorus uptake (56). Much of the magnesium ingested in medicinal form (oxide, hydroxide, chloride, citrate) is poorly soluble and is not absorbed to a great extent. Phosphate and organic chelators (e.g., oxalate, phytate) can delay absorption. Transit time is a major factor in determining the efficiency of magnesium absorption.

c. **Urinary excretion.** The kidney is the major excretory organ. More than two-thirds of absorbed magnesium is excreted in the urine each day. Urinary excretion is about 3% to 5% of the filtered load and is increased in proteinuria. The ascending limb of the tubule absorbs 50% to 75% of the filtered magnesium. so that excretion is reduced to less than 1 mEq/d. Nonetheless, the distal tubule is the major site of magnesium regulation (57). The major regulator is the serum magnesium concentration, and regulation is mediated by Ca/Mg-sensing receptors located on the capillary side of cells of the thick ascending limb. Maximal excretion in response to magnesium loading can exceed 160 mEq/d. Excretion is increased by volume expansion, hypercalcemia, diuretics, alcohol, and phosphate depletion, and is decreased by the action of parathyroid hormone. Because of this tight urinary regulation, magnesium deficiency occurs rarely except when excessive amounts are lost from the body, in intestinal or renal disease.

d. **Parathyroid hormone response.** When hypomagnesemia is mild, parathyroid hormone is released and calcium is released from bone. However, the direct effect of hypomagnesemia on decreasing calcium mobilization from bone blunts this effect (58). When magnesium deficiency is severe and the serum concentration very low, parathyroid hormone secretion is impaired. Along with the direct effect of the hypomagnesemia on bone, calcium flux is lowered and hypocalcemia develops. In this case, hypocalcemia is less a manifestation of depleted calcium stores than of low stores of exchangeable magnesium. Thus, when magnesium deficiency is severe (e.g., in malabsorption), magnesium is required to treat the hypocalcemia.

5. **Deficiency**

   a. **Clinical manifestations.** Magnesium deficiency may not be associated with symptoms. Many of the symptoms of moderate or severe deficiency are nonspecific or are caused by associated electrolyte abnormalities, such as hypocalcemia, hypokalemia, and metabolic alkalosis (Table 7-23). The most common symptoms are muscular twitching and tremor, numbness, and tingling. Less common are muscle weakness, convulsions, apathy, depression, and delirium. Refractory hypokalemia can develop because magnesium plays a role in determining the intracellular–extracellular ratio of the two ions. If magnesium is deficient, potassium supplements can restore serum potassium, but not intracellular potassium (59). Common manifestations include Chvostek's sign and premature ventricular beats.

   b. **Causes.** Most cases of magnesium deficiency arise from gastrointestinal or renal losses (Table 7-24). Hypercalcemia of any cause produces a high filtered load of calcium that competes with magnesium for reabsorption. Any kind of diuresis can decrease the tubular reabsorption of magnesium. In patients with short-bowel syndrome, urinary magnesium levels fell before serum levels and were an early indicator of evolving deficiency (60). Although urinary magnesium is not often useful in diagnosing deficiency, the situation may be different in short-bowel syndrome, in which absorption is so limited.

Table 7-23. Clinical manifestations of moderate/severe magnesium deficiency

Symptoms	Signs	Laboratory abnormalities
Carpopedal spasm	Chvostek	Hypocalcemia
Seizures, tremor	Trousseau	Hypokalemia
Vertigo/ataxia	Arrhythmia	Carbohydrate intolerance
Muscle weakness		ECG: wide QRS complex, prolonged PR interval, inverted T waves, U waves, ventricular arrhythmias
Numbness, tingling		
Depression, psychosis		

ECG, electrocardiogram.

6. **Treatment.** The choice of oral or parenteral magnesium depends on the severity of depletion. However, acute magnesium infusion decreases magnesium absorption in the loop of Henle, so much of the infused parenteral magnesium is excreted. Thus, oral replacement is preferred if the clinical presentation allows. The problem with oral therapy is that most of the salts of magnesium are only poorly soluble.

   a. **Parenteral.** Moderate or severe deficiency should be treated parenterally, especially if tetany or ventricular arrhythmias are present, with 4 to 8 mmol given as an IV loading dose, followed by 25 mmol/d thereafter until the plasma magnesium is above 0.4 mmol/L (57). In patients with normal renal function, up to 20 mmol (2.5 g) can be infused IV over 3 hours in 5% dextrose or 0.9% normal saline solution if deficiency is severe. Magnesium sulfate is incompatible with soluble phosphates, and with alkaline carbonates and bicarbonates, except in dilute solution. For mild deficiency, 1 g can be given IM every 6 hours for a total of four doses. Magnesium has been used parenterally in the absence of deficiency in patients with preeclampsia and ischemic heart disease, although its use in the latter condition is controversial.

   b. **Oral.** Magnesium oxide is commonly used, but it is poorly soluble and can act as a cathartic. Magnesium gluconate is preferred because it is more soluble and is available in a palatable liquid form

Table 7-24. Causes of magnesium deficiency

Gastrointestinal	Renal
Malabsorption	Volume expansion
Diarrhea, especially chronic	Osmotic diuresis
Short bowel syndrome	Diuretics (thiazides, loop diuretics, alcohol,
Enterocutaneous fistulae	aminoglycosides, cisplatin, amphotericin B,
Nasogastric suction, long-term	cyclosporine, foscarnet, pentamidine)
Primary intestinal	Phosphate depletion
hypomagnesemia	Postobstructive nephropathy
Malnutrition, severe	Diuretic phase of acute renal failure
Pancreatitis, acute	Renal transplantation
Prematurity	Hungry bone syndrome
	Hypercalcemia of any cause
	Renal tubular dysfunction

(Table 7-25). Thus, large numbers of tablets can be avoided for long-term therapy. Magnesium chloride is absorbed poorly, less well than magnesium acetate or dietary magnesium (from nuts), and should not be relied on for replacement therapy (61). Magnesium salts can decrease the absorption of some drugs, such as amino-quinolones, digoxin, nitrofurantoin, penicillamine, and tetracyclines. Calcium supplementation of more than 2.6 g/d can lead to a negative magnesium balance. When malabsorption requires supplementation with both calcium and magnesium, they should be given at separate times.

   c. **Supplements for chronic medical diseases.** Magnesium supplements have been used for a variety of medical conditions in which patients are felt to be at risk for deficiency (e.g., diabetes) or in which improved muscular performance is desired (e.g., heart disease). Observational studies in heart disease have provided only a hint that magnesium may be useful for patients with mitral valve prolapse (23). Of course, patients should consume enough magnesium-rich foods or take supplements if their intake is not adequate. Double-blinded placebo-controlled trials of magnesium supplements in hypertension have not demonstrated a reproducible effect. If patients are taking loop or thiazide diuretics, some additional magnesium may be needed to replace that lost in the urine, if one assumes that renal function is normal. Magnesium supplements have not improved glycemic control in either type I or type II diabetes (23). Likewise, evidence does not support magnesium supplements to treat migraine headaches or premenstrual symptoms or to improve exercise tolerance.

7. **Toxicity.** The UL for magnesium is 65 mg/d (children 1 to 3 years old), 110 mg/d (children 4 to 8 years old), and 350 mg/d (all adolescents and adults) (24) (Appendix B). Magnesium supplements are usually not toxic if renal function is normal. Soft stools and diarrhea have been reported after ingestion of more than 500 mg of elemental magnesium (62).

   a. **Hypermagnesemia.** Hypermagnesemia develops when renal excretion is decreased (as in renal failure and eclampsia), in severe diabetic ketoacidosis, and in Addison's disease. Blocking of neuromuscular transmission leads to decreased tendon reflexes (at levels >4 mEq/L) and respiratory paralysis and heart block (at levels >10 mEq/L). Infants of mothers with eclampsia treated with magnesium are at

Table 7-25. Oral magnesium preparations

Preparation	Anion	Tablet size (mg)	Elemental magnesium content (mg per tablet or per 5 mL)[a]
Mag-200	Oxide	400	241
Mag-Ox 400	Oxide	140	83
Magnesium oxide	Oxide	250, 600	130, 360
Uro-Mag	Gluconate	500	29
Magtrate	Gluconate	500	29
Magonate	Gluconate	5 mL	54
Magonate	Gluconate	500	27
Chelated magnesium	Amino acids	500	100
Slow-Mag	Chloride	535	64
Mag-Tab SR	Lactate		84

[a] Assumes equal bioavailability, which is not the case.

risk, as are patients with renal failure receiving magnesium-containing antacids.

Hypermagnesemia does not usually develop until the GFR falls below 13 mL/min. In renal failure, magnesium excretion relative to the GFR is lower than expected from the plasma level. Thus, plasma levels can rise rapidly. At levels of 3 to 5 mEq/L, symptoms include nausea, vomiting, cutaneous vasodilation, and hypertension. At higher levels (5 to 9 mEq/L), drowsiness, hyporeflexia, and muscular weakness occur, and above 10 mEq/L, respiratory arrest is noted, along with prolongation of the QTc interval and atrioventricular block.

   b. **Therapy** of hypermagnesemia involves withdrawal of any oral or parenteral magnesium compounds, hemodialysis or peritoneal dialysis, or infusion of calcium to compete with magnesium on the cellular level. Usually, calcium infusion (1 g of calcium gluconate IV) is not required except for those critically ill.

E. Phosphorus

1. Requirement

   a. **Ratio of phosphorus to calcium.** The recommended ratio of calcium to phosphorus in the diet is between 2:1 and 1:2. Because dietary phosphorus is so abundant and deficiency from decreased intake occurs so rarely, the recommended phosphorus intake is similar to that for calcium except in young infants. In the case of infants ingesting cow's milk with a calcium–phosphorus ratio of 1.2:1, the relative increase in phosphorus intake may contribute to hypocalcemia in early life. Thus, the adequate intake (AI) for phosphorus is set at 100 mg, in comparison with 210 mg for calcium for the first 6 months of life but nearly equal for the next 6 months (Table 7-26).

   b. **DRI.** Data to establish a requirement for phosphorus are not available because, like urinary magnesium excretion, urinary phosphorus excretion does not reflect dietary intake. In general, if the protein intake is adequate, so is the phosphorus intake. About 1 g of phosphorus is needed for each 17 g of nitrogen retained. The DRI exceeds this because of incomplete absorption and obligatory urinary excretion. The efficiency of absorption varies with the source of phosphorus and the ratio of calcium to phosphorus in the diet, so that the recommendation for dietary intake is further confused. The

Table 7-26. Dietary reference intake for phosphorus

Life stage group	Phosphorus (mg/d)	Life stage group	Phosphorus (mg/d)
Infants		Females	
0–6 mos	100[a]	9–13 y	1,250
7–12 mos	275[a]	14–18 y	1,250
Children		19–>70 y	700
1–3 y	460	Pregnancy/lactation	
4–8 y	500	≤18 y	1,250
Males		19–50 y	700
9–18 y	1,250		
19–>70 y	700		

[a] Estimate based on adequate intake (AI). Other values reflect recommended dietary allowance (RDA).
From Standing Committee on the Scientific Evaluation of Dietary Reference Intakes, Food and Nutrition Board, Institute of Medicine. *Dietary reference intakes: calcium, phosphorus, magnesium, vitamin D, fluoride.* Washington, DC: National Academy Press, 1997.

current DRI for adults is 700 mg/d, somewhat below the DRI for calcium (1,000 to 1,200 mg/d); for growing adolescents and pregnant or
lactating women, the DRI is 1,250 mg/d, nearly the same as that for
calcium (1,300 mg/d).

2. Food sources. Phosphorus is a constituent of all cells and is thus present in all foods. The phosphorus content of some foods is listed in Table 7-27. Both organic and inorganic phosphorus (Pi) esters are handled
alike by the alkaline phosphatase present in the intestinal tract.

  a. Milk. The important, relatively low-phosphorus food of animal origin is human milk. In newborns, who cannot respond to the stimulus of low calcium levels by increasing parathyroid hormone output,
this is a perfect food. One liter of human milk contains 150 to 175 mg
of phosphorus, or 25 mg/100 kcal. In contrast, each liter of cow's milk
provides 1,000 mg of phosphorus, or 150 mg/100 kcal. This is an excessive load of phosphorus for a newborn and tends to reduce the
serum calcium level by increasing the serum phosphorus level.

  b. Grains and cereals. A major source of phosphorus in grains and
cereals is inositol hexaphosphoric acid, or phytic acid. Calcium, zinc,
and magnesium phytates are insoluble and are excreted in the stool.
During leavening and baking of bread, some of the phosphorus from
phytic acid is converted to orthophosphate by the action of phytases,
so that some of the phosphorus is absorbed. However, in countries
where unleavened wheat is used, the phytate content of grain
products is increased. If the intake of calcium and vitamin D is also

Table 7-27. Phosphorus content of food

Food	Portion	Phosphorus (mg)
Grains and Cereals		
Bread, white	1 slice	30
Hamburger bun	1 each	44
Cornbread muffins	1 each	128
Rice, cooked	1 cup	74
Bran flakes, 40% cup	½ cup	63
Meat and fish		
Beef, lamb, veal	3 oz	125–300
Beef liver	3 oz	392
Chicken, white meat, roasted	3 oz	183
Fish	3 oz	230–330
Fruits		
Apple, medium	1 each	10
Banana, medium	1 each	22
Cantaloupe	1 cup	27
Orange	1 each	19
Vegetables		
Potato, baked	1 each	115
Tomato	1 each	30
Green peas, frozen	½ cup	69
Dairy products		
Milk, whole	1 cup	227
Cheese	1 oz	200–250
Egg, large	1 each	86
Nuts		
Peanuts, almonds, walnuts	1 cup	520–730
Peanut butter	2 tbs	103

limited, calcium deficiency may develop partly as a consequence of excess dietary phytate.

3. **Assessment.** Phosphorus is well absorbed from the intestine, and the plasma level is carefully regulated by the tubular reabsorption of phosphate. In addition, the movement of phosphorus across cell membranes is rapid and responds to alterations in metabolic activity (e.g., glucose utilization). Thus, neither plasma phosphate nor urinary excretion of phosphate reflects intake or body stores. Abnormal plasma levels can reflect real changes in body stores, but more often they reflect altered renal or metabolic activity.

   a. **Plasma phosphate.** The usual serum assay measures the colored ammonium phosphomolybdate complex. Specimens collected with EDTA or citrate are not acceptable because these compounds interfere with the color reaction of the assay. Hemolysis must be avoided because red cells have a high phosphate content. The normal level is 0.81to 1.29 mmol/L (25 to 45 mg/L) in adults, 1.2 to 2.23 mmol/L (37 to 69 mg/L) in children, and 1.6 to 2.1 mmol/L (50 to 65 mg/L) in infants (20). An assay of fasting serum inorganic phosphate levels is important for meaningful interpretation. The interpretation of serum levels is difficult because many factors influence the phosphorus concentration. The rapid infusion of glucose or insulin can lower levels. In starvation, tissue catabolism releases phosphate, and plasma levels are maintained. When the starving patient is refed, it is essential to provide adequate phosphorus because serum levels can fall precipitously. Table 7-28 lists the major causes of altered plasma phosphate concentrations.

   b. **Urinary phosphate.** The average phosphorus excretion rate in the United States is 600 to 800 mg/d, reflecting a mean intake of 1,500 mg/d for men and 1,000 mg/d for women (20). With phosphate depletion, urinary excretion falls to nearly zero. Urinary phosphate varies with intake but cannot be used to estimate intake because it is regulated largely by parathyroid hormone. However, in the appropriate setting, a low urinary excretion rate can confirm a clinically suspected low dietary intake. Levels above 1,300 mg/d are considered high and reflect high intake.

4. **Physiology**

   a. **Absorption.** Dietary phosphorus is absorbed as the inorganic form and as a component of phosphoproteins, phosphosugars, and phospholipids. In cow's milk, the phosphorus is 70% inorganic, but in cereals and soft tissues of animals, it is largely organic. All the phosphorus must be liberated by phosphatases on the enterocyte brush border and in biliary secretions before absorption can take place. Net absorption is 65% to 75% from cow's milk but exceeds 80% from human milk. In adults and older children ingesting a mixed diet, absorption varies from 58% to 70% and is proportional to intake at all levels of ingestion. Alkaline phosphatase is quite resistant to damage in most diseases of the small bowel; thus, phosphate maldigestion is uncommon. Fecal output of phosphorus is not greater than intake—that is, no obligatory loss occurs in the gut. Digestive juices provide about 200 mg/d in adults. However, because two-thirds of luminal phosphorus is absorbed and the kidney can adjust phosphate excretion over a wide range, deficiency of phosphate from malabsorption rarely occurs.

      Absorption is predominantly by passive diffusion. At low levels of phosphorus intake, active sodium-dependent transport is controlled by 1,25-dihydroxyvitamin D_3. Because of the negative charge on phosphate and paracellular channels, simple diffusion between cells is unlikely. Efflux of phosphate across the basolateral membrane of the enterocyte is probably passive. Absorption is probably stimu-

Table 7-28. Causes of altered plasma phosphate levels

Condition	Mechanism
Hypophosphatemia	
Increased urinary excretion	Urinary loss, decreased replacement on IV therapy, acute alcoholism, vitamin D deficiency, hypophosphatemic rickets, kidney transplantation, volume expansion, renal tubular defects, metabolic or respiratory alkalosis, hyperparathyroidism (decreased tubular reabsorption of phosphate)
Decreased intestinal absorption	Vitamin D deficiency, dietary phosphorus restriction (severe), antacid abuse (phosphate binding), chronic diarrhea
Phosphate compartmentalization	Rapid shift of phosphate between body compartments, TPN, recovery from diabetic ketoacidosis, respiratory alkalosis, sepsis, refeeding syndrome, hormonal therapy (insulin, glucagon, corticosteroids), carbohydrate infusion (glucose, fructose, lactate)
Hyperphosphatemia	
Increased exogenous load	Feeding cow's milk to premature infants, IV infusion, oral supplements, vitamin D toxicity, phosphate enemas
Increased endogenous load	Hemolysis, lactic acidosis, respiratory acidosis, rhabdomyolysis
Decreased urinary excretion	Renal failure, hypoparathyroidism, acromegaly, vitamin D toxicity, bisphosphonate therapy, magnesium deficiency
False (pseudo) hyperphosphatemia	Hemolysis *in vitro,* hypertriglyceridemia, multiple myeloma

TPN, total parenteral nutrition.

lated to some extent by vitamin D and perhaps by parathyroid hormone. Although malabsorption of phosphorus can occur in vitamin D deficiency, sufficient phosphorus is usually absorbed to satisfy daily needs because dietary intake is high and absorption is fairly high, even when somewhat impaired.

b. **Urinary excretion.** Plasma phosphate is derived from input from the intestine and bone. Unlike that of calcium and magnesium, the daily flux of phosphorus to and from bone, the major store of body phosphorus (85%), is quite small. This flux approximates 200 mg/d (3 mg/kg). Plasma levels are regulated mainly via the kidney. The main factor influencing tubular reabsorption of phosphate is parathyroid hormone. However, plasma phosphate levels do not regulate the secretion of parathyroid hormone. It is the calcium level that secondarily regulates phosphate levels. Other hormones—for example, thyroid and growth hormone, estrogens, calcitonin, and vitamin D—all influence plasma phosphate, but much less so than parathyroid hormone does. Finally, phosphorus moves rapidly across cell membranes in response to requirements for intracellular phosphorus and available energy to form high-energy phosphate bonds.

Two different Na/P transporters have been identified in the kidney. Cotransport is regulated both by phosphorus intake and by parathyroid hormone secretion. Parathyroid hormone causes phosphaturia by inhibiting Na/P cotransport in the proximal tubule, acting via both cyclic AMP and the protein kinase C system. During phosphate depletion, the kidney becomes relatively resistant to the phosphaturic effects of parathyroid hormone (57)

c. **Phosphate homeostasis.** Phosphate homeostasis is mainly regulated by the relationship between absorbed phosphorus, plasma inorganic phosphate, and urinary phosphate. Absorbed phosphorus and urinary phosphorus rise with increased intake. Thus, at any given phosphorus intake, the individual adjusts the plasma phosphate to the level at which phosphorus influx into plasma and urinary phosphorus are equal. A high oral phosphate load stimulates parathyroid hormone output by reducing calcium and probably magnesium concentration in the ECF. Parathyroid hormone inhibits tubular reabsorption of phosphate and increases urinary excretion of phosphate. When the serum phosphorus level is reduced by decreased intake or absorption, the serum calcium level increases to inhibit parathyroid hormone output and urinary excretion of phosphate falls. The serum calcium level rises in hypophosphatemia because production of 1,25-dihydroxyvitamin D_3 is stimulated by a low phosphate concentration. Simultaneous vitamin D deficiency does not allow these events to take place; instead, a reduction in calcium absorption and the serum calcium level leads to an increased output of parathyroid hormone and increased urinary phosphate excretion.

d. **Function.** Phosphorus is important for all cells; 80% to 85% is in the bone. The rest is important for energy production (adenosine triphosphate), phospholipid formation, nucleotide formation, buffering systems, and calcium homeostasis.

5. **Deficiency**

a. **Causes.** Most patients who manifest clinical evidence of hypophosphatemia have an underlying wasting disease (63). These commonly include intestinal malabsorption, malnutrition, cancer, chronic and alcoholism. Recovery from severe burns is also associated with hypophosphatemia. Other causes are listed in Table 7-28. Hypophosphatemia at the onset of ketoacidosis probably indicates severe depletion.

b. **Clinical manifestations** occur when plasma phosphorus levels fall below 0.32 mmol/L (10 mg/L). Proximal myopathy and ileus may be the initial symptoms. Severe depletion can be manifested by hemolytic anemia (Pi <0.5 mg/dL), rhabdomyolysis (Pi <1.0 mg/dL), and a variety of complications in less severe depletion (Pi, 1.0 to 1.5 mg/dL). These include impaired chemotaxis, platelet dysfunction, metabolic encephalopathy, metabolic acidosis, peripheral neuropathy, central nervous system dysfunction including seizures, cardiac failure, osteomalacia, and decreased glucose utilization (64). A decrease in Pi leads to decreased levels of 2,3-diphosphogluconate (2,3-DPG), an altered affinity of oxygen for hemoglobin, and tissue anoxia. Renal loss of phosphate is often responsible for clinical phosphate deficiency. In an adult with a plasma phosphate level of 3.5 mg/dL and a GFR of 125 mL/min, filtered phosphate amounts to 6,300 mg/24 h. With an intake of 1,500 mg of phosphorus and 60% intestinal absorption (900 mg), reabsorption of 5,400 mg or 85% of the filtered load is required. In renal tubular disease, loss of phosphate can lead to depletion, evidenced by muscle weakness, malaise, and anorexia. Ingestion of large amounts of aluminum hydroxide or calcium salts can lead to phosphate depletion, even in patients with normal kidneys. Such ingestion causes depletion more rapidly when malabsorption is present.

6. Treatment

  a. **Mild to moderate hypophosphatemia** (15 to 25 mg/L) can be managed without supplemental phosphorus by treating the underlying disorder. When levels fall to 0.32 to 0.48 mmol/L (10 to 15 mg/L) or risk factors for phosphorus depletion are present, replacement is advised with oral supplements—either milk or other oral preparations. Usually, a dosage of 1,000 mg/d corrects phosphorus depletion. Cow's milk contains about 1 mg of phosphorus/mL and is an excellent replacement fluid. Oral supplements as tablets of sodium or potassium phosphate can be given at a dosage of 2 to 3 g/d. Neutrophos (250 mg of phosphorus with 7 mEq of sodium and potassium per capsule) or Phospho-Soda (129 mg of phosphorus with 4.8 mEq of sodium per milliliter) is used most commonly. Uro-KP-Neutral and K-Phos Neutral tablets also contain 250 mg of phosphorus and only 1 mEq of potassium with 250 to 300 mg of sodium. The usual dose is two capsules of Neutrophos or 5 mL of Phospho-Soda given two or three times a day. Oral therapy is limited by the production of diarrhea. These supplements should be used with caution if sodium or potassium restriction is required because they contain significant amounts of these cations.

  Antacids that contain magnesium, calcium, or aluminum can bind phosphate and prevent its absorption. When hypophosphatemia is caused in this way, it can be corrected simply by stopping the antacids. Sometimes, the binding properties of phosphate itself can be used for treatment. Calcium phosphate binds unconjugated bilirubin and has been used to supplement phototherapy in patients with Crigler-Najjar type I disease (65).

  b. **Severe hypophosphatemia** (<1 mg/dL) with symptoms should be treated with IV phosphorus. This form of therapy carries a risk for hypocalcemia and should be used with caution. Commercial solutions are mixtures of monobasic and dibasic sodium or potassium salts and provide 3 mmol of phosphate per milliliter. To avoid confusion, always order in terms of millimoles (mmol) of phosphorus. Initially, the dose should be 0.3 mmol of elemental phosphorus per kilogram of body weight given over 4 to 6 hours in normal saline solution. If the creatinine clearance is below 50 mL/min, this dose should be reduced by half. After serum phosphate and calcium have been checked, subsequent therapy depends on the response. To avoid hypocalcemia or sodium or potassium overload, the dosage of 0.3 mmol/kg of body weight every 6 to 8 hours should not be exceeded. These values must be viewed only as rough guidelines because severe hypophosphatemia may develop with normal body stores of phosphorus. Because phosphate infusion can cause hypocalcemia, IV phosphate should not be used when hypocalcemia is present. Also, calcium and phosphate should not be used in the same IV infusion to avoid precipitation. When renal insufficiency is present, great caution must be exercised in administering Pi by any route.

7. Toxicity.

Hyperphosphatemia develops in patients with renal insufficiency and a marked decrease in GFR. Secondary hyperparathyroidism can ensue with skeletal demineralization. The UL has been set at 4 g/d for adults up to age 70, and at 3 g for those older than 70 years (24) (Appendix B). Treatment entails a low intake of phosphate and ingestion of phosphate binders—aluminum hydroxide, calcium carbonate, or sevelamer hydrochloride (Renagel). Calcium carbonate is preferred initially because it is more palatable and is a more effective antacid in treating the duodenal inflammation commonly associated with chronic renal failure. It is not possible to eliminate dietary phosphorus completely because it is ubiquitous. However, a low phosphorus intake can be achieved and is important in the successful management of chronic renal disease (see Chapter 12).

III. Trace minerals
A. Iron
1. **Requirement.** Unlike those of other minerals, iron stores are not regulated by increased or decreased excretion. The major control mechanism is intestinal absorption, which increases during iron deficiency.
   a. **Daily losses.** In the normal person, iron requirements are determined by the limited and fixed amount of iron excreted. Daily losses are through the gastrointestinal tract, skin, and urine; additional iron is lost from the uterus in women. Fecal iron averages from 6 to 16 mg/d, most of which is unabsorbed dietary iron. Endogenous losses from cells amount to 0.1 to 0.2 mg, and blood loss accounts for 0.3 mg. Biliary secretion is 1 mg/d, but only about 0.20 mg is excreted in the stool. Urinary losses are 0.1 to 0.3 mg/d. Dermal losses in sweat, hair, and nails range from 0.2 to 0.4 mg/d. Total daily losses range from 0.9 to 1.4 mg in males. Additional menstrual losses in women amount to 0.5 to 1.0 mg/d when averaged over a whole month.
   b. **Rate of absorption.** Iron requirements are estimated from the daily losses, and an assumption is based on the amount absorbed from food. The Food and Nutrition Board of the National Research Council and the World Health Organization assume absorption of 10% to 15% provided the percentage of calories from animal sources containing heme iron is high, as it is in industrialized nations.
   c. **Recommended dietary allowance (RDA).** Requirements per kilogram of body weight are highest in infancy (because of low iron stores), during periods of rapid growth, and during menstruation and pregnancy. Table 7-29 outlines the requirements and recommended allowances for iron at various stages. The Standing Committee on the Scientific Evaluation of Dietary Reference Intakes has now assigned an RDA for males of all age groups and for postmenopausal women of 8 mg/d, and for premenopausal women of 18 mg/d (66). During pregnancy, the recommended intake is 27 mg. At birth, the placental supply of iron is replaced by the diet. Even the infant of an iron-deficient mother has normal iron stores at birth. Iron treatment during pregnancy is most beneficial to the mother because the infant

Table 7-29. Dietary reference intakes of iron for individuals

Life stage group	Iron (mg/d)	Life stage group	Iron (mg/d)
Infants		Females	
0–6 mo	0.27[a]	9–13 y	8
7–12 mo	11	14–18 y	15
Children		19–50 y	18
1–3 y	7	51–>70 y	8
4–8 y	11	Pregnancy	
Males		14–50 y	27
9–13 y	8	Lactation	
14–18 y	11	14–18 y	10
19–>70 y	8	19–50 y	9

[a] Estimates based on adequate intake (AI). Other values are recommended dietary allowances (RDAs).
From Standing Committee on the Scientific Evaluation of Dietary Reference Intakes, Food and Nutrition Board, Institute of Medicine. *Dietary reference intakes for vitamin A, vitamin K, arsenic, boron, chromium, copper, iodine, iron, manganese, molybdenum, nickel, silicon, vanadium, and zinc.* Washington, DC: National Academy Press, 2001. Available online at *http://www.nap.edu/ books, Crawler list 0309072794.* Accessed May 30, 2001.

has priority for available iron. Milk is a poor source of iron, but the AI for infants 0 to 6 months of age is based on the daily amount in ingested milk ($\sim$ 0.35 mg/L). Because it is assumed that milk intake and requirements are correlated with body size, the AI may not be adequate for all infants, especially those with a lower intake. In the first 6 to 8 weeks of life, the hemoglobin level falls to 10 mg/dL because increased erythropoiesis is required for oxygen delivery to tissues. Extramedullary hematopoiesis also decreases in this period. During the second 6 to 8 weeks of life, erythropoiesis increases and the hemoglobin level rises to 12.5 mg/dL. In the third 6 to 8 weeks after birth, the dependency on dietary iron increases secondary to growth. The RDA for infants 7 to 12 months of age assumes that by 6 months, feedings complementary to milk are in place. It is at this time during infancy that extra iron is most needed, so that iron deficiency usually occurs at ages 6 to 24 months rather than earlier. Premature infants have decreased stores at birth and use their reserves faster during the growth spurt at 3 to 6 months of age. During adolescence, the hemoglobin level rises 0.5 to 1.0 mg/dL per year. For this reason, adolescents require 50 to 100 mg of iron per year, or a total of about 300 mg during adolescence.

2. **Food sources.** Dietary iron is available in a variety of nuts and seeds and in red meat and egg yolks. About 40% of the iron from these sources is heme iron, absorbed with about 15% to 45% efficiency. This accounts for 7% to 12% of dietary iron in the United States. Milk products, along with potatoes and fresh fruit, are poor in iron. Nonheme iron is absorbed with only about 1% to 15% efficiency. Vegetable iron content varies greatly according to the growing conditions of plants. Many sources of iron, especially inorganic salts and vegetable iron, are not well absorbed without ascorbic acid to reduce ferric to ferrous iron. However, continual ingestion of grams of vitamin C daily can interfere with copper absorption. The sources of nonheme iron often contain unidentified ascorbic acid (e.g., in meat, poultry, and fish) or inhibitors (e.g., tannic acid in tea; phytates in whole grains and legumes; polyphenols in tea, coffee, and red wine; calcium in dairy products or tofu; and zinc in multimineral preparations). In addition, the use of antacids, histamine$_2$ receptor antagonists, or proton pump inhibitors decreases gastric acid secretion and impairs the absorption of inorganic iron.

   a. **Food preparation** is important. Boiling can decrease the iron content of vegetables by 20%, and milling can decrease the iron content of grains by 70% to 80%. The iron content of some foods (e.g., grain products) is enhanced by fortification. Iron-fortified infant formulas and cereals have been widely used, usually with iron sulfate or gluconate. They should contain 4 to 12 mg of iron per liter to prevent deficiency. However, some of the iron salts used for fortification (ferric orthophosphate and pyrophosphate) are absorbed less well than other forms of nonheme iron in the diet. Vegetarians are at risk for iron deficiency because of limited iron availability.

   b. **Average intake** in the United States is 15 mg on a 2,500-kcal diet. The iron content of foods is fairly constant, about 6 mg/1,000 kcal. Heme iron is relatively well absorbed, and the absorption of heme iron is not affected by the composition of the diet. However, heme iron accounts for only 1 to 3 mg/d in the diet. Nonheme iron is less available, and its absorption is influenced by dietary components (e.g., ascorbic acid). Baked goods account for 20% of iron intake in the United States, which is usually added in the form of ferric orthophosphate or sodium acid sulfate salts. The U.S. Department of Agriculture Food Consumption Survey (1989–1991) showed that average diets meet or exceed the RDAs for all life stage groups, except 1- to 2-year-old children (91% of RDA) and women ages 12 to 49 years

(75% of RDA). It is not surprising that these two groups are most at risk for dietary iron deficiency.

Breast milk contains only 0.3 mg/L and cow's milk 0.5 mg/L. Thus, only about 0.25 to 0.85 mg of iron is supplied by milk. If this is the only food source for no more than 3 months, deficiency will not develop. About 50% of iron in breast milk is absorbed, compared with less than 10% of formula iron. Thus, breast milk can be an important source of iron even though the content is low. Iron is added to other infant foods. Electrolytic iron is added to dry cereal at 10 times the normal grain content (45 mg/100 g). This form of iron has a small particle size with a large surface area, but it is not clear how much is absorbed. During the first year of life, it is wise also to provide a meat source of iron to ensure good absorption. Iron deficiency can occur if the iron in enriched foods is poorly absorbed (fortified cereals) and can be avoided if the iron in iron-poor foods is well absorbed (breast milk, vegetables with ascorbic acid). Table 7-30 lists the iron content of selected foods.

   c. **Estimated iron absorption.** An average of 40% of total iron in animal tissues is heme iron; all the rest in the diet is nonheme iron. Thus, in any meal, one calculates the amount of iron from meat, poultry, or fish, multiplies that number by 0.4, and assumes 23% absorption for the heme iron. For the remainder of the iron, 8% absorption is assumed if adequate ascorbic acid (>75 mg per meal) is present. Otherwise, 5% absorption is assumed for an ascorbate intake of 25 to 75 mg, and 3% absorption if less ascorbic acid is ingested (66). On this basis, meals can be categorized according to whether the iron content is of low, medium, or high availability. A low-availability meal provides less than 30 g of meat, poultry, or fish and less than 25 mg of ascorbate. A medium-availability meal provides 30 to 90 g of meat or 25 to 75 mg of ascorbic acid with adequate nonheme iron. A high-availability meal provides more than 90 g of meat or more than 75 mg of ascorbic acid with adequate nonheme iron, or 30 to 90 g of meat plus 25 to 75 mg of ascorbate and nonheme iron.

   Estimates of the available iron in average diets change with age. From infancy to adulthood, dietary iron increases from 3 to 18 mg for males and to 11 mg for females. The available dietary iron is 50 µg/kg of body weight in infancy, 72 µg/kg of body weight in childhood, and 45 µg/kg of body weight in adolescence, falling to 39 µg/kg of body weight for adult men and 27 µg/kg of body weight for adult women.

3. **Assessment.** Because iron absorption is so inefficient and excretion is not regulated, none of the routinely available tests reflect intake but rather assess body stores. They are all used to determine whether iron deficiency or overload syndromes are present. However, the tests for iron deficiency can be especially difficult to interpret. The separation of iron deficiency from anemia of chronic disease is a troubling aspect of nutritional management. A major problem in diagnosis is that iron deficiency often develops slowly, so that the detection of deficiency depends on the stage of iron depletion (67). Thus, no single test is sufficient. In addition, the tests vary in sensitivity. Table 7-31 outlines the various tests available.

   a. **Hemoglobin.** About 60% to 65% of total body iron is in hemoglobin, 4.5% in myoglobin, 10% in nonheme enzymes, and about 30% in storage (ferritin, hemosiderin). Only a small amount (~ 0.15%) is in transport (transferrin) or in cytochromes and other heme enzymes (0.2%). Because the size of the iron pool is related largely to hemoglobin, the size of the total pool varies with body size (and blood volume) and sex, and males have more hemoglobin than females. Table 7-32 lists the

Table 7-30. Iron content of selected foods

Food	Portion	Iron content (mg)	Percentage of RDI (18 mg)
Breads and cereals			
White bread	1 slice	0.7	1–5
Hamburger bun	1 each	0.8	1–5
Saltines	4 each	0.5	1–5
Rice, cooked	1 cup	2.26	10–24
Oatmeal, cooked	1 cup	1.59	10–24
Bran flakes, 40%	½ cup	6.2	25–39
Spaghetti noodles, cooked (enriched)	1 cup	1.96	10–24
Meat and fish			
Beef, lamb, veal	3 oz	2.4–2.6	10–24
Beef liver	3 oz	5.34	25–39
Chicken, white meat roasted	3 oz	0.91	1–5
Fish, cooked	3 oz	0.5–1.0	1–5
Pork, ham	3 oz	0.6–0.8	1–5
Shrimp, boiled	3 oz	2.6	10–24
Sliced meats	1 piece	0.32–0.46	1–5
Vegetables			
Spinach, cooked fresh	1 cup	6.42	25–39
Green beans, frozen	1 cup	1.11	5–12
Peas, frozen	1 cup	2.5	10–24
Potato, baked	1 each	2.75	10–24
Tomato	1 each	0.5	1–5
Dried legumes	1 cup	4–5	10–24
Other vegetables	1 cup	0.8–1.2	5–12
Fruits			
Strawberries	1 cup	0.57	1–5
Apples	1 each	0.25	1–5
Bananas	1 each	0.35	1–5
Orange, small	1 each	0.14	1–5
Apricots, dried	16 halves	2.6	10–24
Dairy products			
Milk, whole	1 cup	0.12	1–5
Cheese	1 oz	0.3	1–5
Eggs, large	1 each	0.72	1–5
Nuts			
Peanuts, pecans, almonds	1 cup	3.3–5.0	25–39
Peanut butter	1 cup	4.3	25–39

RDI, recommended dietary intake.

median values and lower limits for hemoglobin and mean corpuscular volume. Other common causes of low levels of hemoglobin and a low mean corpuscular volume include anemia of chronic inflammation and heterozygous thalassemia trait. The red cell distribution width is usually high (>14.5%) in iron deficiency and tends to be normal in heterozygous thalassemia, but high values are also associated with other conditions, so that red cell distribution width is a poor diagnostic tool for iron deficiency. However, falling values are an early manifestation of a response to oral iron supplementation.
   b. **Serum iron and iron-binding capacity.** Analysis is based on the formation of a colored complex of ferrous iron and dye (20). Hemolysis

Table 7-31. Assessment of functional body iron status

Measurement	Diagnostic use	Reference range (adults)
Functional iron		
Hemoglobin	Assess severity of anemia	13–18 g/dL (M); 12–16 (F)
Red cell indices	Reduced when iron supply or incorporation into Hb is low	MCV 80–94 µm³; MCH 27–32 g/L
RBC zinc protoporphyrin	↑ Protoporphyrin and ↓ RBC ferritin indicate low iron supply to marrow	<70 µg/dL RBC
RBC ferritin	"	3–40 attograms/cell
Serum transferrin receptor	↑ in early iron deficiency; with measure of stores, identifies anemia of chronic disease	8–8.5 mg/L
Tissue iron supply		
Serum iron	Transit compartment, change rapidly	10–30 µmol/L
Serum transferrin	↑ in iron deficiency	47–70 µmol/L
Transferrin saturation	↓ in deficiency if transferrin is high, ↑ in iron overload	16–60%
Iron stores		
Serum ferritin	↓ in deficiency, low normal value is indeterminate in anemia of chronic disease	15–300 µg/L
Response to EPO	If storage iron cannot be used, anemia will respond	NA
Tissue iron	↓ in deficiency, normal in anemia of chronic disease	3–33 µmol/g of dry weight of liver

MCV, mean corpuscular volume; MCH, mean corpuscular hemoglobin; RBC, red blood cell; EPO, erythropoietin.
Modified from reference 68.

Table 7-32. Normal values for hemoglobin and mean corpuscular volume

	Hemoglobin (mg/dL)		MCV (µm³)	
Age (y)	Median	Lower limit	Median	Lower limit
0.5–1.9	12.5	11	77	70
2–4	12.5	11	79	73
5–7	13	11.5	81	75
8–11	13.5	12	83	76
12–14 (females)	13.5	12	85	78
12–14 (males)	14	12.5	84	77
15–17 (females)	14	12	86	79
Adults (females)	14.5	12	87	80
Adults (males)	15.5	14	88	80

interferes with the assay, as does EDTA, citrate, or gross lipemia (>1,000 mg/dL). Serum iron is largely bound to transferrin, a β-globulin with a molecular weight of 80 kDa. Two iron molecules are bound per mole of protein. At any time, 4 to 6 mg of transferrin-bound iron is present in plasma, and transferrin in plasma has the capacity to bind 25 to 30 mg. However, 25 mg of iron passes each day from the reticuloendothelial cells to the plasma, where it is turned over at a rate of 50% hourly. Therefore, the measurement of serum iron is inherently unstable. The daily coefficient of variation can be 30% in the same person. A diurnal variation is seen, with morning values about 30% higher than those in the evening. The value decreases before the menstrual cycle and is increased by the use of oral contraceptives because of progesterone. By the seventh month of pregnancy, the serum iron level reaches a nadir because of dilution and the mobilization of storage iron to the fetus.

(1) **Normal iron levels.** The normal serum iron level in newborns is 150 to 250 μg/dL. This falls in the first few days and then rises again to 130 μg/dL by 2 weeks. In the infant who is not given supplemental iron, the level falls to 80 μg/dL by 6 to 12 months and probably reflects iron deficiency. Normal adult levels range from 65 to 200 μg/dL, with values in men slightly higher than those in women. Mean values for males are 100 ± 35 μg/dL (mean ± SD); for females, they are 90 ± 40 μg/dL.

(2) **Variations in iron levels.** Low iron levels are associated with blood loss, chronic illness and infection, malignancy, and chronic skin disease. The serum iron level is high when outflow from the plasma is decreased, as in aplastic anemia, and when inflow into the plasma is increased, as in megaloblastic anemia with inefficient erythropoiesis. Lysis of cells (hemolytic anemia, acute hepatitis) raises the serum iron level. None of these causes is correlated with increases in body iron stores. In hemochromatosis, alcoholic liver disease, and porphyria cutanea tarda, the increase in body stores is reflected in an elevated serum iron level.

(3) **Normal transferrin levels.** Transferrin is made in the liver and has a half-life of 8 days in plasma. The coefficient of variation is only 8%, less than that for iron. Normal levels for males are 350 ± 50 μg/dL; for females, they are 380 ± 70 μg/dL. Each 500 mL of whole blood contains about 250 μg of iron not incorporated into hemoglobin; most of this is bound to transferrin.

(4) **Variations in transferrin levels.** In pregnancy, levels of transferrin can rise to 400 μg/dL because of the action of progesterone. In infants, the transferrin level is lower, 250 μg/dL (range, 180 to 320 μg/dL). Thus, in infancy, the serum iron level is higher but the transferrin level is lower than in the adult. Transferrin levels are increased during iron deficiency, also during pregnancy even in the absence of iron deficiency. Transferrin levels are decreased by chronic disease, protein deficiency, and hepatic impairment. The usual interpretation of iron, also transferrin levels is based on combined values and the percentage saturation noted, in addition to the individual values.

c. **Free erythrocyte protoporphyrin.** When iron is deficient, protoporphyrins cannot be utilized for heme synthesis and gradually increase during 2 to 3 weeks. They are usually, but not always, elevated (69). Free erythrocyte protoporphyrin levels are often elevated early in iron deficiency, often before anemia develops (>1.24 μmol/L of red blood cells). However, levels rise in most disorders associated with inefficient heme synthesis (e.g., anemia of chronic disease, sideroblastic anemias), so that these increases are nonspecific.

d. Ferritin. Ferritin is the major storage form of iron in the liver, spleen, and bone marrow. It also protects cells from high concentrations of free iron, which can be toxic. Each molecule has 24 subunits, at least two of which are immunologically distinct. Each ferritin complex, with a molecular weight of 450 kDa, has a capacity to bind 2,000 iron molecules or release them in the presence of reducing agents. The source of serum ferritin is unknown but is probably the reticuloendothelial cells. Normally, only very small amounts of apoferritin leak into the serum. The distribution of normal ferritin is skewed to the higher values. Males have larger stores of iron, a finding reflected in their serum ferritin levels. Serum levels reflect reticuloendothelial stores, a compartment that is increased in infection or chronic disease.

(1) **Serum ferritin levels** are proportional to marrow iron and inversely proportional to transferrin levels, which suggests that ferritin levels reflect iron stores. One microgram of ferritin is equivalent to about 8 mg of storage iron, or 120 µg/kg of body weight. Values rise after birth as the destruction of fetal hemoglobin increases stores. Ferritin levels fall later in childhood as adult hemoglobin is produced. Median concentrations of ferritin are about 40 and 170 ng/mL in young women and men, respectively. In anemic, iron-deficient patients, the mean level is less than 10 ng/mL (women) and 15 ng/mL (men).

(2) **Interpretation.** Iron deficiency and decreased stores are associated with levels below 15 ng/mL in adult men, and with levels below 10 ng/mL in women. However, these values are present only about half the time (Table 7-33). The value for diagnosis depends on the stage of iron deficiency, with values in later anemic states falling below 10 ng/mL. Iron overload in patients with hemochromatosis or undergoing transfusion is often associated with high ferritin levels. However, acute liver damage or endogenous ferritin production by tumors elevates ferritin levels without an increase in body iron stores. Cell damage in inflammatory diseases is also associated with falsely high ferritin values. When iron deficiency is combined with reticuloendothelial cell destruction in chronic inflammation, serum ferritin levels are normal and do not reflect true body stores.

(3) **Diagnostic usefulness.** Serum ferritin levels can be abnormal as soon as a lack of iron is detected in bone marrow, but a cutoff value of less than 15 ng/mL is not sufficiently sensitive (Table 7-33). The likelihood of iron deficiency in patients with

Table 7-33. Diagnostic use of the serum ferritin test

Serum ferritin (ng/mL)	Interpretation	Iron-deficiency anemia		Likelihood radio (present/absent)
		present (%)	absent (%)	
<15	Very positive	59	1.1	52
15–34	Moderately positive	22	4.5	4.8
35–64	Nondiagnostic	10	10	1.0
65–94	Moderately negative	3.7	9.5	0.39
>95	Very negative	0.9	75	0.08

Modified from reference 10.

values between 15 to 34 ng/mL is still nearly 5%, and iron deficiency can be present even with higher values. Patients with iron deficiency and ferritin values above 15 mmol/L may be at an early stage of deficiency, or they may have a chronic inflammatory condition that raises the level of serum ferritin, an acute-phase reactant protein. In such cases, values of serum ferritin about twice those in Table 7-33 may be of the same diagnostic significance. Because the "gray" area for serum ferritin is so large (between 15 and 100 mmol/L), it is logical to combine serum ferritin with other measures of the severity of disease. Several tests have been used, none with complete success. The most promising is the soluble plasma transferrin receptor.

   e. **Soluble plasma transferrin receptor (TfR).** The plasma protein is a truncated form of the membrane receptor that is present as a TfR–transferrin complex (71). The TfR number on the cell surface is a reflection of the iron status, increasing as deficiency develops. The log transformation of the ferritin value has been suggested as part of a ratio of TfR/log ferritin (TfR–F index) to normalize TfR values in patients with chronic inflammation (72). It remains to be seen whether this (or any related) measure is robust in repeated studies.

   f. **Direct methods for assessing iron stores.** Iron stores can be assessed directly by three means: phlebotomy, marrow staining, and liver biopsy.

   (1) **Phlebotomy.** If 500 mL is removed per week until the hemoglobin remains below 10 mg/dL for 2 weeks without further bleeding, it can be assumed that iron deficiency has been achieved. The red cell deficit can then be calculated from the hemoglobin content (each 1-g decrease of hemoglobin per deciliter corresponds to a total loss of about 100 mg of iron). Addition to the red cell deficit of 2 mg/d for absorbed iron gives an estimate of the mobilizable storage iron. Normal values in the United States range from 600 to 900 mg for males and from 200 to 300 mg for females. This method is used only when iron overload is present and treated by phlebotomy.

   (2) **Marrow staining** is a qualitative method that distinguishes low iron stores in iron deficiency from other conditions in which stores are normal. In such conditions, low serum measurements of iron deficiency can be caused by chronic disease or a decreased release of iron from the tissues. Marrow staining is not a reliable method for assessing iron overload in hemochromatosis, in which marrow iron is normal.

   (3) **Liver biopsy.** The normal hepatic iron concentration is 70 to 100 µg/g of dry liver weight. In adults, values in hemochromatosis are consistently in excess of 5 g. With values below 70 µg of iron per gram of liver, iron staining is scanty and stores are low.

   (4) **Response to therapy.** The response to therapy is sometimes the best diagnostic approach when iron deficiency occurs in chronic inflammation and test results are indeterminate. Interpretation of the response can be complicated in patients with intestinal disease because oral iron may be poorly absorbed. In some cases, it is appropriate to use IV iron (see below) or erythropoietin (68).

   The response to recombinant human erythropoietin has revealed a new phenotype of iron deficiency in such patients. Iron stores and serum ferritin levels are often normal or elevated, transferrin saturation is often (but not always) below 20%, and mean red cell indices are normal. Such patients may have adequate storage iron but cannot mobilize it rapidly enough to mount a sustained hemoglobin response. In these cases, IV iron may be needed to achieve a good response and reduce the amount of erythropoietin needed (73).

g. Summary of assessment. Iron deficiency is usually sought when anemia is present, although evidence for deficient stores can be found before anemia develops. Iron depletion is progressive, so that the test values diagnostic of deficiency may change during progression from depletion of iron stores without anemia to deficiency with anemia. The best screening test is the serum ferritin level because the only cause of a low value is a decrease in iron stores (74). Values below 15 ng/mL confirm iron deficiency in the presence of anemia, but values between 15 and 100 ng/mL also can indicate deficiency in patients with chronic inflammation. Determinations of serum iron and binding capacity are often ordered at the same time, and if the results are consistent, these help to confirm inadequate iron stores. When iron-binding capacity was elevated, 78% of patients were iron-deficient, but only 26% were deficient when a low transferrin saturation was the parameter used (75). Low serum iron and low binding capacity are the best indicators of anemia associated with chronic inflammation. How to proceed when ferritin values are between 35 and 100 ng/mL is not certain. An elevated red cell distribution width may be helpful in monitoring response to therapy but does not discriminate very well in detecting iron deficiency (76). If confusion still exists, because of the many factors that affect the results of these assays, staining of a bone marrow aspirate can provide a direct measure of iron stores. Histologic staining for iron is only semiquantitative but is good enough to distinguish iron deficiency from disorders of iron metabolism in which tissue iron is normal. Sometimes the iron status is not clear, even after all tests are completed, and the response to therapy must be used.

h. Screening for iron deficiency and overload. The tests available now for iron deficiency can also be used to screen for hereditary hemochromatosis (77). In addition, genotyping can be performed to detect the typical C282Y mutation of the hemochromatosis gene, *HFE*. Table 7-34 summarizes the strategies available for screening populations for iron-related disorders.

4. Physiology. Iron is involved in many reactions: as a redox cofactor for nonheme enzymes (iron–sulfur protein and metalloflavoproteins), as a required cofactor for nonoxidative enzymes (aconitase, ribonucleotide reductase), as a component of heme enzymes involved in electron transport (cytochromes), and as a major constituent of heme as an oxygen-carrying cofactor (hemoglobin, myoglobin). Iron is absorbed differently depending on whether it is ingested as heme (1.5 to 3 mg/d) or in vegetables and nuts (15 to 20 mg/d). The inorganic or nonheme iron is affected by gastric pH and by other salts in the lumen. Heme iron is not affected by luminal factors and is absorbed intact, bound to a putative "heme receptor" on the brush border or intercalated directly into the membrane. Inside the mucosal cell, hydrolysis of heme by heme oxygenase, a microsomal enzyme, liberates free iron. Iron absorption by this route is very efficient (20% to 40%), depending on the state of total body iron stores. When anemia is present, absorption rates are higher. Iron either enters the body or is deposited as ferritin in the mucosal cell. The signal for iron absorption is probably not mucosal ferritin itself, which is increased when the rate of absorption is low. Mucosal ferritin may provide a mechanism of iron excretion into the lumen when the cell is exfoliated.

a. Absorption and body stores. When the size of the iron body pool is decreased, iron absorption increases (78). As much as 5 mg of iron (20% to 30% of intake) can be absorbed each day. When stores are normal (~ 4 to 5 g in adults), absorption varies from 1 mg in males to

Table 7-34. Screening strategies for iron deficiency and hemochromatosis

Parameter	Phenotypic	Phenotypic/ genotypic	Genotypic/ phenotypic
Iron deficiency			
Tests	Tfr or UIBC		
Genetic hemochromatosis			
Initial test	Tfr or UIBC	Tfr or UIBC	C282Y mutation
Secondary test	Fasting Tfr, ferritin	C282Y mutation	Ferritin
Liver biopsy needed	Yes	No	No
Detects all genetic hemochromatosis	No	No	Yes
Detects non-iron overloaded hemochromatosis I	No	No	Yes

Tfr, transferrin; UIBC, unbound iron-binding capacity.
From Adams PC. Population screening for hemochromatosis. *Hepatology* 1999;29:1324.

2 to 3 mg in premenopausal females and matches daily iron losses. Iron overload occurs because excretory capacity is limited. In hemochromatosis, iron absorption is paradoxically elevated. Alcoholics may absorb excess iron from iron complexes in alcoholic beverages and by both paracellular and normal mechanisms.

   b. **Factors affecting absorption.** Iron is absorbed most efficiently in the upper small intestine, especially the duodenum. Gastric acid, hydrogen ions from a reducing agent such as ascorbic acid, or a brush border ferrireductase is needed to reduce nonheme ferric ions to the ferrous form, which is much better absorbed (79). Organic acids (citric, lactic) and amino acids (histidine, lysine, cysteine) form chelates with iron that enhance absorption. Disease or bypass of the proximal small bowel decreases absorption of both heme and nonheme iron. The presence of phytates in grains and of phosphates decreases nonheme iron absorption (80). Inorganic zinc can inhibit the uptake of iron. Humans are unique among mammals in the relatively small amount of dietary iron that is available for absorption and the limited loss of iron from the body.

   The major transmembrane iron transporter is natural resistance-associated macrophage protein 2 (nramp2), now called *divalent metal ion transporter 1* (DMT1) (79). DMT1 is related to nramp1, which is involved in host resistance to intracellular pathogen. DMT1 is expressed mostly in the duodenum, especially the crypts. Expression is markedly increased in diet-induced iron deficiency, which suggests that it is regulated by iron status. An inverse relationship has been found between DMT1 and serum ferritin in normal persons, but not in patients with hereditary hemochromatosis (81).

   c. **Iron loss.** Although the term *iron stores* usually refers to those tissues that contain ferritin and hemosiderin (e.g., liver, spleen), most of the iron in the body is in tissues that require it for function (red blood cells, marrow, muscle). It is also from these functional tissues that iron is lost. Iron can be lost through bleeding because red blood cells contain most of the iron of the body (2,750 mg in 70-kg males and 2,180 mg in females). Bone marrow and muscle contain 610 and 520 mg, respectively, in the two sexes.

d. **Red blood cell production.** Only 20 mg (or 0.5% of a total store of 4 g) is needed for new red cell production each day. This iron comes from the marrow. Only about 5 mg of iron is mobilized per day from storage tissues (liver, spleen), and such mobilization does not provide a rapid buffering for when acute iron loss occurs bleeding (about 250 mg of hemoglobin iron per 500 mL of blood) (82).

e. **Transcellular iron transport.** The mechanism by which iron is released from transferrin involves receptor-mediated endocytosis (79) and release in acidic vesicles when iron–transferrin complexes are involved. Once inside the red cell, ferrous iron is incorporated into the protoporphyrin of hemoglobin by a ferrochelatase. When the red cell dies after about 120 days, the iron in hemoglobin is oxidized and methemoglobin is formed. The iron is reused for hemoglobin synthesis or stored as the ferric ion. High intracellular iron levels down-regulate ferritin synthesis via an iron-responsive element-binding protein (90 kd) that depresses translation (83).

f. **Oxidation of absorbed iron.** The ferroxidase reaction converts ferrous to ferric ion. This conversion is catalyzed by ceruloplasmin and other ferroxidases. When the reaction occurs in serum, the ferric ion is incorporated into transferrin. Another ferroxidase that is different from ceruloplasmin is also found in serum. The conversion of absorbed ferrous to functional ferric ions occurs in tissues and is enzymatically controlled. Iron is brought from storage forms as ferritin in the ferric (Fe_{+++}) form. The release of iron from ferritin occurs via a ferritin reductase system.

5. **Deficiency.** Iron deficiency is characterized mainly by symptoms of anemia—that is, weakness and pallor. In addition, other signs and symptoms are caused by iron deficiency alone: angular stomatitis, atrophic lingual papillae, and koilonychia. Iron deficiency in children is associated with anorexia, decreased resistance to infection, decreased growth, and reversible protein-losing enteropathy. In the absence of anemia in children, iron deficiency can have deleterious effects on behavior and cognitive functions (84). The tests used to diagnose iron deficiency vary according to the stage of the deficiency. Table 7-35 outlines the predictive value of such tests.

Table 7-35. Predictive values of laboratory tests in different stages of iron deficiency

	Stage of iron deficiency[a]			
Test	I	II (predictive value, %)	III	IV
Bone marrow iron stain	100	100	100	100
Serum ferritin (μg/L)	100	100	100	100
Zinc protoporphyrin (μmol/mol of heme)	0	100	100	100
Transferrin saturation (%)	0	71	78	96
Hemoglobin (g/L)	0	0	100	100
MCV (μm$_3$)	0	0	22	100
MCH (pg)	0	0	33	100

[a] The prevalence rates of patients presenting in each stage of deficiency are about 24%, 23%, 15%, and 38%, respectively, for stages I through IV.
Modified from Hastka J, Lassere J-J, Schwarzbeck A, et al. Laboratory tests of iron status: correlation or common sense? *Clin Chem* 1996;42:5.

   a. **Increased utilization.** Iron deficiency is common in children 6 to 24 months old because of increased need and limited body stores.
   b. **Blood loss.** In premenopausal women, anemia is caused by blood loss during menstruation. Iron deficiency in an adult or adolescent male or a postmenopausal woman frequently signifies blood loss from the body, usually from the gastrointestinal tract. Each unit of blood contains approximately 250 mg of elemental iron.
   c. **Inadequate intake.** Iron deficiency is often associated with ingestion of foods in which iron bioavailability is low. It is also associated with other vitamin and mineral deficiencies, most notably with folic acid deficiency in pregnancy and intestinal disease and with zinc deficiency in children that produces anemia, dwarfism, and hypogonadism (85).
   d. **Malabsorption.** Another significant cause of iron deficiency is malabsorption, either in mucosal disease or after bypass of the proximal bowel, as in subtotal gastrectomy with gastrojejunostomy.
   e. **Restless leg syndrome.** Iron deficiency can occur with or without anemia, especially in elderly patients with this syndrome (86). However, in a small, randomized, controlled, double-blind trial of patients, regardless of iron status, iron did not prove to be an effective empiric therapy (87).
6. **Treatment**
   a. **Oral iron** is available in a wide variety of preparations as the only nutrient (Table 7-36) or in combination with other vitamins. The dose of iron given is not crucial provided that it is adequate because the amount absorbed is not linearly related to the dose ingested. In fact, above doses of 10 mg of elemental iron, the increase in milligrams of iron absorbed is rather limited. However, even at high doses of ingested elemental iron (100 mg), 10% can be absorbed by the anemic patient. The ferrous salt is absorbed about three times better than the ferric salt, and all ferrous salts are absorbed equally well. The side effects of iron preparations (nausea, indigestion, diarrhea, abdominal cramping) limit the amount that can be given. The oral route is preferred in virtually all situations, despite the frequency with which side effects occur. Gastrointestinal side effects may be less common with slow-release forms of oral preparations, but the response varies greatly. Some preparations contain tartrazine, which may cause allergic reactions in susceptible patients. Iron absorption may be decreased by antacids, coffee, tea, eggs, or milk. Iron interferes with the absorption of penicillamine and tetracyclines.
      (1) **Length of treatment.** Oral iron preparations should be used for 1 to 3 months until the hemoglobin level is restored to normal and then given for 1 to 3 months longer to allow tissue stores to be replenished. Hemoglobin contains only about 60% of body iron. Thus, it is usually necessary to treat during this second period for nearly as much time as is required to restore hemoglobin levels to normal. Because iron is absorbed better when body stores are low, it is absorbed best during the first month of treatment. Absorption during the second period, when tissue stores are being repleted, is less efficient. The iron deficit can be determined roughly by calculating the amount of iron necessary to replace red blood cell hemoglobin, with 1,000 mg added for an average-sized male adult to replete stores:

$$\text{Iron Deficit (mg)} = \text{Body Weight (lb)} \times [15 - \text{Hemoglobin (g/dL)}] + 1{,}000$$

One can use 13 g/dL as the figure for females. If one assumes an overall absorption rate of 10%, the total elemental iron needed can be estimated by multiplying the iron deficit by 10.

Table 7-36. Selected iron-containing prescription products for oral use[a]

Trade name	Nutrient					
	Fe sulfate (mg)	Fe fumarate (mg)	Fe gluconate (mg)	Fe polysaccharide (mg)	Vitamin C (mg)	Other
Feosol	200 (65)[b]	—	—	—	—	—
Ferancee HP	—	330 (110)	—	—	350	—
Fergon	—	—	435 (50)	—	±200[c]	—
Fer-In-Sol	190 (60)[d]	—	—	—	—	—
Fermalox	200	—	—	—	—	Maalox 200
Fero-Gradumet	525 (105)	—	—	—	±500[c]	—
Ferrofolic	525 (105)	—	—	—	500	Folate 0.8 µg
Ferro-Sequels	—	150 (50)	—	—	—	100 mg of dioctyl Na sulfosuccinate
Hytinic	—	—	—	(150)	—	—
Mol-Iron	390 (78)	—	—	—	±150[c]	—
Niferex-150	—	—	—	(150)	—	—
Niferex + C	—	—	—	(50)	269	—

[a] The content in milligrams is given as the iron salt, with the elemental iron content in parentheses. The percentage of elemental iron provided in salts is ferrous sulfate, 20%; ferrous gluconate, ~12%; ferrous fumarate, 33%. Many of these preparations are available in OTC forms, at doses about half those available by prescription.
[b] Available as elixir, 44 mg of iron per teaspoon.
[c] Preparations available with or without vitamin C.
[d] Available as liquid, 15 mg iron per 0.6-mL drops or 18 mg/tsp of syrup.

The daily tolerated dose, once determined, allows the required duration of therapy to be estimated.

(2) **Dosage.** Oral iron causes nausea and epigastric distress, constipation or diarrhea, and darkened stools. It is taken on an empty stomach unless gastrointestinal side effects occur. In that case, it is usually given after meals two or three times a day. Side effects often dictate the dose that can be tolerated orally. Preparations coated with a wax matrix are available (e.g., Slow FE, which contains 50 mg of Fe per 160-mg tablet) and may be better tolerated. Children should be given iron in a dose of 3 mg/kg per day. Complex vitamin and iron preparations should not be used for symptomatic iron deficiency because other additives can decrease iron availability (88).

(3) **Frequency of dosing.** The concept of intermittent oral iron supplementation is based on the concept of a "mucosal block" of iron absorption (89). The theory suggests that enterocytes down-regulate iron absorption in response to daily exposure to high doses, possibly as a result of increased mucosal ferritin synthesis. Little experimental support for this theory has been found (90). However, despite the lack of supporting evidence, some studies show a similar hemoglobin response to once- or twice-weekly iron dosing in comparison with daily provision (89). The groups studied included children up to age 8, pregnant women, and adolescent girls. No evidence has been found that intermittent dosing is preferred in iron deficiency associated with other clinical presentations.

(4) **Choice of oral iron preparation.** Most products contain ample *iron* to treat iron deficiency, provided that absorption is reasonably normal (Table 7-36). During iron deficiency, net absorption is increased to about 15% to 20% of the ingested dose. Ascorbic acid is included in many preparations, but it is not certain that it enhances absorption to a clinically significant degree. In determining the dose of iron to be given, one should think of the total content of elemental iron, not iron salt. Because the amount of each salt in the tablets varies between manufacturers, one should calculate the elemental iron based on the percentage of iron in each individual salt (Table 7-37).

b. **Parenteral iron**

(1) **Indications.** When bleeding is recurrent and the rate of loss exceeds the capacity to absorb iron, when malabsorption is the cause of deficiency, or when oral iron cannot be tolerated, parenteral iron may be needed. Iron supplements are not included in standard parenteral nutrition therapy but can be safely given when iron deficiency is present (91). Parenteral iron is often given to dialysis patients with or without erythropoietin to prevent iron deficiency, treat iron deficiency, or enhance the response to erythropoietin when iron has been repleted (92). Suggested guidelines for initiating such therapy in dialysis

Table 7-37. Elemental iron content of therapeutic iron preparations

Iron salt	Approximate percentage as elemental iron
Sulfate anhydrous	30
Sulfate, 7·H_2O hydrated	20
Fumarate	33
Gluconate	11.6

patients include a serum ferritin level below 100 μg/L, a transferrin saturation below 20%, and the presence of more than 10% hypochromic red cells. A combination of IV iron and erythropoietin has also been used in chronic inflammatory conditions, such as Crohn's disease. Most patients with Crohn's disease respond to IV iron alone, but erythropoietin can enhance the response (93).

(2) **Preparation and dosage.** Parenteral iron can be given in the form of iron dextran, a complex of ferric hydroxide [$Fe(OH)_3$] and dextran in normal saline solution containing 50 mg iron per milliliter. The complex is dissociated by the reticuloendothelial system and the iron transferred to transferrin. A normal reticuloendothelial system is needed for iron dextran to be useful. The total iron (in milligrams) needed to restore hemoglobin and replace stores is given by the following formula:

$$0.3 \times \text{Body weight (lb)} \times \left(100 - \left[\frac{\text{patient's Hb(g/dl)} \times 100}{14.8} \right] \right)$$

To calculate the dose in milliliters, divide the result by 50. This formula is applicable only for patients with chronic iron-deficiency anemia, not for those who require iron replacement after blood loss. When the patient weighs less than 30 lb, use 80% of the required dose to adjust for a normal hemoglobin value of 12 g/dL in that age group.

(3) **IM route.** First inject a test dose of 0.5 mL IM. Although anaphylactic reactions usually occur within a few minutes, a waiting period of 1 hour is recommended before the treating dose is administered. Each day's dose should not exceed 0.5 mL (25 mg) for infants weighing less than 10 lb, 1 mL (50 mg) for children less than 20 lb, and 2 mL (100 mg) for all others. Injection should be only into the upper outer quadrant of the buttock, placed deeply with a 2- or 3-in needle. If the patient is standing, inject into buttock that is not bearing weight. If the patient is in bed, inject the uppermost buttock. To avoid leakage into subcutaneous tissues, a Z-track method, in which the skin is displaced laterally before injection, is recommended. IM injections can produce brown discoloration at the injection site, sterile abscesses, lymphadenopathy, and local soreness.

(4) **IV route.** The IV route of administration is preferred for parenteral iron because it is better tolerated than repeated IM injections. The test dose (0.5 mL) is given IV, and a delay of 1 hour should elapse before treatment to avoid missing delayed reactions. IV injections of 2 mL or less can be given slowly (<1 mL/min), or the full dose can be diluted in 250 or 500 mL of normal saline solution and infused slowly over 2 to 3 hours. Iron can be provided in low-dose (up to 100 mg per infusion), medium-dose (100 to 400 mg per infusion), or high-dose (500 to 1,000 mg or up to full replacement per infusion) regimens. The total calculated dose of iron replacement can be given safely IV to patients with chronic illness (94) and to patients undergoing dialysis (95). Total dose replacement is more convenient, less expensive, and just as efficacious as divided doses, and it is safe when precautions and observation are adequate.

Anaphylaxis is extremely rare when iron dextran is given in this way. When it occurs, the reaction is usually within the first few minutes after administration and is characterized by respiratory difficulty and cardiovascular collapse. Therefore, iron dextran injections should be administered only to patients with clear indications of iron deficiency who cannot take oral iron. The incidence of all acute hypersensitivity reactions other than anaphylaxis has been estimated to be 0.2% to 0.3%. Such reactions include dyspnea, urticaria, itching, arthralgias, myalgias, and fever. Local phlebitis, vascular flush with too rapid infusion, and hypotension can occur after IV injection. Because of these risks, all patients should be closely supervised. IV iron should be given cautiously to persons with a history of asthma or significant allergy. Epinephrine (0.5 mL of a 1:1,000 solution) should be available for acute hypersensitivity reactions. All iron preparations can induce reactions to what is thought to be "free iron" if the circulating plasma transferrin saturation is exceeded. When more than 2 mL is given IV at one time, patients can experience fever, malaise, arthralgias, headache, nausea, shivering, and flushing, reminiscent of a serum sickness-like illness. Despite concerns about iron overload in patients with chronic diseases who require repeated injections of iron, no evidence of this has been found provided iron is used in conjunction with erythropoietin (92).

  c. Response to iron therapy. Reticulocytosis may be mild initially and usually peaks at 5 to 10 days after the start of therapy. The reticulocyte count or red cell distribution width need be checked only if there is concern about obtaining a response, and then only until it is ascertained that an adequate response has occurred. The reticulocyte count should be corrected for the degree of anemia:

$$\text{Corrected Reticulocyte Count} = \text{Measured Reticulocyte Count} \times \text{Hct}/40$$

    The hemoglobin level usually rises gradually over 1 to 2 months. Failure to respond suggests inadequate intake or absorption of iron, an incorrect diagnosis, or the simultaneous development or detection of folate or vitamin B_{12} deficiency.

7. Toxicity. *Iron overload syndromes* are seen when iron absorption exceeds excretion. This can occur when large doses are ingested or when massive transfusions are administered in diseases of red cell destruction in which iron is not lost in excess from the body. Acute ingestion of less than 20 mg of iron is generally nontoxic to adults. Ingestion of 20 to 50 mg/kg produces gastrointestinal symptoms such as nausea, vomiting, diarrhea, and abdominal pain. The UL is set at 45 mg/d (66). Doses above 60 mg/kg are potentially lethal. Shock, intestinal perforation, oliguria, coagulopathy, acidosis, and lethargy may occur. A serum iron level below 350 µg/dL is not associated with toxicity. Levels above 700 µg/dL are often (50%) associated with toxicity. Chronic overload also develops when iron absorption is excessive but intake is not. This situation arises in genetic hemochromatosis, cirrhosis of the liver, and porphyria cutanea tarda. Tissue damage to the liver, pancreas, heart, joints, and endocrine glands may occur.

  a. Diagnosis of iron overload is best suggested by a high ferritin level and an elevated transferrin saturation and confirmed by liver biopsy.

  b. Phlebotomy (500 mL/mo) can remove 250 mg of iron at a time and reverse some of the tissue damage, especially to the heart and liver. This is the treatment of choice for hemochromatosis. Secondary iron overload after multiple transfusions (as in thalassemia) can be prevented by the use of desferoxamine, best administered subcutaneously by a pump capable of providing a continuous mini-infusion. The range of doses is 20 to 40 mg/kg per day. Adverse effects include local pain and itching, allergic reactions, blurred vision, diarrhea, and tachycardia. For acute symptomatic iron intoxication (serum Fe >350 µg/dL), desferoxamine should be administered IV at a dose of 10 to 15 mg/kg of body weight.

B. Zinc

1. **Requirement.** The body contains between 1.5 and 2.5 g of zinc, so that it is the second most abundant "trace" mineral in the body, after iron. Turnover of body zinc measured by radioisotope studies is about 6 mg/d in adults. Balance studies show that 12.5 mg of dietary zinc is needed per day to maintain a positive balance. Daily loss is estimated at 2.5 mg, mostly in feces. Absorption averages 30% to 40% but has been estimated at 20% for diets containing the highest amounts of fiber. The Standing Committee on the Scientific Evaluation of Dietary Reference Intakes has set the RDAs at 9 and 13 mg/d for adult women and men, respectively. The RDAs for various age groups are outlined in Table 7-38.

   a. **Pregnancy.** The additional amount of zinc needed for fetal development is estimated to be 0.53 to 0.73 mg/d for the last half of gestation. Because zinc is important for the fetus, a liberal allowance of 3 mg of additional zinc is recommended during pregnancy, with the assumption that many diets do not contain much zinc.

   b. **Lactation.** Zinc loss in milk is about 1.2 mg/d and 0.6 mg/d for the first and second 6 months of lactation, respectively (highest in the first month at 2.1 mg/d); the additional recommendation of 4 mg/d during lactation assumes a 20% availability and absorption.

   c. **Infants and children.** Zinc requirements may vary with dietary availability. Assuming that a Western-type diet is ingested with 35% to 40% availability, infants should need 5 mg/d, whereas children ages 1 to 10 years need 10 mg. These amounts may not be enough if a large amount of unrefined cereals containing phytates is ingested or if zinc is lost in sweat or in the intestinal tract.

2. **Food sources.** The average zinc content of diets ingested by adults in the United States has been reported to range from 10 to 15 mg/d or from 6 to 12 mg/d. Whichever figures are correct, the amount of zinc ingested is probably adequate to provide the RDA because clinical zinc deficiency is not common in the United States when the losses of zinc are not excessive.

   a. **Zinc content of food** varies with the content of the soil in which the food is grown and with the content of the fertilizer used. In general,

Table 7-38. Dietary reference intakes of zinc

Life stage group	Zinc (mg/d)	Life stage group	Zinc (mg/d)
Infants		Females	
0–6 mo	2[a]	14–18 y	9
7–12 mo	3	19–>70 y	8
Children		Pregnancy	
1–3 y	3	14–18 y	13
4–8 y	5	19–50 y	11
9–13 y	8	Lactation	
Males		14–18 y	14
14–>70 y	11	19–50 y	12

[a] Estimate based on adequate intake (AI). All others based on recommended dietary allowances (RDAs).

From Standing Committee on the Scientific Evaluation of Dietary Reference Intakes, Food and Nutrition Board, Institute of Medicine. *Dietary reference intakes for vitamin A, vitamin K, arsenic, boron, chromium, copper, iodine, iron, manganese, molybdenum, nickel, silicon, vanadium, and zinc.* Washington, DC: National Academy Press, 2001. Available on line at *http://www.nap.edu/books, Crawler list 0309072794.* Accessed May 30, 2001.

the available zinc is proportional to protein intake because muscle meats and seafood have the highest content and vegetable sources contain zinc-binding anions. In addition, zinc is lost during the process of milling cereals. Breast milk is low in zinc. The risk for zinc deficiency is greater in patients ingesting a lacto-ovo vegetarian diet, but this can be countered by increasing the ingestion of whole grains and legumes (96). An increased rate of growth has been documented in children given modest zinc supplementation in double-blinded, controlled conditions, which suggests a preexisting growth-limiting state of zinc deficiency (97). These findings led to zinc fortification of cow's milk formulas in the mid-1970s. Table 7-39 lists the zinc content of selected foods.

b. Zinc content of diets. The NHANES III was the first study to estimate total nutrient intake, including that in beverages and dietary supplements. Estimates from this survey showed mean intakes of zinc of 5.5 mg in infants and up to about 13 mg in adults, with higher values in male adolescents and adults and values 2.5 to 3.5 mg higher in adults than the mean dietary intake (98). This difference represented supplements taken by 20% of the adult population. Slightly more than half of the population was ingesting more than 77% of the RDA. Those most at risk for inadequate zinc intakes were

Table 7-39. Zinc content of selected foods

Food	Portion	Zinc content (mg)	Percentage of RDI (15 mg)
Grains			
Bread, white	1 piece	0.173	1–5
Bread, rye	1 piece	0.38	1–5
Spaghetti noodles, cooked	1 cup	0.742	1–5
Meat and fish			
Beef, lamb	3 oz	4–6	25–39
Chicken, breast, roasted	1 each	1.05	5–12
Chicken, thigh	1 each	1.75	10–24
Turkey, dark meat	3 oz	3.80	25–39
Turkey, light meat	3 oz	1.73	10–24
Liver, beef	3 oz	4.2	25–39
Clams	1 each	0.5	1–5
Fish	3 oz	0.41–0.53	1–5
Oysters, eastern	1 cup	226	100
Oysters, Pacific	1 cup	41	100
Vegetables			
Vegetables, cooked	1 cup	0.45–0.6	1–5
Peas, green, cooked from fresh	1 cup	1.9	10–24
Fruits, fresh	1 each	0.05–0.09	1
Nuts	1 cup	4.1–4.8	25–39
Dairy products			
Milk, whole	1 cup	0.93	5–12
Yogurt, low-fat, plain	1 cup	2.02	10–24
Cheese	1 oz	0.7–0.93	5–12
Eggs	1 each	0.55	1–5
Beverages			
Cola	1.5 cup	0.28	1–5
Orange juice	1 cup	0.128	1–5

RDI, recommended dietary intake.

children ages 1 to 3 years, female adolescents ages 12 to 19 years, and elderly persons more than 71 years old. A general hospital diet provides 13 to 14 mg of zinc daily. However, a low-protein diet (40 g) contains only 6 to 7 mg. Full liquid diets are marginal in zinc content (8 to 9 mg), and clear liquid diets are quite inadequate (0.3 to 0.4 mg). Vegetarian diets may be limited in bioavailable zinc (99).

3. **Assessment.** None of the available methods reliably and accurately reflects intake and absorption or body stores. Daily losses can be estimated from fecal zinc, but this determination is not routinely available. The plasma zinc determination is the best screening test, but many factors can alter the level that are not associated with a change in body stores. Thus, it is a poor measure of marginal zinc deficiency (100). If zinc deficiency is suspected clinically, it is best diagnosed by a symptomatic response to zinc replacement.

   a. **Plasma.** Changes in plasma zinc do not occur until tissue zinc has been reduced. Thus, plasma zinc is a measure of the exchangeable zinc pool, from which an initial loss of zinc produces deficiency (100). Because plasma zinc can decline after a meal, fasting samples should be used. Most of plasma zinc is bound either tightly to α_2-macroglobulins (30% to 40%) or loosely to albumin. In red cells, 60% of the zinc is in hemoglobin and 20% in the enzyme carbonic anhydrase. About 80% of zinc in blood is in red cells—whole blood contains 8.8 μg/mL and plasma contains 0.7 to 1.4 μg/mL (20). Therefore, minor degrees of hemolysis alter plasma zinc levels. Hypoproteinemia and hyperproteinemia, whether caused by chronic illness or inflammation, stress, or altered protein nutrition, affect plasma zinc levels. Drugs (e.g., glucocorticoids, epinephrine) may alter zinc binding to plasma proteins. Although normal plasma levels (115 ± 12 μg/dL) do not rule out deficiency, low levels (<70 μg/dL) indicate deficiency when unaccompanied by hypoproteinemia, acute stress, or the ingestion of drugs that affect zinc levels. Levels below 50 μg/mL are associated with an increased risk for the development of symptoms, and patients with levels below 30 μg/mL nearly always manifest some aspect of the zinc deficiency syndrome. Neutrophil zinc is theoretically a better assessment of body stores, but because it has not been used frequently, it is not known how much better than plasma zinc it is (20). Normal values are 108 ± 11 μg/1,000 neutrophils. Alkaline phosphatase is a zinc-requiring enzyme, and its activity correlates with plasma zinc levels before and after zinc treatment (101). Low levels can corroborate zinc deficiency.

   b. **Zinc tolerance test.** This test has been used in uremic patients (102). Zinc (25 mg) or zinc sulfate (110 mg) is given in 30 mL of water, and plasma samples are taken hourly for 4 hours. A normal response is a doubling of plasma zinc with a peak at 3 hours. However, the test result is quite variable among subjects in the same group. Its role at present seems limited.

   c. **Urine.** Zinc excretion in urine is relatively low and fixed (i.e., it does not respond to changes in zinc stores). Moreover, it can be affected by altered protein binding in plasma. The major change in obligatory zinc loss in response to varying dietary loads occurs by altering endogenous fecal, not urinary, losses (103). Endogenous fecal excretion is about 1 to 2 mg/d when zinc intake is 5 mg/d. Urine is easily contaminated in some instances with stool; the concentration in stool is higher than that in urine, which ranges from 0.3 to 0.6 mg/d. Thus, urinary zinc levels are not helpful in determining zinc status.

   d. **Hair and nails** contain 90 to 280 parts per million and may reflect zinc intake. Levels of less than 70 parts per million have been associated with poor growth and appetite in children. However, much individual variation is seen because the levels are affected by rate of hair growth and external contamination. Bleaching and cold waving decrease zinc content. Before it is collected, the hair must be washed with water, a nonionic detergent, and EDTA to remove all the easily extractable zinc. It is not clear whether some of the zinc loosely bound to hair is endogenous and should be considered in the total content of the hair. Because collections must be taken with such care, determinations of zinc levels in hair remain a research procedure despite their potential to reflect intake.

  e. **Plasma metallothionein.** Metallothionein is a zinc/copper-binding tissue protein that is reduced in zinc deficiency. Plasma metallothionein levels correlate with hepatic stores, which in turn decline in deficiency. Thus, it has been suggested that low plasma zinc and metallothionein levels denote deficiency. Because metallothionein is an acute-phase reactant, a low plasma zinc level and elevated metallothionein level would suggest a false-positive result for zinc deficiency (104). Metallothionein has also been measured in red blood cells, and low levels were found in red blood cells in a small number of patients on a low-zinc diet while their plasma zinc levels were still normal (103). Thus, red blood cell metallothionein may respond to a labile functional zinc pool. If so, it may prove useful in detecting early zinc deficiency.

4. **Physiology.** Most of the 1.4 to 2.3 g of zinc in the body is bound to zinc-containing enzymes. These include carbonic anhydrase, carboxypeptidases A and B, alcohol dehydrogenase, glutamate dehydrogenase, malate dehydrogenase, glyceraldehyde-3-phosphate dehydrogenase, alkaline phosphatase, RNA and DNA polymerase, and reverse transcriptase. Zinc is required for both catalytic and structural functions. Zinc may activate or inhibit enzymes, modify membrane function, and bind to transcription factors (zinc fingers). In addition, studies of experimental zinc deficiency in animals reveal that zinc regulates other proteins not known to require zinc for activity, including intestinal fatty acid binding protein, cholecystokinin, J chain of immunoglobulins, and ubiquinone oxidoreductases (105). It is easy to imagine how zinc deficiency could lead to alterations in the growth and function of cells.

  a. **Absorption.** About 20% to 30% of ingested zinc is absorbed, particularly in the proximal bowel. Both carrier-mediated and nonsaturable diffusion components have been reported, the former being more active when zinc intake is low. Mucosal metallothionein increases in response to a high intake of zinc (106), but this effect appears to be secondary, perhaps to buffer intracellular zinc. Copper binds to metallothionein more avidly than zinc does. Thus, when zinc is used to treat Wilson's disease, the presumed mechanism involves induction of metallothionein with decreased transfer of copper to the body (107). A series of zinc transporters have been isolated that are thought to function in zinc absorption. ZT-1 is expressed on the basolateral membrane in the intestine and other tissues. Expression is highest in duodenum and jejunum, and in villous rather than crypt cells (108).

Like the absorption of calcium and magnesium, the absorption of zinc is decreased by phosphate and nonphosphate binders in the lumen (109). Calcium availability affects the zinc–phytate relationship because calcium forms a complex in foods such as cereals, corn, and rice. Inositol hexaphosphates and pentaphosphates are the most inhibitory compounds. Release of zinc from the complex can be affected by trace metals (especially copper) and by amino acids. Moreover, the biopotency of phytate is affected by food processing. Thus, the availability of zinc from cereals cannot be predicted (110). Zinc absorption is decreased by a high intake of calcium, phosphate, or both. Zinc oxide, carbonate, and sulfate salts are equally well absorbed by animals, but comparable data are not available in humans. When inorganic zinc is ingested (as sulfate), its absorption is decreased by inorganic iron in the lumen, especially if taken as a separate supplement (111). If either zinc or iron is present as the organic form (food zinc or heme iron), such competition does not occur. Thus, the absorption of zinc from liquid formulas or mineral supplements may depend on the luminal content of iron (or even calcium and phosphate). Cadmium, increasingly found in foods, also inhibits absorption.

Zinc absorption is promoted by animal proteins and by low-molecular-weight organic compounds, such as sulfur-containing amino acids and hydroxy acids (112). Physiologic states that increase the demand for absorbed zinc, such as infancy, pregnancy, and lactation, may affect zinc absorption.

b. Binding. In plasma, zinc is tightly bound to α_2-macroglobin and transferrin. About 60% of plasma zinc is loosely bound to albumin. In the liver, zinc is bound in part to the metal-binding protein metallothionein. It is not clear if this represents a storage form of zinc separate from the functional enzymes, which contain most of the zinc in the body.

c. Excretion. The regulation of excretion is less well understood than control of absorption. The major route of excretion is in the feces (2 to 3 mg/d). About 7.5 to 14 mg of zinc from body stores (1.5 to 2.0g/70-kg person) is secreted daily into the upper intestine. This amount is equal to ingested sources. During passage through the small intestine, an amount equivalent to endogenous loss is usually reabsorbed, but the margin of safety is small. The amount of zinc secreted with each meal is variable, and efficient absorption is required to maintain a normal zinc balance (109). The major normal source of endogenous fecal zinc may be pancreatic juice. Diarrheal fluid may contain more than 11 mg of zinc per liter. Thus, the severity of diarrhea is a good indication of the risk for zinc depletion in patients with gastrointestinal diseases. Urinary excretion is not altered by changes in oral intake, whereas fecal zinc increases in proportion to intake. Another route of excretion is sweat, which has an average concentration of 1.15 mg/L. Thus, during profuse sweating, up to 4 mg can be lost daily. During menses, about 0.4 to 0.5 mg of zinc is lost with the blood. Seminal emissions contain an average of 0.6 mg of zinc per ejaculum. Urinary losses average 0.5 mg/d but are unregulated. Urinary losses can be increased in nephrosis, sickle cell disease, and cirrhosis, and after therapy with penicillamine. Daily loss in normal persons has been estimated at 2.2 to 2.8 mg.

d. Immune function. Zinc deficiency causes a rapid decline in antibody-and cell-mediated immune responses in both humans and animals (113). These defects contribute to the lymphopenia seen in patients with sickle cell anemia, HIV infection, acrodermatitis enteropathica, and chronic renal and gastrointestinal diseases. T cells and B cells are lost from the bone marrow. Because zinc deficiency often accompanies protein–calorie malnutrition, the cause of these defects may be multifactorial. Even in the healthy elderly person with low serum levels of zinc, Th-1 cytokine production by leukocytes may be diminished (114).

5. Deficiency. Zinc deficiency in humans is clearly associated with certain clinical syndromes and has been implicated in others (115).

a. Definite or likely syndromes. As a result of the documentation of these syndromes, the clinical manifestations of zinc deficiency are now better defined (Table 7-40). The symptoms are often nonspecific, but in the appropriate clinical setting, zinc deficiency can be suspected.

(1) Acrodermatitis enteropathica is a hereditary disorder that begins in early childhood. It is characterized by pustular and eczematous lesions on the skin and by diarrhea. Oral, anal,

Table 7-40. Clinical manifestations of zinc deficiency

Degree of deficiency	Cause	Manifestations
Moderate	Diet, alcohol, malabsorption, chronic renal disease, sickle cell disease	Growth retardation, hypogonadism (males), skin rashes, poor appetite, lethargy, taste abnormalities, abnormal dark adaptation
Severe	Acrodermatitis enteropathica, TPN, alcoholism, penicillamine therapy, malabsorption or severe diarrhea	Bullous pustular dermatitis, alopecia, weight loss, neurosensory and psychiatric symptoms, depressed immune function, impaired reproduction

TPN, total parenteral nutrition.
Modified from Prasad AS. Zinc deficiency in women, infants, and children. *J Am Coll Nutr* 1996; 15:113.

and genital ulcers also occur. Irritability and cerebellar ataxia may be present.

(2) Growth retardation, anorexia, lethargy, and hypogonadism have been reported, especially in young males in Iran and Egypt, where available dietary zinc is low.

(3) Acute zinc deficiency has been reported after weeks of total parenteral nutrition, penicillamine therapy, or severe alcoholism. The findings include a rash on the face and limbs; the rash can be pustular, vesicular, bullous, seborrheic, or acneiform. Moist, indolent skin ulcers, when associated with serum zinc levels below 1.0 μg/mL, have been reported to heal with zinc therapy.

(4) Alopecia, confusion, apathy, depression, and loss of taste are associated with zinc deficiency in uremia.

(5) Symptoms suggestive of zinc deficiency can be found in patients with gastrointestinal diseases who have documented or suspected increased fecal losses. Diarrheal disease in infants leads to low serum levels of zinc (116). The rapid transit exacerbates the zinc malabsorption that occurs in diseases of the intestine. These diseases include malabsorption syndromes, inflammatory bowel disease, and other secretory diarrheas. Endogenous losses of up to 20 mg/d have been documented. Malabsorption can lead to a loss of more than 90% of dietary zinc because of decreased transport of zinc across the mucosa and malabsorption of zinc binders, which accumulate in the lumen.

(6) Zinc deficiency associated with protein losses occurs in patients with protein-losing enteropathy and nephrotic syndrome, burns, or trauma. Twenty percent of the total body zinc resides in the skin, so that a severe burn is especially likely to cause zinc deficiency.

(7) Requirements for zinc are increased in periods of growth and during pregnancy, so that any superimposed increased losses accelerate the development of zinc deficiency.

(8) Patients with cirrhosis excrete excess zinc in their urine; testicular dysfunction, anorexia, lethargy, and night blindness responsive to zinc may develop.

(9) Sickle cell anemia leads to urinary losses of zinc. Attributed to zinc deficiency are delayed puberty, hypogonadism, small

stature, anorexia, decreased body hair, chronic leg ulcers, and hypogeusia.

(10) The gonadal function (potency, libido, sperm count) of patients on hemodialysis has been reported to improve after the administration of oral zinc at a dosage of 50 mg/d (115).

   b. **Candidate syndromes**

   (1) Poor wound healing is said by some authors to respond to zinc sulfate replacement. However, others note no change.

   (2) Zinc deficiency can be associated with a diminished response of insulin to glucose, but it is not clear whether zinc plays a role in normal glucose homeostasis or in diabetes.

   (3) Altered taste (dysgeusia) or smell as an isolated finding in nonuremic patients has been said to respond to oral zinc. Other possible causes of an abnormal sense of taste include iron deficiency, candidiasis, psychiatric disorders, and medications (117). The single double-blinded study of the effect of zinc supplements on taste and smell dysfunction did not support a role for zinc (118).

   (4) Acute or persistent diarrhea in children less than 5 years old is prolonged by low weight for age and by decreased cell-mediated immunity, both associated with zinc deficiency in developing countries (119).

6. **Treatment.** Zinc is available as a component of many multivitamin and mineral preparations. It can better be provided as an individual oral supplement in the form of zinc sulfate or gluconate. The 67-mg zinc sulfate tablet provides 15 mg of elemental zinc, equivalent to the RDA, or roughly the amount contained per kilogram of stool. When estimated needs are greater, the patient can be given the 220-mg tablet, which contains 50 mg of elemental zinc. Treatment should continue until the symptoms prompting the use of zinc resolve. Then a maintenance dose (67 mg of zinc sulfate) can be given daily. Zinc sulfate (1 or 5 mg/mL) or zinc chloride (1 mg/mL) is available for IV administration but must be diluted first in saline solution.

   It is difficult to choose a dose for zinc treatment. Zinc is widely available in a Western-type diet. Therefore, if zinc is given in certain disorders (e.g., malabsorption) to prevent the development of deficiency, it is not possible to determine whether the treatment is beneficial. It seems better to reserve treatment for those syndromes that respond to zinc therapy, and for conditions in which zinc has been shown to be beneficial.

   a. **Wilson's disease.** In addition to a diet low in copper, 25 mg of zinc can be given every 4 hours from 7 a.m. to 7 p.m. and 50 mg at 11 p.m., or 50 mg can be given three times a day to decrease copper absorption.

   b. **Macular degeneration.** Preliminary studies have suggested that diets rich in zinc may protect against this condition, although the degree of protection was small (23). Zinc supplements cannot be recommended at this time.

   c. **Decreased dietary intake.** Supplements are indicated when the estimated intake is less than the RDA. However, long-term use of large doses (100 to 300 mg/d) can lead to copper deficiency and elevated levels of cholesterol (23). The results of studies of the effects of zinc supplements on calcium absorption and vice versa have been mixed.

   d. **Diarrhea in children less than 5 years old.** An analysis of seven randomized studies from developing nations showed that mortality was reduced by 15% (acute diarrhea) and by 24% to 42% (continuing or persistent diarrhea) after the addition of 20 mg of elemental zinc, or 3 to 5 mg/kg (119). The greatest effects were seen in male infants less than 1 year old with persistent diarrhea and evidence of wasting or zinc deficiency. It is not clear whether zinc alone or with vitamin A is best, nor whether zinc supplementation will be useful in more developed countries where clinical zinc deficiency is much less common.

e. Conditions in which zinc supplementation is of unproven value. Trials of zinc supplementation for upper respiratory infection continue to provide contradictory results. A metaanalysis of randomized, controlled, double-blinded trials of rhinovirus infection showed no statistical benefit (120). Another review concluded that zinc gluconate lozenges are useful, but that it is important to begin therapy within 48 hours and to have the patient suck the lozenges every 2 hours while awake (121). It further suggested that compounds in the lozenge, such as citric acid or sorbitol, can bind free zinc, so that effectiveness varies. Using the delivery conditions outlined above, a prospective trial administered 12.8 mg of zinc acetate and showed a 40% reduction in the duration of cold symptoms (122). Zinc supplementation had no definite effect in small numbers of trials to modify exercise performance, acne vulgaris, male fertility, or immune function in the elderly (23).

f. Prevention of illness by zinc supplementation. The incidence, prevalence, duration, and severity of diarrhea and pneumonia can be reduced by zinc supplementation of children in the developing world (123). Although the data are not certain, it is likely that intake of bioavailable zinc is low in these populations. Zinc supplementation has also been reported to relieve the diarrhea of acrodermatitis enteropathica, decrease the prevalence of malaria, and improve the neuropsychiatric performance of children at risk for zinc deficiency (124).

7. **Toxicity.** Zinc is relatively nontoxic. Because the zinc content of most foods is low, dietary excess is unlikely. Ingestion of more than 150 mg/d can interfere with copper or iron metabolism, but only if intake of these other ions is limited (125). Impaired immune function and an adverse effect on the ratio of low-density-lipoprotein to high-density-lipoprotein cholesterol have also been reported. All these effects have been reported less frequently with doses between 15 and 100 mg/d. However, the UL for adults is 40 mg/d, based on a reduction in erythrocyte copper/zinc superoxide dismutase activity (66). Very high doses (450 mg/d) have induced copper deficiency with sideroblastic anemia (124). Large acute overdoses (>200 mg) can produce nausea, vomiting, rash, dehydration, and gastric ulceration. Tetracycline absorption may be impaired by zinc.

B. Copper

1. **Requirement.** Copper is a trace element that is essential for humans and many other animals. Estimates of copper requirements are based on balance studies of fecal and other losses and copper absorption for various age groups (66,126). Obligatory losses in adults are about 580 µg/d, and absorption averages about 25%. Intake must be in excess of 35 µg/kg per day to avoid a negative balance. This amounts to between 1.0 and 1.5 mg/d in children and between 1.5 and 2.0 mg in adults. To allow a margin of safety, a daily copper intake of 1.5 to 3 mg is recommended for adults. For children, a daily safe and adequate intake of 0.05 to 0.10 mg/kg is suggested (1). Premature infants are born with low copper reserves and may require more copper. Milk provides about 120 µg of copper per day. Infant formulas may contain copper in a poorly available form (e.g., bound to insoluble anions), and the copper requirement may be higher (~ 0.1 mg/ kg of body weight daily) when these mixtures are used. Copper dietary intakes are listed in Table 7-41.

2. **Food sources.** The richest sources of copper, as of zinc, are crustaceans and shellfish (especially oysters and crabs), and also organ meats (127). The next richest sources are nuts and legumes, dried fruits, and cocoa. Poor sources include dairy products, sugar, and honey. Surveys show that most adults in the United States consume 1 mg of copper or less per

Table 7-41. Dietary reference intakes of copper

Life stage group	Copper (µg/d)	Life stage group	Copper (µg/d)
Infants		Adults (M/F)	
0–6 mo	200[a]	9–13 y	700
7–12 mo	220[a]	14–18 y	890
Children		19–>70 y	900
1–3 y	340	Pregnancy-all ages	1,000
4–8 y	440	Lactation-all ages	1,300

[a] Estimates based on adequate intake (AI). Other values are recommended daily allowances (RDAs).
From Standing Committee on the Scientific Evaluation of Dietary Reference Intakes, Food and Nutrition Board, Institute of Medicine. *Dietary reference intakes for vitamin A, vitamin K, arsenic, boron, chromium, copper, iodine, iron, manganese, molybdenum, nickel, silicon, vanadium, and zinc.* Washington, DC: National Academy Press, 2001. Available online at *http://www.nap.edu/books, Crawler list 0309072794.* Accessed May 30, 2001.

day. A hospital diet may contain less than 1 mg of copper because it includes few copper-rich foods. Full liquid diets provide less than 0.5 mg and clear liquid diets less than 0.1 mg. Table 7-42 lists the copper content of some common foods.

3. Assessment

a. Plasma copper. Most of the copper in the body (80 mg) is in tissues. Red blood cells contain 60% of blood copper as erythrocuprein, a copper and zinc protein that functions as a superoxide dismutase.

    (1) Correlation with intake. In plasma, copper is tightly bound to ceruloplasmin (molecular weight of 160 kDa), which binds 80% of the plasma copper at a ratio of seven copper molecules per molecule of protein. The rest of copper is bound to transcuprein and albumin. The amount of copper exchanged from ceruloplasmin is small compared with the amount absorbed. Therefore, the plasma copper level does not correlate with intake; it only roughly reflects body stores because the plasma compartment comprises such a small percentage of body stores and the turnover of copper within the compartment is slow. Nonetheless, the plasma copper level is a better initial indicator of copper status than is the tissue copper level when deficiency is suspected because tissue copper levels are more stable.

    (2) Normal plasma copper levels for males are 0.91 to 1.0 ± 0.12 µg/mL, and for females they are 1.07 to 1.23 ± 0.16 µg/mL. Oral contraceptives increase the range to 2.16 to 3.0 ± 0.7; this is largely an estrogenic effect. Levels peak in pregnancy at 38 weeks and return to normal within 2 weeks postpartum. Plasma total copper levels can increase in acute and chronic infections and decrease in nephrosis, Wilson's disease, kwashiorkor, or any condition that causes protein malnutrition. Free serum copper values are more instructive than total copper values because the latter are affected by factors that alter binding capacity. Bound copper is estimated to be three times ceruloplasmin levels (µg/dL) because each milligram of ceruloplasmin contains 3.3 µg of copper (128). Free (not bound to ceruloplasmin) copper equals total serum copper minus bound copper. Values below 25 µg/dL are considered within normal range. This calculation is designed to detect elevated levels of free copper, as in Wilson's disease, rather than to detect copper deficiency.

Table 7-42. Copper content of foods

High (>0.2 mg per portion)	Moderate (0.1–0.2 mg per portion)	Low (0.1 mg per portion)
Meat and meat substitutes		
Liver and other organ meats, shellfish, variety meats, lamb, pork, duck, tofu, nuts	Dark meat of chicken, fresh fish, turkey	Beef, veal, bologna, beef frankfurters, eggs
Dairy products		
	Dried skim milk powder, sharp cheeses	Butter, margarine, milk, ice cream, most cheeses, cheese spreads
Vegetables		
Lentils, mushrooms, dried beans, pimientos, french fried potatoes, canned tomatoes	Spinach, sweet potato, squash, beets, asparagus, peas (fresh and canned), baked potato	Green beans, broccoli, cabbage, carrots, cauliflower, corn, brussels sprouts, cucumber, lettuce, green pepper, turnip
Bread and cereal		
Wheat germ and bran, English muffins, bran flakes	Whole wheat bread, pasta, sugar or vanilla wafers	White bread, white rice
Miscellaneous		
Curry powder, nuts, chocolate, molasses, cocoa, Ovaltine, licorice, soup mixes, syrup, canned soup	Pickles, ginger, black pepper, frozen pizza, popcorn, potato chips, pretzels, soda	Hard candy, Jell-O, honey, jelly, white sugar, lemonade, catsup, mayonnaise

From Pennington JT, Calloway DH. Copper content of foods. *J Am Diet Assoc* 1973;63:143.

    b. Ceruloplasmin is a protein that is made in the liver. It functions as a ferroxidase, converting ferrous to ferric ion, and thus affects the flow of iron from cell to plasma. With copper deficiency, ceruloplasmin levels fall, to about 30% in severe deficiency. Iron mobilization is decreased, and a hypochromic, microcytic anemia develops. When ceruloplasmin levels are low in Wilson's disease, other ferroxidases in plasma appear to be able to mobilize iron. Normal levels are 105 to 500 µg/dL. Estrogens increase the levels, and low levels are seen in patients with Wilson's disease (including 10% to 20% of heterozygotes), uremia, and nephrosis and in persons with a low protein intake. Other forms of chronic liver disease associated with a decreased synthesis of plasma protein can produce a low level. In Wilson's disease, ceruloplasmin levels are below 23 µg/dL (129). This value provides an adequate screening test, but false-normal levels may occur in a small percentage of patients. The free serum copper concentration is probably a better measure in Wilson's disease (130).

    c. Hair. A determination of copper in hair entails the same problems as do the determinations for zinc and other trace metals—individual sex- and age-related variations, exogenous contamination, and strict requirements for sample preparation. It cannot be routinely recommended to test body stores.

    d. Urinary copper. From 0.01 to 0.06 mg is excreted daily in the urine. This amount does not usually vary much according to changes in copper intake and reflects free tissue copper and plasma copper loosely bound to albumin. Thus, it does not reflect body stores. In Wilson's disease, free copper in tissues is increased, and urinary excretion can exceed 1.5 mg/d. However, this value is quite variable and can be within the normal range. Values below 50 μg/d, however, virtually exclude Wilson's disease.

4. **Physiology.** About one-third of body copper is in the liver, with large amounts in brain, heart, spleen, and kidneys. Newborns have three times the adult level in their liver, but this falls rapidly after birth and is probably related to immature excretory mechanisms. The newborn has ceruloplasmin in liver but low levels in plasma. Most copper is in the cytosol, bound to enzymes or other copper-binding proteins. The enzymes include cytochrome oxidase, superoxide dismutase, ceruloplasmin, tyrosinase, uricase, lysyl oxidase, and histaminase, among others (128,131). Copper is important for the enzymes mediating the absorption and release of iron from tissues and so is important in hemoglobin production. It is needed for the development and maintenance of blood vessels, tendons, and bones, functioning of the central nervous system, pigmentation of hair, and normal fertility.

   a. **Copper absorption and organ distribution.** Dietary copper is absorbed from the stomach and small intestine. A protein with a high affinity for copper, hCtr1, may transport copper into enterocytes (131). The Menkes' gene protein, MNK, is a membrane-associated P-type adenosine triphosphatase that is required for secretion of copper into the portal vein. Hephaestin is a multicopper oxidase that is deficient in mice with sex-linked anemia. It is a membrane-bound analogue of ceruloplasmin required for iron (but not copper) export from the intestine. In the plasma, copper binds to albumin and perhaps histidine, and is taken up by hCtr1 on the liver membrane. Ceruloplasmin is the major copper-containing protein in plasma and is synthesized in the liver by the Wilson's disease protein, WND. WND is highly homologous with MNK and is defective in patients with Wilson's disease (128).

   b. **Intracellular copper metabolism.** Once hCtr1 mediates copper uptake, a series of small cytoplasmic copper chaperones (e.g., hCOX17, HAH1, and CCS) distribute copper to various cellular compartments or mediate incorporation into proteins (131). In all tissues but liver, MNK transports copper into the Golgi apparatus for incorporation into secreted proteins. MNK then moves to the plasma membrane, where it may mediate copper efflux. In the liver, the protein that is deficient in Wilson's disease, WND, is present in the Golgi and presumably serves a similar function. No chaperone has been isolated for delivering copper to metallothionein.

   c. **Metallothionein,** a small protein (molecular weight of 6 kDa) with tightly bound zinc and copper, is found in many tissues. The high level in fetal liver may allow safe storage of increased liver copper. It may be the initial hepatocyte acceptor for albumin-bound copper from the plasma and may play a role in detoxification. Finally, it has been suggested as a mechanism to block enterocyte absorption of copper. Normally, about 80% of hepatic copper is bound to metallothionein, which is polymerized and insoluble. In Wilson's disease, only about half as much copper is in this form, so that free tissue copper levels rise.

   d. **Hepatic copper content in disease.** In many disorders, especially Wilson's disease, hepatic copper is increased—prolonged cholestasis, Indian childhood cirrhosis, copper poisoning, thalassemia, hemochromatosis, and biliary cirrhosis. However, more stainable copper is demonstrated in the liver in these illnesses than in Wilson's disease, and metallothionein levels may be normal. For this reason, these conditions may not be associated with the same degree of tissue toxicity, presumably secondary to free copper, as Wilson's disease.

    e. Excretion and absorption. Copper from the liver is mainly excreted into bile. This is the major excretory route for copper from the body, and the rate of excretion is 0.5 to 1.3 mg/d. The amount excreted usually balances that absorbed each day from the upper small intestine. Absorption is relatively inefficient (~ 30%), allowing biliary excretion to remove excess copper from the body. The form of inorganic copper affects absorption. The carbonate and nitrate forms are better absorbed than the sulfate, chloride, or oxide. Phytates and ascorbic acid decrease absorption. Copper complexed to amino acids may be better absorbed. Other metals (e.g., Ca, Cd, Zn, Fe, Pb, Ag, Mo) decrease absorption (110).

    f. Other functions. Copper deficiency leads to low serum levels and high tissue levels of iron. This function of copper is carried out by the multicopper ferroxidases, of which ceruloplasmin was the first reported. Ceruloplasmin knockout mice show a severe impairment of iron efflux from reticuloendothelial cells and hepatocytes (132). The multicopper oxidases may bind to iron transport proteins or may be involved primarily in iron export, as is hephaestin. Copper also is necessary to prevent lipid peroxidation, perhaps by playing a role in selenium metabolism. Both humoral and cell-mediated immunity is impaired by copper deficiency in animals.

5. Deficiency. Dietary deficiency is uncommon but may occur in premature infants or in malnourished patients repleted with low-copper diets. Table 7-43 lists the manifestations of copper deficiency in humans.

    a. Premature infants. When milk is the major food source, both copper and iron intakes are low. The copper content of the body increases markedly just before birth, so prematurity is associated with low body stores. Anemia secondary to either iron or copper deficiency can develop. Bone abnormalities have been reported.

    b. Malnutrition. When repletion is high in calories but low in copper content, neutropenia, anemia, diarrhea, and scurvy-like bone changes may occur that are all responsive to copper. Tissue copper levels are often but not always decreased. Osteoporosis has been reported in severe copper deficiency (134).

Table 7-43. Signs and symptoms associated with deficiency of trace metals

Mineral	Signs and symptoms	
	Infants and children	Adults
Cu	Anemia, neutropenia, osteopenia, vascular aneurysms, kinky hair, hypothermia, impaired CNS development	Anemia, neutropenia
Mn	None reported	Hypercholesterolemia, weight loss, change in hair color (one case reported)
Se	None reported	Glucose intolerance, peripheral neuropathy
Se	Cardiomyopathy, chondrodystrophy	Cardiomyopathy, myositis

CNS, central nervous system.
From reference 133.

        c. Menkes' kinky hair syndrome is an inherited disorder caused by a defect in copper absorption (135). The tissue content of copper is always low. Characteristic features are mental deterioration, hypothermia, defective keratinization of hair, metaphyseal lesions, degeneration of aortic elastin, and depigmentation of hair.

        d. Cardiovascular disease. The copper deficiency theory of ischemic heart disease was first proposed in the 1980s, suggested by sudden death in domestic animals with copper deficiency (e.g., "falling disease" of dairy cattle). The evidence is all indirect but nevertheless intriguing. Decreased activity of lysyl oxidase and superoxide dismutase may lead to a failure of collagen and elastin cross-linking (136). Copper deficiency can be associated with low levels of copper in cardiac muscle, increased levels of plasma cholesterol, and electrocardiographic abnormalities. Patients with ischemic heart disease have low cardiac and leukocyte copper concentrations. Short-term copper depletion experiments in humans have produced changes in lipid profiles, electrocardiographic changes, and impaired glucose tolerance (136). The data are not sufficient to recommend replacement therapy at present.

    6. Therapy. Because copper deficiency is uncommon, supplementation is unnecessary with most diets. Despite this fact, copper is included in many multivitamin and mineral preparations. Copper sulfate, the form usually available, contains 0.4 mg of elemental copper per milligram of the anhydrous salt. A daily addition of about 1.0 to 1.5 mg of copper adequately treats deficiency states. However, if oral treatment is used, three times this amount should be given, or about 3 mg of copper as copper sulfate, to allow for the 30% absorption efficiency.

    7. Toxicity

        a. Acute toxicity. The UL for adults is 10 mg/d based on protection from liver damage, which is the critical toxic effect (66). Ingestion of more than 15 mg of elemental copper causes nausea, vomiting, diarrhea, and abdominal cramps resulting from direct mucosal toxicity (137). At larger doses, hemolysis results from inhibition of glucose-6-phosphate dehydrogenase. Gastrointestinal bleeding, azotemia, and hematuria may occur. When ingestion is potentially fatal, jaundice with acute hepatic necrosis and renal tubular swelling are seen. The treatment for acute overdose usually involves gastric lavage. If the dose ingested is very high, penicillamine (1 g/d in adults) can be added to remove excess copper from the body.

        b. Chronic toxicity. In Wilson's disease, free tissue copper and total liver copper (>250 µg/g net weight of liver) are increased. Other diseases are associated with increases in hepatic copper (chronic active hepatitis, primary biliary cirrhosis) but tissue damage related to excess copper has not been seen to develop, perhaps because the level of free tissue copper is not increased. The initial treatment for Wilson's disease consists of a low-copper diet and chelating therapy (penicillamine or trientine). It may be important to combine the diet with chelation therapy initially to reduce the excess copper stores. Zinc supplements also may be helpful for maintenance therapy.

D. Iodine

    1. Requirement. Iodine is a nonmetallic halogen element required for the synthesis of thyroid hormone. About 1 µg of iodine is required per kilogram to prevent goiter in adults. The RDAs are currently based on balance studies (66). Studies of urinary excretion indicate that more than 50 µg is needed per gram of creatinine per day. Goitrogens in the diet (fluoride or rubidium) affect the requirement by decreasing thyroid uptake of iodine. To allow a margin of safety, the RDA for adolescents and adults is set at 150 µg/d. Because the iodine content of human milk is 30 to 100 µg/L, another 70 µg/d is needed during pregnancy, and an additional 70 µg/d (290 µg total) is needed during lactation. The AI for infants 0 to 6 months old is 110 µg/d; for infants 7 to 12 months old, it is 130 µg/d, and it is 90 µg/d for children ages 1 to 8 years. The RDA is 120 µg for children 9 to 13 years old and 150 µg/d for adolescents and children of both sexes 14 years of age or older. The RDA during pregnancy is 220 µg/d, and it is 290 µg/d during lactation.

2. **Food sources.** The iodine content of food and water is closely related to the iodine content of the soil. Areas where the iodine content is likely to be low include glaciated and mountainous regions and areas with heavy rainfall.

   a. **Specific foods.** Seafood is an excellent and consistent source of iodine. The iodine content of dairy products, eggs, and meat depends on the iodine content of the animal feed. The water content varies from 0.1 to 2 µg/L in goitrogenic areas to 2 to 15 µg/L in nongoitrogenic areas. Fruits and vegetables in general are low in iodine. Except for seafood, the source is more important than the type of food in determining iodine content. Shellfish or saltwater fish contain about 70 µg/4 oz. Eggs contain about 4 to 10 µg each, meats about 5 µg/oz, dairy products about 3 to 4 µg/oz, and fruits 1 µg/oz. Breads are low in iodine unless made by the continuous mix process, during which the dough absorbs atmospheric iodine. Some plants contain natural substances that interfere with iodine absorption. These include brussels sprouts and legumes.

   b. **Average iodine intake** in the United States is 250 and 170 µg/d for males and females, respectively. The usual supplement for dietary iodine in the United States is iodized table salt, which contains 76 µg of iodine per gram of salt. The use of 3.4 g of iodized salt per day on average adds 260 µg of iodine to the daily intake. In noncoastal regions, iodized salt should be used. In coastal regions, atmospheric iodine is much higher and provides an extra source of iodine.

3. **Assessment**

   a. The body contains 15 to 20 mg of iodine, 60% to 80% of which is in the thyroid gland. The concentration of inorganic iodine is low, and organic compounds are the usual circulating form (thyroxine, triiodothyronine, diiodotyrosine, and monoiodotyrosine). Measurement of these compounds in blood is a measure of thyroid function, and this measurement correlates with iodine stores in the absence of other thyroid disease. Thyroid-stimulating hormone is regulated by circulating thyroid hormone levels. Because radioimmunoassays and immunochemiluminometric assays for thyroid-stimulating hormone are stable and easily used, this measurement is preferred (20).

   b. **Blood levels.** The inorganic iodine concentration is only 0.08 to 0.6 µg/dL. About 3 mL of serum is required, and the assay depends on the catalytic effect on the reduction of ceric ion by arsenious acid. Thyroxine (T_4) is present at a level of 7 to 11 µg/dL. About 0.5% to 0.07% of this is not protein-bound. The level of free thyroxine therefore is 5.4 ± 1 ng/dL. Triiodothyronine (T_3) resin uptake is a measure of the protein-binding capacity for triiodothyronine and is not a determination of iodine content. Values of thyroid-stimulating hormone are 0.1 to 5.0 mU/L in euthyroid subjects (20).

4. **Physiology.** Food contains mostly inorganic iodide, which is reduced in the gut lumen and nearly completely absorbed. Some iodinated compounds (e.g., thyroid hormones, amiodarone) are absorbed intact. Iodide is handled like chloride and passes easily across membranes, unlike other trace minerals (except for fluoride). It is concentrated in the thyroid and salivary glands. It is secreted as inorganic iodine in saliva and milk but only as the organic form from the thyroid. The iodide pool is replenished from the diet, saliva, gastric juice, and the breakdown of organic thyroxine derivatives. The thyroid gland, kidneys, and salivary and gastric

glands all compete for free iodide. The thyroid must trap about 60 µg of iodide per day to maintain thyroxine levels. Iodide is concentrated by the sodium/iodide cotransporter, a member of the family of cotransporters that use electrochemical sodium gradients to drive coupled uphill transport of sugars, amino acids, vitamins, ions, and water. Iodide is also taken up by stomach, salivary glands, and mammary glands (138). The three pools of body iodide are the circulating inorganic, intrathyroid organic, and circulating organic pools. Iodide is excreted mostly in urine (>50 µg/d), with lesser losses in stool and sweat.

5. **Deficiency.** Iodine deficiency is one cause of hypothyroidism. This deficiency in childhood can result in delayed growth. At all ages, it causes decreases in cellular oxidation and the basal metabolic rate and thus weakness, fatigue, and slow mental responses (139). Depending on the degree of deficiency and age at onset, mental changes can vary from mild intellectual impairment to severe retardation. Iodine deficiency is the most common form of preventable brain damage in the world (140). Hypotension and bradycardia, constipation, pretibial edema, and slow deep tendon reflexes are all seen. Thyromegaly often accompanies dietary iodine deficiency. Because iodide is easily absorbed, malabsorption syndromes do not cause deficiency. Because thyroid hormone production is decreased, the gland becomes hypertrophic in an attempt to compensate, and a goiter develops.

6. **Treatment.** Iodine is a component of many multivitamin and mineral preparations. However, supplementation with 2 g of iodized salt per day provides the full RDA. In the United States, recent trends show a decline in iodine intake, especially among women of reproductive age (141). More than 90 countries currently iodize their salt products, at concentrations from 30 to 100 µg/g of salt. In countries without easily available iodized salt, other iodized vehicles are being tested as a source of supplemental iodine, such as irrigation water and oil. When radioactive iodine therapy is administered, it may be necessary to place patients with a high intake of iodine on a low-iodine diet for 1 to 2 weeks so that the uptake of the radioactive element will be sufficient.

7. **Toxicity**
   a. **Excessive dietary intake.** When intake exceeds 2,000 µg/d, iodide uptake by the thyroid gland is impaired and organic formation falls. These dietary levels can be reached by a large intake of iodine from iodized salt, vitamin and mineral preparations, or iodine-containing coloring dyes and dough conditioners. The margin of safety is great, and toxicity remains unusual at the present level of iodine supplementation. The UL for adults has been set at 1.1 mg/d based on serum thyroid-stimulating hormone concentrations during different levels of iodine intake (66).
   b. **Excessive therapeutic iodine.** Iodine-induced thyrotoxicosis may paradoxically result from excessive iodine therapy given to patients with multinodular goiter or quiescent Graves' disease. Commonly used iodine-containing medications include expectorants and antithyroid medications. The iodine content of these medications far exceeds the normal dietary allowance, as listed in Table 7-44.

      The side effects of potassium iodide include rash, swelling of salivary glands, a metallic taste in the mouth, stomach upset, allergic reactions, and headache. Iodinated glycerols are contraindicated in newborns and nursing mothers because of the possibility of producing hypothyroidism.

E. **Fluorine**
   1. **Requirement.** The protective effect of fluoride on teeth is observed at intakes from 1.5 to 2.5 mg in adolescents. These levels are consistent with the range of fluoride intake in the United States. Therefore, the total AI recommended from food and drinking water is 3 mg/d for adult

Table 7-44. Iodine content of medications

Drug	Iodine or iodide content per therapeutic dose
Glycerol, iodinated	15 mg iodine per tablet or 30 mg per teaspoon of elixir
Calcidrine syrup	152 mg calcium iodide per teaspoon
Potassium iodide syrup	300 mg potassium iodide per teaspoon
Potassium iodide	
Solution	1 g potassium iodide per milliliter
Tablet	320 mg per tablet
Lugol's solution	5% iodine in solution

women and 4 mg/d for men (25). Because fluoride is required for the growth of bone and enamel, these recommendations are based on the prevention of dental caries, not on total body requirements. For children and adolescents, the primary beneficiaries of the prevention of dental caries with fluoride, the AI is 0.7 mg for ages 1 to 3 years, 1.0 mg for ages 4 to 8 years, 2 mg for ages 9 to 13 years, and 3 mg for ages 14 to 18 years. To avoid the danger of mottling of the teeth of infants and children, the UL for infants ages 0 to 6 months is 0.7 mg, and it is 0.9 mg for ages 7 to 12 months. Comparable ULs for children are 1.3 mg for ages 1 to 3 years and 2.2 mg for ages 4 to 8 years. The UL for all others is 10 mg to avoid producing brittle bones.

2. **Food sources**
   a. **Type of food.** Like other anionic trace elements (I, Se), the source of the food (where it is grown) is more important than the type. One exception is ocean fish, each gram of which contains 5 to 10 μg of fluoride. Other foods contain less than 0.5 ppm. Tea is the other food naturally high in fluoride, containing 100 to 200 μg/g. The content of food can be decreased by cooking, during which water is lost, or increased by commercial processing, during which water is added. Cereals contain 1 to 3 μg/g of dry weight and are a major source of fluoride for infants. The availability of cereals for infants has raised the question of the need for water supplements (142). Daily intake in the United States averages about 0.4 mg from food; with water content added, boys average about 0.9 mg/d.
   b. **Water** is the other major source of fluoride. Surface water contains about 1 ppm or less; deep water contains 4 to 8 ppm. The fluoride intake in cities with fluoridated water supplies is from 1.7 to 3.4 mg/d, with a mean of 2.6 mg, exclusive of water ingestion. In nonfluoridated areas, fluoride intake from food averages 0.9 mg/d. The difference represents food preparation. Water intake accounts for 1 to 1.5 mg daily in fluoridated areas and 0.1 to 0.6 mg in nonfluoridated areas. Thus, intake varies from 1 to more than 4 mg/d. Because water supplies most dietary fluoride, either by itself or in foods, it is recommended that water supplies contain at least 1 mg/L, which ensures adequate fluoride intake to decrease the incidence of dental caries. Fluoride-containing dentifrice is ingested (~ 25%) by children less than 5 years old, who may ingest 0.3 mg fluoride per brushing. Thus, daily intake of young children brushing twice daily could be doubled.

3. **Assessment**
   a. **Body stores.** Because fluoride is required for the growth of bone and enamel, these recommendations are based on the prevention of dental caries, not total body requirement. Because most of the fluoride is in bone and enamel and not in extraosseous tissues, no practical method is available for assessing body stores. Bone content ranges from 300 to 600 ppm but is not usually measured.

      b. Urine levels are proportional to intake and average 0.5 to 0.6 ppm. Urine excretion reflects current ingestion or prior exposure to high levels. The efficient renal excretion mechanisms keep blood fluoride at a low narrow range independent of intake.

4. **Physiology.** Fluoride is concentrated in bones and teeth, where it is incorporated into the crystalline structure of hydroxyapatite. This results in increased resistance of the teeth to caries, especially in the preeruptive phase. Fluoride is completely absorbed (90% in the stomach) and is distributed like chloride in soft tissues. Uptake in bone depends on its growth and vascularity. Aluminum, iron, magnesium, and calcium salts can decrease the rate of absorption. About 80% of dietary fluoride is excreted in the urine each day.

5. **Deficiency.** Because fluoride is present in nearly all water supplies, plants, and animals, deficiency does not occur in humans. Fluoride is an essential element for growth in mice and rats but has not been implicated in growth failure in humans.

6. **Treatment.** For children living in a nonfluoridated area, the daily addition of the AI for the appropriate age is adequate to prevent caries. Treatment in adults may prevent further caries. Each 2.2 mg of sodium fluoride contains 1 mg of fluoride. Sodium fluoride is available in chewable tablets (1 mg), lozenges (1 mg), drops (0.125 mg per drop), and solution (0.2 mg/mL). Sodium fluoride has been used to treat osteoporosis (up to 60 mg of fluoride per day alternated in 6-month periods with calcium and vitamin D) in an attempt to stimulate the formation of new bone, which is then hardened by fluoride. No convincing evidence has been found that this treatment is beneficial in the prevention of osteoporosis.

7. **Toxicity.** Fluoride is toxic when ingested in excess.

      a. Mottled teeth have been found in children ingesting water containing more than 8 ppm. Mottling occurs only in permanent teeth and is usually not significant. Eczema, urticaria, gastric distress, and headache have been reported.

      b. Systemic fluorosis. With ingestion of 20 to 80 mg/d for years, a syndrome including osteosclerosis, genu valgum, kyphosis, and spine stiffness can occur. Systemic fluorosis has occurred in areas where a high fluoride intake is endemic (some parts of the Indian subcontinent and South Africa). The UL for adults has been set at 10 mg/d (24).

F. Manganese

1. **Requirement.** Manganese is a trace mineral essential to animals and probably humans. Many problems arise when balance methods are used to estimate trace minimal requirements, and no overt deficiency state exists in humans. Thus, data are insufficient to establish an estimated average requirements (EAR) for manganese, and all the DRIs are based on median AIs. The AI for infants ages 0 to 6 months is 3 µg/d based on total estimated intake from milk. The estimated AIs for other life groups are as follows: 0.6 mg (infants 7 to 12 months old); 1.2 mg (children ages 1 to 3 years); 1.5 mg (children ages 4 to 8 years); 1.9 mg, 2.2 mg, and 2.3 mg (females ages 9 to 13 years, 14 to 18 years, and 19 to 70 years, respectively); 1.6 mg, 1.6 mg, and 1.8 mg (males ages 9 to 13 years, 14 to 18 years, and 19 to >70 years, respectively); 2 mg for pregnancy; and 2.6 mg during lactation. Because the current dietary intake seems adequate, an estimated safe and adequate dietary intake has been set at those levels, 2 to 5 mg for adults (66). Safe intakes are recommended for children and adolescents as follows: 1 to 1.5 mg for ages 1 to 3 years, 1.5 to 2.0 mg for ages 4 to 6 years, and 2 to 3 mg for ages 7 to 10 years. Safe intakes for formula-fed and breast-fed infants are 0.005 mg/d and 0.30 mg/d, respectively (143).

2. **Food sources.** Nuts, dried fruit, cereals and unrefined grains, pineapple, pineapple juice, and tea are very rich in manganese (>1 mg per serving). Legumes, rice, spinach, sweet potatoes, pasta, and whole wheat

bread are good sources of manganese (>0.5 mg per serving). Vegetables and fruits contain only moderate amounts, and dairy products, muscle meats, and seafood contain only small concentrations of the mineral. The average daily intake for adults in the United States is 2.2 mg for women and 2.8 mg for men. Vegetarian diets or diets rich in whole grain products may provide as much as 8 to 10 mg/d. Hospital diets provide about 1 to 2 mg/d, and low-sodium and low-protein diets may supply less than 1 mg/d. Components of the diet can limit manganese absorption or increase excretion, including iron, phosphorus, calcium, copper, phytates, fiber, and polyphenols.

3. **Assessment.** As with other divalent cations, no measurement accurately assesses body stores. Like copper, manganese is excreted mainly in bile, not urine. Therefore, urine does not provide a good measure of recent intake. Red cells contain 13.6 to 16.9 μg/L, but serum/plasma contains only 0.59 to 1.3 μg/L (20). The usual assay is based on atomic absorption spectrometry, which measures total manganese. Radiochemical neutron activation analysis has also been used. Manganese is present in serum as the trivalent form, bound to β_2-globulin. Because this level does not change with altered intake and because deficiency in humans is not recognized, the usefulness of serum levels is small. Urine values vary little, are quite low, and are not useful in assessing manganese status. Hair content varies more among individuals and with such factors as exogenous contamination, color, and season than with manganese status.

4. **Physiology**
   a. **Function.** The body contains about 12 to 20 mg of manganese. The liver and pancreas have the highest content. A few metalloenzymes (superoxide dismutase, pyruvate carboxylase) and many metal–enzyme complexes (hydrolases, kinases, dicarboxylases, transferases) contain manganese.
   b. **Absorption** occurs in the small bowel but is very inefficient. Absorption efficiency is increased in animals when they are deficient. Like the absorption of other cationic metals, the absorption of manganese depends on its form; carbonate and silicate salts are poorly absorbed. Luminal calcium, phosphate, and iron decrease absorption. Excretion varies with bile output, which regulates body content. Manganese activates many enzymes but is an absolute requirement for only a few; thus, deficiency states are rare.

5. **Deficiency.** In animals, neonatal ataxia, retarded skeletal growth, decreased reproductive function, and defects in lipid metabolism are seen. In humans, one case has been reported with weight loss, hypocholesterolemia, dementia, nausea, vomiting, and altered hair color (144). Manganese deficiency was induced in 39 days in young men and caused a fleeting dermatitis (145). Some epileptics have been reported with low blood levels of manganese. Manganese deficiency has not been reported in humans consuming a natural diet, and supplements are not indicated for healthy subjects.

6. **Treatment.** Manganese is a component of some multivitamin and mineral supplements. Therapy for specific deficiency symptoms is indicated very rarely.

7. **Toxicity.** Manganese is relatively nontoxic when ingested, presumably because absorption is low. However, when inhaled as dust, it can produce psychiatric disorders and extrapyramidal signs. Manganese oxide is absorbed across the lungs and is a concern for miners. The UL, set at 11 mg/d, is based on no observable adverse effects on Western-type diets (66). Hypermanganesemia during treatment with total parenteral nutrition (usually 100 to 800 μg/d) can lead to increased signal density in the globus pallidus on magnetic resonance imaging (146). It can been seen in patients with cholestatic liver disease receiving total parenteral nutrition but is not a risk when only the liver disease is present (147). Patients

with cholestasis or neurologic symptoms or who are receiving prolonged total parenteral nutrition should be monitored for hypermanganesemia. If present, the infusion of manganese should be stopped or diminished.

G. Chromium

1. **Requirement.** Chromium is an essential trace mineral that potentiates the action of insulin in certain conditions. A safe intake of chromium would be based on the content of a varied diet that does not lead to deficiency, but deficiency is not readily identified in humans. Thus, the current dietary intake recommendations are based on the median intake of chromium at various ages (AI). The adequate daily intake ranges are listed in Table 7-45. The lower recommendations for younger ages are based on extrapolations of expected food intake. However, the World Health Organization has recommended lower intakes of 25 µg/d to prevent deficiency and 33 µg/d to maintain tissue stores (148) because earlier estimates were based on less accurate measurements of chromium.

2. **Food sources.** Chromium is widely distributed as chromite in the soil. Plants contain between 100 to 500 µg/kg and foods between 20 to 590 µg/kg (149). The form or availability of chromium in specific foods is generally not known. A balanced diet provides chromium with an average availability of 1% to 2%. Spices (>10 µg/g) and brewer's yeast (>40 µg/g) contain the highest concentrations. Meat products (1 to 2 µg/g), dairy products (1 to 1.5 µg/g), and eggs (1 to 2 µg/g) are good sources. Leafy vegetables contain chromium in a relatively unavailable form. Rice and sugar are poor sources. Estimates of daily intake are complicated by the availability of more soluble chromium compounds (picolinate, nicotinic acid) available over the counter in supplements at doses from 50 to 600 µg (23). The best diet to maximize chromium status is one low in simple sugars and rich in unprocessed foods.

3. **Assessment.** Measurement of chromium in tissues is difficult because of the very low levels. Serum levels (2.5 to 5.2 nmol/L) are ten times lower than tissue concentrations and are not in equilibrium with the body stores (20). Serum levels increase rapidly as insulin levels increase and decrease with infection. Urine excretion is 1 to 20 nmol/L, but it correlates poorly with intake because absorption is so poor. Graphite furnace atomic absorption spectrometry is the method most often used. Hair levels are better related to body stores but still are affected by ex-

Table 7-45. Dietary reference intakes of chromium

Life stage group	Chromium (µg/d)	Life stage group	Chromium (µg/d)
Infants		Females	
0–6 mo	0.029/kg	9–13 y	25
7–12 mo	0.611/kg	14–18 y	35
Children		19–50 y	35
1–3 y	11	51–>70 y	30
4–8 y	15	Pregnancy	
Males		14–18 y	29
9–13 y	21	19–50 y	30
14–18 y	24	Lactation	
19–50 y	25	14–18 y	44
51–>70 y	20	19–50	45

Estimates based on adequate intake (AI).
From Standing Committee on the Scientific Evaluation of Dietary Reference Intakes, Food and Nutrition Board, Institute of Medicine. *Dietary reference intakes for vitamin A, vitamin K, arsenic, boron, chromium, copper, iodine, iron, manganese, molybdenum, nickel, silicon, vanadium, and zinc.* Washington, DC: National Academy Press, 2001. Available online at *http://www.nap.edu/books, Crawler list 0309072794.* Accessed May 30, 2001.

ogenous contamination, individual variations, and the other problems that beset this assay in the case of other trace minerals. Normal chromium levels in hair are about 990 ppm at birth; they fall to about 440 ppm after 2 or 3 years of life. The best way to diagnose chromium deficiency is to observe whether symptoms or signs that appear during total parenteral nutrition (hyperglycemia, neuropathy) respond to chromium infusion (149).

4. **Physiology.** Chromium is poorly absorbed (~1% to 2%) regardless of the level of intake or body stores. Oxalates and vitamin C increase and phytates and antacids decrease absorption (150). The hexavalent ion is absorbed better than trivalent chromium. Chromium picolinate and organic complexes from brewer's yeast or with nicotinic acid are absorbed better than the chloride salt. Excretion occurs mainly in the urine. A glucose load or insulin injection increases excretion, especially in diabetics. Trivalent chromium is required for normal glucose metabolism in animals, probably acting as a cofactor for insulin. A low-molecular-weight chromium-binding substance (LMWCr) has been identified as an oligopeptide that binds four chromium ions and activates the insulin receptor (149,151).

5. **Deficiency.** Deficiency has been noted after prolonged total parenteral nutrition (see Chapter 10). Glucose intolerance and impaired release of free fatty acids have been noted, along with increased circulating levels of insulin, neuropathy, encephalopathy, and hypercholesterolemia and hypertriglyceridemia (152). Deficiency is hard to document because no good method is available to assess body stores.

6. **Treatment.** IV administration of 5 to 10 µg of chromium chloride daily for the first few days, followed by 10 µg weekly, is probably adequate therapy. Chromium has been marketed as a weight loss aid and a muscle builder, and as an aid in glucose assimilation. However, no studies have shown a definite benefit in controlling diabetes or blood lipids, increasing lean body mass or decreasing body fat, improving muscle mass in athletes, or improving osteoporosis (23).

7. **Toxicity.** The hexavalent salt is more toxic than the trivalent salt in animals and has been associated with the production of lung tumors. No well-recognized toxic syndrome in humans has been reported. Thus, a UL has not been set (66). Randomized, controlled trials of 175 to 1,000 µg of chromium per day given from 6 to 64 weeks have shown no toxic effects (149). The Environmental Protection Agency has assigned a safety factor of 1,000 to chromium because of no observed adverse effect. This translates to a safe upper limit of 1.47 mg/kg per day. Isolated adverse effects have been reported, but their significance is not clear. Renal failure has been associated with chromium picolinate in two cases (149). Headaches, sleep disturbances, and mood swings have been reported (23).

H. Selenium

1. **Requirement.** Selenium is an essential trace mineral that is a component of the enzyme glutathione peroxidase. Safe selenium requirements for adult Chinese men to prevent deficiency (Keshan disease) have been estimated at 40 µg/d, and two small supplementation studies suggested 70 and 55 µg/d as the intake required to achieve plateau concentrations of plasma glutathione peroxidase (153). To adjust for differences in weight and individual variation, the DRI for adults has been set at 55 µg/d, between the highest and lowest estimates (Table 7-46). Because selenium can be toxic, the ULs have been set not too far above the DRIs. The UL of 400 µg/d for adults is close to the reference dose of 5 µg/kg per day set by the Environmental Protection Agency.

2. **Food sources.** Selenium is present in foods as selenomethionine or selenocysteine. Plant content varies with the soil content. The development of deficiency syndromes in livestock in European countries led to

Table 7-46. Selenium dietary reference intakes and tolerable upper intake levels

Life stage group	DRI	UL	Life stage group	DRI	UL
	µg/d			µg/d	
Infants			Males, Females		
0–6 mos	15[a]	45	9–13 y	40	280
7–12 mos	20[a]	60	14–>70 y	55	400
Children			Pregnancy		
1–3 y	20	90	≤18–50 y	60	400
4–8 y	30	150	Lactation		
			≤18–50 y	70	400

[a] Estimated on adequate intake. All other DRI values represent recommended dietary allowances (RDAs).
From Standing Committee on the Scientific Evaluation of Dietary Reference Intakes, Food and Nutrition Board, Institute of Medicine. *Dietary reference intakes for vitamin C, vitamin E, selenium, and beta-carotene and other carotenoids.* Washington, DC: National Academy Press, 2000.

measures to increase selenium intake, such as top dressing of pasture land with fertilizers to which selenium has been added, which may increase the soil content. Still, selenium intakes in many parts of Europe are lower than in the United States (154). Wheat is a good source of selenium in North America but not in Europe. Much of the selenium in grains is lost in the milling process. The selenium content of animal foods is affected by the selenium content of the animal feed. The best sources of selenium are Brazil nuts and kidney, neither a routine food. Moderately good sources include fish, shellfish, other organ meats, muscle meats, and whole grains. Fruits and vegetables are poor sources. Selenium intakes in the United States average 108 µg/d, with a range from 83 to 129 µg/d. In Europe, comparable values are lower, ranging from 29 to 70 µg/d (154). Food sources supply selenomethionine and selenocysteine, which are incorporated into proteins in place of methionine, but they must be catabolized to an inorganic precursor to form selenophosphate, the precursor for selenocysteine, the active form in selenoproteins. Supplements also provide selenomethionine; however, sometimes the more available selenate and selenite are provided, although they carry the risk for acute toxicity when taken in excess.

3. **Assessment.** Serum levels respond to changes in the diet but can be falsely lowered by any cause of hypoproteinemia. About half of the selenium in serum is incorporated into protein in selenoprotein P. After digestion of serum to remove organic material, a selenium complex is measured fluorometrically (20). Normal serum levels are 0.132 to 0.139 µg/mL. Red cells contain higher amounts (0.23 to 0.36 µg/mL of cells), and hemolysis can alter the serum levels. Low serum levels are not associated with decreased cellular selenium and thus do not reflect body stores. Blood levels range from 3.14 to 3.32 µmol/L. Biologically active selenium can be estimated by measuring glutathione peroxidase in red cells (155). The correlation between these variables (enzyme and serum levels) has been inconstant. This inconsistency has been resolved by the discovery that another protein, selenoprotein P, contains more than 60% of serum selenium in the rat. Hair content correlates with body stores in animals, but the determination is subject to the same problems of contamination and individual variation that arise in measuring the hair content of other trace metals.

4. **Physiology.** Liver and kidney contain the most selenium, with muscle, skin, and nails having the next highest concentrations. Inorganic selenium is poorly absorbed; organic (food) selenium is assimilated best into the body. The absorption rate is not regulated and is highest in the duodenum, varying from 60% to 80% in humans. Feces and urine are the usual excretory routes. Selenium is present in bile in low concentrations. It forms complexes with heavy metals and protects against cadmium and mercury toxicity. Selenium provides a system for intracellular redox regulation. The best-known example of this is its role as a cofactor of glutathione peroxidase, which reduces hydrogen peroxide and protects membranes from oxidative damage. It also plays a role in electron transfer functions and affects drug-metabolizing enzymes. Selenium is included as the selenoamino acid, selenocysteine, in more than 35 proteins, including thioredoxin reductase and the iodothyronine deiodinases that produce active thyroid hormone (154). The exact functional significance of this amino acid is not clear.

5. **Deficiency**
   a. **Definite.** Only a few descriptions of a disorder in humans caused by dietary selenium deficiency have been published, even in areas where selenium deficiency in livestock is widespread. A cardiomyopathy that affected children was described in China (Keshan disease); it can be eliminated with oral selenium (156). Plasma and red cell selenium levels can fall during total parenteral nutrition without causing symptoms for 1 month (157). A chondrodystrophy (Kashin-Beck disease) also occurs in selenium-deficient areas of China (158). Other causative factors are felt to be involved in both these conditions.
   b. **Possible.** Deficiency of selenium is associated with loss of immunocompetency, and supplementation improves laboratory parameters of immune function; however, no clinical syndrome is associated with these changes (23). Deficiency has been linked to infection with some viruses, including HIV and coxsackievirus (154). Selenium is important for reproduction in animals, but the data on humans is inconclusive. Low selenium levels have been associated with depression, and high dietary levels of selenium seem to be associated with fewer such symptoms. Epidemiologic studies linking selenium deficiency to heart disease provide conflicting results. Evidence does not support a role for selenium in improving exercise function (23). Controlled interventions with supplements are needed to determine what role, if any, selenium has in these conditions.

6. **Treatment**
   a. **Deficiency.** If dietary deficiency occurs, 100 to 200 µg daily should be adequate therapy. Areas in the United States rich in selenium are the Great Plains and Rocky Mountain states, especially the Dakotas and Wyoming. If dietary selenium is not considered adequate, a multivitamin/mineral tablet supplying 55 to 70 µg of selenium can be used.
   b. **Gastrointestinal diseases.** In severe malabsorption, a low serum level of selenium was almost always noted (159). Epidemiologic evidence has been found that higher plasma levels of selenium are associated with a decreased prevalence of intrahepatic cholestasis of pregnancy (160).
   c. **Cancer chemoprevention.** In a prospective, double-blinded study, supplementation with 200 µg of selenium per day reduced the incidence of lung, colorectal, and prostate cancers (161). However, the reduction in lung cancer was greater than that expected from smoking cessation. Additional trials are needed to confirm these results (162).
   d. **Toxicity.** A UL for selenium intake has been set at 400 µg/d, and clinical toxicity resulting from much higher intakes in overly potent tablets (>20 mg per tablet) has been reported (153). Nausea, vomiting, fatigue, hair loss, diarrhea, irritability, paresthesias, and abdominal

Table 7-47. Drugs that cause loss of minerals

Drug group	Drug example	Minerals lost	Route of loss Urine	Route of loss Feces	Clinical deficiency produced
Laxatives	Bisacodyl Phenolphthalein Magnesium citrate	K, Ca, Mg, Na	0	+	K, Na
Diuretics	Thiazides Ethacrynic acid Furosemide Mercurials	K, Mg, Zn, Na, P	+	0	Na, K
	Triamterene Spironolactone	Ca, Mg, Zn	+	0	Na
Hormones	Glucocorticoids	Ca	+	+	Osteopenia
		K	+	0	K
	Mineralocorticoids	K	+	0	K
Binding agents	D-Penicillamine	Cu	+	+	None, if diet adequate
	Cholestyramine	Ca	0	+	None
Antacids	Magnesium hydroxide Aluminum hydroxide	P	0	+	P
Alcohol	Liquor, wine, beer	Mg, Zn	+	0	Mg
		P	+	0	P
Minerals	Monobasic and dibasic Na/R phosphates	Ca	0	+	None

cramps have been reported. Ingestion of 5 mg/d in the diet in Enshi County, China, led to loss of hair and nails, skin lesions, tooth decay, and nervous system abnormalities (164). Toxic symptoms are found with blood selenium levels above13.3 μmol/L, but urinary measurements are probably a better indicator of toxicity. Urinary levels should be below 100 μg/L to avoid selenium toxicity (20).

III. Drugs that affect mineral status. A number of drugs cause minerals to be lost from the body in either urine or feces. The use of such drugs may cause or intensify a deficiency of a given mineral. Table 7-47 lists some of these drugs and the minerals affected. The use of laxatives can lead to sodium and water depletion and dehydration, usually with no change in the serum sodium level. Potassium is secreted from the colon under these conditions, and hypokalemia results. Sodium depletion presents clinically when diuretics are used in the absence of sodium overload syndrome. Diuretics can exacerbate hypomagnesemia but usually do not cause it when body stores are normal. Glucocorticoids are associated with osteopenia, which is not a result of decreased calcium stores alone; abnormal vitamin D metabolism is probably also involved. Neutrophos treatment can cause hypocalcemia without a decrease in body calcium stores.

Bibliography

1. National Research Council. *Recommended dietary allowances,* 10th ed. Washington, DC: National Academy Press, 1989.
2. Intersalt Cooperative Research Group. Intersalt: an international study of electrolyte excretion and blood pressure. Results for 24-hour urinary sodium and potassium excretion. *Br Med J* 1988;297:319.

3. Messerli FH, Schmieder RE, Weir MR. Salt. A perpetrator of hypertensive target organ disease? *Arch Intern Med* 1997;157:2449.
4. Cutler JA, Follamnn D, Allendar PS. Randomized trials of sodium reduction: an overview. *Am J Clin Nutr* 1997;65 [Suppl]:643S.
5. Midgley JP, Matthew AG, Greenwood CMT, et al. Effect of reduced dietary sodium on blood pressure. A meta-analysis of randomized controlled trials. *JAMA* 1996; 275:1590.
6. Esslinger KA, Jones PJH. Dietary sodium intake and mortality. *Nutr Rev* 1998; 56:311.
7. Alderman MH, Cohen H, Madhavan S. Dietary sodium intake and mortality: the National Health and Nutrition Examination Survey (NHANES I). *Lancet* 1998; 351:781.
8. McCarron DA. The dietary guideline for sodium: should we shake it up? Yes! *Am J Clin Nutr* 2000;71:1013.
9. Appel LJ, Moore TJ, Obarzenek E, et al. A clinical trial of the effects of dietary pattern on blood pressure. *N Engl J Med* 1997;336:1117.
10. Kaplan NM. The dietary guideline for sodium: should we shake it up? No! *Am J Clin Nutr* 2000;71:1020.
11. McGee S, Abernethy WB, Simel DL. Is this patient hypovolemic? *JAMA* 1999; 281:1022.
12. Consensus statement on the definition of orthostatic hypotension, pure autonomic failure, and multiple system atrophy. *Neurology* 1996;46:1470.
13. Streeten DH. Variations in the clinical manifestations of orthostatic hypotension. *Mayo Clin Proc* 1995;70:713.
14. Adrogue HJ, Madias N. Hyponatremia. *N Engl J Med* 2000;342:1581.
15. Nappert G, Barrios JM, Zello GA, et al. Oral rehydration solution therapy in the management of children with rotavirus diarrhea. *Nutr Rev* 2000;58:80.
16. Alpers DH. Oral rehydration solutions for adults: an underutilized resource. *Curr Opin Gastroenterol* 1998;14:143.
17. ESPAN Working Group. Recommendations for composition of oral rehydration solutions for the children of Europe. *J Pediatr Gastroenterol Nutr* 1992;14:113.
18. Ramakrishna RB, Venkataraman S, Srinivasan P, et al. Amylase-resistant starch plus oral rehydration solution for cholera. *N Engl J Med* 2000;342:308.
19. Adrogue HJ, Madias NE. Hypernatremia. *N Engl J Med* 2000;342:1493.
20. Sauberlich HE. *Laboratory tests for the assessment of nutritional status,* 2nd ed. Boca Raton, FL: CRC Press, 1999.
21. Gennari FJ. Hypokalemia. *N Engl J Med* 1998;339:451.
22. Whelton PK, He J, Cutler JA, et al. Effects of oral potassium on blood pressure: meta-analysis of randomized controlled clinical trials. *JAMA* 1997;277:1624.
23. Sarubin A. *The health professional's guide to popular dietary supplements.* Chicago: The American Dietetic Association,1999.
24. Standing Committee on the Scientific Evaluation of Dietary Reference Intakes, Food and Nutrition Board, Institute of Medicine. *Dietary reference intakes: calcium, phosphorus, magnesium, vitamin D, and fluoride.* Washington, DC: National Academy Press, 1997.
25. Nordin C. Calcium requirement is a sliding scale. *Am J Clin Nutr* 2000;71:1381.
26. Food and Drug Administration. Food labeling: health claims, calcium and osteoporosis. *Federal Register* 1993;58:2665.
27. National Institutes of Health. Optimal calcium intake. *NIH Consensus Statement* 1994;12:1.
28. Miller GD, Heaney RP, Specker BL. Year 2000 dietary guidelines: new thoughts for a new millennium. There should be a dietary guideline for calcium; should there be a dietary guideline for calcium intake? *No Am J Clin Nutr* 2000;71:657.
29. Alexeera L, Burkhardt P, Christiansen C, et al. Assessment of fracture risk and application of screening for postmenopausal osteoporosis. *World Health Organization Technical Report Series 843.* Geneva: World Health Organization, 1994.
30. Canadian Task Force on the Periodic Health Examination. *Canadian guide to clinical preventive health care.* Ottawa: Canada Communication Group, 1994:620.
31. Hodgson SF, Johnston CC. AACE clinical practice guidelines for the prevention and treatment of postmenopausal osteoporosis. *Endocr Pract* 1996;2:155.

32. Kanis J, Devogelaer J, Gennari C. Practical guide for the use of bone mineral measurements in the assessment of treatment of osteoporosis: a position paper of the European Foundation for Osteoporosis and Bone Disease. *Osteoporos Int* 1996;6:256.

33. Bonnick SL. *Bone densitometry in clinical practice: application and interpretation.* Totowa, NJ: Humana Press, 1998.

34. Bone mass measurement act (BMMA). *Federal Register* 1998;63:34324.

35. Bronner F, Pansu D. Nutritional aspects of calcium absorption. *J Nutr* 1999;129:9.

36. Deroisy A, Zartarian M, Meurmans L, et al. Acute changes in serum calcium and parathyroid hormone circulating levels induced by the oral intake of five currently available calcium salts in healthy male volunteers. *Clin Rheumatol* 1997; 16:249.

37. Recker RR. Calcium absorption and achlorhydria. *N Engl J Med* 1985;313:70.

38. Anonymous. Calcium deficiency. *Lancet* 1985;1:1431

39. Arnaud CD, Sanchez SD. The role of calcium in osteoporosis. *Annu Rev Nutr* 1990;10:397.

40. Thacher TD, Fischer PR, Pettifor JM, et al. A comparison of calcium, vitamin D, or both for nutritional rickets in Nigerian children. *N Engl J Med* 1999;341:563.

41. Kalkwarf HJ, Specker BL, Bianchi DC, et al. The effect of calcium supplementation on bone density during lactation and after weaning. *N Engl J Med* 1997; 337:523.

42. Scott EM, Gaywood I, Scott BB. British Society of Gastroenterology: Guidelines for osteoporosis in coeliac disease and inflammatory bowel disease. *Gut* 2000; 46[Suppl 1]:1.

43. Compston JE. Management of bone disease in patients on long-term glucocorticoid therapy. *Gut* 1999;44:770.

44. Andreassen H, Rungby J, Dahlerup F, et al. Inflammatory bowel disease and osteoporosis. *Scand J Gastroenterol* 1997;32:1247.

45. Storm D, Eslin R, Porter ES, et al. Calcium supplementation prevents seasonal bone loss and changes in biochemical markers of bone turnover in elderly New England women: a randomized placebo-controlled trial. *J Clin Endocrinol Metab* 1998;83:3817.

46. Nieves JW, Komar L, Cosman F, et al. Calcium potentiates the effect of estrogen and calcitonin on bone mass: a review and analysis. *Am J Clin Nutr* 1998;67:18.

47. Recker RR, Davies KM, Dowd RM, et al. The effect of low-dose continuous estrogen and progesterone therapy with calcium and vitamin D on bone in elderly women: a randomized, controlled trial. *Ann Intern Med* 1999;130:897.

48. Allender PS, Cutler JA, Follman D, et al. Dietary calcium supplementation on blood pressure: a meta-analysis of randomized clinical trials. *Ann Intern Med* 1996;124:825.

49. Bucher HC, Cook RJ, Gfuyatt GH, et al. Effects of dietary calcium supplementation on blood pressure. A meta-analysis of randomized controlled trials. *JAMA* 1996;275:1016.

50. Bostick RM. Human studies of calcium supplementation and colorectal epithelial cell proliferation. *Cancer Epidemiol Biomarkers Prev* 1997;6:971.

51. Baron JA, Beach M, Mandel JS, et al. Calcium supplements for the prevention of colorectal adenomas. Calcium Polyp Prevention Study Group. *N Engl J Med* 1999;341:101.

52. Rhys-Jacobs S, Starkey P, Bernstein D, et al. Calcium carbonate and the premenstrual syndrome: effects on premenstrual and menstrual symptoms. Premenstrual Syndrome Study Group. *Am J Obstet Gynecol* 1998;179:444.

53. Calcium supplements. *Med Lett* 2000;42:29.

54. Heaney RP. Calcium supplements: practical considerations. *Osteoporos Int* 1991; 1:65.

55. Kelepouris E, Agus ZS. Hypomagnesemia: renal magnesium handling. *Semin Nephrol* 1998;18:58.

56. Levine BS, Coburn JW. Magnesium, the mimic/antagonist to calcium. *N Engl J Med* 1984;310;1253.

57. Weisinger JR. Magnesium and phosphorus. *Lancet* 1998;352:391.

58. Graber ML, Schulman G. Hypomagnesemic hypocalcemia independent of parathyroid hormone. *Ann Intern Med* 1986;104:804.
59. Reinhart RA. Magnesium metabolism. A review with special reference to the relationship between intracellular content and serum levels. *Arch Intern Med* 1988;148:2415.
60. Fleming CR, George L, Stoner GL, et al. The importance of urinary magnesium values in patients with gut failure. *Mayo Clin Proc* 1996;71:21.
61. Fine KD, Santa Ana CA, Porter JL, et al. Intestinal absorption of magnesium from food and supplements. *J Clin Invest* 1991;88:396.
62. Shils ME. Magnesium. In: Shils ME, Olson JA, Shike M, et al., eds. *Modern nutrition in health and disease,* 9th ed. Philadelphia: Lea & Febiger, 1999:169.
63. Knochel JP. The clinical status of hypophosphatemia: an update. *N Engl J Med* 1985;313:447.
64. Knochel JP. The pathophysiology and clinical characteristics of severe hypophosphatemia. *Arch Intern Med* 1977;137:203.
65. van der Veere CN, Jansen PLM, Sinaasappel M, et al. Oral calcium phosphate: a new therapy for Crigler-Najjar disease? *Gastroenterology* 1997;112:455.
66. Standing Committee on the Scientific Evaluation of Dietary Reference Intakes, Food and Nutrition Board, Institute of Medicine. *Dietary reference intakes for vitamin A, vitamin K, arsenic, boron, chromium, copper, iodine, iron, manganese, molybdenum, nickel, silicon, vanadium, and zinc.* Washington, DC: National Academy Press, 2001. Available on line via the Internet at *http://www.nap.edu/ books, Crawler list 0309072794.* Accessed May 30, 2001.
67. Hastka J, Lasserre J-J, Schwarzbeck A, et al. Laboratory tests of iron status: correlation or common sense? *Clin Chem* 1996;42:5.
68. Wormwood M. The laboratory assessment of iron status—an update. *Clin Chim Acta* 1997;259:3.
69. Finch CA, Cook JD. Iron deficiency. *Am J Clin Nutr* 1984;39:471.
70. Sackett DL, Richardson WS, Rosenberg W, et al. *Evidence-based medicine.* New York: Churchill Livingstone, 1997:124.
71. Ahluwalia N. Diagnostic utility of serum transferrin receptors measurement in assessing iron status. *Nutr Rev* 1998;56:133.
72. Baynes RD. Assessment of iron status. *Clin Biochem* 1996;29:209.
73. MacDougall IC, Hutton RD, Cavill I, et al. Poor response to treatment of renal anemia with erythropoietin corrected with iron given intravenously. *Br Med J* 1989;299:157.
74. Guyatt GH, Oxman AD, Ali M, et al. Laboratory diagnosis of iron-deficiency anemia: an overview. *J Gen Intern Med* 1992;7:145.
75. Psaty BM, Tierney WM, Martin DK, et al. The value of serum iron studies as a test for iron-deficiency anemia in a county hospital. *J Gen Intern Med* 1989;2:160.
76. Thompson WG, Meola T, Lipkin M Jr, et al. Red cell distribution width, mean corpuscular volume, and transferrin saturation in the diagnosis of iron deficiency. *Arch Intern Med* 1988;148:2128.
77. Adams PC. Population screening for hemochromatosis. *Hepatology* 1999;29:1324.
78. Cook JD. Adaptation in iron metabolism. *Am J Clin Nutr* 1990;51:301.
79. Andrews NC, Fleming MD, Gunshin H. Iron transport across biologic membranes. *Nutr Rev* 1999;57:114.
80. van Dokkum W. Significance of iron bioavailability for iron recommendations. *Biol Trace Elem Res* 1992;35:1.
81. Zoller H, Pietrangelo A, Vogel W, et al. Duodenal metal-transporter (DMT-1, NRAMP-2) expression in patients with hereditary hemochromatosis. *Lancet* 1999;353:2120.
82. Finch CA, Huebers W. Perspectives in iron metabolism. *N Engl J Med* 1982; 306:1520.
83. Theil EC. The iron responsive element (IRE) family of mRNA regulators: regulation of iron transport and uptake compared in animals, plants, and microorganisms. *Met Ions Biol Syst* 1998;35:403.
84. Lozoff B, Jimenez E, Hagen J, et al. Poorer behavioral and developmental outcome more than 10 years after treatment for iron deficiency in infancy. *Pediatrics* 2000;105:E51.

85. Andrews NC. Disorders of iron metabolism. *N Engl J Med* 1999;341:1986.
86. O'Keefe ST, Gavin K, Lavan JN. Iron status and restless legs syndrome in the elderly. *Age Ageing* 1994;23:200.
87. Davis BJ, Rajput A, Rajput ML, et al. A randomized, double-blind placebo-controlled trial of iron in restless legs syndrome. *Eur Neurol* 2000;43:70.
88. Seligman PA, Caskey JH, Frazier JL, et al. Measurements of iron absorption from prenatal vitamin–mineral supplements. *Obstet Gynecol* 1983;61:356.
89. Beard JL. Weekly iron intervention: the case for intermittent iron supplementation. *Am J Clin Nutr* 1998;68:209.
90. Hallberg L. Combatting iron deficiency: daily administration of iron is far superior to weekly administration. *Am J Clin Nutr* 1999;68:213.
91. Burns DL, Mascioli EA, Bistrian BR. Effect of iron-supplemented total parenteral nutrition in patients with iron deficiency anemia. *Nutrition* 1996;12:411.
92. MacDougall IC. Strategies for iron supplementation: oral versus intravenous. *Kidney Int* 1999;69[Suppl]:S61.
93. Gasche C, Dejaco C, Waldhoer T, et al. Intravenous iron and erythropoietin for anemia associated with Crohn disease: a randomized, controlled trial. *Ann Intern Med* 1997;126:782.
94. Auerbach M, Witt D, Toler W, et al. Clinical use of the total dose intravenous infusion of iron dextran. *J Lab Clin Med* 1988;111:566.
95. Auerbach M, Winchester J, Wahab A, et al. A randomized trial of three iron dextran infusion methods for anemia in EPO-treated dialysis patients. *Am J Kidney Dis* 1998;31:81.
96. Hunt JR, Matthys LA, Johnson LK. Zinc absorption, mineral balance, and blood lipids in women consuming lactoovovegetarian and omnivorous diets for 8 weeks. *Am J Clin Nutr* 1998;67:421.
97. Brown KH, Peerson JM, Allen LH. Effect of zinc supplementation on children's growth: a meta-analysis of intervention trials. In: Sandstrom B, Walter P, eds. *Role of trace elements for health promotion and disease prevention.* Davis, CA: University of California, 1998:76.
98. Briefel RR, Bialostosky K, Kennedy-Stephenson J, et al. Zinc intake of the U.S. population: findings from the Third National Health and Nutrition Examination Survey, 1988–1994. *J Nutr* 2000;130:1367S.
99. Freeland-Graves J. Mineral adequacy of vegetarian diets. *Am J Clin Nutr* 1988;48:859.
100. King JE. Assessment of zinc status. *J Nutr* 1990;120[Suppl 11]:1474.
101. Wiesman K, Hoyer H. Serum alkaline phosphatase and serum zinc levels in the diagnosis and exclusion of zinc deficiency in man. *Am J Clin Nutr* 1985;41:1214.
102. Abu-Hamdan DK, Mahajan SK, Migdal SD, et al. Zinc tolerance test in uremia. Effect of ferrous sulfate and aluminum hydroxide. *Ann Intern Med* 1986;104:50.
103. Wood RJ. Assessment of marginal zinc status in humans. *J Nutr* 2000;130:1350S.
104. Bremner I, Morrison JN. Assessment of zinc, copper and cadmium status in animals by assay of extracellular methionine. *Acta Pharmacol Toxicol* 1986;89[Suppl 7]:102.
105. Blanchard RK, Cousins RJ. Regulation of intestinal gene expression by dietary zinc: induction of uroguanylin mRNA by zinc deficiency. *J Nutr* 2000;130:1393S.
106. Yuzbasiyan-Gurkan V, Grider A, Nostrant T, et al. Treatment of Wilson's disease with zinc: X. Intestinal metallothionein induction. *J Lab Clin Med* 1992;120:380.
107. Cousins RJ. Zinc. In Ziegler EK, Filer LJ. *Present knowledge in nutrition,* 7th ed. Washington DC: ILSI, 1996:293.
108. Cousins RJ, McMahon RJ. Integrative aspects of zinc transporters. *J Nutr* 2000;130:1384S.
109. Krebs NF. Overview of zinc absorption and excretion in the human gastrointestinal tract. *J Nutr* 2000;130:1374S.
110. Mills CF. Dietary interactions involving the trace elements. *Annu Rev Nutr* 1985;5:173.
111. Whittaker P. Iron and zinc interactions in humans. *Am J Clin Nutr* 1998;68:442S.

112. Lonnerdal B. Dietary factors influencing zinc absorption. *J Nutr* 2000;130:1378S.
113. Fraker PJ, King LE, Laakko T, et al. The dynamic link between the integrity of the immune system and zinc status. *J Nutr* 2000;130:1399S.
114. Rink L, Kirchner H. Zinc-altered immune function and cytokine production. *J Nutr* 2000;130:1407S.
115. Prasad AS. Zinc deficiency in women, infants, and children. *J Am Coll Nutr* 1996;15:113.
116. Wapnir RA. Zinc deficiency: malnutrition and the gastrointestinal tract. *J Nutr* 2000;130:1388S.
117. Osaki T, Ohshima M, Tomita Y, et al. Clinical and physiological investigations in patients with taste abnormality. *J Oral Pathol Med* 1996;25:38.
118. Henkin RI, Schecter PJ, Friedewald WT, et al. A double blind study of the effects of zinc sulfate on taste and smell dysfunction. *Am J Med Sci* 1976;272:285.
119. Bhutta ZA, Bird SM, Black RE, et al. Therapeutic effects of oral zinc in acute and persistent diarrhea in children in developing countries: pooled analysis of randomized controlled trials. *Am J Clin Nutr* 2000;72:1516.
120. Jackson JL, Peterson C, Lesho E. A meta-analysis of zinc salts lozenges and the common cold. *Arch Intern Med* 1997;157:2373.
121. Marshall S. Zinc gluconate and the common cold. Review of randomized controlled trials. *Can Fam Physician* 1998;44:1037.
122. Prasad AS, Fitzgerald JT, Bao B, et al. Duration of symptoms and plasma cytokine levels in patients with the common cold treated with zinc acetate. A randomized, double-blind, placebo-controlled trial. *Ann Intern Med* 2000;13:245.
123. Bhutta ZA, Black RE, Brown KH, et al. Prevention of diarrhea and pneumonia by zinc supplementation in children in developing countries: pooled analysis of randomized controlled trials. *J Pediatrics* 1999;135:689.
124. Hambridge M. Human zinc deficiency. *J Nutr* 2000;130:1344S.
125. Fosmire GJ. Zinc toxicity. *Am J Clin Nutr* 1990;51:225.
126. Klevay LM, Medeiros DM. Deliberations and evaluations of the approaches, endpoints and paradigms for dietary recommendations about copper. *J Nutr* 1996;126:2419S.
127. Pennington JT, Calloway DH. Copper content of foods. *J Am Diet Assoc* 1973;63:143.
128. Linder MC, Hazegh-Azam M. Copper biochemistry and molecular biology. *Am J Clin Nutr* 1996;63:797S.
129. Brewer GJ, Yuzbasiyan-Gurkan V. Wilson disease. *Medicine* 1992;71:139.
130. Stremmel W, Meyerrose KW, Niederau C, et al. Wilson disease: clinical presentation, treatment, and survival. *Ann Intern Med* 1991;115:720.
131. Pena MMO, Lee J, Thiele DJ. A delicate balance: homeostatic control of copper uptake and distribution. *J Nutr* 1999;129:1251.
132. Eisenstein RS. Discovery of the ceruloplasmin homologue hephaestin: new insight into the copper/iron connection. *Nutr Rev* 2000;58:22.
133. Triplett WS. Clinical aspects of zinc, copper, manganese, chromium, and selenium. *Nutr Int* 1985;1:60.
134. Danks DM. Copper deficiency in humans. *Annu Rev Nutr* 1988;8:235.
135. Bull PC, Cox DW. Wilson disease and Menkes disease: new handles on heavy-metal transport. *Trends Genet* 1994;10:246.
136. Klevay LM. Cardiovascular disease from copper deficiency—a history. *J Nutr* 2000;130:489S.
137. Bremner I. Manifestations of copper excess. *Am J Clin Nutr* 1998;67[Suppl 5]:S1069.
138. Daniels GH, Haber DA. Will radioiodine be useful in treatment of breast cancer? *Nat Med* 2000;6:859.
139. Kavishe F. Iodine deficiency disorders. In: Sadler MJ, Strain JJ, Caballero B, eds. *Encyclopedia of human nutrition*. London: Academic Press, 1998:1136.
140. Hetzel BS. Iodine and neuropsychological development. *J Nutr* 2000;130:493S.
141. Lee K, Bradley R, Dwyer J, et al. Too much versus too little: the implications of current iodine intake in the United States. *Nutr Rev* 1999;57:177.
142. Rao GS. Dietary intake and bioavailability of fluoride. *Annu Rev Nutr* 1984;9:115.

143. Freeland-Graves JH, Turnlund JR. Deliberations and evaluations of the approaches, endpoints and paradigms for manganese and molybdenum dietary recommendations. *J Nutr* 1996;126:2435S.
144. Burch RE, Sullivan JR. Diagnosis of zinc, copper, and manganese abnormalities in man. *Med Clin North Am* 1976;60:655.
145. Friedman BJ, Freeland-Graves JH, Bales CW, et al. Manganese balance and clinical observations in young men fed a manganese-deficient diet. *J Nutr* 1987;117:113.
146. Fitzgerald K, Mikalunas V, Rubin H, et al. Hypermanganesemia in patients receiving total parenteral nutrition. *JPEN J Parenter Enteral Nutr* 1999;23:333.
147. Wardle CA, Forbes A, Roberts NB, et al. Hypermanganesemia in long-term intravenous nutrition and chronic liver disease. *JPEN J Parenter Enteral Nutr* 1999;23:350.
148. Anderson RA. Nutritional factors influencing the glucose/insulin system: chromium. *J Am Coll Nutr* 1997;16:404.
149. Jeejeebhoy KN. The role of chromium in nutrition and therapeutics and as a potential toxin. *Nutr Rev* 1999;57:329.
150. Ducros V. Chromium metabolism. A literature review. *Biol Trace Elem Res* 1992;32:68.
151. Vincent JB. Quest for the molecular mechanism of chromium action and its relationship to diabetes. *Nutr Rev* 2000;58:67.
152. Anderson RA. Chromium metabolism and its role in disease processes in man. *Clin Physiol Biochem* 1986;4:31.
153. Standing Committee on the Scientific Evaluation of Dietary Reference Intakes, Food and Nutrition Board, Institute of Medicine. *Dietary reference intakes for vitamin C, vitamin E, selenium, and beta-carotene and other carotenoids.* Washington, DC: National Academy Press, 2000.
154. Rayman MP. The importance of selenium to human health. *Lancet* 2000;356:233.
155. Diplock AT. Indexes of selenium status in human populations. *Am J Clin Nutr* 1993;57:256S.
156. Epidemiologic studies on the etiologic relationship of selenium and Keshan disease. *China Med J* 1979;92:477.
157. Jacobson S, Plantin LO. Concentration of selenium in plasma and erythrocytes during total parenteral nutrition in Crohn's disease. *Gut* 1985;26:50.
158. Moreno-Reyes R, Suetens C, Mathieu F, et al. Kashin-Beck osteoarthropathy in rural Tibet in relation to selenium and iodine status. *N Engl J Med* 1998;339:1112.
159. Rannem T, Ladefoged K, Hylander E, et al. Selenium depletion in patients with gastrointestinal diseases: are there any predictive factors? *Scand J Gastroenterol* 1998;33:1057.
160. Reyes H, Baez ME, Gonzalez MC, et al. Selenium, zinc and copper plasma levels in intrahepatic cholestasis of pregnancy, in normal pregnancies and in healthy individuals in Chile. *J Hepatol* 2000;32:542.
161. Clark LC, Combs GF Jr, Turnbull BW, et al. Effects of selenium supplementation for cancer prevention in patients with carcinoma of the skin. A randomized controlled trial. *JAMA* 1996;276:1957.
162. Combs GF, Gray WP. Chemopreventive agents: selenium. *Pharmacol Exp Ther* 1998;79:179.
163. Yang GQ, Wang SZ, Zhou RH, et al. Endemic selenium intoxication of humans in China. *Am J Clin Nutr* 1983;37:872.

III. THERAPEUTIC NUTRITION

8. NUTRITIONAL PLANNING FOR PATIENTS WITH PROTEIN AND CALORIE DEFICIENCY

I. **Definition of nutritional support.** Feeding is not considered medical therapy under ordinary circumstances. When normal diets fail to meet daily requirements or when assessment documents deficiencies, then nutritional planning becomes a part of medical therapeutics. Nutritional support is the specific planning of nutritional therapy when usual diets are inadequate.

   A. **Requirements for protein and calories** are the largest on a daily basis and consequently can be the most difficult to meet. In addition, when protein deficiencies develop, they are corrected slowly. Replacement is limited by a relatively slow rate of accumulation of newly synthesized proteins; only about 5% of the protein deficiency can be restored daily, regardless of the amount of substrate available. Because vitamins and minerals are more easily replaced (see Chapters 6 and 7), nutritional support most often revolves around providing adequate amounts of macronutrients. Deriving a satisfactory, efficient, and acceptable plan for protein–calorie support involves analyzing multiple factors, and no simple algorithm can conveniently direct the health care professional to the best choice of nutritional therapy without such analysis. The final plan utilizes either *enteral* or *parenteral* therapy in a way that best meets the patient's needs.

   B. **Overview of the approach to nutritional support.** Certain *key questions* can be used to help construct an appropriate protein–calorie support plan for most patients. Although nutritional planning is generally approached with the hospitalized patient in mind, it can also be utilized for many outpatients. For any particular patient, one or several of the questions may be more relevant than the others. Consequently, the physician needs to individualize nutritional planning, weighing the various issues appropriately. The first three questions are used to determine the requirements for and urgency of providing macronutrients, whereas the fourth question is used to select the method of protein–calorie support. Obviously, some questions are not listed that might be important in some cases. For example, will any psychological or social factors interfere with delivery of the proper therapy? Is the cost prohibitive to the patient? Are the necessary facilities available locally? However, the purpose of this approach is to outline the questions that most often lead the health care professional to a rational choice of available alternatives. The final choice may be affected by other variables not discussed in this chapter.

   C. **Key questions in planning protein and calorie nutritional support.** These questions direct the clinician in formulating an appropriate support plan. The first three questions are discussed in the following section, and the fourth question is considered in Section IV.

      1. Are current protein and calorie requirements being met?
      2. What is the current degree of body protein and fat depletion?
      3. What is the anticipated length of time that nutritional support will be required?
      4. Is the intestinal tract available and adequate?

II. **Assessing the need for protein and calorie support**

   A. **Are protein and calorie requirements being met?** A complete protein–calorie assessment includes a calculation of energy and protein balance and a determination of the adequacy of the body protein and fat compartments. Providing an estimate of current energy and protein balance completes half of the total assessment. In practice, this estimate is not usually made. However, a case can be made for making the estimate for *all hospitalized patients,* even if a comprehensive assessment of the body compartments does not seem necessary. Two determinations are used to calculate the balance of either protein or energy intake and requirement.

Energy Balance = Energy Intake – Energy Requirement

Protein Balance = Protein Intake – Protein Requirement

Under steady-state conditions (stable weight and good health), intakes meet requirements, and energy balance and protein balance both equal zero.

1. **Determination of protein and calorie requirements.** The formulas used in making these calculations are presented in Chapter 4. Abbreviated methods for estimating protein and calorie requirements are available (see Chapter 5, Section II).

   a. **Rough estimates.** If even these simple calculations seem too complex, at least a rough estimation of requirements should be made for all hospitalized patients. The figures in Table 8-1 can be used for a rapid estimation of the protein and calorie requirements of hospitalized adults if one recognizes the limitations of the method. Besides providing only a crude estimation of the additional requirements for disease, these values assume a linear relationship of basal metabolic rate to body weight, which is actually correct for just a narrow range. Therefore, calorie requirements, as estimated in this way, are accurate only for patients weighing from 60 to 80 kg. The range from 25 to 35 kcal/kg per day provides about 125% to 175% of the recommended basal energy expenditure. To avoid excess provision of macronutrients, goals for glucose should be less than 5 g/kg per day, for lipids less than 1g/kg per day, and for amino acids/proteins 0.75 to 1.5 g/kg per day, the latter based on estimates of protein depletion. However, for many patients, such estimates (as in Table 8-1) provide a sufficiently accurate assessment of protein and calorie needs.

   b. **Situations calling for more precise calculations.** Calculations of calorie requirements in children and in severely underweight or overweight adults must be performed more carefully and can be obtained by using the formulas for metabolic expenditure outlined in Chapter 5. Energy and protein requirements may vary from the estimate in Table 8-1 in certain diseases.

2. **Determination of protein and calorie intake** is easier in hospitalized patients because their diet is controlled and IV fluids are recorded. Chapter 5 (Section VI) includes methods for assessing the caloric intake by nutrition history. Caloric counts by a dietitian for 24-hour periods should be used to make an accurate determination of calorie intake during a period of hospitalization if inadequate intake is not obvious. The best use of the calorie count requires a sampling of three 24-hour periods. Tables 5-7 and 11-2 list the caloric and protein content of commonly used prepared foods. The caloric content of formulas for enteral supplementation is discussed in Chapter 9 and of parenteral nutrition solutions in Chapter 10.

Table 8-1. Rapid estimation of protein and calorie requirements of adult patients

Degree of stress	Calorie requirements (kcal/kg[a] per day)	Protein requirements (g/kg[a] per day)
None–mild	25	0.75
Moderate–severe metabolic stress	35	1.0–1.5

[a] Desired body weight.

3. **Remedial causes of appetite suppression** should be treated. Hunger is a complex feeling, and the exact regulatory mechanisms of food intake have not been determined. Multiple factors are involved in producing the sensations of hunger and satiety, including hypothalamic signals, changes in gastrointestinal motility, gastric distention, metabolic factors, taste, and psychological and social influences. Significant derangements in any of these areas are likely to alter overall appetite for food. The appetite of the hospitalized patient is often obvious after several days of inpatient observation. Evaluation of methods of food intake will indirectly evaluate appetite. By generating a sampling of recent food intake, a nutrition history will indicate food likes and dislikes, average caloric intake, and sources of specific nutritional deficiency. Dietitians are well educated in this technique. A suppressed appetite should not be accepted without evaluation of the cause. At times, a correctable reason for appetite suppression can be determined. Remediable causes for decreased appetite include the following:

   a. **Side effects of medication or toxicity.** Many medications can alter appetite, often because of effects on the central nervous system or gastrointestinal tract. Common medications that are frequently incriminated include narcotic analgesics, oral antibiotics, iron preparations, aspirin-containing compounds, and other nonsteroidal antiinflammatory agents. The list of medications occasionally producing nausea or interfering with appetite is endless. Consequently, the ordered medications should be carefully reviewed and possible offending agents discontinued.

   b. **Disease of the upper gastrointestinal tract.** The mouth should be examined for the presence of significant oral, dental, or pharyngeal disease, especially in severely debilitated or immunosuppressed patients. Poorly fitting dentures commonly limit the intake of solid food. Some patients with undiagnosed peptic ulcer disease or esophagitis have a poor appetite as their major symptom. Careful questioning may elicit symptoms of dysphagia, odynophagia, dyspepsia, epigastric pain, or postprandial nausea and vomiting, which should prompt further investigation of the gastrointestinal tract and institution of appropriate therapy.

   c. **Depression.** One of the more common causes of unplanned weight loss is depression. Although depression may cause an increased appetite and weight gain, a decreased appetite is a more common symptom. Associated symptoms of fatigue, decreased activity, insomnia or early awakening, and dysphoric mood help the examiner to make the diagnosis. Supportive psychotherapy, antidepressants, and psychiatric consultation should be used appropriately, but rapid improvement in appetite should not be expected routinely.

4. **Therapeutic decisions based on energy and protein balance.** If calculations show that the patient is in positive nitrogen (protein) and energy balance, then the current nutritional support plan is satisfactory to prevent further loss of body proteins. When a negative balance is determined, then the remaining key questions must be answered. The urgency of nutritional support for hospitalized patients in negative balance can be determined by answering the first three questions, and suitable guidelines for making such decisions are given in Tables 8-2 and 8-3.

B. **What is the current degree of body protein and fat depletion?** Many of the decisions regarding the urgency of instituting protein and calorie nutritional support, especially the intensive forms of support (i.e., forced enteral feeding and total parenteral nutrition), revolve around the answer to this question. In fact, it is usually in response to an abnormal laboratory value that the physician begins to consider nutritional therapy. Clinical, anthropometric, and laboratory data are used to formulate a general opinion regarding the degree of depletion; the difficulties of arriving at a meaningful nutritional

Table 8-2. Nutrition planning for patients with moderate to severe protein–calorie malnutrition

Protein and calorie balance	Nutrition plan
Negative	
Long period of support anticipated	Increase intake now.
Short period of support anticipated	Delay intensive therapy; minimize losses until acute illness subsides; reevaluate frequently.
Zero	Delay intensive therapy; minimize losses until acute illness subsides; reevaluate frequently.
Positive	Try to maintain current caloric and protein intake.

assessment are described in Chapter 5, but no formula is sufficiently satisfactory to be used routinely. The parameters used in both minimal and comprehensive evaluation are outlined in Chapter 5, Tables 5-18 to 5-21, and Fig. 5-4, and the clinical applications of the evaluations are discussed in the text. By using current techniques, the physician can divide patients into two main clinical groups: (a) those with normal protein and fat body compartments or mild deficiencies and (b) those with moderate to severe deficiencies.

C. **What is the anticipated length of time that nutritional support will be required?** Assessment of balance and body compartments provides a database of objective parameters and calculated requirements. This third key question is the first of several that help the health care professional apply the database to patient situations. Anticipating the length of time that energy and protein requirements will not be satisfied by normal diets (i.e., the cumulative result of negative balance) helps determine the urgency of instituting protein–calorie support.

1. Estimation of the cumulative result of negative balance for the anticipated length of illness puts into perspective the end result of persistent negative energy balance.

   a. Representative estimates of weight losses incurred—depending on the degree of negative balance and the length of illness—are given in Table 8-4. This estimate is based on the assumption that a negative balance of 3,400 kcal represents a loss of 1 lb of body weight. (The derivation of this relationship is presented in Table 5-11.)

   b. In situations of metabolic stress, such a relationship is not as accurate as it is in situations of slow weight gain or loss, and this rela-

Table 8-3. Nutrition planning for patients with mild malnutrition or normal nutritional status[a]

Protein and calorie balance	Nutrition plan
Negative	
Long period of support anticipated	Increase intake as soon as possible; reevaluate frequently.
Short period of support anticipated	No change from current plan necessary.
Zero	No change from current plan necessary.
Positive	No change from current plan necessary.

[a] As estimated by history, physical examination, and laboratory tests.

Table 8-4. Estimated cumulative effect of negative balance

Estimated balance (kcal/d)	Cumulative weight loss during illness (illness length in days)											
	2	4	6	8	10	12	14	16	18	20	22	24
−4,000	2.4[b]	4.7	7.1	9.4	11.8	14.1	16.5	18.8	21.2	23.2	25.9	28.2
−3,500	2.1	4.1	6.2	8.2	10.3	12.4	14.4	16.5	18.5	20.5	22.6	24.7
−3,000	1.8	3.5	5.3	7.1	8.8	10.6	12.4	14.1	15.9	17.6	19.4	21.2
−2,500	1.5	2.9	4.4	5.9	7.4	8.8	10.3	11.8	13.2	14.7	16.2	17.6
−2,000	1.2	2.4	3.5	4.7	5.9	7.1	8.2	9.4	10.6	11.8	12.9	14.1

−5%[a] −10%[a]

[a] Percentage weight change for a 154-lb (70-kg) patient.
[b] Estimated weight loss in pounds.

tionship does not remain constant as weight loss progresses. Also, the relationship does not take into account the adaptive processes that occur during starvation. However, it does help the clinician make a crude estimate of expected losses.

  c. It is clear from Table 8-4 that the well-nourished patient with large caloric deficits (3,000 to 3,500 kcal/d) will accumulate a significant weight loss within 1 to 2 weeks, and in 2 to 4 weeks with modest deficits (2,000 to 2,500 kcal/d). It is not always possible to make reasonable estimates of the time that a hospitalized patient will maintain a large negative balance—that is, show an inability to meet protein and calorie needs on a hospital diet. However, conceptualizing the cumulative effect of negative balance helps determine the urgency of nutritional support. At least one can decrease the degree of protein and calorie losses, even if achieving positive balance is not feasible.

  d. The anticipated need for nutritional support is arbitrarily considered to be *long* if more than 7 to 10 days of significantly negative balance is expected.

 2. The initial degree of depletion is relevant. Certainly the majority of well-nourished patients tolerate well the negative nitrogen and energy balance that occurs with brief medical illnesses or after routine surgical operations. The fat stores that are maintained in normally nourished persons allow for such periods of negative energy balance. Protein does not have a storage depot; consequently, negative protein balance implies loss of structural and functional proteins from the outset. In situations of increased catabolism, such as during illness or in the postoperative period, protein losses are accelerated, and measurable protein deficiency becomes apparent more rapidly than does calorie deficiency. The importance of additional deficiency incurred during the period of anticipated negative balance depends on the initial degree of protein and fat depletion.

III. Guidelines for determining the urgency of protein and calorie support. The following guidelines (Tables 8-2 and 8-3) assume that protein and calorie balances parallel each other—that is, that the degree of negative protein balance is similar to the degree of negative energy balance. This is not always the case, and at times, protein requirements exceed basal requirements by more than do simultaneously calculated energy requirements. Replacement always requires both calories and protein to support the protein needs most effectively. The support plan at times must be modified to include a larger percentage of protein for patients with large protein losses.

 A. Patients with consistently moderate or severe deficiencies according to a comprehensive assessment of nutritional status and patients who give the impression of significant protein–calorie malnutrition on a minimal assessment are approached according to the guidelines in Table 8-2.

  1. For patients with established deficiencies, optimal nutritional support should exceed the calculated daily requirements so as to replete the deficiencies. If support is initiated during an acute illness in the moderately to severely depleted patient, it may not achieve a positive balance initially, but it should be continued after illness resolves until reassessment reflects improvement of nutritional status out of the severe range or until it is apparent that the patient is meeting calorie and protein requirements with an oral diet.

  2. These patients also may benefit from 1 to 3 weeks of protein–calorie support that exceeds the estimated requirements to achieve an anabolic state (with replacement of concomitant vitamin or mineral deficiencies) before they undergo any surgical procedure, if the delay is feasible. Alterations in muscle function can develop with subtle nutritional changes that are not reflected in other measures of nutritional status (1). One must be cautious not to overfeed severely catabolic patients because it is often not possible to achieve positive calorie or protein balance, especially if they are infected. Such patients are also more susceptible to adverse effects of nutritional support (Table 5-24). Although it has not been shown convincingly that replacement improves overall morbidity or mortality, patients starting with better nutritional status (or less severe disease, as these two interpretations cannot be separated by available methods) appear to fare better postoperatively.

B. Patients with normal protein–calorie nutritional status or mild deficiencies can be managed according to Table 8-3. By definition, a long illness anticipates that 10% or more of the current weight will be lost. Although intake need not be increased immediately for these patients based on this anticipation, the physician should not wait until deficiencies become clinically apparent. However, review of prospective, randomized trials of parenteral or enteral feeding perioperatively shows no clear benefit (2). It seems clear that perioperative parenteral or enteral feeding should not be given routinely to surgical patients who are not nutritionally depleted. For selected patients who are marginally depleted in nutrients and who are expected not to be able to tolerate oral feedings, nutritional supplements can be considered. For patients who are clearly depleted by history, nutritional support should be seriously considered.

C. Patients with specific disorders. The data for providing nutritional support in many diseases are not very robust and are based mostly on studies other than randomized, controlled, double-blinded trials (Tables 5-22 and 5-23). The use of nutritional support should be individualized and considered a part of overall disease management rather than as specific therapy for a particular condition.

IV. Determining the method of delivery for protein and calorie support

A. Choosing between enteral and parenteral support. The usual guideline for choosing between enteral and parenteral nutritional support is to use enteral support wherever possible. Parenteral nutrition should be used in patients who are or will become malnourished and who do not have sufficient gastrointestinal function to restore or maintain an adequate nutritional status (3). The feasibility of enteral support is determined by whether or not the intestine is available for use and is functioning adequately. The consensus of nutrition experts is that the gastrointestinal tract is more physiologically and metabolically effective than the parenteral route for nutrient utilization (4,5). Enteral nutrition is preferred over parenteral nutrition for several reasons.

1. Enteral nutrition provides nutrients to the gastrointestinal mucosa that are not provided by parenteral nutrition. The foremost of these nutrients are short-chain fatty acids provided to the colonic mucosa by the bacterial degradation of fiber. Short-chain fatty acids are an important source of energy for the colonic mucosa (6).

2. Nutrients in the intestinal lumen may protect the integrity of the gastrointestinal tract. Prolonged parenteral nutrition in rodents is associated with atrophy of the gastrointestinal tract. However, atrophy may not be so important a finding in humans on parenteral feeding (7).

3. Enteral nutrition is safer, more convenient, and less expensive than parenteral nutrition. One of the relative benefits proposed for enteral nutrition is that it is associated with fewer septic complications compared than is parenteral nutrition. In most of these comparison studies, the parenterally and enterally fed groups did not receive diets that were equivalent in terms of calories and protein. These studies raise the question of whether the increased number of septic complications in the parenterally fed group were a consequence of the route of administration or of the associated overfeeding and hyperglycemia (8–10).

B. Is the intestinal tract available and adequate? This question, the fourth of the key questions previously mentioned, is pivotal in determining the method of delivering the protein and calorie requirements. Many times, the best method will seem obvious. However, in certain situations, more careful analysis is necessary to make the most reasonable decision. The therapeutic methods available at an institution may dictate the most feasible plan, and in such cases, theoretical analysis will not necessarily indicate the most suitable method of nutritional therapy.

1. **Types of nutritional support.** The two broad categories of nutritional support (i.e., not relying on table foods) are enteral therapy and parenteral therapy. Details of these feeding techniques are covered in Chapters 9 and 10, respectively.

   a. **Enteral therapy** can be divided into *oral feeding* and *forced enteral feeding,* or tube feeding. Forced enteral feeding includes both nasoenteric tube feeding and gastrostomy or enterostomy feeding.

   b. **Parenteral therapy** can be divided into *partial parenteral nutrition* and *total parenteral nutrition* via a peripheral or central vein. The general use of the terms *total parenteral nutrition* and *hyperalimentation* to refer only to central vein parenteral nutrition is incorrect because the provision may be neither total nor above normal requirements. As a rule, enteral support is preferred to parenteral forms of nutritional therapy because morbidity and expense are less.

2. **Factors in assessing adequacy of the intestinal tract.** In many situations, the intestinal tract is unavailable, at least transiently, to accept food products. Having intestinal disease *per se,* however, does not necessarily preclude the use of enteral nutrition. Various factors are involved in assessing the availability and adequacy of the intestinal tract. Estimating the adequacy of the gastrointestinal tract for enteral nutrition requires a consideration of basic physiology. The ultimate determination in clinical practice often must be made by trial and error.

   a. **Motility requirements**

      (1) **Deglutition.** Normal deglutition is necessary for *oral* enteral therapy and can be impaired in severe local oropharyngeal disease and bulbar central nervous system disease. Severe abnormalities do not prevent use of the stomach and small bowel for enteral therapy with tube feeding techniques.

      (2) **Esophageal motility.** Most esophageal motility disorders do not interfere with nutrition, especially on an acute basis in hospitalized patients. Severe achalasia can result in impaired delivery of food to the small bowel. Esophageal clearance of solids is gravity-dependent. Poor clearance of pills and food cubes has been demonstrated in supine patients, but the problem resolves with upright posture.

      (3) **Gastric motility.** Satisfactory gastric motility is necessary for successful oral or nasogastric enteral therapy. Gastric emptying is not gravity-dependent but rather relies on gastric neuromuscular integrity and gastroduodenal coordination. The causes of gastric retention are many (Table 8-5). Gastric motility disturbances, in contrast to obstructive causes of gastric retention, do not always preclude the use of oral or nasogastric tube feeding, especially when the disturbance is mild.

      (4) **Small-bowel motility.** Assessment is more difficult than for the esophagus and stomach. The detrimental effects of abnormal small-bowel motility are also more difficult to anticipate in estimating small-bowel adequacy. Even a very prolonged radiographic small-bowel transit time (>6 hours), which can be associated with celiac disease, amyloidosis, or pseudoobstruction syndromes, does not necessarily prevent enteral therapy. A complete absence of bowel sounds or a failure to pass flatus in diffuse ileus is the best indicator that small-bowel motility is unsatisfactory.

   b. **Intestinal length.** The minimum length of small bowel to provide an adequate absorptive surface is variable and depends on the de-

Table 8-5. Causes of gastric retention

Mechanical obstruction	Altered motility
Duodenal ulcer	Ileus (e.g., postoperative, metabolic)
Pyloric channel ulcer	Anticholinergic drugs
Gastric carcinoma	Vagotomy (retention of solid foods)
Proximal small-bowel carcinoma	Diabetes mellitus and other
Adhesions	autonomic neuropathies
Pyloric stenosis	Spinal cord injury
Pancreatitis	Acute central nervous system disease
Pancreatic carcinoma	Chronic degenerative central nervous
	system disease
	Hypocalcemia
	Hypothyroidism
	Pain
	Opiates
	Severe protein deficiency
	Pseudoobstruction syndromes

gree of adaptation of the remaining intestine, the presence or absence of the ileocecal valve, and the presence of intrinsic pathology in the remaining bowel. A general guideline is that at least 2 ft of jejunum (radiographically) beyond the ligament of Treitz is required to provide sufficient absorptive surface that ordinary table foods can be tolerated.

- **(1)** Patients with considerably more small bowel than this still require specific nutrient supplementation and dietary modification. Ileal adaptation cannot replace the absorptive capacity of the duodenum and jejunum because of the smaller initial surface area. Consequently, loss of the proximal small bowel results in profound malabsorption even when most of the ileum is preserved.
- **(2)** The proximal small bowel cannot provide active transport of bile acids and vitamin B_{12}, even when the mucosa becomes hypertrophic. Specific management of the short-bowel syndrome is covered in Chapter 9.

- c. **Surface area.** Diffuse mucosal small-bowel diseases (e.g., nontropical sprue, Whipple's disease, lymphangiectasia, lymphoma) readily produce malabsorption by decreasing the available functional mucosal surface. The mucosal absorptive area is normally amplified by the plicae circulares ($\times 3$), villi ($\times 10$), and microvilli ($\times 20$). Altogether, these factors increase the surface area of the intestinal cylinder 600-fold. Some interference with absorption can be predicted by the radiographic pattern and peroral small-bowel biopsy findings, but the degree of impairment can best be estimated by the resulting degree of malabsorption (fecal fat determination) during a therapeutic trial or test period. Suspecting surface area inadequacy should not prevent an attempt at using the intestinal tract for nutritional support, but it may be preferable to use a modified diet (Chapter 11), enteral supplementation (Chapter 9), or parenteral nutrition (Chapter 10).

3. Situations and disorders interfering with enteral feeding

- a. **Severe diarrheal illnesses,** regardless of the cause, interfere with enteral feeding. These include acute infectious enteritis and other secretory diarrheal illnesses. If fecal output increases with enteral feeding, then such support is interfering with overall patient management. Moderate diarrheal illnesses sometimes may be controlled with antidiarrheal medication, which may also control the diarrhea that occurs with enteral feeding.

b. **In extensive Crohn's disease** of the small bowel, enteral therapy may be feasible and is not contraindicated, especially if the patient does not become markedly symptomatic with the administration of food. Providing parenteral nutrition and not placing any food products into the intestinal tract ("bowel rest") have not proved beneficial but may help some patients. Prolonged administration (>3 weeks) of parenteral nutrition with bowel rest is usually required if this technique is expected to assist in remission of disease. Enteral feeding is feasible in patients with (a) a lack of symptoms (mainly pain) after feeding and (b) adequate absorption to meet protein and energy requirements. Placing food in the intestinal tract does not worsen the disease process itself. In children, but not adults, enteral feeding compares favorably with glucocorticoids for the management of symptoms.

c. **Severe active inflammatory colonic diseases.** Colonic disease *per se* does not imply a need for parenteral support. Low-residue diets ensure little ileal volume for delivery to the colon. Colonic integrity is not necessary for intestinal absorption of protein and calories. However, motor activity of the colon responds, probably through both neural and hormonal mechanisms, to the introduction of food into the upper intestinal tract. Consequently, patients with severe colonic disorders, such as those listed below, may become more symptomatic (diarrhea and pain) during enteral feeding.
   1. Acute extensive ulcerative colitis or Crohn's colitis
   2. Diverticulitis
   3. Extensive pseudomembranous colitis

d. **Acute gastrointestinal bleeding.** During the early evaluation of upper or lower gastrointestinal bleeding, enteral feeding is not indicated. Feeding will interfere with radiographic and endoscopic investigation and any surgical intervention that may be necessary.

e. **Imminent abdominal surgery.** Concern for nutritional support should not override one's judgment regarding the best management of patients with undiagnosed abdominal disorders that will probably require surgical intervention.

f. **Obstructing lesions of the small bowel or colon.** Enteral feeding is not strictly contraindicated in patients with chronic obstruction. Minimal-residue products fed through a tube can be adequately absorbed through a short length of small bowel above an obstruction. If the patient requires suction for decompression and symptomatic relief, then enteral feeding should be withheld. If the introduction of enteral products precipitates symptoms by enhancing small-bowel or colon motility, then this method must be abandoned.

g. **Ileus.** Diffuse postoperative ileus, in association with severe medical illness or intraabdominal pathology, generally prevents the use of enteral feeding. The absorptive capacity remains intact, but retention of the food products and secretions in the proximal intestine and stomach leads to vomiting and possibly pulmonary aspiration. Determining that the motility disturbance is severe enough to prevent enteral therapy may require a therapeutic trial. The trial should be terminated if vomiting or gastric retention occurs. A trial should not be attempted if bowel sounds are completely absent and no stool or flatus is passed.

h. **Acute inflammation of the pancreas or biliary tract.** Hormonal stimulation of these structures by feeding may exacerbate symptoms. No evidence has been found that feeding prolongs an episode of acute cholecystitis or pancreatitis. Evidence does indicate that nasogastric suction (which is performed only without feeding) decreases pain in acute pancreatitis, but it does not appear to alter the course of the illness. Recognizing that the reason for withholding feeding in these situations is to prevent or reduce symptoms of the primary disease process or a resulting ileus, the physician should attempt to resume enteral feeding as soon as the clinical picture allows. Recent changes in the approach to the patient with acute pancreatitis have resulted in earlier enteral feeding.

4. **Available methods in the intact intestinal tract.** Three general methods are available to deliver food to the alimentary tract. Each has advantages and disadvantages. All allow balanced, nutritionally complete diets to be delivered and utilize the natural absorptive mechanisms of the intestinal tract.

   a. **Oral feeding** is always the preferred form of support. Nutritional needs can be met with standard diets and commercially available supplements (see Chapter 9).

      (1) **Advantages**
          (a) Physiologic
          (b) Least expensive
          (c) Socially well accepted
      (2) **Disadvantages.** None.

   b. **Nasogastric or nasoduodenal tube feeding** is a method of utilizing the intestinal tract when requirements for successful oral feeding cannot be met. Small-caliber feeding tubes are commercially available that can be placed into the stomach or proximal small bowel with little morbidity and satisfactory patient acceptance. Techniques of placement and a description of the available tubes are presented in Chapter 9, Section IV, as are the advantages and disadvantages of the various forms of forced enteral feeding.

      Patients with advanced *dementia* are one of the largest groups receiving tube feeding. These patients often have difficulty eating, and food-related problems increase as dementia progresses. They may resist eating, experience dysphagia, or aspirate. For these reasons, gastrostomy tubes are frequently placed in patients with dementia. However, a review of the literature revealed no evidence that tube feeding prolonged life in these patients (11).

      (1) **Advantages**
          (a) The need for adequate appetite or deglutition is circumvented.
          (b) Inexpensive nutrition is provided; several commercially available products are satisfactory and complete.
          (c) This provides a safe method of forced feeding (see Chapter 9, Section IV, for a description of complications).
      (2) **Disadvantages**
          (a) An indwelling tube that causes nasopharyngeal irritation is required, and the patient is deprived of the various pleasant sensations associated with eating. Tubes with diameters of 3 mm or less are much less irritating than larger, stiffer tubes and can be tolerated for long periods.
          (b) It is less psychologically and socially acceptable, especially for outpatient use.

   c. **Tube gastrostomy or enterostomy feeding** requires placement of a feeding tube through the abdominal wall into the stomach or a loop of proximal jejunum. The two types of tubes are compared in Chapter 9, Section IV.

      (1) **Advantages**
          (a) A completely obstructing lesion of the proximal intestinal tract does not preclude placement of a jejunostomy tube distal to the obstruction.

        (b) Bolus feeding through a large-bore tube allows an ambulatory patient more freedom.

        (c) Certain patients may find this method more psychologically or socially acceptable than a nasal tube.

    (2) Disadvantages

        (a) Surgery, endoscopy, or interventional radiology is required, usually with sedation.

        (b) More tube care is needed than with nasally placed tubes.

5. Management when the intestinal tract is not available and adequate

  a. Methods of feeding. If the entire calculated requirements cannot be given enterally, then parenteral support can be used either to supplement enteral feeding or to meet the determined requirements totally. Parenteral nutrition can be provided through a central or a peripheral vein. *Total parenteral nutrition* by either method is reserved for situations in which therapy is deemed urgent or when the intestinal tract remains completely unusable. *Partial parenteral nutrition* can be offered to complete requirements when enteral nutrition alone is not satisfactory. Because of the potential morbidity associated with *central vein parenteral nutrition* (usually total parenteral nutrition), this method of therapy is not generally instituted if the duration of need is anticipated to be less than 7 to 10 days (see Section IIC). However, the anticipation is an estimate, and severely malnourished patients can be candidates for central vein parenteral nutrition even when new deficits are expected to be small. Advantages and disadvantages of central and peripheral parenteral nutrition are discussed in the next section.

  b. Parenteral nutrition by central venous route

    (1) Advantages

        (a) The catheter can be left in place for long periods.

        (b) High-osmolarity solutions can meet protein and calorie requirements.

    (2) Disadvantages

        (a) Complications of the central IV line may develop.

        (b) High-osmolarity solutions may cause metabolic complications.

  c. Parenteral nutrition by peripheral venous route

    (1) Advantages

        (a) A central line is not required.

        (b) Fewer metabolic complications develop than with high-osmolarity solutions.

    (2) Disadvantages

        (a) Frequent catheter changes are required.

        (b) Severe thrombophlebitis is common.

        (c) Volume limitations can prevent protein and calorie requirements from being met.

        (d) Peripheral line placement may limit patient mobility.

  d. Limitations of parenteral nutrition. Parenteral nutrition may not easily supply all protein and calorie requirements because of (a) osmolarity limitations of IV solutions and (b) volume limitations in a 24-hour period. This is particularly true when peripheral veins are used. Examples of typical base solutions used for peripheral parenteral nutrition are given in Chapter 9, Section IV. *Regarding peripheral parenteral nutrition:*

    (1) Even with the supplemental use of fat emulsions, more than 3,000 mL/d is required to provide 2,500 nonprotein calories. Osmolarity limitations make it difficult to achieve the large nonprotein calorie–nitrogen ratios desired in parenteral nutrition to ensure optimal use of delivered amino acids.

(2) If estimated calorie and protein requirements are incompletely met by oral feeding and oral supplements, additional calories and protein can be delivered by the peripheral parenteral route without exceeding the volume and osmolarity limitations.

C. **Total parenteral nutrition and complete bowel rest as primary therapy.** Certain patients qualify for total parenteral nutrition with complete bowel rest (nothing by mouth) regardless of their current nutritional status. These are rare circumstances overall (e.g., refractory Crohn's disease, enterocutaneous fistulae), and the primary indications are outlined in Chapter 9, Section I. Because few patients fit into this category, the key questions included in usual nutrition planning do not consider this possibility.

V. **Formulating a final protein and calorie support plan.** The final plan is designed according to the previously mentioned considerations. The key questions lead to decisions regarding the urgency of support and methods of protein and calorie delivery. More than one suitable method of support are usually available. An appropriate plan does not interfere with usual medical care but rather is an effective adjuvant to medical and surgical therapeutics. Of importance to the clinician is the appropriate selection of patients for intensive nutritional support (forced enteral feeding and total parenteral nutrition). The key questions can help select these patients. Figure 8-1 presents an algorithm based on the key questions that are useful in selecting patients with negative protein and calorie balance for intensive nutritional support. The following examples refer to the algorithm.

A. **Example 1**

1. **History.** A 26-year-old man with a 7-year history of Crohn's disease and two prior small-bowel resections enters the hospital because of an exacerbation of symptoms. Despite outpatient therapy with immunosuppressive medications, he has continued to experience fatigue, a poor appetite, crampy postprandial abdominal pain, diarrhea, and low-grade fevers, but he does not appear dehydrated. His weight has dropped from 142 lb (usual) to 130 lb (8.5% decrease) in the past 3 months. Physical examination reveals a thin man with a tender abdominal mass in the right lower quadrant. Laboratory data include the following values: hemoglobin, 12.2 g/dL; white blood cell count, 16,000/mm^3 (he is receiving corticosteroids); 9% lymphocytes (total lymphocyte count, 1,440/mm^3); serum albumin, 3.2 g/dL; and total iron-binding capacity, 270 mg/dL. A small-bowel radiographic study shows multiple skip lesions typical of Crohn's disease in the remaining ileum with a very narrowed distal segment proximal to the prior anastomosis.

2. **Impression and plan.** Although the degree of recent weight loss suggests that significant protein–calorie malnutrition may be present, screening laboratory tests indicate that the degree of depletion is probably not severe. Despite the favorable assessment, total parenteral nutrition may be indicated in this situation because of the patient's poor appetite and to lessen his discomfort during the management of refractory extensive Crohn's disease of the small bowel. The planned course of therapy will probably exceed 3 to 4 weeks.

B. **Example 2**

1. **History.** A 49-year-old alcoholic man is admitted with acute epigastric pain boring through to the back, nausea, and vomiting of 24 hours' duration. The diagnosis of acute pancreatitis is made; nasogastric suction and IV fluids are initiated. Although the patient denies significant weight change in the past 6 months, the admitting physician reports that the patient appears somewhat wasted. Initial laboratory values include serum albumin, 2.7 g/dL; total lymphocyte count, 1,000/mm^3; and total iron-binding capacity, 200 mg/dL. Mumps and streptokinase-streptodornase (SKSD) skin tests are placed as controls for a tuberculin skin test, but the patient fails to react to any of these skin-test antigens.

2. **Impressions and plan.** Laboratory data support the clinical impression of significant (moderate to severe) protein–calorie malnutrition and

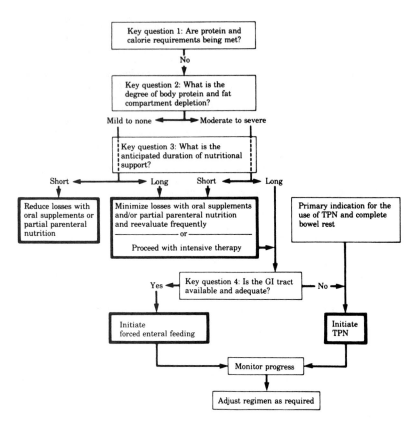

FIG. 8.1. A flow diagram useful for selecting patients in negative protein and calorie balance for intensive nutritional support. TPN, total parenteral nutrition; GI, gastrointestinal.

severe disease. Failure to react to the skin tests also may be a consequence of malnutrition. The established deficiencies are suspected to be a result of chronically poor intake accompanying alcoholism. Although the protein and calorie balances are negative while the patient is receiving IV 5% dextrose in water, the current illness is expected to be short. The current illness prevents use of the intestinal tract, and peripheral vein dextrose–amino acid solutions can be used to minimize further losses in this already depleted patient pending resolution of his illness.

C. **Example 3**

1. **History.** Fever and a productive cough have developed in a 72-year-old woman in previously good health. Because her appetite is poor and her fluid intake inadequate, she is admitted for therapy. She appears acutely ill and mildly dehydrated. Radiographic examination of the chest confirms the diagnosis of lobar pneumonia. Laboratory studies reveal normal hemoglobin and albumin levels and a normal lymphocyte count. Nutritional history estimates a recent daily intake of 650 kcal and 20 g of protein.

2. **Impression and plan.** No historical features suggest protein–calorie malnutrition in this patient, and the laboratory data support the impression. Remember, however, that albumin levels are affected by hydration.

Current intake does not match calculated requirements, but the illness is expected to be short. Oral liquid supplements are offered to improve fluid, protein, and calorie balance until the pneumonia resolves and a regular diet is tolerated.

D. Example 4

1. **History.** Progressive respiratory failure has developed in a 58-year-old man with chronic obstructive lung disease and several recent acute respiratory infections. He is admitted and requires mechanical ventilation. His weight has fallen from 166 to 156 lb (6% decrease) in the past 6 months. Laboratory values include a serum albumin level of 3.0 g/dL, total iron-binding capacity of 240 mg/dL, and total lymphocyte count of 1,100/mm^3. Anthropometric data obtained in the intensive care unit revealed both the triceps skinfold measurement and midarm muscle circumference to be below the tenth percentile for the population of individuals with the patient's usual body weight. Current treatment includes 150 g of IV dextrose per day as the only calorie source.

2. **Impression and plan.** Clinical, laboratory, and anthropometric data suggest a moderate degree of protein–calorie malnutrition. In this case, the anticipated duration of nutritional support is unclear. Because of the existing deficiencies, it is reasonable to proceed with intensive support. Forced enteral feeding with a small-caliber nasoduodenal tube is initiated.

E. Example 5

1. **History.** A 52-year-old woman is transferred from another hospital after a complicated postoperative course. Within the past 8 weeks, she has undergone a vagotomy and pyloroplasty for peptic ulcer disease and then reoperation for gastric outlet obstruction with creation of a gastrojejunostomy. The stoma is functioning poorly. She continues to require nasogastric suction because of vomiting, and a revision of the anastomosis will be necessary. She appears to be overweight (height of 65 in), but her weight has fallen from 220 to 192 lb (13% decrease) in the past 2½ months. She states that she is very weak. Laboratory values include a white blood cell count of 5,200/mm^3, 12% lymphocytes (total lymphocyte count of 620/mm^3), serum albumin level of 2.13 g/dL, and total iron-binding capacity of 180 mg/dL (estimated transferrin level, 100 mg/dL).

2. **Impression and plan.** The history of recent operations and weight loss suggests that significant protein–calorie malnutrition may be present. In this case, initially excessive fat stores have prevented the appearance of wasting despite persistent negative balances and concomitant protein losses. Laboratory data (albumin, transferrin, total lymphocyte count) support the suspicion that severe body protein depletion has developed. Based on the current degree of negative balance (her only intake is IV 5% dextrose) and the fact that another laparotomy is necessary, it is felt that the anticipated duration of support may be long. The patient is appropriately selected for intensive nutritional support; because the intestinal tract is not readily available for use, total parenteral nutrition is instituted. It is decided to give the patient 3 weeks of total parenteral nutrition before her third laparotomy.

F. Example 6

1. **History.** A 66-year-old woman is admitted because of diarrhea, a poor appetite, and a 5% weight loss in the past 23 months. Twelve months ago, she completed a course of radiation therapy for carcinoma of the cervix. Small-bowel series reveals several long areas of fold thickening and spiculation in the distal ileum, consistent with radiation enteritis. Laboratory values include a serum albumin of 3.0 g/dL, serum transferrin level (estimated from the total iron-binding capacity) of 190 mg/dL, and total lymphocyte count of 1,200/mm^3. A creatinine–height index of 68% is calculated from a 24-hour urinary creatinine collection, originally ordered for determining creatinine clearance. Inpatient calorie counts reveal a daily intake of 800 to 900 kcal and 20 to 30 g of protein.

2. Impression and plan. At least a mild degree of protein–calorie malnutrition is suggested by the history and screening laboratory tests. Protein losses may be occurring from the intestinal tract, and these losses would accelerate the rate of protein depletion. The nearly normal serum transferrin level may be a result of concomitant iron deficiency secondary to persistent gastrointestinal blood loss. The anticipated length of negative balance is uncertain, and attempts are made to increase oral intake with low-fat, high-protein commercial supplements. Antidiarrheal medications are also used. Although the diarrhea abates, repeated calorie counts suggest that the negative balance of about 500 kcal/d is persisting because of poor appetite. Forced enteral feeding with similar formulas via a nasoduodenal tube is offered to the patient, but she chooses to continue to try oral supplements; she wishes to be discharged and be reevaluated in several weeks.

Bibliography

1. Rochester DF. Malnutrition and the respiratory muscles. *Clin Chest Med* 1986;7:91.
2. Klein S. Enteral and parenteral nutrition. In: Sleisenger M, Fordtran J, eds. *Gastrointestinal disease,* 5th ed. Philadelphia: WB Saunders, 1993:2085.
3. Matarese LE. Enteral feeding solutions. *Gastrointest Endosc Clin N Am* 1998;8:593.
4. Klein S, Kinney J, JeeJeebhoy K, et al. Nutrition support in clinical practice: review of published data and recommendations for future research directions. *JPEN J Parenter Enteral Nutr* 1997;21:133.
5. Lord L, et al. Enteral nutrition implementation and management. In: *The ASPEN nutrition support practice manual.* Silver Spring, MD: American Society for Parenteral and Enteral Nutrition, 1998:5.
6. Klein S. Short-chain fatty acids and the colon. *Gastroenterology* 1992;102:364.
7. Moore FA, Feliciano DV, Andrassy RJ, et al. Early enteral feeding, compared with parenteral, reduces postoperative septic complications. *Ann Surg* 1991;216:172.
8. Reynolds JV, Kanwar S, Welsh FKS, et al. Does the route of feeding modify gut barrier function and clinical outcome in patients after major upper gastrointestinal surgery? *JPEN J Parenter Enteral Nutr* 1997;21:196.
9. Raff T, Hartmann B, Germann G. Early intragastric feeding of seriously burned and long-term ventilated patients: a review of 55 patients. *Burns* 1997;23:19.
10. Hochwald SN, Harrison LE, Heslin MJ, et al. Early postoperative enteral feeding improves whole body protein kinetics in upper gastrointestinal cancer patients. *Am J Surg* 1997;174:325.
11. Finucane TE, Christmas C, Travis K. Tube feeding in patients with advanced dementia: a review of the evidence. *JAMA* 1999;282:1365.

9. ENTERAL NUTRITIONAL THERAPY

I. **General principles.** This chapter outlines methods of providing the major nutrients (protein and calories) if usual diets are inadequate or ineffective. Enteral protein and calorie therapy includes *supplementation* with usual foods and commercially available products and *enteral feeding*. The Board of Directors of the American Society of Parenteral and Enteral Nutrition has published *Guidelines for the Use of Parenteral and Enteral Nutrition in Adult and Pediatric Patients* (1), a very useful reference.

A. **Forced enteral feeding** is an intensive form of enteral nutritional support in which tube feeding techniques are used. Diets of forced enteral feeding are nutritionally complete and provide not only protein and calories but also all other essential nutrients.

B. **Modification of the basic diet** is often necessary in the nutritional management of certain diseases. Modified diets for specific diseases may or may not incorporate commercial supplements; these diets are covered in Chapters 11 and 12. Techniques used in managing two special problems of protein and calorie absorption (pancreatic insufficiency and short-bowel syndrome) are outlined in Sections VI and VII of this chapter.

C. **Micronutrient deficiencies** are often also present in patients who require protein and calorie support. Many of the supplements recommended are fortified with vitamins and minerals. The replacement of isolated micronutrient deficiencies is covered in Chapters 6 and 7.

D. **Essential fatty acid (EFA) deficiency** is uncommon as an isolated deficiency; it is seen most often in patients who are severely deficient in protein and calories or who are being treated with parenteral nutrition without EFA supplementation. EFA requirements and replacement are covered in Sections II and IV of Chapter 10.

II. **Indications for enteral therapy**

A. **Indications for oral supplementation.** Hospitalized patients are often placed on modified-consistency diets (see Chapter 11, Section II) with inadequate protein or calorie content to meet daily requirements. Supplements improve daily intake. More frequently, protein and calorie supplements are used to bolster usual diets in a reliable way. It is often as easy, if not easier, to instruct a patient to take one or two cans of a supplement with a defined nutritional content as it is to suggest a selection of foods that may be unfamiliar or unappealing to the patient. Many commercial supplements are now available in multiple flavors to avoid taste monotony in long-term use. Certain groups of people are particularly good candidates for dietary supplements.

1. **Persons with a daily energy deficit by calorie count,** including the following:

a. **Patients chronically ill with anorexia,** who may not be meeting requirements. Weight loss can be diminished by adding nutritional supplements.

b. **Persons with an increased energy expenditure of activity (EEA)** may have a daily deficit despite a relatively normal appetite. Examples follow:

(1) **Athletes** may have an increased EEA during training and be in daily negative caloric balance.

(2) **Patients with anorexia nervosa** often have an increased EEA despite a relatively normal-appearing caloric intake.

(3) **Patients with chronic inflammatory diseases** may have increased energy requirements because of inflammation but maintain only a usual caloric intake for their size.

2. **Patients preparing for tests,** specifically radiographic studies, are subjected to a negative caloric balance day after day in the hospital. Nutritional supplements, particularly in combination with a clear liquid

diet, can minimize nutritional losses. Many low-residue commercially available supplements can be used in conjunction with the clear liquid diet. In most cases, low-residue supplements added to the diet while the colon is being prepared do not compromise the quality of a barium enema or colonoscopy.

3. **Patients with specific dietary needs** benefit from the special characteristics of many commercially available supplements.

   a. **Most supplements are low in residue** because they contain no vegetable or meat fiber. Supplements containing no fiber and no fat probably add the least to the volume entering the colon. Blenderized foods contain greater amounts of indigestible fiber. Soy polysaccharide has been added to several supplements to increase their fiber content. *High-fiber products* may be beneficial to patients with altered bowel habits resulting from functional motor disorders.

   b. **Many lactose-free supplements are available.** Corn syrup solids, sucrose, glucose, and other sugars serve a source of carbohydrate; casein, soy protein, egg whites, or amino acids (or a combination of these) serve as a source of protein, so that the need for milk additives or lactose is avoided.

   c. **Supplements high in carbohydrate content** as a calorie source are useful for patients on low-fat diets. Supplements low in carbohydrate may be beneficial to patients with severe respiratory disease (see Section IVA).

   d. **Patients requiring liquid or soft diets** because of an inability to chew foods, painful oral lesions, strictures of the esophagus, or poor gastric antral motor activity may prefer commercially prepared supplements to usual dietary liquids or blenderized and puréed foods. Usual dietary liquids alone are deficient in the vitamins and minerals normally delivered by dietary vegetables and meats. Commercial supplements can guarantee satisfactory vitamin and mineral allowances along with protein and calorie supplementation.

   e. **Supplements with modified amino acid profiles** have been developed for patients with renal failure, chronic liver disease, and increased metabolic stress.

      (1) **For patients with renal failure,** essential amino acids added to a diet low in total protein content help to promote a positive nitrogen balance without causing unacceptable increases in blood urea nitrogen (BUN). The amino acid profiles in these supplements are designed to meet and exceed by several times the normal essential amino acid requirements, but the optimal supplementation of essential amino acids is unknown. Supplementation of a diet containing 18 to 20 g of protein with 13 to 26 g of essential amino acids daily may prolong the period of conservative treatment in patients with chronic renal failure and postpone the start of regular dialysis (2).

      (2) **Patients with chronic liver disease and hepatic encephalopathy** also have consistently abnormal plasma amino acid profiles, with an increase in aromatic amino acids (phenylalanine, tyrosine, tryptophan) and decreased proportions of branched-chain amino acids (isoleucine, leucine, valine). Protein supplements rich in branched-chain amino acids can be added to the protein-restricted diet to assist in establishing a positive nitrogen balance without precipitating encephalopathy. Disease-specific protein supplements are covered in Section IIIB.

      (3) **The rationale for supplementing branched-chain amino acids** in cases of increased metabolic stress is given in Sections III and VI of Chapter 10. In general, these formulas are reserved for forced enteral feeding.

B. Indications for enteral feeding

1. **Patients selected for intensive protein and calorie support** (as discussed in Chapter 8) are those who are severely malnourished or are expected to become protein-depleted because of persistent negative nitrogen balance. Once a patient is selected for intensive nutritional support, the availability and adequacy of the intestinal tract must be evaluated. Forced enteral feeding is generally preferred to total parenteral nutrition (TPN) if the intestinal tract can be used for the reasons outlined in Section III of Chapter 8. Patients who qualify for forced enteral feeding often have one or several of the following problems:

   a. Existing severe protein or protein–calorie malnutrition

   b. Anorexia

   c. Fractures of the head and neck or neurologic disorders preventing satisfactory oral feeding

   d. Coma or depressed mental state

   e. Need for prolonged assisted ventilation

   f. Serious medical or surgical illnesses (e.g., burns) in which metabolic requirements are very high

2. **Specific indications for the use of enteral feeding**

   a. Enterocutaneous fistulae have been reported to close with the continuous use of defined formula diets in up to 70% of cases; however, series reporting the use of enteral feeding for the primary treatment of enterocutaneous fistulas are small and uncontrolled. Complete bowel rest with the use of TPN has been employed more commonly as a nonsurgical attempt to close fistulae before definitive surgery. Primary treatment of fistulae with enteral feeding or TPN may require several months to be effective, but fistulae usually recur with the resumption of oral feeding (3).

   b. Small-bowel adaptation following massive intestinal resection and subsequent short-bowel syndrome occurs when intraluminal nutrients are again presented to the remaining small-bowel mucosa. The introduction of hydrolyzed amino acids and concentrated carbohydrates in the form of elemental diets has been used to encourage small-bowel recovery and adaptation and hasten conversion to regular oral feedings; however, no convincing data support this approach. Because many elemental products are unpalatable, enteral feeding with them may be more effective while the transition is made to oral feeding in patients with short-bowel syndrome. Enteral nutrition can be used even if diarrhea occurs in this setting.

   c. Preparation of the bowel for surgery has been carried out with a low-residue, chemically defined diet. In patients who are seriously ill or seriously malnourished, this may be accomplished most effectively with enteral feeding of low-residue formulas.

   d. Crohn's disease of the small bowel can be managed with total bowel rest and TPN if feeding causes intolerable symptoms. Many symptoms of Crohn's disease of the small bowel are exacerbated by feeding. In some patients, however, feeding of a low-residue, highly absorbed formula does not produce intestinal symptoms yet allows adequate nutritional support pending clinical remission of the inflammatory bowel disease. Data are insufficient to estimate the effectiveness of forced enteral feeding in inducing remission of inflammatory bowel disease. Forced enteral nutrition with an elemental diet has been proposed as an approach to reduce inflammation in Crohn's disease. Controlled trials have compared elemental diets with prednisone. Some trials found them equally effective, whereas others found prednisone to be superior (4). Studies supporting this use of an elemental diet as primary therapy included patients who had to be force-fed or did not analyze those who could not tolerate oral feedings. Metaanalyses of these studies found prednisone to be superior to elemental diets (5,6). It is possible, however, that ordinary diets stimulate inflammation in certain patients. If this concept is correct, then TPN with nothing by mouth or elemental diets may be useful in a subset of patients as primary therapy.

  e. Severe acute pancreatitis was for years considered an indication for TPN. Enteral nutrition was considered contraindicated because it was thought that it would worsen pancreatic damage. Recent studies have demonstrated that a partially elemental diet administered through a nasoenteral tube is well tolerated in acute pancreatitis (7,8).

  f. Dementia as an indication for enteral nutrition is discussed in Section IV of Chapter 8.

III. Supplementation of the diet with protein and calories

  A. Feeding modules. Almost all the familiar commercial products for oral supplementation or tube feeding are "complete" formulas that provide a mixture of macronutrients and micronutrients. These products supply a person's nutritional needs completely if taken in sufficient quantity. In addition to the "complete" formulations, commercial sources produce feeding modules that provide a single macronutrient. Feeding modules for protein, carbohydrate, and fat are available (Table 9-1), as are modules for vitamins and minerals. These modules can be used to alter commercial formulas or as an oral supplement, to tailor both tube feedings and oral diets to a patient's unique nutritional requirements. Feeding modules are more expensive than "complete" formulations.

  B. Protein supplementation can be with the usual dietary constituents or with commercially available supplements. Protein sources can differ in taste and effectiveness. Foods and commercial products that are high in protein can be unpalatable to the patient with anorexia. Amino acids and oligopeptides have a particularly medicinal aroma and taste. The quality of a protein supplement as a source of amino acids for growth is referred to as the *biologic value of the protein*. The protein content of various foods is listed in Table 11-19.

  1. Protein supplementation with table foods. Patients with normal appetites who are not meeting daily protein requirements or who require additional protein supplementation for protein compartment depletion may benefit from dietary alterations with table foods. Table 9-2 lists the usual foods that can serve as dietary protein supplements. Certain characteristics of these foods may limit their use depending on coexisting intestinal disorders.

  a. Milk products. The lactose content is high; hard cheeses contain the least lactose per serving. The fat content is at least 4 g per serving (serving sizes are listed in Table 9-2) except for skim and nonfat dry milk, both of which have less than 1 g/cup. Most cheeses are high in fat, but a selection made with skim milk is available.

  b. Eggs. Egg whites contain protein without lipid. The cholesterol is in the yolk.

  c. Peanut butter contains 8 g of fat per tablespoon (50% of its weight is fat).

  d. Fish. Flat fish are lowest in triglyceride, whereas steaklike fish has a fat content quantitatively similar to that of beef.

  3. Supplementation with commercially available products. Although the use of table foods as protein sources would seem ideal, the use of commercial supplements is probably more reliable in most cases. Table 9-1 classifies modular nutritional products depending on the type of nutrient provided. Isolated protein supplements (Casec powder, ProMod) are concentrated but expensive for daily use. Supplements that provide both protein and nonprotein calories (e.g., Ensure) may be the most convenient and palatable for the majority of patients who require additional protein (Table 9-3). The most appropriate protein supplement for an individual

Table 9-1. Feeding modules

Product	Manufac-turer	Major nutrient source	Protein (g/100 g)	CHO (g/100 g)	Fat (g/100 g)	Calories (kcal/100 g)	Na (mg/100 g)	K (mg/100 g)	Cl (mg/100 g)	Ca (mg/100 g)	Phosphate (mg/100 g)
Protein modules											
Casec	Mead	Calcium caseinate	90	NA	2	380	100	10	300	1,400	800
ProMod	Ross	Whey protein	76	<10	<9	424	<227	<985	NA	<667	<500
Carbohydrate modules											
Moducal	Mead	Glucose	0	95	0	380	70	5	170	NA	NA
Polycose liquid	Ross	Glucose polymers	0	2.5/5 mL	0	10/5 mL	Trace	Trace	<7/5 mL	<1/5 mL	Trace
Polycose powder	Ross	Glucose polymers	0	94	0	380	<110	<10	<223	<30	<5
Fat modules											
MCT Oil	Mead	Coconut oil	0	0	NA	830	NA	NA	NA	NA	NA

NA, not applicable; CHO, carbohydrate; MCT, medium-chain triglyceride.

Table 9-2. Common foods that can serve as supplemental sources of protein for the usual diet

Protein source	Biologic value	Food	Serving size	Approximate protein content (g per serving)
Milk	85	Whole milk	1 cup	8.5
		Skin milk	1 cup	9
		Nonfat dry milk	1 tbs	2.7
		Ice cream	1 cup	6
		Ice milk	1 cup	6
		Cottage cheese	1 cup	30
		Yogurt (low-fat)	1 cup	8
		Cheese slice	1 oz	6–8
Egg	85	Egg	1 large	7
		Eggnog	1 cup	12
Vegetable	70–75	Peanut butter	1 tbs	4
Meat	75–90	Lean beef	1 oz	7
		Fresh fish	1 oz	7
		Tuna	1 oz	7
		Chicken/turkey (without skin)	1 oz	8

patient will meet the desired and calculated requirements together with dietary sources of protein, be palatable, and comply with any dietary restrictions.

3. **Disease-specific protein supplements** (Table 9-4) contain amino acids in proportions thought to be beneficial in the dietary management of renal and hepatic disease (see Section IIA) and severe catabolic states. Specific nutritional characteristics of these supplements are given in Tables 9-3, 9-5, and 9-6.

   a. Several products have a negligible *electrolyte content*; water used in reconstituting the powders may add considerably to the final electrolyte content. (The sodium content of water varies from 0 to 500 mg/L. The average sodium content of local tap water is available from the water utility company. St. Louis tap water contains on average 35 to 50 mg of sodium per liter.)

   b. The usual daily supplement of Amin-Aid varies from two to four packets per day and provides approximately 15 to 30 g of amino acids. Modification of the protein requirement in *renal disease* is outlined in Section II of Chapter 12. Patients on dialysis do not require a special renal formula; they can be managed on standard enteral preparations, which are much less expensive.

   c. Oral branched-chain amino acid supplements are less likely than dietary protein to precipitate hepatic encephalopathy in patients with *chronic liver disease*. Hepatic-Aid and NutriHep are oral supplements that are rich in branched-chain amino acids. Supplementation with 10 to 60 g of protein as amino acids is the suggested daily range, which should be adjusted to the patient's metabolic needs and protein tolerance. It is not yet clear whether these products will prove to be clinically useful. The special hepatic formulas are very expensive and can be justified only for patients who become encephalopathic on conventional formulations. Most disease-specific protein supplements do not provide vitamins and minerals in the quantities needed to maintain normal nutrition.

   d. **High-nitrogen products** (Alitra Q, TraumaCal) with increased proportions of branched-chain amino acids are available. These products are promoted for use in patients with catabolic stress. Unfortunately, the renal function of many patients in catabolic stress is impaired, and they cannot tolerate the high nitrogen load. The practical advantages of products with modified amino acid profiles over other protein and calorie products in typical hospitalized patients are unclear. In one study, nitrogen retention appeared to be better in patients with moderate to severe stress who were given products rich in branched-chain amino acids (8).

C. Calorie supplements

1. **Calorie supplementation with table foods** is conceptually attractive but often practically unfeasible. A normal diet with adequate calorie content restores glycogen and fat stores in the patient who has voluntarily or involuntarily starved. However, a lack of available calorie sources is not usually the reason for negative calorie balance and fat store depletion in the United States. If increasing the usual diet with good calorie sources satisfies the daily requirements, then this is the ideal way of managing calorie deficiency. The caloric value of some common foods is given in Table 5-7. An extensive listing of the nutritional values of foods available in the United States is published in the United States Department of Agriculture Handbook No. 456 (*The Nutritive Value of American Foods in Common Units.* Washington, DC: Agriculture Research Service, U.S. Department of Agriculture, 1975), in *Bowes and Church's Food Values of Portions Commonly Used* (New York: Harper and Row, 1985), and in E. S. Hand's *Food Finder,* 2nd ed. (Salem, Oregon: ESHA Research, 1990). See Table 1-8 for additional resources.

2. **Commercially available supplements with a high caloric content.** Table 9-5 lists supplements that are good sources of calories and proteins. An 8-oz glass of a commercial supplement with a caloric density of 1 kcal/mL increases the daily caloric intake by 240 kcal. Detailed nutritional information about these supplements is listed in Table 9-3. The ideal caloric supplement for an individual patient should be both palatable and compatible with any dietary restrictions necessary for management.

   a. If the product is to be taken orally and the patient tolerates lactose, the *milk-based formulations* should be considered; they taste better and are less expensive than other enteral products.

   b. Many patients are lactose-intolerant or prefer the taste of standard formulas to that of milk-based formulas. Most patients find one or more flavors of the standard formulas tolerable, especially if they are served cold.

   c. For patients with special dietary requirements, the choice of an oral formula is much like that of tube feedings, described below.

3. **Carbohydrate modules** are usually composed of glucose polymers formed by the partial hydrolysis of starch. Modules with smaller polymers are sweeter and have a higher osmolality than those with large polymers.

4. **Fat modules** consist of medium-chain triglycerides (e.g., MCT oil). MCTs contain fatty acids with chains that have 6 to 12 carbon atoms, whereas long-chain triglycerides, the predominant lipid in both vegetable and animal fats, contain fatty acids with chains that have 14 or more carbon atoms.

   MCT oil is an interesting calorie supplement derived from coconut oil (Table 9-1). Because of their greater solubility in water, MCTs can be hydrolyzed and absorbed with minimal amounts of pancreatic enzymes and without bile salts. The medium-chain fatty acids appear in the portal bloodstream (rather than the lymphatics) without being reesterified to triglycerides. The chains of 97% of the fatty acids in the oil have 8 or 10 carbon atoms, and no linoleic acid is present. The the-

(*text continues on page 319*)

Table 9-3. Nutrient analysis of various commercially available protein and/or calorie

Product	Manu-facturer	Oral (O) Tube (T)	Macronutrient major sources Protein	CHO	Fat	Caloric distribution (%) Protein	CHO	Fat	Caloric density (kcal/mL)	Osmolality[a] (mOsmol/kg)	Fiber (g/1,000 kcal)
Alitra Q	Ross	O,T	S,M,AA	CS,S,F	MCT,SA	21	66	13	1.0	575	0
Amin-Aid	Rand D	O	AA	MD,S	S	4	74.8	21.2	2.0	700	0
Boost	Mead	O	M	CS,S	CA,C,SU	17	67	16	1.0	N/A	0
Boost HP	Mead	O	C	CS,S	S	24	55	21	1.0	650–690	0
Boost Plus	Mead	O	C	CS,S	C	16	50	34	1.52	630–670	0
Boost with Fiber	Mead	O	C,S	MD,S	C,CA,MCT	17	53	30	1.06	480	10
Carnation Instant Breakfast	Clintec	O	M	MD,S,L	MF	19	63	18	0.93	640	0
Carnation Instant Breakfast (no sugar)	Clintec	O	M	MD,L	MF	25	52	23	0.70	524	0
Choice dm	Mead	O,T	M	MD,S	CA,SA,C,MCT	17	40	43	1.06	300–440	13.6
Comply	Sherwood	O,T	C	CS,S	C	16	48	36	1.5	410	0
Crucial	Clintec	T	CH,AR	MD,CS	MCT,FI,S	25	36	39	1.5	490	0
Deliver 2.0	Mead	T	C	CS	S,MCT	15	40	45	2.0	640	0
Diabeti-Source	Mead	O	C,P	MD,S	CA,SU	17	53	30	1.06	480	10
Ensure	Ross	O,T	C,S	CS,S	C	14	54.5	31.5	1.06	470	0
Ensure Plus	Ross	O,T	C,S	C	CS,S	15	32	53	1.5	600	0
Ensure Plus HN	Ross	O,T	C,S	C	CS,S	17	30	53	1.5	650	0
Ensure with Fiber	Ross	O	C,S	FOS,CS,S	C	14.5	55	30.5	1.1	480	14
Fibersource	Clintec	T	C	CS	CA,MCT	14	56	30	1.2	390	8
Forta Shake	Ross	O	M	S,L	MF	24	54	25	1.0	N/A	0
Glucerna	Ross	O,T	C	CS,F	SA,S,F	16.7	33.3	50	1.0	370	14.4
Glytrol	Clintec	O,T	C	MD,CS,F	CA,SA,MCT	18	40	42	1.0	380	15
Hepatic-Aid II	McGaw	O	AA	MD,S	S	15	57.3	27.7	1.2	560	14
Immun-Aid	McGaw	O,T	L,AA	MD	MCT, CA	32	48	20	1.0	460	0
Impact	Novartis	T	C,AR	CS	FI	22	53	25	1.0	375	0
Impact with Fiber	Novartis	T	C,AR	CS,GV	FI	22	53	25	1.0	375	10
Isocal	Mead	T	C,S	MD	S,MCT	13	50	37	1.06	300	10
Isocal HN	Mead	T	C,S	MD	S,MCT	17	47	36	1.06	300	0
Isosource	Novartis	O,T	CS,C,S	CS	CA,MCT	14	56	30	1.2	490	0
Isosource 1.5	Novartis	T	C	CS,S	CA,MCT,S	18	44	38	2.0	650	8.0
Isosource HN	Novartis	O,T	CS,C,S	CS	CA,MCT	18	52	30	1.2	330	0
Jevity	Ross	T	C	CS	MCT,C,S	16.7	53.3	30	1.06	310	13.6
Lipisorb	Mead	O,T	C	CS,S	MCT,C	14	46	40	1.0	320	0
Nepro	Ross	O,T	C	FOS,CS,S	SA,S	14	43	43	2.0	635	0
Nova-Source 2.0	Novartis	O,T	C	CS,S	CA,MCT	18	43	39	2.0	790	0
NuBasics	Clintec	O	C	CS,S	CA,C	14	53	33	1.0	500–520	0
NuBasics Plus	Clintec	T	C	CS,S	CA,C	14	47	39	1.5	620–650	0
Nutren 1.0	Clintec	T	C	MD,CS	MCT,CA	16	51	33	1.0	412	0
Nutren 1.0 with Fiber	Clintec	T	C	MD,CS	MCT,CA, C	16	51	33	1.0	310–370	14
Nutren 1.5	Clintec	T	C	MD,CS	MCT,CA,C	16	45	39	1.5	430–530	0
NutriHep	Clintec	T	AA,HP	MD,CS	MCT,CA,C	11	77	12	1.5	620–650	0
NutriVent	Clintec	O	C	MD,S	CA,MCT	18	27	55	1.5	450	0
Optimental	Ross	T	S,C	FOS,MD,S	F,MCT,CA	20.5	55	24.5	1.0	540	0
Osmolite HN	Ross	T	C,S	G	C,S,MCT	16.7	53.3	34.8	1.06	300	0
Osmolite	Ross	T	C,S	G	MCT,C,S	14	54.6	31.4	1.06	300	0
Oxepa	Ross	O,T	C	MD,S	CA,MCT,F	16.7	28.1	55.2	1.5	493	0
Peptamen	Clintec	O,T	M	MD,ST	MCT,SU	16	51	33	1.0	270	0
Perative	Ross	T	C,L,AR	CS	CA,MCT	20.5	55	25	1.3	425	0
ProBalance	Clintec	T	C	MD,CS	MCT,C,CA	18	52	30	1.2	350–450	8.3
Promote	Ross	O,T	C,S	CS,S	CA,MCT	25	52	23	1.0	340	0

supplements and diets (see Table 9-5 for major classifications)

Non-protein calorie/ nitrogen ratio	Protein (g/1,000 kcal)	CHO (g/1,000 kcal)	Fat (g/1,000 kcal)	per 1,000 kcal											Nutri- tionally complete[e]
				Na (mg)	K (mg)	Cl (mg)	Ca (mg)	P (mg)	Mg (mg)	Fe (mg)	I (µg)	Cu (mg)	Zn (mg)	Mn (mg)	
120:1	52.5	165	15.5	1,000	1,200	1,300	733	733	267	15	100	1.3	20	3.4	Yes
NA	10	187	24	<173	<117	NA	NA	NA	NA	NA	NA	NA	NA	NA	NA
125:1	43	170	18	550	1,690	1,440	1,270	1,060	420	15.2	161	1.7	19	3	Yes
78:1	60.4	140	22.8	921	2,079	1,465	1,000	921	326	16.7	138	2	13.8	2.8	Yes
134:1	40.1	125	137.5	559	974	836	559	559	224	10	84	1.1	11.1	1.6	Yes
120:1	43.4	131.1	33	679	1,311	1,311	792	660	264	12	99	1.3	13.1	1.7	Yes
NA	48	160	20	880	2,400	NA	1,600	1,200	400	18	180	2	15	NA	NA
NA	63	132	26	1,105	3,158	NA	2,105	1,579	632	23.7	237	2.63	19.7	NA	NA
122:1	42.5	100	48.1	802	1,717	1,198	1,000	1,000	396	17.9	150	2	19.8	13.6	Yes
134:1	40	120	40	733	1,233	1,133	667	667	267	12	100	1.3	20	3	Yes
67:1	62.5	90	45	779	1,248	1,160	667	667	267	12	100	2	24	2.7	Yes
145:1	37.5	100	51	400	840	590	505	505	200	9.1	74	1.0	10	1.5	Yes
120:1	50	90	49	1,000	1,400	1,100	670	870	270	12	100	1.3	15	3.3	Yes
153:1	35.2	137.2	35.2	800	1,480	1,240	500	500	200	9	75	1	11.25	2.5	Yes
146:1	36.6	133.2	35.5	704	1,296	1,296	470	470	189	8.5	70	0.96	10.6	2.34	Yes
125:1	41.7	133.2	33.2	786	1,265	1,066	705	705	282	12.7	106	1.42	15.9	3.52	Yes
148:1	36	147	34	786	1,265	1,066	705	705	282	12.7	106	1.42	15.9	3.52	Yes
151:1	36	140	34	940	1,500	940	560	560	220	10	83	1.1	14	2.8	Yes
82:1	59	128	28	827	2,793	N/A	1,897	1,552	272	15.5	129	1.72	18.1	2.07	Yes
140:1	41.8	93.7	55.7	928	1,561	1,435	704	704	282	12.7	106	NA	1.5	15.9	Yes
114:1	45	100	47.5	740	1,400	1,200	720	720	286	12.8	120	1.5	15	3	Yes
148:1	38	144	31	<288	<196	NA	NA	NA	NA	NA	NA	NA	NA	NA	NA
53:1	80	120	22	575	1,055	888	500	500	200	9	75	0.76	2	25	Yes
71:1	56	132	28	110	1,300	1,300	800	800	270	12	100	NA	1.7	15	Yes
71:1	56	140	28	1,100	1,300	1,300	800	800	270	12	100	NA	1.7	15	Yes
71:1	32	125	42	500	1,245	1,000	595	500	200	9	75	1	10	2.5	Yes
125:1	42	117	42	877	1,500	1,360	800	800	320	14	120	1.6	12	4.3	Yes
148:1	36	140	34	1,000	1,400	940	560	560	220	10	83	1.1	14	2.8	Yes
116:1	45.3	113.3	43.3	867	1,400	1,067	733	733	287	12.7	107	1.4	21.3	1.4	Yes
116:1	44	130	34	1,000	1,400	940	560	560	220	10	83	1.1	14	2.8	Yes
125:1	42	144	35	880	1,480	1,240	860	716	286	12.9	107	1.44	16.1	3.56	Yes
157:1	35	117	48	734	1,251	1,168	701	701	200	9.2	93.8	1.25	12.5	1.9	Yes
157:1	34.9	107.6	47.8	415	518	505	686	343	105	9.5	78.9	1.1	11.8	2.63	Yes
116:1	45	110	44	380	800	550	500	550	210	9.5	80	1.1	8.0	1.1	Yes
154:1	35	132	37	876	1,248	1,200	500	500	200	9	75	1	10.5	2	Yes
154:1	35	117	43	780	1,248	1,160	500	500	200	9	75	1	10.5	2	Yes
131:1	40	127	38	876	1,248	1,200	668	668	268	12	100	1.4	14	2.7	Yes
131:1	40	127	38	876	1,248	1,200	668	668	268	12	100	1.4	14	2.7	Yes
131:1	40	113	45	500	1,253	1,000	693	693	333	12	100	1.3	13.3	2.7	Yes
209:1	26	193	14	213	880	1,000	667	667	267	12	101	1.3	10.1	2.7	Yes
116:1	45	67	63	415	528	505	686	343	105	9.5	78.9	NA	1.1	11.8	Yes
97:1	51.3	138.5	28.4	1,060	1,760	1,340	1,060	1,060	425	13	160	1.9	16	3.6	Yes
125:1	42	133.6	34.8	880	1,480	1,360	715	715	286	12.86	107.2	1.43	16.08	3.57	Yes
153:1	35.2	137.2	36.4	600	960	800	500	500	200	9	75	1	11.5	2.5	Yes
125:1	45	100	47.5	872	1,308	1,125	703	703	287	12.7	107	1.4	16	3.7	Yes
131:1	40	127	39	500	1,252	1,000	800	700	400	12	100	1.4	14	2.7	Yes
97:1	51	136	29	800	1,330	1,269	667	667	267	12	100	NA	1.34	15	Yes
14:1	45	130	34	637	1,300	1,080	1,042	833	333	15	125	1.7	20	3.3	Yes
75:1	62.5	130	26	928	1,980	1,263	960	960	320	14.4	120	1.6	18	4	Yes

(continued)

Table 9-3. (*Continued*)

Product	Manu-facturer	Oral (O) Tube (T)	Protein	CHO	Fat	Protein	CHO	Fat	Caloric density (kcal/mL)	Osmolality[a] (mOsmol/kg)	Fiber (g/1,000 kcal)
			Macronutrient major sources			Caloric distribution (%)					
Promote with Fiber	Ross	O,T	C,S	CS,S	CA,MCT	25	50	25	1.0	380	14.4
Protain XL	Sherwood	T	C	MD	MCT,C	22	51	27	1.0	340	8
Pulmocare	Ross	O,T	C	S,CS	C	16.7	28.1	55.2	1.5	465	0
Reabilan	Clintec	T	M,C	MD,T	MCT, S,F	12.5	52.5	35	1.0	350	0
Reabilan HN	Clintec	T	M,C	MD,T	MCT,S,F	17.5	47.5	35	1.33	490	0
Renalcal	Clintec	T	AA,HP	MD,CS	MCT,CA,C	17	58	35	2.0	600	0
Replete	Clintec	T	C	MD,CS	CA, MCT	25	45	30	1.0	290	0
Resource	Novartis	O	C	MD,CS	CA,MCT	25	45	30	1.0	300	0
Resource Plus	Novartis	O	C,S	CS,S	C	15	53	32	1.5	600	0
Subdue	Mead		HP	MD,CS	CA,MCT	20	50	30	1.0	330–525	0
Suplena	Ross	O,T	C	CS,S	SA,S	6	51	43	2.0	600	0
TraumaCal	Mead	O,T	C	CS,S	S,MCT	22	38	40	1.5	490	0
TwoCal HN	Ross	O,T	C	CS,S	C,MCT	16.7	43.2	40.1	2.0	690	0
Ultracal	Mead	T	C	MD	S,MCT	17	46	37	1.06	310	13.6
Vital HN	Ross	O,T	P,AA	CS,S	MCT,SA	16.7	73.9	9.4	1.0	500	0
Vivonex T.E.N.	Novartis	T	AA	MD,S,T	SA	15	82	3	1.0	630	0

Formulations may have changed since the preparation of this table. Consult manufacturer's literature.

Protein sources: AA, amino acids; AR, arginine; C, casein salts; CH, casein hydrolysate; DL, delactosed lactalbumin; E, egg white solids; HP, hydrolyzed proteins other than casein; L, lactalbumin; M, milk proteins; P, mixed protein sources; S, soy protein. **Carbohydrate sources:** CS, cornstarch or corn syrup solids; F, fructose; FOS, fructose oligosaccharides; G, glucose; GO, glucon oligosaccharides; L, lactose; M, mixed carbohydrate sources; MD, malt dextrin; MS, monosaccharides; S, sucrose; SP, soy polysaccharides; T, tapioca starch. **Fat sources:** C, corn; CA, canola oil; F, mixed fat sources; FFA, free fatty acids; FI, fish oil; MCT, medium-chain triglycerides; MF, milk fat; S, soy oil; SA, safflower oil; SU, sunflower. **Other abbreviations:** CHO, carbohydrates; NA, not available.

[a] When served full strength prepared in the usual way or diluted to suggested caloric density. The supplement or diet is said to be nutritionally complete if 2,000 mL or less meets the recommended dietary allowance (RDA) of all vitamins and minerals for average adult.

Table 9-4. Disease-specific enteral products

Disease	Products	Characteristics
Renal failure	Amin-Aid Nepro Suplena Renalcal	Very low protein, enriched in essential amino acids, most products have low electrolyte content.
Hepatic failure	Hepatic-Aid II NutriHep	Low protein, low in aromatic amino acids, high in branched-chain amino acids, low sodium.
Pulmonary failure	NutriVent Pulmocare Oxepa	High fat, low carbohydrate.
Glucose intolerance	Glucerna Choice Glytrol DiabetiSource	High fat, low carbohydrate, may contain fructose, contain fiber.
Immune compromise	Impact Crucial	Contain RNA, high in ω-3 fatty acids, arginine-enriched.

Non-protein calorie/ nitrogen ratio	Protein (g/1,000 kcal)	CHO (g/1,000 kcal)	Fat (g/1,000 kcal)	per 1,000 kcal											Nutri-tionally complete[a]
				Na (mg)	K (mg)	Cl (mg)	Ca (mg)	P (mg)	Mg (mg)	Fe (mg)	I (µg)	Cu (mg)	Zn (mg)	Mn (mg)	
75:1	62.5	139	28	928	1,980	1,263	960	960	320	14.4	120	1.6	18	4	Yes
93:1	55	138	30	860	1,500	1,350	800	800	320	21.6	120	NA	2.4	36	Yes
125:1	41.7	70.4	61.4	873	1,155	1,126	704	704	282	12.7	106	1.4	1.4	15.9	Yes
175:1	31.5	131.5	38.9	699	1,251	2,000	499	499	251	10	74.7	1.6	10	2	No
125:1	44	119	39	752	1,249	1,880	339	375	248	10	76.2	0.95	10	2	No
338:1	17	145	41	0	0	0	0	0	0	0	0	0	7	0	No
75:1	62.5	113	34	500	1,560	1,000	1,000	1,000	400	18	160	NA	2	24	Yes
154:1	35	140	35	840	1,500	950	500	500	200	9	75	1	15	2	Yes
146:1	37	130	35	850	1,400	1,100	470	470	210	9.6	70	1.1	16	1.4	Yes
100:1	50	127	34	1,110	1,610	1,390	850	850	340	15.2	127	1.7	16.1	2.5	Yes
392:1	15	128	48	392	558	463	693	364	105	9.5	78.9	NA	1.05	11.8	Yes
91:1	55	95	45	787	927	1,067	500	500	133	5.9	50	NA	1	9.9	Yes
125:1	41.7	108.2	45.3	653	1,221	821	526	526	211	9.5	78.9	1.05	11.85	2.63	Yes
128:1	42	116	43	865	1,495	1,337	787	787	315	14	118	1.6	16	2.4	Yes
125:1	41.7	185	10.8	566	1,400	1,032	667	667	267	12	100	1.4	15	3.4	Yes
149:1	38	210	2.8	460	780	820	500	500	200	9	75	1	10	0.9	Yes

oretical caloric value is 8.3 kcal/g. The entry of MCTs into mitochondria is independent of carnitine, and they rapidly undergo β-oxidation. The average serving size is 1 tbs (15 mL), which contains 14 g of fat. The caloric value per serving is estimated at about 110 kcal/tbs (15 mL). MCT oil can be used as a caloric supplement in patients with fat malabsorption of any cause. However, for practical purposes, 3 to 4 tbs (approximately 400 kcal) is the largest daily dose that does not cause some diarrhea. For this reason, its use is limited to patients with fat malabsorption and an inadequate daily caloric intake who might benefit from the addition of only 300 to 400 calories. It is clear that even in these patients, most dietary calories must come from the carbohydrate sources and longer-chain triglycerides that are included in their low-fat diet. If MCT oil is the only source of fat in the diet, the patient is at risk for the development of EFA deficiency because no EFAs are found in MCT oil. A cookbook with recipes including MCT oil is available from Mead Johnson, Evansville, Indiana. Supplementation with MCT oil leads to high levels of uncleared MCTs in patients with severe liver disease or portal–systemic shunts. However, these levels do not appear to have a deleterious effect on the clinical parameters of encephalopathy.

IV. Enteral feeding

A. Formulas for enteral feeding

1. **Kitchen-prepared diets** are still used in some cases.

    a. **Disadvantages.** The expenditure of time required, with little, if any, monetary savings, makes these diets less appealing now that many nutritionally complete diets for tube feeding are commercially

Table 9-5. Classification of commercially available complete enteral nutrition products

Standard	Volume-restricted	High in protein	Intact protein Disease-specific	Critical care	With fiber	Milk-based	Elemental or chemically defined
Nutren 1-0	Nutren 1.5 or 2.0	Boost HP	Glytrol	Immun-Aid	Ensure with Fiber	Carnation Instant	Crucial
Isocal	Comply	Ensure Plus HN	Choice	Impact	Boost with Fiber	Carnation Instant (no sugar)	Alitra Q
Isosource	Deliver 2.0	Isocal HN	Glucerna	Impact with Fiber	Nutren 1.0 with Fiber	Forta Shake	Peptamen
Osmolite	Isosource 1.5	TwoCal HN	DiabetiSource	Perative	Ultracal		Reabilan
NuBasics	NuBasics Plus	Osmolite HN	NutriHep	Replete	Fibersource		Reabilan HN
Lipisorb	NuBasics 2.0	Isosource HN	Hepatic-Aid II	TraumaCal	ProBalance		Vivonex T.E.N.
Boost	Boost Plus		NutriVent	Promote	Jevity		Vital HN
Resource	Resource Plus		Oxepa	Protain XL	Promote with Fiber		Subdue
Ensure	Ensure Plus		Pulmocare				Optimental
	NovaSource 2.0		Renalcal				
			Amin-Aid				
			Nepro				
			Suplena				

Table 9-6. Categories of enteral products

Intact protein:	Amino acids provided in intact protein rather than in hydrolyzed proteins or as free amino acids. Requires normal digestive and absorptive abilities.
Standard:	Intact protein, caloric density 1.2 kcal/mL or less, ratio of nonprotein calories to nitrogen greater than 130:1. These are the products of choice for the vast majority of patients on enteral nutrition.
Volume-restricted:	Intact protein, caloric density greater than 1.2 kcal/mL. These products may be useful when fluid overload is a problem, as in renal failure, ascites, or congestive heart failure.
High in protein:	Intact protein, ratio of nonprotein calories to nitrogen of less than 130:1. These products may be useful for patients with high requirements for protein synthesis (e.g., severe trauma, protein losing enteropathy, decubitus, healing wounds). They are much less effective in severe inflammatory illness characterized by enhanced catabolism.
Disease-specific:	Intact protein, products promoted to meet needs of patients with specific diseases.
Critical care:	High protein supplemented with arginine; may contain MCT oil or fish oil.
With fiber:	Formulas with fiber produce more fecal residue. Use of these formulas will increase stool bulk and may help relieve constipation or diarrhea. In most of the enteral formulations that contain fiber, the fiber source is soy-polysaccharide fiber (SPF), which is largely insoluble and serves to increase stool bulk. Fructooligosaccharides, which are degraded by colonic bacteria to form short-chain fatty acids, have been added to some formulations.
Milk-based:	Dietary supplements designed to be mixed with milk. Nutritional data in Table 9-3 include the nutritional contributions of the milk. These products are used primarily as oral supplements rather than tube feedings. As a group, they are better tasting and less expensive than any of the other enteral products. However, many patients do not tolerate them because of their lactose content.
Elemental or chemically defined:	In elemental diets, calories are supplied primarily as free amino acids and oligosaccharides. Chemically defined diets are similar but contain partially hydrolyzed proteins. These formulas are promoted for patients with diminished capacity to digest and absorb foods. In view of the tremendous functional reserve of the pancreas and intestine, very few patients are incapable of digesting and absorbing standard enteral formulations. Moreover, elemental and chemically defined diets may be hyperosmolar and cause gastric retention and diarrhea. Elemental and chemically defined diets are usually more expensive than polymeric diets.

available. Kitchen-prepared diets are not recommended for infusion through the small-caliber tubes commonly in use today because they do not have the excellent flow characteristics of the highly dispersed commercial products. Bacterial contamination is more likely to be a problem with kitchen-prepared diets than with canned commercial formulations.

b. **Example** of a kitchen-prepared diet with 1,800 kcal/1,800 mL; yield: nearly 2 qt.

(1) **Recipe**

Food	Measure	Weight (g)
Milk, whole	¾ cup	200
Strained meat	1¾ cup	400
Strained vegetables	1 cup	200
Nonfat dried milk	¾ cup	45
Orange juice	1¼ cup	300
Cream	1¼ cup	300
Corn syrup	8 tsp	—

(2) **Partial composition**

Nutrient	Amount	Percentage RDA[a]
Kilocalories	1,805	[b]
Protein	89 g	160
Fat	78 g	—
Carbohydrate	186 g	—
Calcium	1,240 mg	155
Phosphorus	1,395 mg	170
Iron	12 mg	120
Sodium	1,420 mg	—
Potassium	3,320 mg	—
Vitamin A	5,680 IU	114
Vitamin B$_1$	0.7 mg	50
Vitamin B$_2$	1.3 mg	80
Niacin	16.4 mg	90
Vitamin C	261 mg	435

[a] For a 50-year-old 70-kg man.
[b] See Chapter 5 for calculation of the calorie requirement.

2. **Commercial enteral formulations** (Tables 9-3, 9-4, and 9-5) are available with many variations in specific characteristics and nutritional content. A very large number of commercial enteral formulations are available, and new formulations are introduced frequently. Because of the rapid turnover of commercial enteral formulations, Table 9-3 will be out of date in the near future. The addresses, phone numbers, and Internet addresses of the leading manufacturers are given in Table 9-7. Each of these companies has technical personnel who will answer questions about new formulations and mail appropriate literature. The most suitable diet for an individual patient is one that provides the planned, desired allowances of macronutrients and micronutrients and also is appropriately restricted and varied according to any intestinal or metabolic disorders that are present. Seldom is a single preparation clearly the best one for any given patient. Many commercially available products have similar features with minor alterations. Tables 9-5 and 9-6 group commercial diets by major features, and Table 9-3 provides detailed nutritional information and the special characteristics of these diets. The following are definitions of some terms used in the tables:

   a. **Low-residue.** This term is applied to diets that contain no meat or vegetable fiber.

   b. **Caloric density.** The caloric densities of commercial enteral products range from 0.5 to 2.0 kcal/mL; those of most standard formulations are about 1.0 kcal/mL. The more dense formulas (1.5 to 2.0 kcal/mL) are used in patients for whom fluid overload may be a problem (e.g., renal failure, congestive heart failure, ascites). Denser formulas are frequently hypertonic; the added osmolar load may cause diarrhea (al-

Table 9-7. Major manufacturers of enteral nutrition products

Clintec Nutrition Company
Affiliated with Baxter Healthcare
  Corporation and Nestles S.A.
Three Parkway North, Suite 500
P.O. Box 760
Deerfield, IL 60015-0760
1-800-422-2752
www.baxter.com

B. Braun (McGaw)
2525 McGaw Ave.
P.O. Box 19791
Irvine, CA 92713
714-660-2000
1-800-854-6851 (technical assistance)
www.braunusa.com

Mead Johnson Nutritionals
A Bristol-Myers Squibb Company
2400 West Lloyd Expressway
Evansville, IN 47721
1-800-457-3550
www.meadjohnson.com

Novartis Nutrition (formerly Sandoz)
5100 Gamble Drive
St. Louis Park, MN 55416
1-800-999-9978
www.novartis.com

Ross Laboratories
Division of Abbott Laboratories
625 Cleveland Ave.
Columbus, OH 43215
614-227-3333
1-800-544-7495
www.abbott.com

though hypertonicity is not a common cause of the diarrhea seen with enteral feeding). Calorically dense formulas can be diluted with water to reduce diarrhea and maintain fluid balance, but this maneuver may complicate fluid balance.

   c. **Osmolality.** Whole proteins and complex polysaccharides contribute a large number of calories to a formulation but relatively few milliosmoles. In contrast, free amino acids and monosaccharides contribute many more milliosmoles for the same number of calories. As a result, the osmolalities of elemental and chemically defined diets tend to be higher than those of standard formulations with intact proteins and complex carbohydrates. The electrolyte content of the formulation also contributes to the osmolality without affecting caloric density. Isotonic formulations have an osmolality of about 300 mOsmol, which is similar to that of blood. Some commercial enteral formulations are hypertonic (Table 9-3). Hypertonic solutions can cause delayed gastric emptying with nausea, vomiting, and distention. Hypertonic solutions entering the small bowel cause intestinal fluid secretion; if this fluid is not reabsorbed in the intestine, diarrhea and dehydration develop.

   d. **Ratio of nonprotein calories to nitrogen.** For most patients receiving forced enteral nutrition, the quantity of amino acids provided in standard enteral formulas is large enough to provide for protein synthesis so long as enough formula is given to provide for caloric needs. In a few patients (e.g., those who have sustained severe trauma), the requirements for protein synthesis are so great that a lower ratio of calories to protein may be optimal. This ratio is expressed as nonprotein calories to nitrogen (kilocalories per gram of nitrogen). The conversion of nitrogen to protein and vice versa is as follows:

Grams of Nitrogen = (Grams of Protein) / 6.25

All manufacturers of enteral formulations offer high-nitrogen products, even though the number of patients who are likely to benefit from these formulations is small. Patients given high-nitrogen formulas are likely to use amino acids for energy and so increase their urea production. As a result, these formulations should be given with caution to patients with renal failure. These formulations also may be associated with increased ammonia production and should be given with caution to patients with hepatic disease.

    e. Nutritionally complete. This term is applied to diets that in themselves (except possibly for an additional water requirement in some patients) provide 100% of the recommended dietary allowances (RDAs) for average adults. The volume of the formula necessary to meet the RDAs varies from person to person. In general, the amount of formula necessary to meet the calculated daily calorie requirement comes close to providing 100% of the RDAs, including vitamins, for average adults. The needs of patients with excessive losses or requirements may not be satisfied by these formulas alone. In Table 9-3, the column labeled "Nutritionally Complete" indicates whether 2,000 mL of the enteral formula meets the RDA for the average adult. With some of the newer formulations, even smaller volumes meet the RDA.

    f. Satisfactory for small-caliber tube feeding. The formula is highly dispersed and should not occlude a feeding tube with a 2-mm inner diameter. Formulas containing milk or fiber from meat or vegetables are not recommended for use through small-caliber tubes because they clog the tubes.

  3. Choosing an enteral product for tube feeding

    a. Proteins provide 4% to 32% of the calories in enteral products. High-protein formulations are given to patients with protein deficiency or large requirements for protein. High-protein formulations increase urea excretion by the kidney, so that fluid volumes must be increased. Most patients who receive high-protein formulations would be just as well served by standard formulations. Amino acids can be in enteral formulas as free amino acids (monomeric), partially hydrolyzed proteins (oligomeric), or intact proteins (polymeric) (9). Partially hydrolyzed proteins contain some free amino acids, dipeptides, and tripeptides, but larger peptides predominate. Free amino acids and partially hydrolyzed protein are found in *elemental diets*; intact proteins are found in standard formulations. Intact proteins and partially hydrolyzed proteins must be digested to amino acids, dipeptides, and tripeptides to be absorbed; dipeptides and tripeptides are more easily absorbed than free amino acids. However, few data support the contention that amino acids are better absorbed when presented as free amino acids or partially hydrolyzed protein than as intact protein in most patients, although oligopeptides may be of some advantage in patients with small-bowel disease (10,11). The evidence supporting the use of elemental diets is quite thin. Balance studies in patients who have undergone intestinal resections have failed to establish advantages of these formulations over standard polymeric formulations (12). Formulas containing free amino acids and oligopeptides have several disadvantages in comparison with those containing intact proteins. They are more expensive and less palatable; they are also hypertonic and, as a result, more likely to cause cramps and diarrhea.

    b. Most patients can be managed nicely on one of the *standard formulations* (Table 9-5). Several products are available for oral or tube administration.

c. Patients who have problems with *diarrhea* or *constipation* on a standard formula may benefit from a standard formula with *fiber*. The most commonly used source of fiber in enteral formulations is soy polysaccharide. Fiber is fermented by colonic bacteria to short-chain (butyric, acetic, and propionic) fatty acids that serve as energy sources for colonocytes. Fiber also decreases the rate of gastric emptying and delays the absorption of dietary glucose.

d. Patients with *fluid overload* may benefit from a volume-restricted (more calorically dense) formula. The sodium content of the formula is also important in these patients. Adults require 1 mL of water per kilocalorie or 30 to 35 mL/kg of their usual body weight. Tube-fed patients may not get enough free water, especially when nutrient-dense formulas are used.

e. Lipids provide 3% to 55% of the calories in enteral formulas. Most formulas provide 30% to 40% of calories as lipids, usually from corn, safflower, sunflower, or soy oils. MCT oil is commonly used because it is more easily absorbed and does not require bile salts for absorption. Linoleic acid should provide 2% to 4% of calories to prevent EFA deficiency. Some research suggests that linoleic acid at higher doses suppresses the immune response. Formulations designed to bolster the immune response may include MCT oil or fish oil to reduce the linoleic acid content.

f. Disease-specific formulations (Table 9-4)

　(1) Pulmonary disease. When a calorie of carbohydrate is metabolized, more carbon dioxide is produced than when a calorie of fat is metabolized. The rapid administration of a large carbohydrate load to a patient with severe pulmonary disease may increase the carbon dioxide tension. Several companies make calorically dense enteral formulas that are low in carbohydrate and high in fat for patients with severe pulmonary disease. These formulas also have a high caloric density and are low in sodium for volume restriction. The differences in carbon dioxide production per kilocalorie among the various enteral formulas are modest, and probably these small differences are significant for only a few patients with pulmonary disease. It is important to remember that the amount of carbon dioxide produced is more a function of the number of calories consumed than of the macronutritient source of the calories. Patients with pulmonary disease should not be overloaded with calories.

　(2) Hepatic disease. Patients with chronic liver disease are likely to be intolerant of enteral protein because of encephalopathy secondary to portal–systemic shunting. Chronic liver disease is also associated with an abnormal pattern of circulating amino acids; the concentrations of aromatic amino acids (phenylalanine, tyrosine, and tryptophan) are increased, and the concentrations of branched-chain amino acids (leucine, isoleucine, and valine) are decreased. It has been postulated that this imbalance contributes to encephalopathy because it leads to the production of false neurotransmitters. Several commercial enteral nutrition products are specially formulated for patients with chronic liver disease. These products have low levels of total protein, high concentrations of branched-chain amino acids, and low concentrations of aromatic amino acids. A number of trials have compared these special formulas with conventional formulas in patients with hepatic encephalopathy. On the whole, the differences were small, and only in the largest trial was the hepatic formulation clearly better (13). The special hepatic formulations are very expensive, and their use can be justified only in patients who are encephalopathic when given standard formulations in quantities sufficient to achieve positive nitrogen balance (see Chapter 11, Section IIID). *Alcoholism,* the most frequent cause of chronic liver disease, is associated with other nutritional problems, including deficiencies of thiamine, folate, vitamin C, zinc, and magnesium. Dietary supplementation with a standard enteral formulation accelerated clinical improvement in alcoholic liver disease (14). Chronic liver disease is frequently associated with ascites and edema. Control of salt and water balance is an important component of the management of chronic liver disease. The sodium content of enteral formulas varies considerably (Table 9-3); for many patients with liver disease, the sodium content of the enteral product is more important than the amino acid composition. Hyponatremia frequently accompanies ascites and edema in chronic liver disease; a calorically dense (1.5 to 2.0 kcal/mL), low-sodium formula allows the intake of both salt and water to be controlled in such patients.

(3) **Renal disease.** In chronic renal failure, the ability of the kidney to excrete urea and electrolytes is limited. An important part of the management of chronic renal disease is the adjustment of dietary and fluid intake to accommodate for the diminished functional capacity of the kidneys. One estimate of the demands placed by a nutritional product on the kidneys is the renal solute load, which is determined primarily by the protein and electrolyte content of the formula. The major contributors to the renal solute load are urea, the end-product of protein digestion, and the electrolytes (sodium, potassium, and chloride). The greater the renal solute load, the greater the obligatory water loss through the kidneys. As the degree of renal functional impairment increases, the ability of the kidney to concentrate solutes is diminished. Thus, the greater the impairment of renal function, the greater the obligatory water loss for a given solute load. A number of commercial enteral formulas have been developed specifically for patients with chronic renal disease. These formulas have a relatively low protein content with a high percentage of essential amino acids. The diminished protein content is designed to limit urea production, and the high percentage of essential amino acids is designed to allow for adequate protein synthesis with minimal urea production. Most of these formulas have a low electrolyte content to minimize the renal solute load. Potassium is especially problematic in renal disease; patients with renal disease have difficulty excreting large potassium loads. Some renal formulas have no added vitamins and minerals; others contain vitamins and minerals in reduced amounts. Particular care needs to be taken with minerals, such as chromium, that are excreted in the urine. Metabolic complications are fairly frequent in patients on enteral nutrition. These problems are much more common in patients with chronic renal disease because their capacity to regulate fluid and electrolytes through adjustments in renal excretion is greatly diminished. For this reason, patients with renal disease on enteral nutrition should be monitored more frequently and more carefully than patients without renal disease. Particular attention should be given to serum electrolytes, daily weights, and inputs and outputs. As can be seen in Table 9-3, some of the formulas for the tube feeding of patients with renal failure contain only

small amounts of electrolytes or none at all. These formulas may need to be supplemented with electrolytes to prevent severe electrolyte imbalance. Frequently, vitamin supplements are also necessary. Special renal enteral formulations are most useful for patients who have significant renal impairment but are not yet on dialysis. Patients who have milder degrees of renal impairment can be managed with standard formulas; patients on dialysis can also be managed with standard formulas (see discussion of the dietary management of renal disease in Chapter 12).

(4) **Critical care and immune deficiency.** A number of studies have evaluated the supplementation of enteral formulations with nucleotides, glutamine, arginine, and ω-3 fatty acids to enhance immune function. In one of them, an immune-enhancing diet improved cell-mediated immunity but had no effect on hospital stay or mortality (15). A study of infectious complications in trauma patients found that patients fed an immune-enhancing diet had fewer major infectious complications than did those receiving an isocaloric isonitrogenous diet (16). Despite the positive results of this study, the benefits of immune-enhancing ingredients are inconclusive (17). The results of a recent review of nutrition in the critically ill suggest that immunonutrition is associated with a lower rate of infection, fewer days on ventilation, and shorter hospital stays, but no improvement in mortality (18).

(5) **Other nutrients in commercial enteral formulas**

(a) **Glutamine.** Glutamine, a nonessential amino acid that accounts for about 8% of the amino acids in dietary protein, is the most abundant amino acid in plasma. It performs important functions as the principal carrier of nitrogen from the periphery to visceral organs and as a source of energy for enterocytes. In catabolic states, glutamine is released from skeletal muscle and is taken up by the intestine, where it is burned for fuel. Depletion of plasma glutamine is associated with loss of intestinal integrity, villous atrophy, ulcerations, and necrosis. Parenteral nutrition formulations do not include glutamine because it is not an essential amino acid and because it may break down in solution. TPN is associated with atrophy of the intestine and pancreas in rats, and these effects can be attenuated by glutamine supplementation (19). Villous atrophy and the loss of intestinal integrity would be especially undesirable in severely ill patients, but evidence is scarce that this occurs in humans (20). In rats, mucosal atrophy predisposes to bacterial translocation and the development of sepsis. In rat studies, glutamine-enriched diets were found to be trophic for the gut. Glutamine supplementation increases the adaptive response of the intestine to resection, improves the survival of patients with peritonitis, and reduces the damage sustained by the intestine in response to radiation (21) and 5-fluorouracil. Thus, some data (mostly in animals) support a role for glutamine supplementation. However, human data on glutamine supplementation only suggest an effect on disease outcome (20). All enteral formulas contain glutamine; however, several commercial companies have recently released products that contain especially high levels. The glutamine content of standard commercial formulations is given in Table 9-8. Alitra Q

Table 9-8. Estimated glutamine content of selected defined enteral formulas

Formula	Glutamine content (g/1,000 kcal)
Alitra Q	15.5
Carnation Instant Breakfast with milk	3.7
Ensure	2.9
Ensure HN	3.4
Impact	3.5
Isocal	2.8
Jevity	3.4
Nutren 1.0	3.2
Osmolite	2.9
Osmolite HN	3.4
Peptamen	2.1
Pulmocare	3.3
Reabilan HN	2.8
TraumaCal	4.4
Vital HN	2.0
Vivonex T.E.N.	4.9

contains 15.5 g of glutamine per 1,000 kcal; in comparison, a standard formula, such as Ensure, contains 2.9 g of glutamine per 1,000 kcal. Supplementation with high levels of glutamine is used because some investigators believe that glutamine is a conditional essential amino acid in catabolic states. Even though humans have the capability of synthesizing glutamine, the synthetic capacity may be exceeded by the demand for glutamine in catabolic states. The benefits of supplementation with high levels of glutamine in catabolic states in humans remain to be demonstrated. Similarly, the ability of glutamine supplementation to preserve gastrointestinal structural and functional integrity in humans during prolonged forced enteral nutrition is yet to be established.

(b) **Dietary fiber and short-chain fatty acids.** Several standard enteral formulations are now available with fiber added. Fiber-containing enteral formulas are more viscous and may require a larger-diameter feeding tube for adequate flow. In most cases, soy polysaccharide is the fiber added to enteral formulas to increase stool bulk and regulate transit time. Fiber-containing enteral formulations are most commonly used in patients who are not critically ill on long-term forced enteral nutrition. In these patients, the addition of fiber diminishes the incidence of both constipation and diarrhea. Fiber retains water in the colon, and thus the addition of fiber may require the addition of free water to prevent constipation and dehydration. The utility of fiber-containing enteral formulations in critically ill patients remains to be demonstrated.

Short-chain fatty acids are an important fuel for the colonic mucosa in health and disease. Short-chain fatty acids are produced in the colon during bacterial fermentation of undigested carbohydrates. Dietary fiber is the major substrate for the production of short-chain fatty acids by colonic bacteria. Theoretically, a reduction of the levels of short-chain fatty acids in the colonic lumen may be associated with adverse effects on the function of the colonic epithelium. Long-term ingestion of an elemental diet in rats results in diminished production of short-chain fatty acids in the colonic lumen and atrophy of the colonic mucosa. Animal studies suggest that short-chain fatty acids are important for epithelial cell proliferation and wound healing in the colon. The addition of fiber to enteral formulations increases the levels of short-chain fatty acids in the colon. A significant reduction in inflammation was noted in the defunctionalized colon when short-chain fatty acids were instilled in the affected portion of the colon of patients with diversion colitis (22). In view of the important role of short-chain fatty acids in the maintenance of colonic structural and functional integrity, the use of fiber-containing formulations should be seriously considered in any patient for whom tube feedings are expected to be the sole source of nutrition for an extended period of time, especially patients with intestinal disease or injury. Recently, some manufacturers have added *fructo-oligosaccharides* to enteral nutrition formulations. Fructo-oligosaccharides are mixtures of oligomers composed primarily of β-D-fructose monomers linked by β2-1 osidic bonds. Fructo-oligosaccharides are fermented by bacteria in the colon to form short-chain fatty acids (23) (see Section IID of Chapter 11).

B. **Feeding techniques for forced enteral feeding.** *Forced enteral feeding* is defined as the direct instillation of nutrients into or just proximal to the organ of absorption (small bowel) through a tube placed nasally or through a surgically or endoscopically created ostomy. Nasogastric and nasoduodenal tubes are more commonly used for forced enteral feeding than are feeding gastrostomy and feeding enterostomy tubes. Rapid bedside placement of nasogastric and nasoduodenal tubes makes this form of intensive nutritional support very easy to initiate. The increased experience with nasoduodenal tubes has, in many situations, reduced the need for enterostomy. Once a patient is selected for forced enteral feeding, the appropriate form of tube feeding should be selected. Characteristics of feeding tubes are reviewed elsewhere (24,25).

1. **Advantages and disadvantages of various forced enteral feeding techniques**
   a. **Nasogastric technique**
      (1) **Advantages.** The tube is easily placed. Large quantities can be fed intermittently, so that the patient is free between feedings. The stomach tolerates large volumes of hyperosmolar feeding without cramping, distention, or vomiting. This technique uses the physiology of normal gastric emptying to prevent intestinal overload. Equipment requirements are minimal (no pump), and the method is easily learned.
      (2) **Disadvantages.** Intermittent feeding can lead to reflux and tracheobronchial aspiration. Gastric retention occurs when gastric emptying is not normal. The tube is uncomfortable in the nose and is visually displeasing. It is not recommended for long-term use.
   b. **Nasoduodenal technique**
      (1) **Advantages.** This technique can overcome problems of gastric retention. Gastroesophageal reflux of formula and subsequent risk for tracheobronchial aspiration are reduced. The proper use of a nasoduodenal tube reduces the risk for aspirating the tube feeding, but the patient is still at risk for aspirating gastric

contents. Infusion of the formula is constant, and small-caliber tubes are used. Use of this type of tube may help determine if delayed gastric emptying is the reason for an inability to sustain oral feeding.

(2) **Disadvantages.** It may be difficult to place the tube tip in the small bowel properly. Tube placement may have to be confirmed radiographically, which raises the cost. The duodenum does not tolerate large volumes, especially large volumes of hyperosmolar formulas. Gastrointestinal side effects are more frequent—specifically cramping, distention, vomiting, and diarrhea. The tube is uncomfortable in the nose and is visually displeasing. The requirement for a pump increases the expense and technical complexity. The tube can migrate or be inadvertently pulled back into the stomach, so that the patient is exposed to an increased risk for aspiration. The use of a nasoduodenal tube with a pump also raises the risk for enteral feeding running on "automatic pilot" without adequate monitoring. We have seen a number of patients from nursing homes who aspirated when enteral feedings were pumped through a nasoduodenal tube that had been dislodged into the stomach.

c. **Gastrostomy technique**

(1) **Advantages.** This technique allows for intermittent feeding and normal gastric emptying. The tube can be placed with the patient under sedation or local anesthesia. The esophageal irritation of a nasally placed tube is avoided. A large-caliber tube can be used for medications. Small-caliber tubes can be placed through the gastrostomy into the small bowel.

(2) **Disadvantages** are similar to those for nasogastric tube feeding except for visual and nasal discomfort. Large-bore tubes can ulcerate the gastric mucosa. Local skin care is required.

d. **Jejunostomy technique**

(1) **Advantages.** This technique bypasses an obstructive lesion or motor abnormalities involving the gastrointestinal tract proximal to the jejunum. The advantages are the same as for nasoduodenal tubes. Additionally, the tube position in the small bowel is certain.

(2) **Disadvantages.** Intestinal side effects are frequent, as with nasoduodenal tubes. General anesthesia is required for placement. Local skin care is necessary. No commercially available permanent jejunostomy tubes are really adequate, so that this is a technically difficult approach. It is possible to place a jejunostomy tube percutaneously, but this approach entails greater risk (26,27).

2. **Choosing a technique for forced enteral feeding**

a. **Nasogastric tube.** Choose a nasogastric tube if the tube will be in place for less than 4 weeks, problems with gastric retention or aspiration are not anticipated, and the patient is unlikely to pull the tube out.

b. **Nasoduodenal tube.** Choose a nasoduodenal tube if the tube will be in place less than 4 weeks, the patient is unlikely to pull the tube out, and problems with gastric emptying or aspiration are anticipated (although nasoduodenal tubes can migrate back into the stomach and cause aspiration). One can choose a nasoduodenal tube rather than a nasogastric tube even for a patient with normal gastric emptying because the nasoduodenal tube is smaller in diameter, softer, and more comfortable. The disadvantage of this approach is that intermittent feedings are not possible with a nasoduodenal tube.

c. **Gastrostomy.** Choose a gastrostomy if the tube will be in place longer than 4 weeks, the patient has no problems with gastric retention or aspiration, and the patient is likely to pull out a naso-gastric tube.

   d. Jejunostomy tube. Choose a jejunostomy tube if the tube will be in place longer than 4 weeks, the patient has problems with gastric retention or aspiration, and the patient is likely to pull out a naso-duodenal tube. Intermittent feedings are not possible with jejunostomy tubes.

3. **Tubes for nasogastric and nasoduodenal feeding.** Forced enteral feeding can be accomplished through a standard nasogastric tube or a Salem sump. However, smaller-caliber tubes (either nasogastric or nasoduodenal) of softer materials are better tolerated for long feeding periods. In addition, if continuous-infusion feeding techniques are planned, a longer feeding tube that reaches the distal duodenum is preferable. Most continuous-infusion forced enteral feeding, however, is performed through small-bore tubes designed specifically for nasoduodenal intubation. Table 9-9 lists the characteristics of several commercially available tubes for nasogastric or nasoduodenal feeding.

4. **Techniques of nasoenteral tube placement**
   a. Place patient in a sitting position or with the head of the bed elevated more than 45 degrees.
   b. Stiffen the tube by cooling it in ice water, and advance the lubricated tip to the posterior nasopharynx. The wooden end of an applicator swab may be gently inserted into a distal feeding hole and used as a guide to advance the tube through the nasal passage. A stiffener provided for this purpose also may be used.
   c. Ask the patient to swallow to open the upper esophageal sphincter and allow the tube with tractor to enter the esophagus. Gentle encouragement with a stiffener may be necessary to enter the upper esophageal sphincter of a patient who is uncooperative or comatose.
   d. Stiffeners that can be used to position the tubes include angiography catheter guidewires and commercially available stylets provided with some feeding tubes. If any type of stiffener is used, care must be taken to prevent the stiffener from protruding through one of the infusion holes. A "corkscrew" technique with use of a commercial stylet can assist in tube passage. The use of stiffeners or stylets also increases the risks associated with tube placement. We have seen tubes with stylets perforate the esophagus and lung when inadvertently introduced into the trachea.
   e. If a nasogastric tube is used, the position in the stomach can be confirmed by aspirating the gastric contents. Injecting air through a tube, especially a small-bore tube, while auscultating the abdomen helps determine that the tube is in a hollow viscus. This can be deceiving, however, and injection of air through a tube that has entered the tracheobronchial tree in an unconscious patient also may produce a gurgling noise. If the tube is passed too far into the stomach, it will bend so that the tip is not in the most dependent portion of the stomach. In that case, aspiration can give a false estimate of the gastric contents. The position of the tube can be confirmed radiographically.
   f. A variety of techniques can be used for passing nasoduodenal tubes. We use a 10F 100-cm Corpak tube with stylet. Metoclopramide (10 mg) is given IM, and the tube is introduced 10 minutes later. We auscultate over the stomach test for gastric residual and then advance to 95 cm and check the pH. We do not place the patient on the right side, nor do we wait for the tube to migrate beyond the ligament of Treitz before use. Other approaches include placing the patient on the right side to promote passage of the tube out of the stomach and the use of fluoroscopy to assess tube position. At some institutions, a plain film of the abdomen is routinely obtained to document tube

Table 9-9. Characteristics of several small-caliber tubes for forced enteral feeding

Manufacturer (brand name)	Tube material	Length[a]	Gauge[a] (French)	Bolus material	Other features
Argyle (Duo-Tube)	Polyurethane	20,36,42 in	5,6,8	Tungsten or silicone	Tip is 15–17F caliber; outer sheath for tube placement.
Kendall (Entriflex, Dobbhoff)	Polyurethane	36,43,55 in	8,10,12	Tungsten	Straight or bulbous tip; separate stylet available. Flow-through feature of stylet allows sampling of gastric and enteral contents to help establish position.
Clintec	Polyurethane	20,37,43 in	6,8,10,12	Tungsten	Available with and without stylet.
Corpak (Silk, Corsafe)	Polyurethane	22,36,43 in	5,6,8,10,12	Tungsten	Stylet; pill-shaped tip on Corsafe tubes; nonweighted tips available.
Ross (Flexiflo)	Polyurethane	36,45 in	8,10,12,14,16	Tungsten	Available with and without tips and optional stylet.
Sherwood (Kangaroo)	Silicone, polyurethane	43 in	8,12	Tungsten spring	Flow-through tip; stylet.

[a] Representative lengths and gauges provided; others may be available.

position before use; however, we do not routinely the check tube position radiographically.

g. Ideally, the most distal portion of a small-bowel tube approaches or passes the ligament of Treitz. *Reflux* into the stomach of fluids instilled into the small bowel is less likely when the feeding ports are in this location. However, this complication is still likely in patients who have previously aspirated gastric reflux, even with an appropriately placed tube.

h. The proximal end of the tube can be taped to the forehead or pinned to a gown to prevent accidental dislodgement. Tight taping of feeding tubes to the nose results in skin ulceration over the alar cartilage because these feeding tubes are often in place for long periods of time.

5. **Percutaneous techniques of feeding tube placement** have expanded and simplified the use of tube feeding when nasogastric or nasoduodenal tube placement fails or is impractical. Patients who require long-term forced enteral feeding (e.g., after a cerebrovascular accident involving the swallowing center) are often candidates. Percutaneous techniques have advantages over surgical gastrostomy and jejunostomy in that they are less expensive and do not require general anesthesia. Complication rates also may be lower. These tubes generally can be used for feeding within 24 to 48 hours of placement.

   a. In percutaneous endoscopic gastrostomy, a 16- to 18-gauge latex or silicone catheter is placed through the abdominal wall directly into the stomach. The endoscope is used to help localize a site at which the stomach is in close apposition to the anterior abdominal wall. Three techniques are commonly used. In the Ponsky-Gauderer technique, a needle is placed through the abdominal wall into the stomach; a string is placed through the needle and pulled out of the mouth with an endoscope; finally, a gastrostomy tube is tied to the string and pulled through the stomach and out the anterior abdominal wall. In the Sachs-Vine technique, a guidewire is placed through a needle in the abdominal wall into the stomach; the end of the guidewire is then pulled out of the mouth with an endoscope; finally, a gastrostomy tube is pushed over the guidewire into the stomach and out the hole in the abdominal wall. In the Russell technique, a tube is placed over a guidewire that has been inserted through the abdominal wall and stomach. The success rates and complication rates with the three techniques are similar.

      (1) Basic requirements for use of the percutaneous endoscopic gastrostomy technique include the following:

         (a) Ability to pass the endoscope (not possible in some patients with severe neurologic disease)

         (b) Ability of the patient to tolerate sedation

         (c) An unobstructed esophagus if the pull-through technique is to be used

         (d) Absence of excessive obesity

         (e) No history of a complicated surgical procedure in the upper abdomen that may have caused bowel loops to adhere between the stomach and abdominal wall

      (2) Complications are relatively common. Early reports of low complication rates were related to patient selection and short duration of follow-up. The rate of complications is influenced by the advanced age and debility of the patients who generally undergo this procedure. Death occurs in 0.5% of patients. Major complications (peritonitis, necrotizing fasciitis, severe hemorrhage) occur in 1%. Lesser complications (tube extrusion or migration, gastrocolic fistula, aspiration) occur in 8%. Wound infection occurs in 2% to 5%. The likelihood of this complication is reduced if a single dose of a first-generation cephalosporin such as cefazolin is given before the procedure (28).

b. **A percutaneous gastrostomy placed with radiologic guidance** also has been described. A site is localized with fluoroscopy and ultrasonography. The tube is advanced over a guidewire that has been inserted through the abdominal wall with the stomach inflated. A nasogastric tube is required for gastric insufflation. This technique also has a low complication rate and is advantageous for patients who cannot undergo endoscopy or who may have trapped bowel loops.

c. **A percutaneous pharyngostomy** technique has been described that simplifies previous surgical procedures (29). A needle is used to gain access to the piriform sinus. A small-caliber gastric or duodenal feeding tube can then be pulled through the pharyngostomy. This approach is rarely needed but may be useful in patients who are not candidates for percutaneous endoscopic gastrostomy or radiologic or surgical placement of tubes yet require long-term forced enteral feeding.

6. **Technique of nasoduodenal or jejunostomy tube feeding**
   a. **An appropriate feeding formula** should be selected.
   b. Nasoduodenal and jejunostomy tubes have small internal diameters, and as a result, a pump is required to force formulas through them. Initiate feeding at a *slow, constant infusion rate* of 20 to 30 mL of isotonic or slightly hypotonic solution per hour. The rate is then increased 10 mL/h every 4 hours until the goal rate is achieved. A typical goal for the final infusion rate is 80 to 100 mL/h. The final infusion rate is calculated from the desired daily provision of calories and protein.
   c. **Maintain a 30-degree elevation** of the head of the bed during constant infusion to prevent tracheobronchial aspiration. It is good practice to keep the head elevated even when feeding ports are near or distal to the ligament of Treitz.
   d. **Feeding formulas in cans do not need to be refrigerated.** If they are refrigerated, they should be brought to room temperature before infusion. Formulas in bags should be kept refrigerated until used and should be allowed to hang no more than 4 hours in a feeding solution administration set. The longer the formula hangs in the bag at room temperature, the higher the level of bacterial contamination (30). If a longer infusion time for each bag is needed, feeding sets that keep the formula chilled while hanging are available. The feeding bag should be changed or washed thoroughly every 24 hours to prevent bacterial contamination. Theoretical complications related to *bacterial growth* in the feeding formula rarely develop into true clinical problems. However, small outbreaks of nosocomial enteric infection have been documented. Commercial formulas may have an advantage in this regard over blenderized foods because they are sterile.
   e. **Tube flushes** with at least 30 mL of water or dark carbonated soda every 4 hours are needed to keep the tube open.
   f. **Intermittent or gavage feeding** directly into the small bowel through nasoduodenal or jejunostomy tubes is not recommended because of the secretory osmotic response of the small bowel to hypertonic bolus feedings.

7. **Technique of nasogastric tube or gastrostomy tube feeding.** Constant-infusion techniques used with nasoduodenal tubes also can be used for gastrostomy and nasogastric tube feeding. Constant infusion into the stomach may be advantageous in a few conditions, including short-bowel syndrome. However, in most cases, because of the possibility of gastric retention of the infusate, intermittent feeding

through tubes with feeding ports in the stomach is the recommended technique. Additionally, rates of oxygen consumption appear to be lower and cumulative nitrogen balance appears to be better with intermittent feeding than with the continuous-infusion technique. Intermittent feeding can be carried out by bolus with a 60-mL syringe or by intermittent drip with or without a pump. A satisfactory technique for initiating intermittent feeding through a nasogastric or gastrostomy tube is the following:

a. **An appropriate feeding formula** should be selected.

b. **Elevate the head of the patient's bed** at least 30 degrees from the horizontal before the feeding is begun, and leave the patient in this position for at least 2 hours after the feeding has been completed.

c. **Aspirate** through the nasogastric or gastrostomy tube before initiating the feeding to determine whether retained gastric secretions are present. Although almost all centers use the residual volume as a guide to managing tube feedings, the recommended cutoff volume varies considerably, and few data are available on which to base a recommendation. At most centers, intermittent tube feedings are delayed if the residual volume is more than 100 mL (150 mL at some centers); however, the best study suggests that residual volumes up to 200 mL may be seen in patients who tolerate tube feedings (31). If the residual volume is too large, delay feeding for an hour or two and recheck the residual volume. One can attempt to reduce residual volumes with the use of prokinetic agents, feeding formulations lower in fat, and intermittent rather than continuous feeding.

d. **Begin a feeding schedule** of 100 to 150 mL of isotonic or slightly hypotonic formula every 4 hours. Isotonic fluids empty most rapidly from the stomach.

e. **Increase the formula amount** by 50 mL every one or two feedings up to a maximum of 450 mL every 4 hours. If bloating or abdominal discomfort develops with a bolus, the patient should be encouraged to wait 10 to 15 minutes before administering the next bolus. Patients with normal gastric function tolerate 450 mL per bolus feeding. Three or four bolus feedings per day provide the daily nutrient requirements for most patients. Flush with at least 30 mL of water or dark carbonated soda after each feeding to keep the tube open.

f. **Be certain to aspirate residual** from the stomach before giving the next feeding to ensure that the feeding rate is tolerated. Normal gastric emptying of liquids is strongly influenced by osmolarity of the liquid. Because emptying is fastest when the liquid is isosmotic, increasing the formula concentration to full strength further reduces the rate of gastric emptying when hyperosmotic formulas are used.

g. **Gastric motor disorders** seldom interfere with the emptying of liquids. Vagotomy increases intragastric pressure and actually increases the gastric emptying of liquids. Persistent gastric retention of feeding formula indicates gastric outlet obstruction, proximal small-bowel obstruction, or ileus involving the stomach and proximal small bowel.

h. **Ambulatory patients** requiring intermittent nasogastric or gastrostomy feeding may tolerate larger volumes of formula delivered less often. Normal people consume two or three large meals per day, with gradual emptying of the stomach contents into the small bowel during 3 to 5 hours. It is important that patients receiving tube feedings not recline for at least 2 hours after instillation of a feeding, even one as small as 100 mL. Regurgitation is possible with a nasogastric tube because it interferes with the function of the upper and lower esophageal sphincters, which normally prevent tracheobronchial aspiration during recumbency.

8. **Gastrostomy and jejunostomy stoma care**
    a. **Skin protection.** Many patients do not require a dressing around the tube. Dressings should be used if drainage is present or if it is feared that the tube will become dislodged. If a dressing is required, a simple 4 × 4-in dressing and tape suffice in most cases. A few patients have problems with the skin around the opening. When necessary, Squibb Stomahesive paste can be applied directly around the tube where it exits from the skin. If a clear plastic Op-Site adhesive dressing or a 4-in square of Stomahesive or Hollihesive is placed over the paste and ostomy site (without causing the tube to kink), the tube and stoma can be visualized and the patient can take a bath or shower. This type of protective dressing prevents skin irritation from gastrointestinal fluids. Stomahesive and Hollihesive are expensive and should be used only as required for skin breakdown or other problems.
    b. **A 1 × 4-in strip of Squibb Stomahesive skin barrier** or the equivalent placed near the stoma site provides an irritation-free attachment site for adhesive tape if it is needed to stabilize the tube.
    c. **If tape and gauze dressings** are used, they should be changed when they become soiled or every 2 to 3 days so that the skin and stoma site can be examined.
    d. **Standard gastrostomy tubes,** in particular percutaneous gastrostomy tubes, can be replaced with a short silicone post ("The Button," Wilson-Cook, Winston Salem, NC). The intragastric component of the post is a mushroom tip, and the external part is a small, tablike cross-piece. An attached flap closure provides a flush surface. During feeding, a tube is inserted into the open post. This device, which can be placed 4 to 6 weeks or more after the gastrostomy procedure, allows a better cosmetic effect and the regression of granulation tissue from the original tube in some patients, and it reduces skin irritation. The Button is designed as a one-way antireflux valve. A special adapter is needed to cannulate the valve and check the residual volume or detect decompression.
    e. **Specialized therapists.** Consultation with the local enterostomal therapist or a nurse with special interest in stoma therapy can be very helpful. These specialists can help design individual dressings according to the location of the stoma, nature of the tube, and the patient's daily activities, and they can also manage skin problems and any technical difficulties that may arise.
9. **Monitoring forced enteral nutrition.** Patients on forced enteral nutrition must be monitored to detect complications and evaluate the efficacy of the nutritional support (Table 9-10). Daily surveillance for complications includes assessment of vital signs, number of bowel movements, and patient complaints. Patients must be observed carefully for the most common complications: dehydration, fluid overload, aspiration, and electrolyte abnormalities. Weight loss, a rising BUN, and declining urine output are signs of dehydration. Rapid weight gain, edema, and intake greatly in excess of output are signs of fluid overload. Cough, fever, and increased breath sounds are signs of aspiration. Positive signs of the efficacy of nutritional support come slowly. Weight gain and an increase in albumin may not be seen until after weeks of nutritional support. On the other hand, negative signs of efficacy of nutritional support develop rapidly. A patient whose albumin level and lean body mass continue to fall after initiation of nutritional support is not receiving the expected benefits. This may represent an inability to absorb the enteral formula because of mucosal abnormalities or increased motility. Alternatively, the patient's caloric requirements may have been underestimated.

Table 9-10. Monitoring patients receiving forced enteral nutrition

Assessment	Frequency
Nursing	
Gastric residuals (gastric feedings only)	Before each feeding
Vital signs	Daily
Weight	Daily
I/O	Daily at first, then as needed
Electrolytes	
Serum sodium, potassium, chloride, bicarbonate	Baseline, then twice a week
Renal function	
BUN, creatinine	Twice a week
Other laboratory	
Calcium, phosphorus, magnesium, albumin	Baseline, then once a week
Triglycerides, cholesterol	As indicated
Glucose	For nondiabetics: daily for 3 days, then three times a week
	For diabetics: Every 4–6 hours until blood sugar and insulin dose are stable, then less often
Hematocrit	Twice a week
Prothrombin time	As needed

I/O, in and out; BUN, blood urea nitrogen.

Many tube-fed patients receive less than their entire prescribed intake (32). Common reasons include the following:
    a. Tube dislodgement
    b. Gastrointestinal intolerance
    c. Medical procedures that interrupt feeding
    d. Problems with the position of the feeding tube

C. Complications of forced enteral feedings

    1. Metabolic complications. Fluid and electrolyte problems are common in patients receiving tube feedings, and in many cases, the formula must be modified to solve these problems. Hypokalemia, hyponatremia, hypophosphatemia, and hyperglycemia are among the most frequent metabolic complications. Some of the complications result from the use of commercial products, all of which have a fixed electrolyte content. This disadvantage is easily outweighed by their convenience of use and modest expense.

        a. Electrolyte disturbances. The mineral contents of the formulas are given in Table 9-3 and are based on the usual requirements (see Chapter 7). Some patients may require additional supplements or may not tolerate the preestablished amounts of individual minerals. Problems are especially likely to develop in patients with renal, hepatic, or cardiac disease. Periodic monitoring of serum levels of sodium, potassium, chloride, calcium, phosphorus, and magnesium detects the most frequent electrolyte abnormalities.

        b. Deficiencies of trace minerals may appear in patients on longterm forced enteral feeding. Formulas based on egg albumin provide the most selenium, whereas the selenium contents of many other formulas are less than the proposed safe and adequate range of intake. Clinically relevant zinc deficiency also has been noted. Zinc deficiency is especially likely in patients with zinc loss from the gastrointestinal tract, as in active Crohn's disease. Patients receiving defined formulas as their only source of nutrition for prolonged periods must be observed for micronutrient deficiencies.

c. **Volume overload.** The formula volume to provide 2,000 kcal delivers 40 to 80 mEq (1 to 2 g) of sodium in most cases. The amount of sodium given per day in the tube feeding diet may not be readily appreciated by the physician. Refer to Table 9-3 for the sodium content of the various formulas, and note that some formulas have a considerably lower sodium content than others. If hyponatremia is significant in a patient with sodium and water retention, the total daily volume can be decreased by selecting a formula with greater caloric density while still restricting sodium.

d. **Hyperosmolarity syndrome** is an uncommon complication resulting from inadequate intake of free water despite continuous ingestion of a high osmotic load. The clinical syndrome includes lethargy, obtundation, appearance of dehydration, and at times fever. Serum electrolytes reveal hypernatremia and hyperosmolarity. The *treatment* includes increasing daily free water by supplementing the usual routine with water or by diluting the formula. IV 5% dextrose in water or 0.45% sodium chloride solution may be necessary, as in the management of hypernatremia, if changes in mental status are significant.

e. **Refeeding syndrome** may develop when patients who are severely malnourished are begun on enteral (or parenteral) nutrition (33). With refeeding, phosphate and magnesium move from the extracellular to the intracellular space, causing hypophosphatemia and hypomagnesemia (34). Patients who are hypophosphatemic before the start of feeding should be depleted. Serum magnesium and phosphate levels should be monitored carefully in all patients who are being refed (Table 5-25).

f. **Warfarin resistance** may result from the unsuspected delivery of vitamin K in enteral supplements or feeding formulas. The estimated safe and adequate daily intake of vitamin K is 70 to 140 μg, yet the average diet in the United States contains 300 to 500 μg of this vitamin. Warfarin resistance is an uncommon development with the vitamin K content of currently available products.

2. **Nonmetabolic complications**

a. **Diarrhea and gastrointestinal discomfort** (nausea, abdominal pain, bloating) are the most common complications of enteral feeding, occurring in as many as 20% of patients. The incidence of diarrhea in tube feeding depends on the definition of diarrhea. If diarrhea is defined broadly (one or more liquid stools per day), the incidence in tube-fed patients is more than 70%; if a more stringent definition is used (four or more liquid stools per day or five or more stools per day), the incidence falls to 21% (35). Diarrhea in a tube-fed patient is the result of interactions between the patient and the tube feeding; diarrhea does not develop in normal volunteers given conventional tube feedings (36). The reasons for diarrhea are variable but often can be categorized as follows:

(1) Drug-induced diarrhea may be related to antibiotics (37), antacids, or laxatives.

(2) Diarrhea may be induced by sorbitol or other nonabsorbable sugars in elixirs and other medications (38). Elixirs of cimetidine, acetaminophen, and theophylline (among others) contain large amounts of sorbitol.

(3) In the past, when many enteral formulations contained lactose, intolerance to lactose was a common cause of diarrhea in tube-fed patients. Now only a few commercial formulas contain lactose (Table 9-3).

(4) Infection should be considered as a potential cause of diarrhea—in particular, pseudomembranous colitis in patients who have received antibiotics (37).

(5) Improper matching of the enteral formulation to the patient can lead to diarrhea. If a high-fat diet is given to a patient with pancreatic insufficiency or bile salt deficiency, diarrhea will develop.

(6) Hypertonicity of the formula is commonly invoked as a cause of diarrhea, although it is seldom the culprit. Nonetheless, it may be worth switching from a hypertonic to an isotonic formula.

(7) Reduction of the flow rate may relieve the diarrhea.

(8) Patients on a fiber-free enteral formula may benefit from switching to a fiber-containing formula; however, fiber-containing formulas are more likely to clog the feeding tube (39).

(9) Bacterial contamination of the enteral formula in the bag is possible, especially if it has been hanging at room temperature too long (40). Culture the formula and switch the bag.

(10) Hypoalbuminemia is associated with a higher rate of diarrhea in tube-fed patients (41).

(11) If none of the listed problems appears to be a cause of the patient's diarrhea, a trial of an antidiarrheal agent is indicated (6 to 10 drops of deodorized tincture of opium every 6 to 12 hours, 30 mg of codeine sulfate every 6 hours, 10 mL of diphenoxylate liquid every 6 hours, or 10 mL of loperamide elixir every 6 hours).

b. Esophagitis or esophageal ulcer. Nasally placed tubes can cause esophagitis, by directly irritating the esophageal mucosa and by interfering with normal protective mechanisms against esophageal damage by gastric acid. Competence of the lower esophageal sphincter, normal esophageal stripping by primary and secondary peristalsis, and swallowing of saliva all appear to help prevent reflux esophagitis in normal persons, and all these mechanisms may be impaired in patients with feeding tubes.

(1) Esophagitis has been reported uncommonly in patients with small-caliber tubes; this may be because the tube caliber is smaller or because the newer tubes, which are not made of rubber, do not become brittle with time. Symptoms include heartburn and possibly dysphagia and odynophagia. Gastrointestinal bleeding from the lesion can be discovered during aspiration before a feeding or by checking the stool for occult blood.

(2) Treatment. It may be difficult to heal the lesion with the tube in place. Elevation of the head of the bed and switching from intermittent feedings to small, frequent feedings are helpful from a mechanical standpoint. Histamine$_2$-receptor antagonists and proton pump inhibitors reduce gastric acidity and may be more conveniently delivered to these patients than antacids.

c. Tracheobronchial aspiration is a serious complication that can be prevented by taking several precautions. Aspiration is especially likely to occur in patients who have an altered gag reflex, a swallowing disorder, or an altered level of consciousness. A lower incidence of aspiration in patients in intensive care units compared with those on medical or surgical wards suggests that adequate nursing care and pulmonary precautions can reduce the incidence of aspiration (42). Patients with nasally placed tubes can be particularly susceptible because the tube can interfere with normal functioning of the upper and lower esophageal sphincters—important barriers to the reflux of gastric contents. The placement of a tube within the proximal small bowel bypasses the problem of gastric retention, but reflux into the stomach is possible. If the feeding ports are beyond the ligament of Treitz, reflux is less likely; however, aspiration has occurred from jejunostomy tubes. Although theoretical reasons favor the placement of tubes in the small bowel over placement in the stomach, available data do not clearly demonstrate a lower incidence of aspiration with small-bowel tubes (43). The patient with pulmonary aspiration may be asymptomatic or may present with gagging, fever, tachycardia, tachypnea, or respiratory distress. Aspirated formulas can be detected by examining pulmonary secretions with glucose strips. (The presence of blood in the sputum can cause a false-positive result of a test for glucose.) This sensitive technique indicates that tracheobronchial aspiration may accompany more than one-third of nasogastric feedings, but that clinically significant sequelae are most likely when aspiration is continually detected. One common misconception is that the presence of a tracheostomy or an endotracheal tube eliminates the possibility of aspiration. In fact, many patients aspirate around tracheostomy tubes and endotracheal tubes. Precautions that reduce the occurrence of aspiration are the following:

    (1) **Establish correct placement of the tube,** particularly a soft, small-caliber tube, before initiating feeding. The correct position of a soft, small-caliber tube can be confirmed radiographically.

    (2) **Keep the head of the bed elevated** at least 30 degrees at all times for the patient receiving a continuous infusion and for at least 2 hours after a feeding for the patient receiving intermittent feeding.

    (3) **The ambulatory patient should not be allowed to lie down** for at least 2 hours after a feeding.

    (4) **Aspirate** contents from the stomach via the nasogastric tube before each feeding when intermittent feedings are given to check for gastric retention, and delay the subsequent feeding if necessary (see Section IVB7c).

    (5) **Delayed gastric emptying** may be approached pharmacologically with prokinetic agents (44).

  d. Clogging of the tube occurs most frequently when small-caliber (<2 mm ID) tubes are used. Obstruction occurs from the instillation of poorly crushed medication into the tube or from intraluminal buildup of formula residue. Aluminum-containing antacids may interact with some nutritional formulas to produce plugs. Most blenderized diets and those containing meat or vegetable fiber are not recommended for use through small-diameter tubes. Highly dispersed commercial tube diets are less likely to clog tubes, but clogging of small-bore tubes occurs with some frequency even with commercial diets, especially if the tubes are not irrigated regularly. Another cause of tube clogging is failure to adequately dissolve enteral formulas that come in powder form. The use of a blender in preparing formulas from powdered material can avoid clumping. Clogged tubes should be irrigated with water or sugar-free carbonated beverages.

  e. Very rare complications have included small bowel perforation, pneumatosis intestinalis, rupture and division of the feeding tube, and inadvertent IV administration of the formula. Bronchopulmonary complications, including perforation of the lung, can occur if a stylet is used and inadvertently enters the trachea. This complication can occur even in the presence of an inflated tracheostomy tube cuff.

V. Administering medications through feeding tubes. For many patients with feeding tubes, especially those at home or in extended-care facilities, the tube is the only practical avenue for administering medications. Liquid medications are pushed through the tube; tablets are crushed, mixed with water, and pushed through the tube. However, not all medications can be administered successfully by feeding tube. Some general guidelines have been developed, but the guidelines may not be applicable to certain combinations of drugs, enteral formula, and feeding tube.

A. General guidelines

1. **The tube.** The location of tube must be considered. Drugs administered beyond the pylorus are absorbed more rapidly. Antacids and carafate should not be delivered beyond the pylorus. The diameter of the tube must be considered. The smaller the diameter, the more likely it is to become clogged. Thick liquids such as antacids should not be administered through a tube with a diameter smaller than 10F.

2. **The drug**

   a. Slow-release drugs (e.g., Calan SR, Cardizem, Isordil Tembid) and enteric-coated drugs (e.g., MI-Cebrin, Azulfidine EN-tabs) should not be crushed because crushing may increase the rate of absorption (for slow-release formulations), expose the drug to degradation in the stomach, or cause gastric upset.

   b. Pancreatic enzymes (e.g., Pancrease) are usually enteric-coated. If they are crushed and administered by nasogastric tube, they can be inactivated by gastric acid.

   c. The use of liquid preparations is generally preferable to crushing and dissolving tablets. A liquid formulation of a drug should be used if it is available.

3. **Administration**

   a. Crushed tablets should be reconstituted in at least 10 to 15 mL of water.

   b. Hard gelatin capsules should be opened and the powder dissolved in at least 10 to 15 mL of water.

   c. Drugs that are hypertonic or that irritate the gastrointestinal mucosa should be dissolved in larger volumes of water before administration.

   d. Drugs should not be added to the enteral formula.

   e. The enteral formula should be stopped before medication is administered.

   f. The feeding tube should be flushed with water to remove residual formula before medication is administered.

   g. The feeding tube should be flushed with water (10 to 30 mL) after the drug is administered.

   h. For patients on intermittent gastric feeding schedules, the timing of administration of medications that should be taken on a full or empty stomach should be adjusted according to the patient's feeding schedule.

B. Drugs with specific requirements

1. **Phenytoin.** The absorption of phenytoin may be diminished when it is given to patients on continuous tube feedings, although this is not the case with all tube feedings (45). Blood levels should be checked and the dose of phenytoin adjusted accordingly. Similarly, the dose of phenytoin may need to be reduced when a patient is switched from continuous feedings to intermittent tube feedings or oral feedings. In patients on intermittent tube feedings, phenytoin should be given as far as possible from the time of feeding. We hold tube feeding for 1 hour before and after phenytoin is administered.

2. **Warfarin.** The vitamin K in tube feedings interacts with warfarin and decreases its effects. The prothrombin time should be monitored when tube feedings are initiated, discontinued, or interrupted.

3. **Theophylline.** The absorption of theophylline may be impaired with continuous tube feedings; blood levels should be monitored.

4. **Carbamazepine suspension (Tegretol).** Drug is often lost when undiluted suspension adheres to polyvinyl chloride feeding tubes.

5. **Potassium chloride syrup** becomes viscous and gelatinous and clogs the tube.

6. **Ciprofloxacin.** We hold tube feedings for 1 hour before and after ciprofloxacin is administered.

VI. Pancreatic insufficiency. In the United States, chronic pancreatitis secondary to alcoholism is the most common cause of exocrine pancreatic insufficiency in adults. Fat malabsorption does not become significant until lipase output is less than 10% of normal, and consequently, a considerable portion of the gland must be destroyed before insufficiency is clinically recognized. Other causes of pancreatic insufficiency include cystic fibrosis, hereditary pancreatitis, other types of chronic pancreatitis, surgical resection, and obstruction of the pancreatic duct by calculi, inflammation, stricture, or cancer. Steatorrhea and creatorrhea result from inadequate secretion of lipase and proteases, respectively. However, as in most cases of malabsorption, the severity of intestinal symptoms is related to the degree of steatorrhea. Nutritional support does not reduce disease activity in pancreatitis and should not be viewed as primary therapy. Management is directed toward relief of symptoms, restoration of nutritional status, and then maintenance of protein and calorie balance. Returning the efficiency of fat absorption to normal should not be a goal.

A. Diet. A low-fat diet with 50 to 70 g of triglycerides per day should be tried initially to control symptoms. The intake of fat can be liberalized as control with supplemental enzymes is achieved. Protein supplementation is recommended because the intake of dietary protein is restricted along with the intake of fat. The daily allotment of fat and protein should be equally distributed in three or more meals per day.

B. Enzyme replacement. Large doses of supplemental enzymes are required to reduce steatorrhea in many patients. Lipase activity *in vitro* varies considerably, depending on the preparation (Table 9-11), as does the cost. Commercial preparations are of two types: pancreatin and pancrelipase. Pancreatin is an extract of hog pancreas standardized for amylase and trypsin activity, and pancrelipase is a lipase-enriched extract. Tablets, capsules, and enteric-coated preparations all may be effective in reducing or abolishing steatorrhea if adequate amounts of enzymes are supplied. Approximately 30,000 IU of lipase must be taken with each meal to eliminate steatorrhea completely, and even then enzyme is inactivated by gastric acid. Taking all the tablets at once with a meal is as effective as taking them intermittently with and after a meal. The usual doses of products with *in vitro* enzyme activity that can be given to reduce steatorrhea are given in Table 9-11.

C. Measures to enhance the effects of supplemental enzymes. Patients who are hypochlorhydric or achlorhydric usually respond well to enzyme preparations alone. Maintaining the intragastric pH above 4 in patients with normal gastric secretion or hypersecretion improves the response to administered enzymes. Proton pump inhibitors or histamine$_2$-receptor antagonists, in addition to enzymes, reduce steatorrhea in some patients. Concomitant administration of sodium bicarbonate (1.3 g orally) or aluminum hydroxide gel (30 to 60 mL) with the enzymes also may be effective. Magnesium hydroxide, aluminum hydroxide, and calcium carbonate may actually worsen steatorrhea and are not useful adjuncts to enzyme replacement.

D. Vitamin supplementation. Fat-soluble vitamin supplementation is rarely needed once the previously mentioned measures are taken to reduce steatorrhea because the concentrations of bile acids required to solubilize the fat-soluble vitamins are usually normal. Moreover, the fat-soluble vitamins do not depend on pancreatic hydrolysis for absorption. Identified deficiencies at the outset of therapy should be corrected. Vitamin B deficiency can result from pancreatic insufficiency. Pancreatic proteolytic enzymes are needed to digest haptocorrins and so liberate ingested cobalamin and to bind to intrinsic factor. Enzyme supplementation corrects this error.

VII. Short-bowel syndrome. This disorder, which usually results from extensive small-bowel resection, is not strictly defined. In some cases, the loss of small-bowel surface area is so great that intolerable losses of fluids and electrolytes occur with feeding, whereas in others, maintenance of adequate protein and calorie balance is the only major problem. These examples illustrate the extremes of the spectrum of clinical features. Massive surgical resection

Table 9-11. Pancreatic enzyme preparations

Product	Lipase (units)	Amylase (units)	Protease (units)	Company
Cotazyme S capsule	5,000	20,000	20,000	Organon
Cotazyme capsule	8,000	30,000	20,000	
Creon 5 capsule	5,000	16,600	18,750	Solvay
Creon 10 capsule	10,000	33,200	37,500	Pharmaceuticals
Creon 20 capsule	20,000	66,400	75,000	
Donnazyme tablet	1,000	12,500	12,500	Robbins Pharmaceutical
KU-Zyme capsule	75 mg	30 mg	6 mg	Schwartz
KU-Zyme HP capsule	8,000	30,000	30,000	
Pancrecarb MS 4	4,000	25,000	25,000	Digestive Care, Inc.
Pancrecarb MS 8	8,000	40,000	45,000	
Pancrease capsule	4,500	20,000	25,000	McNeil Pharmaceutical
Pancrease MT 4	4,000	12,000	12,000	
Pancrease MT 10	10,000	30,000	30,000	
Pancrease MT 16	16,000	48,000	48,000	
Pancrease MT 20	20,000	56,000	44,000	
Ultrase capsule	4,500	20,000	25,000	Scandipharm
Ultrase MT 12	12,000	39,000	39,000	
Ultrase MT 18	18,000	58,500	58,500	
Ultrase MT 20	20,000	65,000	65,000	
Viokase powder ¼ tsp	16,800	70,000	70,000	Robbins Pharmaceutical
Viokase tablet	8,000	30,000	30,000	
Zymase capsule	12,000	24,000	24,000	Organon

of diseased, ischemic small bowel (arterial or venous occlusion, strangulation in hernia, volvulus) is the leading cause of the most severe form of the syndrome. Gradual "whittling away" of small intestine with multiple resections for Crohn's disease, on the other hand, is a common cause of the less severe clinical picture. Short-bowel syndrome with severe malabsorption is usually associated with resection of at least part of the more proximal small bowel. After massive resection, it is often unclear whether adequate bowel remains for satisfactory enteral management. As a general rule, a resection of 2-ft segment of jejunum (beyond the ligament of Treitz), in addition to the entire duodenum, is necessary.

A. During adaptation after massive resection. In the first 2 weeks to 2 months, adaptive responses include an increase in caliber of the remaining bowel and epithelial hyperplasia. Supportive measures must be taken while adaptation is taking place.

    1. Initiate TPN (see Chapter 10). Nutritional deterioration is prevented during the restoration of electrolyte and water balance and attempts at gradual feeding while the functional capacity of the remaining bowel is assessed. TPN is such an important measure after sudden massive resection that patients should be transferred to institutions capable of performing this nutritional technique in the stable postoperative period.

    2. Monitor serum electrolytes, calcium, and magnesium regularly. Large amounts of parenteral minerals are necessary to make up for intestinal losses. Zinc losses also can be profound (see Chapter 7).

    2. Control gastric hypersecretion. About 50% of patients who have undergone massive resection have transient gastric hypersecretion that can result in severe peptic ulcer disease. The mechanism is unclear but is felt to be hormonal (loss of an inhibitory control mechanism). Proton pump inhibitors or histamine$_2$-receptor antagonists are the treatments of choice.

4. **Begin feeding** with small amounts of low-fat, low-lactose, isosmolar supplements as soon as possible. Oral feeding or a nasogastric tube is better than a nasoduodenal tube in these patients, who must make maximal use of the gut they have left. Intraluminal nutrients help to promote adaptation. Gradually increase intake while monitoring fecal output.

B. **Following adaptation after massive resection, or for long-term management of less severe short-bowel syndrome**

1. **Diet therapy**
   a. **Low-fat, low-residue diets** (see Chapter 11) and **low-fat supplements** (see Table 9-5) are used if the colon is present.
   b. **Patients with ileostomy or jejunostomy** may benefit from a high-fat diet with more than 50% of calories as fat in each meal (see Chapter 11). This technique capitalizes on the delay in gastric emptying induced by dietary fat. A trial-and-error approach may be necessary to determine the most beneficial diet for this subgroup of patients with short-bowel syndrome.
   c. **Lactose is restricted** initially until the symptoms are under best control. Liberalization with monitoring of the clinical response is then appropriate.
   d. **Enteral feeding** (see Section IV) during both the adaptation and postadaptation periods with low-residue, low-fat, low-lactose, isosmolar formulas (Table 9-3) can be attempted in patients who cannot take oral supplements. However, infusion directly into the small bowel is likely to exacerbate diarrhea severely, at least transiently.

2. **Vitamin and mineral supplementation.** Supplementation of fat-soluble and often water-soluble vitamins is necessary (see Chapter 6 for assessment and therapy). Vitamin B$_{12}$ (500 μg/mL IM) must be given if the distal ileum has been resected. Calcium and magnesium supplementation (see Chapter 7) is usually required. Calcium supplementation may be necessary to reduce oxalate absorption. Calcium and magnesium supplements may be necessary to make up for the intestinal loss of these minerals in the form of soaps. Iron supplementation is necessary if the duodenum has been resected or if persistent occult bleeding is present.

3. **Antidiarrheal therapy** is helpful in reducing food-induced diarrhea in the postadaptation stage.
   a. Frequent small meals are better than two or three large meals.
   b. If drugs are required to control diarrhea, we begin with 2 mg of loperamide two or three times daily and gradually increase the dosage up to 40 mg/d if needed. If this is ineffective, we use 6 to 10 drops of deodorized tincture of opium and 6 to 15 drops of tincture of belladonna (10%) before each meal, or give a capsule formulated from 30 mg of powdered opium and 15 mg of powdered belladonna before meals. This effectively retards gastric emptying, interferes with normal motor activity, and reduces diarrhea. The liquid preparations may be most easily absorbed.

4. **Nutritional assessment** may be periodically necessary to determine the effectiveness of therapy (see Table 5-25 for evaluation of nutritional status). Calorie counts alone are not adequate unless the coefficient of malabsorption is known. See Chapter 5 for a discussion of the assessment of protein and calorie status.

C. **Home TPN** (see Section IX of Chapter 10). A small number of patients with short-bowel syndrome cannot be managed with enteral therapy. Either adequate intake produces intolerable diarrhea with unmanageable fluid and electrolyte losses, even after maximal adaptation, or protein and calorie status gradually deteriorates despite careful attention to the previously discussed management measures. Home TPN can be a lifesaving nutritional support system for this small group of patients.

Bibliography
1. American Society of Parenteral and Enteral Nutrition. Guidelines for the use of parenteral and enteral nutrition in adult and pediatric patients. *JPEN J Parenter Enteral Nutr* 1993;17[1 Suppl]:1S.
2. Alvestrand A, Ahlberg M, Bergstrom J. Retardation of the progression of renal insufficiency in patients treated with low-protein diets. *Kidney Int Suppl* 1983; 16:S268.
3. Klein S, Kinney J, Jeejeebhoy K, et al. Nutrition support in clinical practice: review of published data and recommendations for future research directions. *JPEN J Parenter Enteral Nutr* 1997;21:133.
4. Lindor KD, Fleming CR, Burnes JU, et al. A randomized prospective trial comparing a defined formula diet, corticosteroids, and a defined formula diet plus corticosteroids in active Crohn's disease. *Mayo Clin Proc* 1992;67:328.
5. Griffiths AM, Ohlsson A, Sherman PM, et al. Meta-analysis of enteral nutrition as a primary treatment of active Crohn's disease. *Gastroenterology* 1995;108:1056.
6. Fernandez-Banares F, Cabre E, Esteve-Comas M, et al. How effective is enteral nutrition in inducing clinical remission in active Crohn's disease? A meta-analysis of the randomized clinical trials. *JPEN J Parenter Enteral Nutr* 1995;19:356.
7. Lobo DN, Memon MA, Allison SP, et al. Evolution of nutritional support in acute pancreatitis. *Br J Surg* 2000;87:695.
8. Cerra FB, Shronts EP, Konstantinides NN, et al. Enteral feeding in sepsis: a prospective, randomized, double-blind trial. *Surgery* 1985;98:632.
9. Olree K, et al. Enteral formulations. In: *The ASPEN nutrition support practice manual.* Silver Spring, MD: American Society for Parenteral and Enteral Nutrition, 1998:4.
10. Rees RG, Hare WR, Grimble GK, et al. Do patients with moderately impaired gastrointestinal function requiring enteral nutrition need a predigested nitrogen source? A prospective crossover controlled clinical trial. *Gut* 992;33:877.
11. Brinson RR, Hanumanthu SK, Pitts WM. A reappraisal of the peptide-based enteral formulas: clinical applications. *Nutri Clin Pract* 1989;4:211.
12. McIntyre PB, Fitchew M, Lennard-Jones JE. Patients with a high jejunostomy do not need a special diet. *Gastroenterology* 1986;91:25.
13. Cerra FB, Cheung NK, Fischer JE, et al. Disease-specific amino acid infusion (F080) in hepatic encephalopathy: a prospective, randomized, double-blind, controlled trial. *JPEN J Parenter Enteral Nutr* 1985;9:288.
14. Kearns PJ, Young H, Garcia G, et al. Accelerated improvement of alcoholic liver disease with enteral nutrition. *Gastroenterology* 1992;102:200.
15. Moore FA, Moore EE, Kudsk KA, et al. Clinical benefits of an immune-enhancing diet for early postinjury enteral feeding. *J Trauma* 1994;37:607.
16. Kudsk KA, Minard G, Croce MA, et al. A randomized trial of isonitrogenous enteral diets after severe trauma. *Ann Surg* 1996;4:531.
17. Keith ME, Jeejeebhoy KN. Enteral nutrition. *Curr Opin Gastroenterol* 1998;14:151.
18. Beale RJ, Bryg DJ, Bihari DJ. Immunonutrition in the critically ill: a systematic review of clinical outcome. *Crit Care Med* 1999;27:2799.
19. O'Dwyer ST, Smith RJ, Hwang TL, et al. Maintenance of small bowel mucosa with glutamine-enriched parenteral nutrition. *JPEN J Parenter Enteral Nutr* 1989; 13:579.
20. Alpers D. Is glutamine a unique fuel for small intestinal cells? *Curr Opin Gastroenterol* 2000;16:155.
21. Souba WW, Klimberg VS, Hautamaki RD, et al. Oral glutamine reduces bacterial translocation following abdominal radiation. *J Surg Res* 1990;48:1.
22. Harig JM, Soergel KH, Komorowski RA, et al. Treatment of diversion colitis with short-chain fatty acid irrigation. *N Engl J Med* 1989;320:23.
23. Roberfroid MB, Delzenne N. Dietary fructans. *Annu Rev Nutr* 1999;18:117.
24. Guenter P, et al. Delivery systems and administration of enteral nutrition. In: Rombeau JL, Rolandelli RH, eds. *Clinical nutrition: enteral and tube feeding.* Philadelphia: WB Saunders, 1997:240.
25. Kirby DF, et al. Enteral access and infusion equipment. In: *The ASPEN nutrition support practice manual.* Silver Spring, MD: American Society for Parenteral and Enteral Nutrition, 1998:3.

26. Gorman RC, Morris JB. Minimally invasive access to the gastrointestinal tract. In: Rombeau JL, Rolandelli RH, eds. *Clinical nutrition: enteral and tube feeding.* Philadelphia: WB Saunders, 1997:174.
27. Shike M, Bloch AS. Enteral nutrition. *Gastrointest Endosc Clin N Am* 1998;8:529.
28. Jain NK, Larson DE, Schroeder KW, et al. Antibiotic prophylaxis for percutaneous endoscopic gastrostomy. A prospective, randomized, double-blind clinical trial. *Ann Intern Med* 1987;107:824.
29. Bucklin DL, Gilsdorf RB. Percutaneous needle pharyngostomy. *JPEN J Parenter Enteral Nutr* 1985;9:68.
30. Kohn CL. The relationship between enteral formula contamination and length of enteral delivery set usage. *JPEN J Parenter Enteral Nutr* 1991;15:567.
31. McClave SA, Snider HL, Lowen CC, et al. Use of residual volume as a marker for enteral feeding intolerance: prospective blinded comparison with physical examination and radiographic findings. *JPEN J Parenter Enteral Nutr* 1992;16:99.
32. Abernathy GB, et al. Efficacy of tube feeding in supplying energy requirements of hospitalized patients. *JPEN J Parenter Enteral Nutr* 1989;13:387.
33. Havala T, Shronts E. Managing the complications associated with refeeding. *Nutr Clin Pract* 1990;5:23.
34. Hayek ME, Eisenberg PG. Severe hypophosphatemia following the institution of enteral feedings. *Arch Surg* 1989;124:1325.
35. Bliss DZ, Guenter PA, Settle RG. Defining and reporting diarrhea in tube-fed patients—what a mess. *Am J Clin Nutr* 1992;55:753.
36. Kandil HE, Opper FH, Switzer BR, et al. Marked resistance of normal subjects to tube-feeding-induced diarrhea: the role of magnesium. *Am J Clin Nutr* 1993;57:73.
37. Guenter PA, Settle RG, Perlmutter S, et al. Tube feeding-related diarrhea in acutely ill patients. *JPEN J Parenter Enteral Nutr* 1991;15:277.
38. Edes TE, Walk BE, Austin JL. Diarrhea in tube-fed patients: feeding formula not necessarily the cause. *Am J Med* 1990;88:91.
39. Scheppach W, Burghardt W, Bartram P, et al. Addition of dietary fiber to liquid formula diets: the pros and cons. *JPEN J Parenter Enteral Nutr* 1990:14:204.
40. Belknap DC, Davidson LJ, Flournoy DJ. Microorganisms and diarrhea in enterally fed intensive care unit patients. *JPEN J Parenter Enteral Nutr* 1990;14:622.
41. Brinson RR, Kolts BE. Diarrhea associated with severe hypoalbuminemia: a comparison of a peptide-based chemically defined diet and standard enteral alimentation. *Crit Care Med* 1988;16:130.
42. Mullan H, Roubenoff RA, Roubenoff R. Risk of pulmonary aspiration among patients receiving enteral nutrition support. *JPEN J Parenter Enteral Nutr* 1992; 16:160.
43. Lazarus BA, Murphy JB, Culpepper L. Aspiration associated with long-term gastric versus jejunal feeding: a critical analysis of the literature. *Arch Phys Med Rehabil* 1990;71:46.
44. Annese V, Janssens J, Vantrappen G, et al. Erythromycin accelerates gastric emptying by inducing antral contractions and improved gastroduodenal coordination. *Gastroenterology* 1992;102:823.
45. Marvel ME, Bertino JS Jr. Comparative effects of an elemental and a complex enteral feeding formulation on the absorption of phenytoin suspension. *JPEN J Parenter Enteral Nutr* 1991;15:316.

10. PARENTERAL NUTRITIONAL THERAPY

I. **General principles.** Parenteral nutrition can be used to supply all the essential nutrients without use of the intestinal tract. In most cases, parenteral nutrition is reserved for hospitalized patients who are temporarily unable to meet nutritional requirements through enteral routes. Although an effective form of therapy, total parenteral nutrition (TPN) is expensive and raises the cost of hospital care (1).

   A. **The successful establishment of a positive nitrogen balance and growth by means of TPN** was demonstrated successfully more than 30 years ago. Since then, patients have been maintained on TPN at home and have survived for many years. TPN can be provided through either a central or a peripheral vein, although a central line is almost always preferred.

   B. When parenteral nutrition is used to provide only part of the daily requirements, it is referred to as *partial parenteral nutrition.* Many hospitalized patients receive partial parenteral nutrition in the form of dextrose solutions or dilute amino acid solutions as part of their routine hospital care.

   C. Most of this chapter deals with TPN administered through a *central venous access.* The principles and specific applications of parenteral nutrition therapy administered through peripheral veins are covered in Section IVC. TPN can be delivered in many ways, and considerable variations in technique are noted between investigators and institutions. The techniques offered in this chapter have been employed satisfactorily at Barnes-Jewish Hospital and the Washington University School of Medicine.

   D. **Indications for TPN**

      1. **Patients who are selected for intensive nutritional therapy** are severely malnourished at the outset or are in marked negative nitrogen balance and are not expected to be able to meet nutritional requirements soon. The factors used in selecting patients for intensive nutritional therapy are covered in Chapter 8. Unless bowel rest is directly indicated, the intestinal tract should be used for intensive nutrition therapy if it is available and adequate. Evaluation of the adequacy and availability of the intestinal tract is covered in Sections IVA and IVB of Chapter 8. The choice of patients for TPN depends on clinical judgment, and guidelines still remains vague (2). Many reports document that TPN improves the nutritional status of malnourished patients; fewer reports document that it improves clinical outcomes. The Veterans Affairs Trial, a large multicenter trial of perioperative TPN in patients undergoing major surgery, found that fewer complications developed in patients who were severely malnourished (loss of ~15% of body weight) if they received TPN (3). A review of 13 prospective, randomized, controlled trials involving more than 1,250 "malnourished" (defined by weight loss, low plasma proteins, or prognostic indices) patients with gastrointestinal cancer showed that TPN given 7 to 10 days before surgery decreased postoperative complications by about 10% (4). However, TPN used routinely postoperatively in similarly "malnourished" general surgical patients was associated with an increase in complications of about 10%.

      2. **Patients with certain gastrointestinal disorders** have been treated with *complete bowel rest* as a primary form of therapy along with TPN. Bowel rest is based on the notion that excluding all oral intake minimizes trauma to and contractile activity in the diseased bowel. The gastrointestinal tract maintains a cyclic motility pattern even during fasting. Periodic surges of pancreatic and gastric secretion also occur in relation to the migrating motor complex, which in humans cycles at approximately 2-hour intervals. TPN does not alter this periodic activity in laboratory animals. Despite continued motor and secretory activity between periods of digestion, most experience supports the idea that

limiting oral intake reduces symptoms of abdominal pain and diarrhea in patients with gastrointestinal disorders, at least for the duration of the therapy. Satisfactory data to support the careful use of bowel rest and TPN as primary therapy have been obtained in the following disorders, particularly inflammatory bowel disease (5).

a. **Crohn's disease** of the small bowel remits with complete bowel rest, so that most patients experience symptomatic improvement, but the effect is not specific. Four studies have compared short-term remission rates in patients treated with parenteral nutrition (and bowel rest) with enteral nutrition. All these studies found similar remission rates in the two groups (Table 10-1).

Total parenteral nutrition or enteral nutrition improves the nutritional status of these patients, including those eventually requiring surgical intervention. The success rate of nutritional support in sustaining subsequent remission in patients with active Crohn's disease is no greater than that in control subjects, and less than that in patients on glucocorticoid treatment. Three metaanalyses examining the results of prospective, controlled, randomized trials concluded that enteral nutrition is not as effective as corticosteroids, with a pooled odds ratio of 0.35 in all studies and overall short-term remission rates of 60% and 80% for enteral nutrition and steroid treatment, respectively (10–12). Moreover, the pooled studies found no difference in the response rates for elemental and intact protein supplements. Enteral nutrition alone may be of some benefit, although no study has directly compared enteral nutrition alone with drug therapy alone. The reported short-term remission rates of about 60% in the enteral nutrition plus steroid groups are greater than the earlier reported remission rates of 20% to 40% on no therapy (4).

Many of the studies reporting the effect of TPN in Crohn's disease have been retrospective, but about 64% of cases of "refractory" disease respond to 2 to 3 weeks of TPN. However, the 1-year relapse rate has been reported to be from 28% to 85%, and long-term remission rates for steroids plus TPN are no different from those for steroid treatment without nutritional support (13). Crohn's disease of the colon is less responsive than small-bowel disease. No studies have compared TPN alone with steroid treatment alone.

No prospective studies have been carried out to test the efficacy of nutritional support in closing fistulae. However, a retrospective analysis of small-bowel fistulae of all causes found a lower mortality rate (8% vs. 33%), a higher spontaneous closure rate (56% vs. 27%), and a higher surgical closure rate (92% vs. 59%) in patients on nutritional support (14).

b. **Crohn's disease with growth retardation** can be managed without corticosteroids with either enteral nutrition or TPN. If steroids are necessary because of symptomatic, active Crohn's disease, nu-

Table 10-1. Incidence of short-term remission in patients receiving parenteral nutrition plus bowel rest versus enteral nutrition in Crohn's disease

Study	PN + bowel rest	EN
Lochs et al. (6)	7/10 (70%)	8/10 (80%)
Jones (7)	14/19 (88%)	11/17 (85%)
Greenberg et al. (8)	12/17 (71%)	11/19 (58%)
Wright and Adler (9)	4/5 (80%)	3/6 (50%)
Total	38/51 (75%)	32/52 (62%)

PN, parenteral nutrition; EN, enteral nutrition.

tritional support may be the treatment of choice for patients who can tolerate a long period of forced enteral feeding. In most situations, growth retardation in Crohn's disease can be managed with enteral feeding or oral supplementation to the usual diet, without recourse to TPN.

c. **Colitis in inflammatory bowel disease.** Two prospective, randomized trials with small numbers of patients (9 and 16) compared TPN and bowel rest with regular diet in patients on steroids for acute inflammatory colitis. No differences in short-term remission rates or frequency were found (15,16). One other study found no difference in remission rates for patients treated with enteral nutrition or TPN when both were used as adjunctive therapy to steroids (17). However, TPN is quite useful to replete the nutritional deficits of malnourished patients with ulcerative colitis who are being prepared for surgery.

d. **The adaptation period after intestinal resection in short-bowel syndrome** can be managed successfully with TPN. Fluid and electrolyte balance is maintained, and nutritional depletion prevented during the 1- to 2-month adaptation period before complete enteral nutrition is successfully reestablished. Patients who have undergone resection of up to 50% of the small bowel usually can be managed without permanent parenteral support. Patients who have undergone resection of more than 75% of the small bowel usually require long-term parenteral nutrition at home to avoid malnutrition; however, even patients who have had a massive resection may eventually demonstrate a degree of adaptation that allows parenteral nutrition to be discontinued.

e. **Severe pancreatitis** is sometimes an indication for TPN and bowel rest. Neither enteral nutrition nor TPN alters the outcome of mild or moderate pancreatitis (4). Patients with severe nutritional depletion at the outset benefit from parenteral nutritional repletion during the time the intestinal tract cannot be used. TPN can also be useful if oral feeding cannot be tolerated for a prolonged period, usually more than 2 weeks, by patients with an initially normal nutritional status. TPN can be useful in patients with complications such as abscess, pseudocyst, fistula, and ascites, but enteral feeding can be tolerated more often than has been appreciated. TPN is not always required in pancreatitis, and recently, the trend has been to treat patients with pancreatitis enterally with a tube placed beyond the ligament of Treitz. Pancreatitis is sometimes accompanied by hypertriglyceridemia. When patients with pancreatitis are given TPN, lipid emulsions should not be part of the TPN formulation if the serum triglyceride levels are above 400 mg/dL. The administration of lipids to patients with normal triglyceride levels has no adverse effects. TPN may be required to prevent nutritional deterioration when feeding induces symptoms, but in most cases of pancreatitis, this form of therapy is not required.

f. **Pediatric gastrointestinal disorders,** including congenital gastrointestinal anomalies and protracted nonspecific diarrhea, have been managed with bowel rest and TPN. Nonspecific diarrheas generally abate shortly after initiation of TPN, so that further evaluation can be undertaken while existing malnutrition is corrected.

II. **Nutrient requirements during parenteral nutrition.** The calculation of calorie and protein requirements in disease is covered in Chapter 5. Dietary vitamin and mineral requirements are discussed in Chapters 6 and 7. Certain modifications must be made in calculating the requirements when the nutrient replacement is to be given through a parenteral route. Table 10-2 summarizes the essential nutrients delivered in a TPN plan and the usual method and frequency of administration.

Table 10-2. Method and usual frequency of nutrients delivered during total parenteral nutrition

Nutrient	Route of delivery	Formulation for delivery	Frequency of delivery
Water	IV	Base solution	Daily
Protein (amino acids)	IV	Crystalline amino acids in base solutions or three-in-one admixtures	Daily
Calories			
Carbohydrates	IV	Dextrose in base solution of three-in-one admixtures	Daily
Fat	IV	Lipid emulsion or three-in-one admixtures	Daily[a]
Essential fatty acids	IV or topical skin application	Lipid emulsion or three-in-one admixtures	Daily to weekly
Vitamins			
A,D,E	IV	Multivitamin preparation	Daily or every other day
B complex	IV	Multivitamin preparation	Daily
B_{12}	IV or IM	B_{12} for injection	Monthly or daily
C	IV	Multivitamin preparation or ascorbic acid for injection	Daily
K	IM or SC injection	Aqueous colloidal solution	Weekly
Minerals			
Na,K,Cl,Mg,Ca,P	IV	Electrolyte additive to base solution or three-in-one admixtures	Daily
Fe	IV or IM	Iron dextran	Monthly or as titrated to iron needs
Zn,Mn,Cr,Cu	IV	Trace mineral solutions	Daily
Co	IV or IM	Provided by B_{12}	Monthly or daily
Se,I,Mb	IV	Solution for injection	Daily

[a]Often provided daily, but not required to meet calorie requirements.

A. Calorie requirements can be calculated in various ways, as outlined in Chapter 5. The rapid estimation of calorie requirements for hospitalized patients is described in Section IIB of Chapter 5. The question of whether the amino acids administered in TPN should be considered as a calorie source continues to be debated. Some clinicians do not count them as a calorie source, based on the expectation that some of the amino acids will be incorporated into new protein rather than metabolized. We count amino acids as a calorie source in the expectation that more will be metabolized than incorporated into new protein. This assumption helps prevent overfeeding. Most calories in central venous TPN base solutions come from concentrated dextrose. In commercially available IV solutions, dextrose is measured as the monohydrate; this reduces its caloric value to 3.4 kcal/g. Lipid emulsions for parenteral nutrition therapy are even more concentrated sources of calories. A 10% lipid emulsion provides 1.1 kcal/mL, and a 20% emulsion approximately 2 kcal/mL. Excessive calories result in overfeeding and hyperglycemia (see Section VIIIA1).

B. Protein requirements can be very high during intensely catabolic states. A positive nitrogen balance may not be feasible during the first few days of severe catabolic stress. The calculation of protein requirements in disease is described in Chapters 5 and 8. The intake of protein should remain moderate and not exceed 1.0 to 1.2 g/kg for most patients. This level of protein delivery should be exceeded only in the absence of severe underlying disease or a catabolic state (i.e., when the body is able to increase its protein synthetic rate in proportion to the increased provision).

  1. A positive caloric balance is necessary to establish a positive nitrogen balance. For delivered amino acids to be incorporated into new protein rather than catabolized, the ratio of nonprotein calories to grams of nitrogen should approach 150:1. This ratio is based on the fact that 10% to 15% or more of required calories during catabolism are derived from protein breakdown. A positive nitrogen balance can be established when the calorie-to-protein ratio is less than 150:1; however, the delivered amino acids are best utilized when the ratio of nonprotein calories to nitrogen is higher.

  2. The protein requirement of patients on parenteral nutrition may be difficult to calculate because of *nonmeasurable protein losses* from wounds or draining body fluids and because of increased needs resulting from inflammation, immobilization, or other conditions. *Periodic reassessment* of the nutritional status by means of anthropometric or biochemical measurements or both may be required to determine whether or not nutritional delivery is satisfactory.

C. Water requirements vary depending on the capacity of the patient to excrete an osmotic load. The usual requirement is 30 mL/kg in the normal adult, or approximately 1 mL/kcal delivered. An additional 360 mL/d is recommended for each degree centigrade of temperature elevation. Also, 300 to 400 mL of water per day may be necessary for new intracellular fluid if anabolism is being induced.

Restriction of water is necessary during volume overload and in the presence of hyponatremia. Patients who become hyperosmotic may need additional free water on a daily basis. Regular laboratory monitoring and the daily measurement of weight detect abnormalities of water metabolism.

D. Vitamin requirements during parenteral therapy are *uncertain* because they are not based on balance studies. (Refer to Chapter 6 for a discussion of specific vitamin requirements and monitoring for vitamin deficiencies.) Recommendations for parenteral vitamin therapy have been made by the American Medical Association Nutrition Advisory Group. These recommendations are listed in Table 10-3 but are considered, in part, controversial. It is important to recognize that deficiencies may appear even if these guidelines are followed. The blood levels of vitamins in patients maintained on long-term TPN according to these guidelines are generally normal.

Table 10-3. Guidelines for daily parenteral vitamin supplementation (children 11 years of age or older and adults)

Vitamin	Daily IV dose
A	3,300 IU
D	200 IU
E	10 IU
B$_1$ (thiamine)	3.0 mg
B$_2$ (riboflavin)	3.6 mg
B$_3$ (niacin)	15.0 mg
B$_5$ (pantothenic acid)	40.0 mg
B$_6$ (pyridoxine)	4.0 mg
B$_7$ (biotin)	60.0 mg
B$_9$ (folacin)	400.00 µg
B$_{12}$ (cobalamin)	5.0 µg
C (ascorbic acid)	100.0 mg
K	2.5 mg[a]

[a] Parenteral vitamin K supplementation is not included in the official recommendations because some patients are receiving anticoagulants.
From American Medical Association Nutrition Advisory Group guidelines. *JPEN J Parenter Enteral Nutr* 1979;3:258, with permission.

1. **Vitamin A** has been shown to undergo photodecomposition if the TPN bag is exposed to bright sunlight. Additionally, adsorption of this vitamin to the bag and tubing may reduce the actual infusion by as much as 50%. Whether this effect applies to other vitamins is not known. It is recommended that vitamin solutions be added shortly before infusion is begun.
2. **The correct dosing of vitamin D** is currently unknown. For short-term TPN, the dosage listed in Table 10-3 is satisfactory. However, the development of metabolic bone disease during long-term TPN has been reported; it responds to removal of vitamin D from the TPN solution (see Section VIIIA7).
3. **Vitamin E** is provided by lipids in lipid emulsions and in some multivitamin preparations. The quantity contained in lipid emulsions is not enough to prevent deficiency in some patients on long-term TPN.
4. **An additional 500 mg of ascorbic acid is often given daily** to the average adult patient during periods of increased metabolic stress.

E. **Mineral requirements** vary considerably from patient to patient and for an individual patient during a course of TPN therapy. Ranges of major mineral requirements for patients receiving central vein TPN are listed in Table 10-4. For optimal nitrogen repletion, adequate supplementation of these minerals is required.

1. **Variations in the potassium requirement** result from changes in cellular flux during glucose infusion and from reversal of the catabolic state. As metabolic stress decreases, potassium requirements decrease during the course of TPN. Potassium requirements are also affected by drugs (e.g., diuretics) and renal function.
2. **The phosphate requirement** varies with the number of calories provided. Hypophosphatemic patients should be repleted before TPN is initiated. When it is initiated, supplementation with 7 to 9 mmol/1,000 kcal is the initial recommendation, with modification depending on serum levels. Refeeding after starvation can induce hypophosphatemia (18). In this circumstance, the serum phosphate level must be measured frequently and additional phosphate given. In contrast, the amount of phosphate in the TPN formula of patients with renal failure may need to be reduced because clearance is impaired.

Table 10-4. Ranges of major mineral requirements during total parenteral nutrition

Electrolyte	Daily requirement range (mEq)
Sodium	50–250
Potassium	30–200
Chloride	50–250
Magnesium	10–30
Calcium	10–20
Phosphorus	10–40

3. **The acid–base balance** of the patient is influenced by the chloride and acetate content of the TPN formula. Acetate can be converted to bicarbonate, which raises the pH. In cases of metabolic acidosis, the acetate content of the formula should be increased and the chloride content decreased. Increasing the acetate content of the TPN solution is also useful in cases of large bicarbonate loss, as in pancreatic fistula. In contrast, the chloride content should be increased in metabolic alkalosis. The chloride content should also be increased when nasogastric tube drainage results in a significant loss of stomach acid.

4. **Requirements for other minerals.** Certain minerals are required in smaller amounts, and daily supplementation is probably not routinely necessary during short courses of TPN. However, syndromes have been caused by the omission of zinc, chromium, and copper from long-term TPN. Recommendations for parenteral supplementation of these minerals were established by the American Medical Association Nutrition Advisory Group. These recommendations are listed in Table 10-5. The maintenance dose for copper may be too high; 0.3 mg/d for the stable adult and 0.4 to 0.5 mg/d in cases with intestinal losses may be more appropriate. The additional supplementation of *selenium* (40 µg/d) and *molybdenum* (20 µg/d) is becoming routine for patients on long-term TPN because likely deficiency syndromes have been reported for these minerals. Supplementation of *iodine* (1.0 to 1.5 µg/kg) prevents deficiency of this mineral. Transdermal absorption of iodine from iodine-containing solutions used to cleanse the catheter site contributes to the total daily intake.

F. **Linoleic acid,** an 18-carbon essential fatty acid (EFA), must be supplied for all patients receiving TPN. Although a large amount of adipose storage fat is linoleic acid (8% to 10%), fatty stores are largely inaccessible during the

Table 10-5. Selected daily IV delivery of certain essential trace elements to adults

Element	Stable adult	Comments
Zinc	2.5–4.0 mg	Increase dose with catabolic state; increase dose with intestinal fluid losses.
Copper	0.5–1.5 mg	Reduce dose with biliary disease.
Chromium	10–15 µg	Increase dose to 20 µg with intestinal losses, reduce in renal disease.
Manganese	150–800 µg	Reduce dose with biliary disease.
Iodine	100–140 µg	
Iron	0.5 mg	
Molybdenum	20–130 µg	Reduce dose with renal disease.
Selenium	20–40 µg	Reduce dose with renal disease.

infusion of concentrated carbohydrate solutions. High plasma levels of insulin, resulting from the infusion of concentrated glucose, prevent the release of the EFAs into the circulation.

Isolated linoleic acid deficiency is uncommon in situations other than long-term TPN but has been reported in patients on glucose-based TPN without lipids for as little as 2 weeks.

1. **Manifestations of EFA deficiency,** which often appear 3 to 4 weeks after the initiation of TPN, include the following:
   a. Dry, cracked, scaling skin with impetigo and oozing in intertriginous folds
   b. Coarsened hair
   c. Hair loss
   d. Impaired wound healing
   e. Mild diarrhea (a possible manifestation)

2. **Tests for deficiency** include measuring the triene–tetragena ratio in tissue lipids. Deficiency is present when the ratio exceeds 0.4. The ratio of linoleic acid to arachidonic acid also can be measured. Normal values average 1.67 ± 0.62. Ratios of approximately 1.2 are seen in EFA deficiency.

3. **Although the exact requirement for EFAs** is unclear, it has been estimated that 4% to 5% of the daily energy requirement should consist of linoleic acid. An additional 1.5% should be added during pregnancy and 0.7% during lactation. The requirement can be met by providing the fatty acid on a daily or weekly basis.

4. **Sample calculation of EFA requirement:**

   Daily Energy Requirement = 2,000 kcal

   $$2,000 \text{ kcal} \times 0.05 = 100 \text{ kcal/d to be met by EFAs}$$

   $$100 \text{ kcal} \times \frac{1 \text{ g of EFA}}{9 \text{ kcal}} = 11 \text{ g of EFA per day}$$

5. **Linolenic acid** is another 18-carbon fatty acid; it has one more unsaturated bond than linoleic acid. A functional requirement for linolenic acid had not been demonstrated previously in humans, but a clinical syndrome with features of episodic numbness, paresthesias, weakness, pain in the legs, and blurred vision developed in a child after 5 months on a TPN regimen in which the lipid emulsion was low in linolenic acid. The symptoms resolved when the regimen was changed to include a lipid emulsion with a higher content of linolenic acid. It has been estimated that the requirement for linolenic acid is about 0.5% of total calories. Currently, it is unclear whether linolenic acid is a necessary component in any but very long courses of TPN because only one possible case of human deficiency has been reported.

III. **Nutrient solutions for parenteral nutrition**
   A. **Base solutions.** The base solution is the amino acid and dextrose combination to which electrolytes, vitamins, and minerals are added. The dextrose–amino acid combination must be prepared in the hospital pharmacy with sterile technique by combining concentrated dextrose solutions with commercially available amino acid preparations. Characteristics of various commercially available amino acid solutions are given in Tables 10-6, 10-7, and 10-8.
      1. **Note the variations in electrolyte content** of the various commercial products (Table 10-6). This becomes important when the final electrolyte content of combined solutions is calculated. Many of the 3% to 5% solutions are used in peripheral vein parenteral nutrition. Higher concentrations of electrolytes have been added to these solutions so that they can be ordered without additional electrolyte supplementation.

Most of the more concentrated amino acid solutions have a low concentration of electrolytes so that individualized combinations of total daily electrolytes can be prepared.

2. **The osmolarity** of a base solution can be estimated from a weighted average of the dextrose and amino acid constituents. Tables 10-6 and 10-9 list the osmolarity and caloric content of concentrated amino acid and dextrose solutions. The estimate of osmolarity in the final solution does not include osmoles provided by added electrolytes and other supplements.

3. **The caloric content** is calculated on the basis of the dextrose and amino acids; the dextrose monohydrate used in IV solutions provides 3.4 kcal/g. One liter of a typical base solution prepared from 500 mL of an 8.5% amino acid solution and 500 mL of 50% dextrose contains 250 g of dextrose. This provides 850 kcal from glucose and 42.5 g of amino acids per liter. The protein equivalent of such a solution is approximately 40 g/L (one molecule of water is removed when an amino acid is added to a protein; thus, 42.5 g of amino acid is the equivalent of a somewhat smaller amount of protein). Not all the amino acids are used for protein synthesis; some are metabolized and thus contribute to the caloric content of the solution. The nonprotein calorie-to-nitrogen ratio of solutions prepared in the typical way is approximately 125:1. The overall nonprotein calorie-to-nitrogen ratio can be further increased by adding lipid emulsions to the daily caloric input. *The rate of glucose administration should be kept below 7 mg/kg per minute.* More rapid administration results in hyperglycemia and fatty liver.

4. **The amino acid profiles** of many commercially available solutions are presented in Tables 10-7 and 10-8. The profiles of solutions for standard use (Table 10-7) are based on amino acid concentrations in normal serum with modifications to stimulate anabolism. Solutions with different amino acid compositions are available for specific metabolic needs (19). The modifications noted in Table 10-9 include the following:

   a. **The concentrations of essential amino acids are increased** in the formulas designed for patients with renal failure (Aminess, Aminosyn-RF, Nepyramine, RenAmin) (see Section VA). Patients on dialysis do not need increased amounts of essential amino acids and can be given standard amino acid solutions. The formulations enriched with essential amino acids are much more expensive than standard solutions, and their use can be justified only in the small group of patients with significant renal failure who are not on dialysis. Some of the essential amino acid formulations are available only in low concentrations (e.g., RenAmin 6.9%) and can cause problems of fluid overload.

   b. **Concentrations of the branched-chain amino acids (BCAAs)** (leucine, isoleucine, and valine) are increased in several specialized solutions (Aminosyn-HBC, BranchAmin, FreAmine-HBC, HepatAmine). These amino acids are grouped together because of their structural similarities and because the first two steps in the sequence of reactions by which they are degraded are the same for all three. Solutions with increased BCAAs are intended for use in situations of increased metabolic stress and in hepatic failure with encephalopathy (see Section VB). The BCAAs are oxidized outside the liver, in skeletal muscle, heart, and kidney, and they serve as a fuel source for muscle in the injured state. These amino acids also appear to have a regulatory role in preventing protein degradation and stimulating amino acid synthesis (particularly leucine) in both liver and muscle. Standard amino acid solutions have total BCAA concentrations of 20% to 25%. The optimal concentration of BCAAs to improve nitrogen balance in severe metabolic stress is twice this (*text continues on page 360*)

Table 10-6. Electrolyte and nitrogen content of crystalline amino acid solutions for parenteral nutrition

Product	Sodium (mEq/L)	Potassium (mEq/L)	Magnesium (mEq/L)	Acetate (mEq/L)	Chloride (mEq/L)	Phosphorus (mmol of P per liter)	Nitrogen (g/L)	Osmolarity (mEq/L)	pH
Standard									
Aminosyn 10%	0	5.4	0	148	0	0	15.7	1,000	5.3
Aminosyn 8.5% w/o lytes	0	5.4	0	90	35	0	13.4	850	5.3
Aminosyn 8.5% + lytes	70	66	10	142	98	30	13.4	1,160	5.3
Aminosyn II 10%	45	0	0	72	0	0	15.3	873	5.0–6.3
Aminosyn II 8.5%	33	0	0	61	0	0	13	742	5.0–6.5
FreAmine 10%	10	0	0	89	<3	10	15.4	950	6.5
FreAmine III 8.5%	10	0	0	72	2	10	13.0	810	6.6
Novamine 15%	0	0	0	151	0	0	23.7	1,388	5.2–6.0
Procalamine 3%	35	24	5	47	41	3.5	4.6	735	6.8
Travasol 10%	0	0	0	87	40	0	16.5	1,000	6.0
Travasol 8.5% w/o lytes	3	0	0	73	34	0	9.3	520	6.0
Travasol 8.5% + lytes	70	60	10	141	70	30	14.3	1,160	6.0
Travasol 3.5% M	25	15	5	54	25	7.5	5.9	525	6.0

Catabolic state								
Aminosyn-HBC 7%	7	0	70	42	0	NA	665	5.2
BranchAmin 4%	0	0	0	0	0	4.43	316	6.0
FreAmine HBC 6.9%	10	0	57	<3	0	9.7	620	6.5
Hepatic failure								
HepatAmine 8%	10	0	62	<3	10	12.0	785	6.5
Renal failure								
Aminess 5.2%	0	0	50	0	0	6.6	416	6.4
Aminosyn-RF 5.2%	0	0	105	0	0	7.7	475	5.2
Nephramine 5.4%	5	0	44	<3	0	6.5	435	6.5
RenAmin 6.5%	0	0	60	31	0	10	600	5.0–7.0
Pediatric								
Aminosyn-PF 10%	3.4	0	46	0	0	15.2	834	5.0–6.5
Trophamine 10%	5	0	97	<3	0	15.5	875	5.0–6.0

Formulations may have changed since the preparation of this table. Consult prescription information.

Table 10-7. Amino acid profiles of standard crystalline amino acid solutions for parenteral use[a]

Amino acid	Aminosyn 10%	Aminosyn II 10%	FreAmine III 10%	Novamine 15%	Procalamine 3%	Travasol 10%
Essential amino acids (g/dL)						
Lysine	0.72	1.05	0.75	1.18	0.31	0.58
Tryptophan	0.16	0.20	0.15	0.25	0.05	0.18
Phenylalanine	0.44	0.30	0.56	1.04	0.17	0.56
Methionine	0.40	0.17	0.53	0.75	0.16	0.40
Threonine	0.52	0.40	0.40	0.75	0.12	0.42
Leucine	0.94	1.00	0.91	1.04	0.27	0.73
Isoleucine	0.72	0.66	0.69	0.75	0.21	0.60
Valine	0.80	0.50	0.66	0.96	0.20	0.58
Nonessential amino acids (g/dL)						
Histidine	0.30	0.30	0.28	0.89	0.08	0.48
Glutamate	—	0.74	—	0.75	—	—
Proline	0.86	0.72	0.63	0.89	0.34	0.68
Aspartate	—	0.70	—	0.43	—	—
Serine	0.42	0.53	0.59	0.59	0.18	0.50
Arginine	0.98	1.02	0.95	1.47	0.29	1.15
Alanine	1.28	0.99	0.71	2.17	0.21	2.07
Glycine	1.28	0.50	1.40	1.04	0.42	1.03
Tyrosine	0.04	0.27	—	0.04	—	0.04
Cysteine	—	—	<0.02	—	<0.02	—

Formulations may have changed since the preparation of this table. Consult prescribing information.
[a] Values are given for a single concentrated solution available in each product line.

Table 10-8. Amino acid profiles of modified crystalline amino acid solutions for specialized parenteral use

Amino acid	Catabolic state				Renal failure			Hepatic failure	Pediatric growth formulas	
	Aminosyn-HBC 7%	Branch-Amin 4%	FreAmine HBC 6.9%	Aminess 5.2%	Aminosyn-RF 5.2%	Nephramine II 5.4%	Ren-Amin 6.5%	Hepat-Amine 8%	Aminosyn-PF 10%	Trophamine 10%
Essential amino acids (g/dL)										
Lysine	0.25	—	0.41	0.60	0.54	0.64	0.45	0.61	0.47	0.49
Tryptophan	0.09	—	0.09	0.19	0.16	0.20	0.16	0.07	0.12	0.12
Phenylalanine	0.23	—	0.32	0.82	0.73	0.88	0.49	0.10	0.30	0.29
Methionine	0.21	—	0.25	0.82	0.73	0.88	0.50	0.10	0.12	0.20
Threonine	0.27	—	0.20	0.38	0.33	0.40	0.38	0.45	0.36	0.25
Leucine	1.58	1.38	1.37	0.82	0.73	0.88	0.60	1.10	0.83	0.84
Isoleucine	0.79	1.38	0.76	0.52	0.46	0.56	0.50	0.90	0.53	0.49
Valine	0.79	1.24	0.88	0.60	0.53	0.64	0.82	0.84	0.45	0.47
Nonessential amino acids (g/dL)										
Histidine	0.15	—	0.16	0.41	0.43	0.25	0.42	0.24	0.22	0.29
Glutamate	—	—	—	—	—	—	—	—	0.58	0.30
Proline	0.45	—	0.63	—	—	—	0.35	0.80	0.57	0.41
Aspartate	—	—	—	—	—	—	—	—	0.37	0.19
Serine	0.22	—	0.33	—	—	—	0.30	0.50	0.35	0.23
Arginine	0.51	—	0.58	—	0.60	—	0.63	—	0.86	0.73
Alanine	0.66	—	0.40	—	—	—	0.56	0.77	0.49	0.32
Glycine	0.66	—	0.33	—	—	—	0.30	0.90	0.27	0.22
Tyrosine	0.03	—	—	—	—	—	0.04	—	0.04	0.14
Cysteine	—	—	<0.02	—	—	<0.02	<0.02	—	—	<0.02
Taurine	—	—	—	—	—	—	—	—	0.05	0.02

Formulations may have changed since the preparation of this table. Consult prescribing information.

Table 10-9. Osmolarity and caloric content of concentrated dextrose solutions

Dextrose concentration (wt/vol)	Osmolarity (mOsmol/L)	Caloric content[a] (kcal/dL)
5%	250	17
10%	500	34
20%	1,000	68
50%	2,500	170
70%	3,500	237

[a] Based on the caloric value of dextrose monohydrate used in commercial preparations (3.4 kcal/g).

amount. BranchAmin is mixed with standard solutions to supplement the BCAA content. The other specialized solutions have total BCAA concentrations ranging from 35% to 45%. All the BCAA formulations are extremely expensive, and their use can best be justified in the small group of patients with liver disease who become encephalopathic when given standard amino acid mixtures. Some of the BCAA formulations are available only in low concentrations (e.g., BranchAmin 4%) and can cause problems of fluid overload.

  c. **Solutions intended for pediatric use,** but not restricted to pediatric patients, include *taurine,* dicarboxylic amino acids, and tyrosine (Trophamine, Aminosyn-PF). The formulas are based on the amino acid profiles of breast-fed infants. Taurine is involved in bile acid conjugation, calcium flux in brain and muscle, and the regulation of endocrine secretion by the pituitary and adrenal cortex. The concentration is also high in retina. Taurine has not been considered essential for humans, but it may be a requirement for neonates.

  d. None of the standard amino acid solutions for TPN contains *glutamine* because it is thought to be unstable and its breakdown products are toxic. The stability of glutamine in solution is influenced by temperature, pH, and the other constituents of the solution (20). During catabolism, intracellular levels of glutamine fall. Animal studies have shown that glutamine-supplemented enteral or parenteral nutrition decreases intestinal damage and improves survival in sepsis (21). However, prolonged TPN supplemented with glutamine has resulted in apparent hepatic toxicity and no improvement in intestinal absorptive toxicity (22). One study in humans demonstrated improved clinical outcomes with glutamine-supplemented TPN in bone marrow transplantation (20), but a more recent study shows no short-term benefit from either oral or parenteral glutamine supplementation (23). Prolonged home TPN supplemented with glutamine resulted in apparent hepatic toxicity and no improvement in intestinal absorptive activity (22).

B. Lipid emulsions. Milky emulsions of soybean or safflower oil in combination with glycerol and emulsifiers are available in 10%, 20%, and 30% concentrations. The emulsified particles are about the same size as chylomicrons. The 10% emulsions provide 1.1 kcal/mL, the additional nonfat calories coming largely from glycerol. After they enter the bloodstream, the lipid particles become coated with apoproteins and are metabolized like chylomicrons. Various amounts of linoleic acid and linolenic acid are present in the emulsions depending on the parent oil. Characteristics of several commercially available lipid emulsions are given in Table 10-10.

  1. Lipid emulsions can be used to *supply EFAs* (see Section IIF) and as a *concentrated source of calories.* Because the emulsions are isotonic, administration together with the base solution reduces the overall osmo-

Table 10-10. Characteristics of lipid emulsions for parenteral use

Product	Parent oil	Average droplet size (µg)	Osmolarity (mOsmol/L)	Caloric content (kcal/mL)	Linoleic acid % total fat	Linolenic acid % total fat
Intralipid 10%	Soybean oil	0.5	260	1.1	50	9
Intralipid 20%	Soybean oil	0.5	268	2.0	50	9
Intralipid 30%	Soybean oil	0.5	200	3.0	50	9
Liposyn II 10%	Soybean and safflower oils	0.4	320	1.1	66	4
Liposyn II 20%	Soybean and safflower oils	0.4	340	2.0	66	4
Liposyn III 10%	Soybean oil	0.4	284	1.1	54	8
Liposyn III 20%	Soybean oil	0.4	292	2.0	54	8

larity of the infused fluids, an advantage in peripheral vein parenteral nutrition. Fats have a lower respiratory quotient than carbohydrates do, which is the rationale for using lipids to provide a larger proportion of the daily nonprotein calories in patients with respiratory failure. The ideal percentage of total calories to be delivered as fats is unknown. Although problems have been associated with very high rates of lipid administration (>1 kcal/kg per hour), the upper limit of the acceptable range for the contribution of lipids to total calories is not established. We routinely use 25% to 50% but have few data to support this approach. A component of glucose must be included (500 to 900 kcal/d for adults) for brain and other tissues that require oxygen. If not provided, the glucose is derived from amino acids by gluconeogenesis. TPN formulations that include lipid emulsions are associated with less hyperglycemia, lower serum levels of insulin, and less hepatic damage than formulations in which glucose is the only major source of calories. However, toxic effects associated with lipid emulsions have been reported. These include impaired neutrophil function and increased risk for infection (24). The toxic effects of lipid emulsions are primarily associated with rapid infusion at rates that exceed resting energy expenditure. *Limiting the rate of lipid administration to 0.03 to 0.05 g/kg per hour has been recommended* (25).

2. **Administering the emulsion.** Lipid emulsions can be given separately from the base solution, together with the base solution in a single bag (see Section IIIC), or together with the base solution in a separate bag. A Y-tube arrangement of the two bags is used to mix the base solution and lipid emulsion just before they enter the patient. Just a few years ago, all hospitals used separate administration or Y-tube arrangements for TPN; now, however, more and more are using total nutrient admixtures (three-in-one bags) as the standard method for administering TPN. Issues of stability have become more important as home TPN has become more common and delays between the preparation and use of TPN formulas are longer. In general, admixtures are less stable than base solution and lipids in separate bags. A new product has the base solution and lipid in separate compartments of one bag. The compartments are separated by a zipper, which is opened just before use. If the Y-tube arrangement is used, it is important to avoid "cracking" the emulsion; mixing the lipid emulsion with the base solution as short a time as possible before insertion of the IV catheter helps prevent cracking. Lipid emulsions are infused through tubing sets provided by the manufacturer; the tubing sets must not contain the plasticizer di-2-ethylhexylphthalate (DEHP). This potentially toxic plasticizer is gradually eluted by the emulsion and is found in some other commercially available IV tubing. A test dose of 1 mL of a 10% emulsion per minute for 5 minutes is recommended for adults at the initiation of lipid emulsion therapy.

C. **Total nutrient admixture (three-in-one system).** In a total nutrient admixture, the lipid emulsion and base solution are combined in a single bag (26). This approach allows a hospital pharmacy to combine all the components of a patient's TPN formula for a whole day in a single 3-L bag. Physical manipulation of the central line is reduced, as is the risk for infection. Reduced requirements for nursing time and equipment (bags, tubes) lead to cost savings. However, certain problems are associated with total nutrient admixtures.

1. Lipid droplets (0.33 to 0.5 μm) can clog filters. This problem can be overcome by using filters with larger pores (≥1.2 μm). The Food and Drug Administration guidelines recommend the use of filters.

2. Some of the drugs that are compatible with base solutions are incompatible with total nutrient admixtures. These include amikacin, tetracycline, methyldopa, and iron dextran. A major study of the stability of 106 different drugs in many different parenteral nutrition formulations

is of considerable interest (27). More drugs are compatible with a separate base solution and lipid emulsion than with a nutrient admixture. The range of concentrations of divalent cations compatible with total nutrient admixtures is smaller than the range of concentrations compatible with base solutions.

3. Parenteral formulations containing lipids are more likely to be contaminated with bacteria and fungi for two reasons: fat is a good medium for growth, and lipid emulsions cannot be given with the small-pore filters (0.22 mm) that are best for trapping organisms.

4. It is more difficult to see particulates, such as precipitated salts.

5. The emulsion may break down, with fat droplets combining to form larger fat droplets and, if deterioration progresses, the fat and water components separating. The safe use of total nutrient admixtures requires visual inspection for signs of deterioration before administration. Deterioration takes place in stages.

   a. **Aggregation.** Larger fat droplets form and are distributed throughout the solution. Aggregation can be reversed by gently shaking the bag.

   b. **Creaming.** Creaming is the formation of a thin (1- to 2-cm) layer of aggregated fat droplets on the surface of the solution. Creaming is reversible with gentle shaking.

   c. **Coalescence.** Coalescence is the further fusion of fat drops to create a thicker (10-cm), dense layer at the surface. If coalescence develops, the infusion must be discontinued.

   d. **Oiling out.** Oiling out occurs when fat droplets separate from the solution and appear as a clear layer on the surface. If oiling out is observed, the infusion should be discontinued. The likelihood that a lipid emulsion will deteriorate increases with time and temperature. Total nutrient admixtures should not hang at room temperature for more than 24 hours.

6. In pediatric patients, three-in-one admixtures tend to occlude the catheter progressively as they are deposited (28).

D. **Electrolyte and trace mineral preparations for parenteral use.** These should be added to base solutions for parenteral nutrition in pharmacy IV additive rooms under controlled, aseptic conditions. The use of laminar flow hoods has reduced the incidence of contaminated fluids. Most electrolyte additives are ordered individually by the prescribing physician. Occasionally, premixed electrolyte formulations can be used. Rather than depend on commercially prepared solutions, the physician is advised to base electrolyte prescriptions on calculated requirements and the results of laboratory monitoring. Combination solutions are also available to provide trace minerals.

E. **Comprehensive vitamin preparations for parenteral nutrition** contain the amounts of fat- and water-soluble vitamins listed in Table 10-3 and are available through hospital pharmacies that prepare TPN solutions. Among the commercially available vitamin mixtures that provide the required amounts of all the vitamins listed in Table 10-3, except vitamin K, are Berocca Parenteral Nutrition (Roche), MVC 9 + 3 (LyphoMed), and MVI-12 (Rorer). Ascorbic acid can be provided separately. The water-soluble component in combination multivitamins can be given alone if signs of fat-soluble vitamin excess are detected. Note that vitamin K is not provided by combination multivitamin preparations that match the guidelines given in Table 10-3.

IV. **Techniques of parenteral nutrition.** The following sections outline techniques for the use of parenteral nutrition through either central or peripheral venous access. It has been suggested that parenteral nutrition is administered most successfully in institutions with well-defined teams (25). A parenteral nutrition team usually consists of an interested physician, dietitian, nurse, and pharmacist. Whether or not specific persons are identified as members of a team, each of these services must actively participate if parenteral nutrition is to be effective and safe.

Parenteral nutrition can be administered in several ways to result in a positive nitrogen and calorie balance and repletion of defined deficiencies. The techniques used by the author are outlined in the following sections.

A. Central venous catheter insertion and care

1. **Careful insertion of a central venous catheter** is the first step in initiating central vein TPN. The decision to initiate central venous TPN is never made on an emergency basis, and consequently, a central venous catheter should be inserted under aseptic conditions with adequate assistance. Standard technique for placement of a subclavian catheter should be used. Although the internal jugular vein provides satisfactory access to the superior vena cava, it is much more difficult to maintain an occlusive dressing when the catheter is placed in the neck.

   a. **For short-term TPN, triple-lumen catheters or Hohn catheters are used.** These catheters are introduced percutaneously into the subclavian or jugular vein. *For longer-term TPN, Raaf and Hickman catheters are used.* These and other long catheters are burrowed through the subcutaneous tissue in the anterior chest wall and exit away from the site of subclavian or jugular vein puncture. Both are made of Silastic and may be less damaging to the endothelial lining of the vein than polyethylene catheters. In addition, the catheters have a rough outer coat along a short segment of their subcutaneous portion. The rough coat promotes fibrin deposition, and theoretically, infectious complications are reduced by the formation of a tight fibrin sheath. The burrowed catheters are recommended for patients with a tracheostomy or other conditions in which the skin entry site would seem likely to become contaminated. Burrowed catheters are also recommended for patients whose TPN will be administered at home or will be prolonged (>4 weeks).

   b. Regardless of the type of catheter used, the following basic rules should be followed in caring for the central venous line:

      (1) Always use strict aseptic technique in handling the catheter, tubing connections, and the dressing over the catheter.

      (2) To avoid the possibility of an air embolus, never disconnect the tubing from an unclamped catheter with the patient in an upright position.

      (3) Always obtain a chest roentgenogram after insertion of the catheter or a change of position before any TPN fluid is instilled.

   c. **Avoid drawing blood from the TPN line,** and avoid infusing medications or blood products by piggyback technique if possible. In a small number of patients with limited venous access, we have been forced to use the same line for cycled TPN, blood products, and medications. We have not had problems with infection in these patients when the lines were properly managed. Similar complication rates have been noted in oncology patients with central lines used for multiple purposes and in those with lines used exclusively for TPN, a finding that supports judicious use of the TPN catheter for other purposes when required.

   d. **Do not piggyback medications** or blood products into the parenteral nutrition line. If this rule must be broken, compatibility of the solutions must be established before the piggybacked solution is started. If medications are piggybacked, they should be administered above the filter.

2. **Tubing should be changed** with careful attention to aseptic technique to avoid contamination of the tubing hubs. The frequency of tubing changes varies from every 24 hours to every 72 hours, depending on hospital policy.

   a. Use of unnecessary tubing and extension sets is discouraged. A stopcock should not be part of the tubing assembly because it is easily contaminated.

b. The tubing–catheter junction should be wiped with alcohol before being disconnected to avoid inadvertent contamination of the catheter hub.

c. The Food and Drug Administration recommends the use of in-line filters with both base solutions and three-in-one admixtures. This recommendation was prompted by two deaths caused by calcium phosphate precipitates in three-in-one admixtures. Although filters with 0.22-μm pores effectively filter bacterial and particulate contamination, they also interfere with the free flow of concentrated carbohydrate solutions. Albumin and lipid emulsions cannot be administered through small-pore filters. Insertion of the filter creates an additional opportunity for contamination in the tubing assembly. Despite their filtering capabilities, in-line filters do not appear to reduce catheter infection rates significantly. Filters reduce the infusion of particulate matter in the solution. Filters with larger pores (≥1.2 μm) are used with three-in-one admixtures; 5-μm filters are less expensive and must be changed less often than 1.2-μm filters.

3. An occlusive dressing is an important part of central venous catheter maintenance. The dressing must be occlusive on all sides to prevent catheter contamination. Gauze dressings are usually changed every 48 hours—more often should the dressing become wet or obviously soiled. Alternatively, transparent dressings of a porous synthetic material (Op-Site) can be left in place for longer periods, up to 7 days. A transparent dressing does not have to be removed so that the catheter entry site can be inspected, and the number of dressing changes can be reduced. The technique of a standard occlusive gauze dressing is outlined below.

a. Supplies necessary for gauze dressing change
   (1) Four packages of 4 × 4-in gauze pads
   (2) Acetone
   (3) Povidone-iodine (Betadine) solution and ointment (ointment is optional)
   (4) Tincture of benzoin (optional)
   (5) Sterile gloves
   (6) Silk tape, 2-in width.
   (7) Masks (optional)

b. Technique of catheter change (Fig. 10-1)
   (1) Put on mask to minimize chance of airborne contamination (optional).
   (2) Open supplies and apply povidone-iodine and acetone solutions to the 4 × 4-in pads.
   (3) The patient's head should be turned away from the site.
   (4) Remove the old dressing down to the catheter insertion site. Dressings are discarded according to total body substance isolation.
   (5) Inspect the insertion site and area for inflammatory signs and appropriate position of the catheter. Note any markings on the catheter that indicate the length of the catheter inserted into the patient. Do not use a temporary catheter if less than 10 to 12 cm remains in the patient.
   (6) Put on sterile gloves.
   (7) Clean the area around the site thoroughly with acetone on sterile 4 × 4-in pads.
   (8) Repeat this procedure with acetone and then with povidone-iodine.
   (9) Allow the povidone-iodine to dry for 30 seconds, and then apply a dab of povidone-iodine ointment (optional) to the catheter insertion site and to any suture sites (Fig. 10-1A).
   (10) Apply tincture of benzoin to the skin where the tape will be applied (optional).

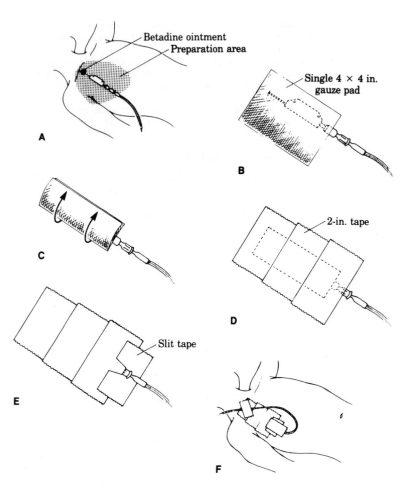

FIG. 10.1. Technique of applying an occlusive central venous catheter dressing. **A:** The preparation area extends from above the skin entry site to below the catheter–tubing junction. **B:** A single 4 × 4-in sterile gauze pad is placed over the exposed catheter to avoid a bulky dressing. **C:** The gauze pad is folded in half lengthwise. **D:** Single strips of 2-in-wide tape are applied to the folded pad. The dressing should be occlusive all around the pad, and the catheter hub should be partially exposed. **E:** A slotted tape secures the dressing at the catheter hub site. **F:** Additional short pieces of tape should be used to secure and protect the catheter–tubing junction and direct the tubing over the patient's shoulder. (From Clouse RE, et al. *The Barnes Hospital parenteral nutrition handbook,* 2nd ed. St. Louis: Barnes Hospital, 1985, with permission.)

(11) Fold one 4 × 4-in pad in half and apply lengthwise to cover the area from the insertion site up to the catheter hub (Fig. 10-1 B,C).

(12) Apply 2-in silk tape as shown in Figure 10-1D.

(13) Complete the dressing by making the hub area occlusive with slotted tape (Fig. 10-1E).

(14) Tape the catheter–hub junction and secure the tubing to the skin (Fig. 10-1F).

(15) Note the dressing change and describe the insertion site in the medical record.

4. **Aseptic maintenance of the catheter and tubing system** cannot be emphasized enough for the safe administration of long-term TPN through a central venous catheter. The following precautions should be followed in addition to the techniques mentioned above:

   a. Avoid a bulky dressing. A single folded 4 × 4-in pad should be adequate.

   b. Make sure the dressing is occlusive on all sides.

   c. Tape all connections to avoid accidental disconnection or contamination.

   d. Clean all connections, including the catheter–tubing connection, with alcohol or povidone-iodine before any tubing changes are made.

   e. Change the catheter dressing if it is wet. If the replaced dressing also becomes damp, then the catheter–tubing junction and exposed catheter should be examined carefully. Under no circumstances should this examination be performed in a casual way without adhering to the usual aseptic technique. If the catheter dressing must be removed, then the same sterile precautions should be taken as during dressing change to avoid accidental contamination of the catheter insertion site.

   f. Once infusion from a solution bag is started, the bag should not hang for more than 24 hours so that bacterial growth is minimized.

B. **Ordering TPN through a central vein.** Orders for TPN must be carefully written because of the multiple additives needed on a daily basis. A special order form is recommended to avoid transcription errors and accidental omission of important nutrients. Figure 10-2 is an example of a central venous TPN order form. According to this order form, TPN bags are sequentially numbered throughout a patient's course of therapy. Note that all the additives are ordered on the same order form so that the daily prescription of nutrients can be seen easily. An entire day's orders can be written on a single sheet one day in advance so that the pharmacy additive room is not rushed in preparing the TPN solutions.

   1. **Selection of a TPN formula** depends on the protein and calorie requirements of the patient. The formula should contain the appropriate quantities of nitrogen and calories to meet the daily requirements and restore nutritional status. At Barnes-Jewish Hospital, three-in-one admixtures are the standard form of TPN; however, in many hospitals, base solutions, with or without lipid emulsions in a separate bag, are the standard form of TPN.

      a. The form in Fig. 10-2 lists four standard solutions for central parenteral nutrition: intermediate-nitrogen, high-nitrogen, very-high-nitrogen, and low-nitrogen. The intermediate-nitrogen formulation is suitable for the majority of patients. High-nitrogen and very-high-nitrogen formulations are suitable for highly stressed patients (e.g., major trauma) with normal renal function. The low-nitrogen formulation is suitable for patients with renal dysfunction.

      b. **Administered amino acids are best utilized** when the daily nonprotein calorie provision matches the daily energy requirement. Fewer calories may prevent positive nitrogen balance; more calories may contribute to overfeeding and hyperglycemia (see Section VIIIA1). At any level of caloric delivery (below, at, or above the total daily energy requirement), the provision of additional nitrogen as amino acids improves nitrogen balance. For many hospitalized patients, TPN solutions with nonprotein calorie–nitrogen ratios of 150 : 1 are appropriate. At Barnes-Jewish Hospital, the standard (intermediate-nitrogen) TPN formula contains 1,000 kcal in 786 mL, and the caloric distribution is 60% glucose, 16% protein, and 24% fat. It contains 40 g of amino acid (6.3 g of nitrogen) per 1,000 kcal (840 nonprotein calories).

BARNES-JEWISH HOSPITAL

A-2

BJC HEALTH SYSTEM

PARENTERAL NUTRITION ORDER FORM

TPN cut-off time for ordering is **1400**

DATE
DUE: _____ BAG #: _____ Calories to the nearest 100 Kcal per 24 hours: _____ . Hang time is **2000**.

Check One	STANDARD SOLUTIONS	% Total Kcals Provided As			GM / 1000 Kcal			Approx. Vol. Per 1000 Kcal
		Amino Acid	Dextrose	Fat	Amino Acid	Dextrose	Fat	
	a) Intermediate Nitrogen	16%	60%	24%	40	176	27	786 ml
	b) High Nitrogen	20%	55%	25%	50	162	28	843 ml
	c) Very High Nitrogen	24%	56%	20%	60	165	22	946 ml
	d) Low Nitrogen	12%	65%	23%	30	191	26	680 ml
	e) Modified (Approval Required)	__%	__%	__%	----	----	----	----------
	f) Peripheral	16%	32%	52%	40	94	58	1429 ml
	g) Amino Acid / Dextrose	10% Amino Acid _____ ml			70% Dextrose _____ ml			
	Lipids (as separate infusion)	circle one: 100 ml, 250 ml, 500 ml, 20% Intralipid rate _____ ml/hour						

ELECTROLYTES	Suggested Daily Amount	Quantity Ordered
Sodium	60-120 mEq	mEq
Potassium	30-80 mEq	mEq
Chloride	80-140 mEq	mEq
Acetate*	*	BALANCE
Calcium	4.6-9.2 mEq	mEq
Magnesium	8.1-24.3 mEq	mEq
Phosphorus	12-24 mMol	mmol
MICRONUTRIENTS		
MVI-12	10 ml/day	ml
Trace Elements - 5	1 ml/day	ml
Vitamin K	10 mg/Monday	mg
MEDICATIONS		
Regular Insulin	Reg. Humulin only	units

WEIGHT: _____ HEIGHT: _____
(Used for nutritional calculation)

Serum Electrolytes

Na+   Cl⁻   BUN
                        glu
K+   HCO₃   Cr

Mg++ _____
PO₄ _____

Comments _____

_____

_____

Date _____ Time _____ Physician Signature _____

Beeper # _____

Print Physician Name

BJ 3418-877 REV. 4/97   **Page NSS at 790-4677 for assessment prior to initiating TPN**

FIG. 10.2. Sample order form for ordering total parenteral nutrition through a central vein.

The nonprotein calorie–nitrogen ratio is 133 : 1. This formula delivers more nitrogen than is necessary for many patients when 3 L/d is given. The most accurate method is to calculate the energy and protein requirements independently and provide appropriate amounts of each macronutrient (see Chapter 5). The characteristics of amino acid solutions are given in Table 10-6. The use of formulas with modified amino acid profiles in renal and liver failure is discussed in Section V.

    c. Note that amino acid solutions contain various amounts of electrolytes (Table 10-6). Be certain that the pharmacy takes the electrolyte content of the amino acid solution into account when filling the final electrolyte prescription. Keep in mind that the electrolyte concentrations (in the amino acid solutions) are reduced when the amino acid solution is combined with concentrated dextrose and lipid in the final formula.

2. **Electrolyte additives.** Major minerals can be added by specifying the actual additive (e.g., sodium chloride, sodium acetate, potassium chloride, magnesium sulfate, calcium gluconate) or, ideally, by specifying the final content of the individual cations and anions. The form in Fig. 10-2 allows the physician to order the final content of the individual ions; this includes the electrolyte content of the amino acid solution. The usual ranges of electrolyte requirements during TPN for the average adult patient are listed in Table 10-4.

    a. If more than one TPN bag is used per day, electrolytes should be divided evenly among the bags. This practice avoids *electrolyte incompatibilities.*

    b. In general, no more than 12.2 mEq of magnesium should be added per liter.

    c. The calcium–phosphate solubility product can be exceeded easily. Coadministration of these two minerals will be successful if no more than 15 mmol of phosphorus as potassium phosphate or sodium phosphate is added to a 1-L solution containing 4.6 mEq of calcium, or no more than 10 mmol of phosphorus is added to a liter containing 9.2 mEq of calcium. Calcium phosphate solubility is affected by pH; the higher the pH, the lower the solubility. In compounding TPN solutions, it is important that solubility of calcium be calculated based on the volume at the time it is added rather than the final volume. Calcium phosphate solubility is a very real problem, and deaths have been caused by calcium phosphate precipitates in TPN solutions.

3. **Vitamins** are ordered daily or every other day from the outset of parenteral nutrition therapy. Vitamin K is not part of standard multivitamin preparations because of the needs of patients on warfarin; for this reason, vitamin K must be provided separately. We add 10 mg of vitamin K to the TPN solution once a week for all patients except pregnant women, who get 1 mg daily. Additional ascorbic acid may be provided during intense catabolic stress. A *suitable vitamin prescription* for the average adult is 10 mL of MVI-12 per day (contains the quantities listed in Table 10-3).

4. **Trace mineral** supplements may be ordered as additives to the TPN solution.

    a. Zinc is added as zinc sulfate according to the requirements outlined in Table 10-5. The addition of 4 mg of elemental zinc meets the average daily requirements of most patients who do not have additional intestinal losses of zinc.

    b. Iron deficiency can be corrected with the administration of parenteral iron (e.g., iron dextran) IM or IV (see Chapter 7). The IM administration of iron dextran rarely has been associated with pain, the formation of sterile abscesses, and tissue atrophy. As a result, IV administration is the preferred route. The usual daily requirements are met by the monthly administration of 1 mL of iron dextran (50 mg of elemental iron), which may be added directly to a base solution but not to a total nutrition admixture. If abnormal amounts of iron are being lost from the gastrointestinal tract or other sites of bleeding, larger replacement doses are necessary. Iron replacement should be titrated to laboratory indices of iron status. The parenteral administration of iron dextran is associated with anaphylaxis. The precautions to be taken in administering parenteral iron as outlined in Section IIIA of Chapter 7, and these must be carefully observed. The parenteral administration of iron, whether for replacement or maintenance, is associated with a series of potential problems. Establishing the appropriate dose can be difficult; requirements depend on daily losses, which may be difficult to assess. Iron deficiency results in anemia; chronic iron overload can cause cirrhosis. Because of the large stores of iron and the low rate of turnover in iron-repleted patients, the problems associated with iron administration can be avoided in many cases by not giving parenteral iron at all. If a patient has normal stores before TPN, and if TPN is to be given for less than 2 months, no iron need be given during the course of TPN.

   c. **Other trace elements** may be added individually to the TPN formula daily. Commercial trace metal solutions provide *chromium, copper, zinc, manganese, selenium, iodide,* and *molybdenum* in various combinations to provide the recommended daily adult dose in 0.8 to 3 mL of solution, depending on the manufacturer.

   d. **Iodine and selenium deficiencies** have been described in patients on long-term TPN. Either element must be ordered individually— iodine as sodium or potassium iodide and selenium as selenous acid; the suggested daily dose is 1.0 μg of iodine per kilogram and approximately 40 μg of selenium as selenous acid. *Molybdenum* (20 μg) also may be given daily. These trace minerals are often reserved for patients receiving long-term TPN therapy. One commercial combination solution, MTE-7, contains iodine, selenium, and molybdenum in addition to chromium, copper, iodide, and zinc.

5. **Other additives** may be included directly in the TPN formula or administered safely in piggyback fashion with the base solution or three-in-one admixture. Compatibility is a complex issue that is influenced by the exact components of the nutrient solution (including electrolytes, vitamins, and minerals), pH, concentration of the additive, and mixing sequence. Thus, a statement that an additive is compatible with TPN formulations may not be applicable to a particular TPN formulation. Lack of compatibility may result in failure to deliver the additive, precipitation of electrolytes from the TPN solution, or damage to the lipid emulsion. Most pharmacies have a short list of medications that are commonly added directly to TPN formulations (histamine$_2$-receptor antagonists, insulin, vitamins). Other additives are better given piggyback fashion. Table 10-11 lists the additives reported to be compatible with base solutions or three-in-one admixtures. Some of these additions are compatible with either base solution or three-in-one admixtures, whereas others are compatible with base solution but not three-in-one admixtures. References for the compatibility of specific additives appear in the following publications: Teasley-Strausburg KM, ed. *The Nutrition Support Handbook* (Cincinnati: Harvey Whitney Books, 1992), available from Clintec, and Dickerson RN, et al. "Parenteral Nutrition Solutions." In: Rombeau JL, Caldwell MD, eds. *Parenteral Nutrition* (Philadelphia: WB Saunders, 1993). Current information about compatibility is available in *Trissel's Handbook on Injectable Drugs* (Bethesda, Maryland: American Society of Hospital Pharmacists, 1994).

   a. **Regular insulin** reduced hyperglycemia when added directly to the TPN solution. Hypoglycemia is less apt to result from a decrease in the fluid rate or inadvertent interruption of the TPN fluid if the insulin is added directly to the fluid rather than given by SC injection. Insulin is not routinely added to all TPN solutions. For patients who required insulin before the initiation of TPN, add one-third to one-half the usual total daily dose of insulin as regular human insulin to the TPN bag, and then supplement with additional SC insulin as

Table 10-11. Compatibility of total parenteral nutrition and piggybacked medications

Additive	TPN base[a]	Three-in-one	Additive	TPN base[a]	Three-in-one
Albumin	C	I	Hydrocortisone	C	X
Amikacin	C	I	Imipenem	X	X
Aminophylline	C	C	Insulin	C	C
Amphotericin B	I	I	Iron dextran	C	I
Ascorbic acid	C	C	Isoproterenol	C	C
Carbenicillin	C	X	Kanamycin	C	C
			Lidocaine	C	C
Cefazolin	C	C	Meperidine	C	X
Cefoxitin	C	C	Methicillin	C	X
Cephalothin	C	X	Metronidazole	I	I
Cephapirin	C	C	Methyldopate	C	I
Chloramphenicol	C	X	Mezlocillin	C	X
Cimetidine	C	C	Morphine	C	X
Clindamycin	C	C	Multivitamins	C	C
Cyanocobalamin	C	X	Nafcillin	C	X
Cyclosporine	C	X	Norepinephrine	C	C
Cytarabine	C	X	Octreotide	I	I
Dexamethasone	C	C	Oxacillin	C	C
Digoxin	C	C	Penicillin G	C	C
Dopamine	C	C	Potassium		
Doxycycline	C	X	Phenytoin	I	I
Erythromycin	C	C	Phytonadione	C	C
Famotidine	C	C	Piperacillin	C	C
Folic acid	C	C	Ranitidine	C	C
Furosemide	C	C	Ticarcillin	C	C
Gentamicin	C	C	Tobramycin	C	C
Heparin	C	C	Vancomycin	C	C

C, compatible; I, incompatible; X, not recommended or no information.
[a] TPN base refers to a mixture of amino acid solution, dextrose, and electrolytes.

dictated by the blood glucose level (29). Oral hypoglycemics are discontinued when TPN is initiated, and insulin is administered SC as required. Insulin should be given to patients who have not previously been on insulin but whose blood sugars are consistently above 200 mg/dL on TPN. The usual starting dose is 5 to 10 U of regular insulin per liter of TPN fluid containing 25% dextrose (final concentration). Synthetic human insulin (Humulin) is recommended to avoid an allergic reaction.

   b. **Corticosteroids** can be added directly to the TPN fluid for patients with inflammatory bowel disease or other disorders requiring steroid therapy. It may be advantageous to use steroid preparations with less mineralocorticoid activity (dexamethasone or methylprednisolone) to avoid undesired fluid and salt retention.

   c. **Heparin** has been advocated by some as an additive to prevent fibrin plugging of the central venous catheter. Sodium heparin is compatible at all concentrations with the TPN solution but probably is of little benefit and is not currently recommended for routine TPN use.

6. **Nutrients not added to the TPN solution**

   a. **Linoleic acid (EFA)** requirements are met either with three-in-one admixtures or the periodic administration of IV lipid emulsions (see Section IIIB). EFA requirements are calculated as outlined in

Section IIF, and the linoleic acid content of the lipid emulsion is listed in Table 10-10. For the average adult patient, 500 mL of a 10% lipid emulsion administered twice a week meets the EFA requirement. Linoleic acid also can be supplied by the oral administration of various oils if oral intake is permitted. Corn oil and safflower oil contain 7.2 and 9.8 g of linoleic acid per 15 mL, respectively. The daily oral administration of 1 to 2 tbs of either of these oils satisfies the EFA requirement of most patients if intestinal absorption is satisfactory, but some patients on TPN may require larger oral amounts of EFA to prevent deficiency. Topical administration also may be effective in unusual situations, although this route is not recommended to correct an established deficiency. (Peanut oil contains only 3.9 g and olive oil 0.9 g of linoleic acid per 15 mL.) *Linolenic acid supplementation* may be essential during long courses of TPN (see Section IIF5). Soybean oil emulsions (Intralipid) contain satisfactory amounts of this fatty acid to prevent deficiency, whereas safflower oil preparations do not.

b. Vitamin K, as already mentioned, may or may not be part of the daily IV nutrient regimen. Vitamin K deficiency is a frequent inadvertent complication of TPN therapy. A suitable schedule of vitamin K replacement is outlined in Section IVB3. The vegetable oils in lipid emulsions contain small but significant amounts of vitamin K that must be considered in the vitamin K status of the patient (30).

7. Initiating TPN. The decision to begin TPN is never an emergency. TPN should be initiated under controlled conditions and according to a defined protocol. In the past, we introduced the TPN solution slowly and gradually increased volume during 2 to 3 days. More recently, we have initiated TPN with the full volume (up to 3 L/d) and have not had problems with patient tolerance. The presence of hyperglycemia or a history of glucose intolerance requires slower advancement of the rate of infusion to allow for control of the blood glucose level. A set of specific orders pertaining to the initiation of TPN should be written for nursing personnel. These include the following:

a. Check vital signs, including temperature, every 4 to 6 hours.

b. Record daily weight.

c. Record intake and output.

d. Perform an Accucheck for blood sugar every 6 hours for 48 hours and then every morning as long as TPN is administered. For patients with diabetes, the frequency is every 4 hours until blood sugar levels are stabilized.

e. Change IV tubing according to TPN protocol.

f. Change the central catheter dressing every 48 hours according to TPN protocol. For surgically placed tubes, change the dressing at the operation site every 7 days.

g. Notify physician if temperature rises above 38°C.

8. The appropriate protocol for discontinuing TPN has been controversial, and practice patterns vary from hospital to hospital. Some investigators have recommended infusing 10% dextrose to avoid hypoglycemia if TPN is interrupted and slow tapering of TPN solutions to avoid hypoglycemia when TPN is discontinued. In these circumstances, the potential for hypoglycemia is thought to be related to the continued secretion of insulin when the infusion of high-glucose solutions is stopped. Others have suggested that, in most cases, TPN solutions can be stopped abruptly without causing hypoglycemia (31). We have switched from slow tapering to abrupt discontinuation without problems. Hypoglycemia is more apt to develop in patients who have received IV or SC insulin, and in this circumstance, gradual tapering of the TPN solution and frequent measurements of blood sugar are indicated.

9. Cyclic TPN is a method of parenteral nutrition in which the base solution or three-in-one admixture is infused over a 12- to 16-hour period, usually at night. One guideline for deciding the duration of the infusion during cycling is that the patient should not receive more than 0.5 g of glucose per kilogram of body weight per hour. Cycling has no physiologic disadvantage over continuous infusion and may actually be better. The fluids are discontinued in the morning so that the patient is free to perform the usual daily activities. This method of TPN delivery is used for patients who will ultimately be sent home on TPN and is also suitable for selected patients expected to undergo long courses of TPN in the hospital (e.g., patients receiving bone marrow transplantation). Cyclic TPN may not be suitable for patients with diabetes, especially those requiring insulin, because of the risks for hypoglycemia. Cyclic TPN also may be unsuitable for patients with heart failure, who cannot tolerate the higher rates of fluid administration.

  a. A period of stability (>24 hours) on conventional TPN therapy (24-hour infusions) should be demonstrated prior before cyclic TPN is initiated. The technique is not advisable for patients who are persistently hyperglycemic or who have erratic insulin requirements.

  b. Long-term catheters (e.g., Hickman or Raaf) are utilized so that the catheter can be clamped when the fluid is disconnected. Special modification of the externalized portion of several long-term catheters allows for frequent clamping without damage to the catheter.

  c. In the past, we converted to cyclic therapy according to a schedule for gradual conversion from constant to cycled TPN, and many hospitals still follow such a schedule. More recently, we have switched directly from constant infusion to cycling without gradual conversion and have not had any problems.

  d. The use of a volumetric infusion pump is required. Cyclic TPN is facilitated by using a single 2- or 3-L bag for the entire night's infusion. The three-in-one system (see Section IIIC) is ideal for cyclic infusion if lipid emulsions are required.

  e. Monitor the blood glucose level by Accucheck during the infusion until a safe, daily infusion schedule is verified.

  f. Use sterile technique each time the catheter is handled to connect or disconnect the tubing. A sterile cap should be placed over the catheter tip when it is not in use. Be certain to clamp the catheter before disconnecting it from the solution tubing.

  g. Flush the catheter port with heparinized saline solution immediately before beginning an infusion and when discontinuing the infusion. We use 1:100 heparinized saline solution for permanent catheters and 1:10 for temporary catheters. The volume of the flush varies from 1 to 5 mL and is determined by the length and internal diameter of the catheter.

C. Ordering parenteral nutrition through a peripheral vein

  1. General principles

  a. Providing TPN through a peripheral vein is more difficult than through a central vein because peripheral veins tolerate concentrated hypertonic solutions poorly. Daily volume limitations in combination with the requirement for less concentrated solutions prevent delivery of the desired number of calories. Protein, vitamin, and mineral requirements can be met more easily. However, positive balance for both calories and protein is difficult to establish in any patient with more than mild metabolic stress. In most institutions, central TPN is viewed as the procedure of choice for almost all patients requiring TPN; however, some investigators advocate an increased use of peripheral TPN (32,33).

  b. The administration of IV dextrose in dosages as small as 400 to 500 kcal/d significantly reduces, but does not eliminate, negative nitrogen balance. Amino acid solutions in concentrations of 3.0 to 3.5 g/dL without any additional nonprotein calorie source also reduce negative nitrogen balance. This form of *protein sparing* has its place in the management of certain patients in whom continued severe nitrogen loss would be detrimental. The approach is only temporizing, and more intensive therapy should be considered if parenteral nutrition is necessary.

   c. Uses of peripheral vein parenteral therapy. Parenteral nutrition through a peripheral vein can be used for the following purposes:

   (1) To diminish negative nitrogen balance

   (2) To meet nitrogen and calorie requirements partially, with the balance of the total requirements supplied by oral feeding

   (3) Occasionally to meet total daily requirements

2. **Basic rules to follow in planning peripheral parenteral nutrition**

   a. Keep the osmolarity of the final infusate below 800 to 900 mOsmol/L (see Tables 10-6 and 10-9 and Section IIIA for estimation of osmolarity) and the dextrose concentration at 10% or less.

   b. Utilize lipid emulsions to increase the nonprotein calories delivered per day and decrease the osmolarity of the final infusate. At Barnes-Jewish Hospital, the standard peripheral parenteral formula is a three-in-one admixture with a caloric distribution of 32% dextrose, 16% protein, and 52% fat and a caloric density of 0.7 cal/mL. Three liters of this three-in-one admixture contains 84 g of protein, a total of 2,100 calories, and 1,763 nonprotein calories. Possible immunosuppressive effects have been associated with formulations in which lipids provide such a high portion of the calories.

   c. Do not allow fats to provide more than 60% to 70% of the total daily nonprotein calories (>2.5 g/kg of body weight per day).

   d. Make sure that both the physician and the pharmacist understand the electrolyte content of the ordered solution. Many of the 3.0% to 3.5% amino acid solutions for peripheral venous administration contain significant amounts of electrolytes. The ordering physician should be aware of the electrolyte content before adding additional electrolytes to the daily parenteral nutrition prescription (Table 10-6).

   e. Change the IV infusion site regularly and at the first sign of thrombophlebitis.

   f. If TPN is being attempted through a peripheral vein, all the nutrient requirements described in Section II must be delivered on a regular basis.

3. **Base solutions for peripheral vein parenteral nutrition** are prepared by combining amino acid solutions and concentrated dextrose as described for central vein TPN. Three-in-one admixtures for peripheral administration are also prepared as for TPN.

   a. Osmolarity limitations prevent the use of final dextrose concentrations in excess of 10%. See Table 10-6 for characteristics of amino acid solutions and Table 10-9 for the osmolarity and caloric content of concentrated dextrose. Keep in mind that any devised combination base solution consisting of commercially prepared amino acid solutions and concentrated dextrose will reduce the final electrolyte content depending on the volume of the two constituents.

   b. Two examples of base solutions in which 3.5% *M* Travasol is used are given below. Neither of these base solutions alone provides an ideal nonprotein calorie–nitrogen ratio. In combination with lipid emulsions or oral intake or both, they can deliver sufficient protein and calories to meet the requirements of a patient with no more than mild metabolic stress.

(1) **Example 1.** A moderate-protein, low-osmolarity solution that would be helpful in combination with oral intake:

500 mL of 3.5% *M* Travasol
500 mL of 10% dextrose
_____

1,000 mL
Nonprotein calories: 170 kcal/L
Osmolarity: 475 mOsmol/L
Amino acid content: 17.5 g/L

(2) **Example 2.** A higher-protein, higher-calorie, higher-osmolarity solution that, in combination with lipid emulsions, might meet total daily protein and calorie needs:

800 mL of 3.5% *M* Travasol
200 mL of 50% dextrose
_____

1,000 mL
Nonprotein calories: 340 kcal/L
Osmolarity: 860 mOsmol/L
Amino acid content: 28 g/L

This formula should be infused together with a lipid emulsion to reduce overall osmolarity of the infusate.

4. **Lipid emulsions** (Table 10-10) are used in peripheral parenteral nutrition not only to prevent EFA deficiency but also to supply a large percentage of the daily nonprotein calories (see Section IIIB).

   a. **Lipids provide a source of daily calories.** When 1,000 mL of a 10% lipid emulsion is administered together with 3,000 mL of a base solution, as in Example 1, 1,600 nonprotein kilocalories (68% provided by lipid) and 52.5 g of amino acids are provided in a 24-hour period. Likewise, 1,000 mL of a 10% fat emulsion in combination with 3,000 mL of a base solution, as in Example 2, provides 2,100 nonprotein kilocalories (52% from lipid) and 84 g of amino acids per day. In both these examples, the administration of 4 liters of fluid is required per day to achieve only modest caloric delivery.

   b. **Lipids may prevent thrombophlebitis** by reducing osmolarity when infused together with the base solution. However, some evidence indicates that lipids do not prevent this complication. It is difficult to maintain a positive balance for a prolonged period with peripheral TPN because of the frequent development of thrombophlebitis. In-line filters and the addition of a combination of heparin and hydrocortisone to the base solution may be of some benefit in difficult cases. Additional electrolyte and mineral additives further increase the osmolarity of the base solution.

D. **Monitoring metabolic function during parenteral nutrition.** Every institution has its own standard schedule of laboratory tests for monitoring patients on parenteral nutrition. An example is given in Table 10-12 in many institutions, routine tests are scheduled more frequently. Metabolic complications occur frequently, and the results of routine monitoring should be used not only to adjust the TPN formula but also to regulate the frequency of monitoring. Thus, if a patient is found to be hypokalemic on routine monitoring, the appropriate response is not only to increase the potassium content of the TPN formulation but also to monitor the serum potassium level more frequently.

   1. **A series of laboratory tests** should be obtained regularly to detect the metabolic complications of parenteral nutrition.

      a. Measure electrolytes, creatinine, blood urea nitrogen (BUN), complete blood cell count, alkaline phosphatase, aspartate aminotransferase, bilirubin, albumin, prealbumin, calcium, phosphate, and magnesium at the start of TPN and at 48 hours. If all values are normal, these parameters are then measured weekly except for electrolytes and BUN, which are measured three times per week.

Table 10-12. Suggested laboratory monitoring during total parenteral nutrition therapy[a]

At start of TPN
Electrolytes, BUN, creatinine, CBC count, calcium, magnesium, phosphate,[b] alkaline phosphatase, AST, total bilirubin, albumin, prealbumin, and triglycerides

48 hours after TPN initiation
Electrolytes, BUN, CBC count, calcium, magnesium, phosphate, alkaline phosphatase, AST, total bilirubin, albumin, prothrombin time, and triglycerides

Every Monday
Electrolytes, BUN, creatinine, CBC count, calcium, magnesium, phosphate, alkaline phosphatase, AST, total bilirubin, albumin, prealbumin, and triglycerides

Every Wednesday and Friday
Electrolytes and BUN

AST, aspartate aminotransferase; BUN, blood urea nitrogen; CBC, complete blood cell; TPN, total parenteral nutrition

[a] In addition to the laboratory studies listed here, an Accucheck for blood sugar is performed at the start of TPN, every 6 hours for 48 hours, and every morning as long as the patient receives TPN.

[b] Electrolytes are sodium, potassium, chloride, and bicarbonate.

   b. Blood glucose levels are determined by Accucheck every 6 hours for 48 hours and then each morning as long as TPN is continued. The blood glucose level is monitored more frequently in diabetes.

   c. Monitor triglycerides at baseline, at 48 hours, and once a week thereafter to make sure that the patient is clearing the lipids administered in the TPN admixture.

   d. Monitor weight daily for fluid overload. A weight gain of 1.5 kg/wk or less is expected during intensive parenteral nutrition therapy. A faster rate of weight gain probably indicates fluid and salt retention.

   e. Once the course of parenteral nutrition is stable, a schedule that minimizes venipuncture can be followed (Table 10-12). All attempts should be made to limit venipuncture to once a day, to reduce not only unnecessary blood loss but also the chance of infecting the central catheter. Blood should not be drawn directly from the TPN catheter line for routine laboratory studies.

2. **Monitoring for the adequacy of protein and calorie therapy** is also an important part of TPN management.

   a. **Weight change** is the simplest indicator of successful nutritional repletion, but weight gain can indicate accumulation of fat or water without a similar effect on lean body cell mass. Twenty-four–hour urine collections for urinary urea nitrogen (UUN) can be used to determine nitrogen balance (see also Section VIIIA of Chapter 5). These studies are not performed routinely but may be useful in selected conditions. Nitrogen balance studies are most helpful when the adequacy of TPN is uncertain. This test can be repeated daily or every other day until a positive nitrogen balance is ascertained. Thereafter, if a satisfactory positive balance is unclear, UUN determinations can be repeated on a weekly basis or more often if changes in the regimen are necessary.

   b. **Improvement in the levels of circulating proteins** (e.g., albumin, prealbumin, transferrin, and retinol-binding protein) slowly reflects gradual improvement in this compartment of body proteins.

   c. **Anthropometric measurements of skeletal muscle mass** are not expected to change during the usual course of parenteral nutrition in the hospital. Only in research situations are these tests commonly performed.

Improved muscle strength is a more sensitive indicator of improved skeletal muscle function. The adjunctive use of *physical therapy* for bedridden patients is helpful in restoring muscle mass and muscle function.

d. **Immunocompetence testing** with skin test antigens (Table 5-19) should be repeated no more frequently than every 10 to 14 days if the patient was initially anergic. Demonstrating the restoration of immunocompetence is not usually clinically important in routine TPN administration. Underlying disease (e.g., AIDS) or therapy (e.g., immunosuppressive agents) may make the results of immunocompetence testing uninterpretable.

e. **At some institutions, indirect calorimetry** is used to follow the adequacy of nutritional supplementation in critically ill patients at the bedside. Oxygen and carbon dioxide levels in respired gas samples are measured. The caloric equivalent of the oxygen consumed within a period of time can be calculated. The calories consumed can then be compared with the calories administered.

V. **Modification of parenteral nutrition for patients with organ failure**

A. **Parenteral nutrition in renal failure**

1. **Basis for using modified base solutions**

a. **BUN levels** correlate well with the symptoms of uremia, and the major contributor to urea synthesis is dietary protein. BUN may be a good marker for other waste products involved in the uremic syndrome. The restriction of dietary protein may reduce the BUN. However, to maintain a positive nitrogen balance, the restriction should be to no less than 0.5 to 0.6 g/kg per day, or approximately 40 g of dietary protein in the average adult. Even this level of protein restriction is indicated only in patients whose BUN is above 100 mg/dL and in whom no other cause can be identified. In patients with lower BUN values and in those on hemodialysis, protein is not restricted to this extent. Hemodialysis patients are given 0.8 to 1.0 g/kg per day.

b. **Abnormal plasma amino acid profiles** have been observed in patients with chronic renal failure. A reduction in the levels of essential amino acids has been noted consistently. The cause is not known, but a reduction is also seen in patients with protein–calorie malnutrition and may represent the catabolic state of uremia.

c. BUN levels are reduced and a positive nitrogen balance is still attained when a larger percentage of dietary protein is supplied as essential amino acids. At one time, the reutilization of urea nitrogen to form nonessential amino acids from essential amino acids was thought to be the mechanism of this beneficial effect. However, the reduced BUN is a consequence of decreased urea synthesis (34). Despite the theoretical implications, the use of parenteral nutrition formulations rich in essential amino acids has not consistently resulted in improved outcomes in patients with acute renal failure. These parenteral nutrition formulas are very expensive. Because of their cost and the absence of data to indicate that they affect clinical outcomes, formulas rich in essential amino acids should be reserved for the small group of patients with elevated BUN and creatinine levels who are not candidates for dialysis. Other patients with renal failure should receive standard amino acid formulations.

2. **Characteristics of renal failure solutions** (Nephramine, Aminosyn RF, RenAmin, Aminess) are given in Tables 10-6 and 10-8 (note the minimal electrolyte content of these amino acid solutions). The modified amino acid profiles provide the following:

a. The minimum daily nitrogen requirement to maintain a positive nitrogen balance

b. A much larger proportion of essential amino acids in the amino acid profile

3. **Typical base solutions and three-in-one admixtures for patients with renal failure** combine amino acid solutions for renal failure with concentrated dextrose. To achieve a greater reduction in the overall volume delivered per day, 70% dextrose can be substituted for the usual 50% dextrose, so that a more concentrated solution is provided.
   a. **Specific solutions**
      (1) **Example 1**
         500 mL of 5.4% Nephramine
         500 mL of 50% dextrose
         _____

         1,000 mL
         Nonprotein calories: 850 kcal/L
         Osmolarity: 1,470 mOsmol/L
         Amino acids: 27 g/L
      (2) **Example 2.** Volume is less because 70% dextrose is used (Table 10-11).
         500 mL of 5.4% Nephramine 5.4%
         300 mL of 70% dextrose
         _____

         800 mL
         Nonprotein calories: 714 kcal/800 mL
         Osmolarity: 1,590 mOsmol/L
         Amino acids: 27 g/800 mL
   b. **Use of base solutions or three-in-one admixtures.** Two liters of the solution in Example 1 or 1,600 mL of the solution in Example 2 would meet the caloric and protein requirements of many stable patients with chronic renal failure without causing undue increases in BUN. This is particularly applicable to patients not on long-term hemodialysis. A more liberal use of formulas with standard amino acid profiles is appropriate for patients on dialysis.

   Instead of the base solutions described in Example 1 and Example 2, one can use a three-in-one admixture for patients with renal failure. A low-nitrogen admixture (Fig. 10-2) with a standard amino acid solution makes it possible to deliver large numbers of calories without raising the BUN excessively and without causing fluid overload. The use of fat as a source of calories provides an advantage in renal failure. The low-nitrogen three-in-one admixture has a caloric density of 1.5 kcal/mL; in comparison, the base solution in Example 1 has a caloric density of 0.85 kcal/mL, and that in Example 2 has a caloric density of 0.89 kcal/mL. The use of fat as a source of calories allows the total fluid load to be reduced. Periodic monitoring for metabolic complications, including elevated triglycerides, and for adequacy of protein and calorie therapy is necessary to determine whether the TPN formula is satisfactory.
4. **Electrolyte modifications** include restrictions of potassium, phosphate, magnesium, sodium, and chloride in comparison with the usual daily requirements of patients whose renal function is normal. Daily monitoring of the blood levels of these minerals is usually necessary until the appropriate daily formula has been determined. Omit an electrolyte or reduce its concentration in the formula if the serum level is elevated. Patients with normal serum electrolyte levels who are not on dialysis require daily mineral supplementation on the low side of the average range. Serum potassium, phosphate, and magnesium levels may fall precipitously with the initiation of TPN.
5. **The vitamin schedule** used for patients with normal renal function may be satisfactory for patients with renal failure, although deficiencies of water-soluble vitamins tend to develop in uremic patients. Additional folic acid, pyridoxine, and vitamin D (as an oral supplement) may be necessary. Some institutions use vitamin B complex plus vitamin C sup-

plemented with 1 mg of folic acid per day instead of MVI-12 as the routine TPN vitamin supplement for patients with renal failure. Increased requirements for water-soluble vitamins have been observed in both predialysis and dialysis patients (the dialysate reduces vitamin levels). Vitamin A supplementation is not recommended initially because serum retinol-binding protein and vitamin A levels are often elevated. Assessment for deficiencies of these vitamins is described in Chapter 5.

   6. Patients with renal failure may not require some trace elements that are cleared by the kidneys (e.g., selenium and chromium).

B. Parenteral nutrition in liver failure

   1. TPN is limited in liver failure for the following reasons:

     a. Potential hepatotoxicity of the infused solutions or detrimental effects of fatty infiltration

     b. Exacerbation of encephalopathy during protein feeding

   2. Alterations in blood amino acid profiles have been observed consistently in patients with liver failure and encephalopathy, with an increase in the proportion of aromatic amino acids (phenylalanine, tyrosine, tryptophan) and a decrease in the proportion of BCAAs (isoleucine, leucine, valine). Encephalopathy can be reversed and a positive nitrogen balance restored simultaneously with the oral feeding of dietary supplements high in BCAAs, although the outcome of the illness is unchanged. The efficacy of similar formulas for parenteral nutrition (e.g., HepatAmine or BranchAmin plus a standard formula; Table 10-9) in improving overall clinical outcome is not yet firmly established. Some prospective, controlled trials suggest that parenteral nutrition with BCAAs is more effective than treatment with lactulose and neomycin in reversing encephalopathy (35). The use of special hepatic amino acid formulations can be most easily justified in patients who become encephalopathic when given standard amino acid formulations at rates that meet their minimum amino acid requirements.

   3. Patients with stable liver disease may be given TPN with a base solution consisting of the usual combination of amino acids and dextrose.

     a. To prevent encephalopathy, the minimum daily requirement for protein should be administered. Forty to fifty grams of crystalline amino acids daily satisfactorily meet the basal nitrogen requirement of patients with mild or no metabolic stress.

     b. Base solutions with higher nonprotein calorie–nitrogen ratios than the usual half-and-half combination of 8.25% amino acids and 50% dextrose are appropriate if protein restriction is important to prevent encephalopathy.

     c. Restriction of free water and sodium restriction is generally necessary in patients with severe liver disease and volume overload.

     d. Mild liver disease (noncirrhotic disease) is not a contraindication to parenteral nutrition, especially if the patient otherwise would have been selected as a candidate for intensive nutritional support.

     c. **Evidence of deteriorating liver disease** (e.g., onset of encephalopathy, development of portal hypertension) mandates a reevaluation of the need for parenteral nutrition and generally an immediate reduction in the amount of protein delivered per day. With mild elevations of liver enzymes alone (see Section VIIIA9), parenteral nutrition need not be discontinued. Carbohydrates also may be poorly handled in the failing liver; in severe liver failure, hypoglycemia may be a problem. Lipid emulsions are poorly metabolized by the abnormal liver and must be given with caution in the presence of any liver disease. Lipid emulsions are thought to be contraindicated in the presence of severe liver disease.

C. Parenteral nutrition in heart failure. Volume limitations require the formulation of a base solution that is more concentrated in caloric content so that no more than 2,000 mL needs to be delivered in a 24-hour period to meet the calorie and protein requirements of a patient with heart failure. A three-in-one admixture, such as the low-nitrogen formula in Fig. 10-2, delivers a large number of calories in a small volume. When this formula is ordered for a patient with heart failure, it is necessary to specify a low-sodium content. Parenteral nutrition must be delivered with care if significant ventricular failure is present because even 2,000 mL of concentrated TPN solution can precipitate pulmonary edema.

D. **Parenteral nutrition in respiratory failure.** The progression of respiratory failure is related to the function of the muscles of respiration. A poor nutritional state is associated with a loss of muscle mass and function (36). Carbon dioxide production rapidly increases when patients who have been fasting are fed a high-carbohydrate diet. Increased carbon dioxide production can become a problem when TPN is initiated in patients with respiratory failure and carbon dioxide retention. Modification of the TPN plan so that 30% to 50% of the daily nonprotein calories is provided by lipid emulsion reduces the carbon dioxide production that results from carbohydrate feeding alone. The reduction in carbon dioxide production associated with fat feeding is related to the lower respiratory quotient of fat than of carbohydrate. However, the major determinant of carbon dioxide production is not the relative amounts of fat and carbohydrate but rather the total caloric load. Reducing the total number of calories should reduce carbon dioxide production.

1. **Lipid emulsions are indicated on a daily basis** as a source of calories, not just of EFAs, in patients with severe respiratory disease and carbon dioxide retention. The improvement in the respiratory quotient and the reduction in carbon dioxide production are most notable if lipids are infused continuously over a 24-hour period. Although mildly detrimental effects on pulmonary function testing are noted in association with the use of lipid emulsions, the beneficial effect of reducing carbon dioxide production appears to outweigh the detrimental effects of carbon dioxide retention on pulmonary function in adults. This may not be true in infants, especially neonates with hyaline membrane disease.

2. **Modification of volume and sodium delivery** may be necessary in respiratory failure, as in other situations of fluid overload, such as cardiac failure.

E. **Parenteral nutrition in cancer**

1. **Reasonable expectations for the benefits of TPN** in cancer patients are the following (2):

   a. Reversal of nutritional deficiencies that have developed (as in other illnesses)

   b. Improved tolerance to tumor therapy

   c. Little or no effect on tumor growth

2. **Individual nutrient abnormalities** detected by laboratory tests may be related to poor recent intake, are probably not directly related to the cancer, and usually can be corrected by oral supplementation.

3. **Cancer patients medically suited for TPM can be selected** according to the same guidelines as patients with other illnesses (see Section V of Chapter 8). The best candidates for TPN include the following:

   a. Patients who meet the criteria for malnutrition and have a reasonable chance of responding to appropriate oncologic therapy.

   b. Patients who have previously undergone oncologic therapy and are incapable of adequate enteral nutrition because of malnutrition that developed during previous treatment.

   c. Nutritionally intact patients whose treatment plan necessitates multiple courses of chemotherapy, possibly combined with radiation treatment or surgery, when optimal nutritional status during treatment is a necessary goal. Enteral and parenteral nutrition is associated with better clinical outcomes in patients undergoing bone marrow transplants.

  4. Specific modification of parenteral nutrition solutions is necessary only if concomitant organ failure is present. TPN prevents nutritional deterioration when a tumor or tumor therapy makes use of the gastrointestinal tract impossible, but instituting it often entails an ethical rather than a medical decision.

VI. Modification of parenteral nutrition in severe metabolic stress. The catabolism mediated by catecholamines, cortisol, glucagon, and other mechanisms during metabolic stress resists reversal. It may be impossible to correct a negative nitrogen balance under such circumstances (37).

 A. Effects of nutrient delivery in this setting include the following:

  1. Increased delivery of amino acids improves nitrogen balance, but the beneficial effect plateaus, so that a positive balance is not attained even with adequate delivery of nonprotein calories.

  2. Increased delivery of energy may be poorly tolerated. Loads high in glucose are handled ineffectively (even if the total amount of glucose is less than the daily energy requirement). Lipid oxidation continues as part of the stress response to provide endogenous calories. Infused glucose, in part, may be shunted to glycogenesis and can become an additional metabolic stress. Infusion of approximately 800 kcal/d as glucose is useful in stress for the glucose-dependent tissues (mainly brain).

  3. BCAAs are directly metabolized by skeletal muscle and can serve as a source of energy during the stress response. These amino acids (particularly leucine) also play a regulatory role in protein catabolism (see Section IIIA4). Both protein synthesis and catabolism are increased during metabolic stress. A reduction in excessive catabolism improves the nitrogen balance, and BCAAs may be beneficial by this mechanism. However, BCAAs have not been shown to influence the clinical outcome favorably in critically ill patients.

 B. Therapeutic implications

  1. The clinical outcome is more directly related to successful management of the underlying disease than to nutrition.

  2. Total caloric provision should be near the calculated energy requirement.

  3. Lipids should be given as a component of the daily caloric source (30% of total provision) to avoid the potential stress of excessive glucose infusion. Lipids also reduce the likelihood of severe hyperglycemia, which can be induced by glucose infusion in this setting.

  4. Increased proportions of BCAAs (leucine, isoleucine, valine) in the amino acid solution are provided in several commercially available products (Table 10-8). Little evidence has been found that they improve clinical outcomes in these patients. Aminosyn-HBC and FreAmine-HBC are formulated with approximately 45% BCAAs. BranchAmin 4% contains only BCAAs and can be combined with standard amino acid solutions to increase the proportion of BCAAs in the final base solution. The nitrogen-sparing effects of BCAAs appear to be maximal when their total concentration approximates 45% to 55%. In view of their cost and the lack of evidence of a better clinical outcome, the use of these products may be difficult to justify. Standard amino acid solutions are appropriate for almost all these patients.

VII. Modification of parenteral nutrition techniques for pediatric patients. Nearly all the principles and practices outlined in the preceding sections apply to pediatric patients. However, the techniques are sufficiently different, especially for neonates, that a reference source specifically addressing pediatric nutrition should be consulted (38).

VIII. Complications of parenteral nutrition. The morbidity associated with parenteral nutrition is the greatest deterrent to its use in many institutions. Complication rates are effectively reduced when teams that include physicians, dietitians, nurses, and pharmacists are organized to administer parenteral nutrition. The assignment of specific persons to a team may not be necessary to keep the complication rate at an acceptable level. However, cooperation by all the named services is certainly important. Serious complications develop in fewer than 5% of patients treated with TPN at institutions where a team approach has been implemented. The complications of parenteral nutrition can be categorized as metabolic or nonmetabolic depending on whether they are related to the nutritional formula or the mechanical technique of delivery.

A. Metabolic complications

1. **Hyperglycemia and hyperosmolarity.** A common complication resulting from the delivery of concentrated dextrose, hyperglycemia is more likely to develop during periods of intense catabolic stress. The ability to handle the glucose load may improve as parenteral nutrition continues. Hyperosmolarity results from the insufficient administration of free water or from persistent glycosuria and free water diuresis. The insidious development of hyperglycemia and glycosuria during an apparently stable course of TPN can indicate the onset of a new catabolic stress, such as catheter sepsis. Hyperglycemia secondary to insulin resistance is seen in chromium deficiency. Hyperglycemia is also seen in patients who are being overfed and receiving more calories than they need. Short-term overfeeding causes hyperglycemia; long-term overfeeding causes fatty liver and can result in impaired immune function. Overfeeding with resultant hyperglycemia is one of the most common and most serious problems associated with TPN. Caloric intakes of more than 30 kcal/kg per day in nondiabetic patients receiving TPN results in significant hyperglycemia (39). The concern for the metabolic complications of overfeeding has led to growing support for hypocaloric feeding (40).

   a. **Detection.** Blood glucose levels should be determined by Accucheck every 6 hours for 48 hours after initiation of TPN therapy and then daily during stable TPN therapy. For patients with diabetes, an Accucheck is performed every 4 hours until the blood sugar level is stable.

   b. **Treatment.** The most straightforward treatment is to reduce the number of calories administered. Reducing the number of carbohydrate calories while increasing the number of lipid calories may also be useful. Another approach is to add insulin to the TPN bag or to give insulin IM or SC.

2. **Hypoglycemia.** High levels of insulin that develop during the continuous infusion of concentrated dextrose can precipitate hypoglycemia if the TPN is inadvertently interrupted or abruptly discontinued. This is very uncommon in normal adults, although it does occur in children and in adults receiving insulin. The fear of inducing hypoglycemia with rapid cessation of glucose infusions has led some to suggest that TPN solutions be tapered rather than abruptly stopped; however, others have found that abrupt cessation is not associated with hypoglycemia (31). In patients who receive insulin, hypoglycemia is less likely if regular insulin is added to the TPN fluid rather than given SC when additional insulin is necessary.

   a. **Detection.** The complication is suspected when hypoglycemic symptoms develop (e.g., sweating, palpitations, mental status changes, lethargy or agitation, hunger, faintness, confusion) and is confirmed by measuring the blood glucose level.

   b. **Treatment** involves initiation of peripheral 5% or 10% dextrose if the central line is discontinued and maintenance of this infusion for 2 hours. If a too-rapid decrease in the TPN infusion rate is the cause, increase the rate, then taper more gradually.

3. **Abnormalities of any serum electrolyte concentration** can develop during TPN; requirements vary considerably from patient to patient and during an individual patient's course of therapy. Potassium requirements may be high initially because of fluxes from the extracellular to

intracellular space (secondary to insulin and glucose administration) and because of reversal of the catabolic state. This initially high requirement is likely to decrease during the course of TPN. Hyperchloremic acidosis was once a frequent complication of parenteral nutrition because of the high chloride content of early amino acid solutions. Currently available solutions are low in chloride, and this complication is now less frequent. Still, one should *keep the chloride content equal to or below the sodium content in the daily prescription to prevent hyperchloremia* unless unusual chloride losses are occurring. Phosphorus requirements increase with the initiation of protein anabolism. Inadvertent omission of phosphate results in hypophosphatemia shortly after TPN is initiated.

   a. **Detection.** Watch for signs or symptoms of electrolyte abnormalities; regular laboratory monitoring of serum electrolytes (Table 10-12) may detect a problem before it becomes clinically apparent.

   (1) **Sodium**

      (a) **Signs and symptoms of hyponatremia:** confusion, irritability, lethargy, seizures

      (b) **Signs and symptoms of hypernatremia:** thirst, oliguria, decreased skin turgor, mild irritability, mental depression

   (2) **Potassium**

      (a) **Signs and symptoms of hypokalemia:** weakness, hyporeflexia, paresthesias, flaccidity, paralysis (in extreme cases), respiratory depression, arrhythmias, T-wave flattening, irritability, stupor, nausea, ileus

      (b) **Signs and symptoms of hyperkalemia:** weakness, paresthesias, depressed reflexes, paralysis, bradycardia, ventricular arrhythmias (often bradyarrhythmias), hyperacute T waves, cardiac arrest

   (3) **Calcium**

      (a) **Signs and symptoms of hypocalcemia:** circumoral paresthesias, tetany (carpopedal spasm, Chvostek's sign, Trousseau's sign), irritability, confusion, seizures, ventricular arrhythmias, prolongation of QT interval

      (b) **Signs and symptoms of hypercalcemia:** confusion, lethargy, psychosis, coma, anorexia, nausea, abdominal pain, constipation, vomiting, dehydration

   (4) **Magnesium**

      (a) **Signs and symptoms of hypomagnesemia:** weakness, fasciculations, tremors, confusion, seizures, symptoms of hypocalcemia and hypokalemia

      (b) **Signs and symptoms of hypermagnesemia:** nausea, vomiting, lethargy, hyporeflexia, weakness, respiratory depression, coma

   (5) **Phosphate**

      (a) **Signs and symptoms of hypophosphatemia:** weakness, paresthesias, paralysis, hemolysis, weakness of respiratory muscles, rhabdomyolysis (symptoms usually not present unless phosphate level <1 mg/dL)

      (b) **Signs and symptoms of hyperphosphatemia:** few symptoms; metastatic calcification possible

   b. **Treatment** involves appropriate modification in subsequent bottles. If more urgent correction is necessary, appropriate IV fluids should be given by peripheral vein to avoid exceeding solubility limitations or making rapid rate changes in the base solution. To correct deficiencies in calcium, phosphate and magnesium, take the following measures:

   (1) Parenteral calcium is usually given at a rate of 1 to 2 g/h. Calcium chloride should be administered only into a central vein

because of the risk for inducing thrombophlebitis in peripheral veins. A patient with symptomatic hypocalcemia (tetany) can be given 1 g of calcium gluconate over 10 minutes.

(2) Parenteral phosphate should be diluted in a large (250 mL) volume of fluid.

Parenteral phosphate

For a serum phosphorus level of 1 to 2 mg/dL, give 0.2 mmol/kg over 4 to 6 hours.

For a serum phosphorus level below 1 mg/dL, give 0.3 mmol/kg over 4 to 6 hours.

Oral phosphate

Neutra-phos powder provides 250 mg (8 mmol) per packet.

(3) For patients with normal renal function, up to 16 mEq (2 g) of magnesium can be given IV over 4 to 6 hours; it is mixed in 50 to 100 mL of normal saline solution or 5% dextrose.

4. **Induced vitamin or mineral deficiencies.** Vitamin deficiencies are unlikely if a regular schedule of vitamin supplementation is followed (see Section IVB3). However, vitamin K deficiency is common because this vitamin is not included in most commonly available multivitamin preparations for parenteral use. Certain trace mineral deficiencies also have appeared during long-term parenteral nutrition. These deficiencies can be prevented by supplying trace minerals (see Section IVB4), especially for severely malnourished patients and those expected to receive TPN for more than a month.

   a. **Detection.** Results of routine laboratory monitoring (Table 10-12) suggest certain vitamin or mineral deficiencies. The clinical syndromes produced by vitamin and trace mineral deficiencies are described in Chapters 5 and 6.

   b. **Treatment** involves appropriate replacement.

5. **Elevation of the BUN** is common with the institution of TPN. Increased urea synthesis is responsible for modest increases in BUN. Inordinate increases in BUN may represent hyperosmolar dehydration with insufficient administration of free water. A BUN value exceeding 75 to 100 mg/dL indicates a need to modify TPN therapy in most cases.

   a. **Detection** is by determination of the BUN.

   b. **Treatment.** Increased amounts of free water must be given in the form of 5% dextrose via a peripheral vein if dehydration and hyperosmolarity are present. Free water without dextrose also may be given directly in the TPN bag. Insulin therapy for hyperglycemia may be necessary. Free water should be increased in subsequent TPN bottles. If hyperosmolar dehydration is not present, a reduction in the TPN infusion rate decreases the BUN.

6. **Hyperammonemia.** With currently available amino acid solutions, this is not a clinical problem in adults. Arginine supplementation included in the amino acid formula provides adequate substrate in the urea cycle for urea synthesis from ammonia.

   a. **Detection.** Lethargy, twitching, generalized seizures in infants, and a high blood ammonia level are noted

   b. **Treatment.** Arginine supplementation is provided at a rate of 0.5 to 1.0 mmol/kg per day.

7. **Metabolic bone disease.** In some patients receiving long-term TPN (>2 to 3 months), severe pain develops in the periarticular regions, lower extremities, and back despite apparent improvement in the overall nutritional status. Bone biopsies reveal patchy osteomalacia and decreased mineralization, although serum levels of calcium, phosphorus, parathyroid hormone, and total 25-hydroxyvitamin D are normal. Low serum levels of 1,25-dihydroxyvitamin D have been reported in patients on long-term TPN; thus, an altered vitamin D metabolism may be involved in the pathogenesis of the syndrome. Symptoms resolve and 1,25-dihy-

droxyvitamin D levels normalize after TPN is discontinued. Abnormalities have also been found in the bone biopsy specimens of asymptomatic patients. Other factors contributing to bone disease include hypercalciuria during the TPN infusion (likely related to glucose loading or an increased burden of organic sulfate) and possibly improper administration of trace minerals.

    a. Detection. The pathogenesis is not well understood; no good serum marker is available at this time. Symptoms usually include pain in the periarticular regions, lower extremities, and back. Bone biopsy is required for diagnosis.

    b. Treatment. Temporary or permanent discontinuance of TPN and removal of vitamin D from the solution are the only currently known therapies.

8. Hypercapnia. The increase in carbon dioxide production during concentrated carbohydrate feeding may be detrimental to patients with severe lung disease and carbon dioxide retention. It may be difficult to wean such patients from ventilators during concentrated carbohydrate TPN feeding (see Section VD).

    a. Detection. Respiratory acidosis is revealed by measurement of the arterial blood gases.

    b. Treatment involves a reduction in the carbohydrate infusion and the substitution of carbohydrate with lipid emulsions to provide 30% to 60% of daily nonprotein calories. It is also important to make sure that the patient is not being overfed. If that is the case, the total number of calories administered should be reduced.

9. Liver dysfunction. Elevated transaminases (aspartate aminotransferase, alanine aminotransferase) are common with the initiation of TPN (41–44). The elevations often resolve with continued parenteral therapy, although persistence of the abnormalities for 4 to 6 weeks is recognized. Delayed elevations or persistent elevations (>20 days) may represent toxic hepatitis, thought to be related to the amino acid infusion (possibly from products of tryptophan degradation). A reduction in liver enzyme levels has been reported with the use of metronidazole. A retrospective review also suggested that liver enzymes are less likely to be elevated in patients receiving metronidazole (45). This effect is possibly related to a reduction in the anaerobic bacterial overgrowth in the small bowel that occurs during TPN. Such organisms may produce hepatotoxic substances—for example, endotoxins, or lithocholic acid. Levels of alkaline phosphatase up to twice normal have been noted in half of patients receiving TPN for more than 20 days. (See Section VB for a discussion of TPN in liver disease.) In some patients, elevated liver enzymes and painful hepatomegaly result from acute fat accumulation during carbohydrate feeding. The administration of glucose at rates above 7 mg/kg per minute is associated with the development of fatty liver. A recent study of liver disease in patients on home TPN found high rates of liver disease in patients on long-term TPN (46). Chronic cholestasis developed in 65% of patients after an average of 6 months of TPN. The prevalence of complicated liver disease was 26% after 2 years of TPN and 50% after 6 years.

    a. Liver function is detected by regular monitoring of liver enzymes and bilirubin (Table 10-12). Fatty liver sometimes can be detected by computed tomography of the liver.

    b. Treatment. Elevated liver enzymes *per se* are not an indication for discontinuation of TPN. The onset of hepatic encephalopathy requires a reduction in protein delivery and possibly discontinuance of amino acid infusion if significant hepatic toxicity is suspected (see Section VB). Fatty liver often resolves with a reduction of the daily carbohydrate load.

10. Gallbladder disease. Cholelithiasis or gallbladder sludge has been detected unexpectedly frequently in patients on long-term TPN. Changes in bile composition and decreased gallbladder contractions may be responsible.

  a. **Detection** is usually by ultrasonographic examination of the gallbladder.

  b. **Treatment** may require cholecystectomy in symptomatic patients. Prevention of this complication with cholecystokinin injections has been reported.

11. **Adverse reactions to lipid emulsions**

  a. **Early or immediate reactions** occur in fewer than 1% of cases. These include dyspnea, cyanosis, cutaneous allergic phenomena, nausea, vomiting, headache, back pain, flushing, sweating, fever, dizziness, and local inflammation at the infusion site. Some lipid formulations include egg proteins, which may be the basis of the allergic reactions.

   (1) **Hyperlipidemia** develops during the infusion but should resolve within 2 to 4 hours after the infusion.

   (2) **Poor lipid clearance** is common in renal or hepatic failure.

   (3) Rarely, hypercoagulability and thrombocytopenia have been described.

   (4) Complications of lipid emulsions are related to the rate of administration. Complications are more likely if the rate of lipid administration exceeds the resting metabolic rate. Limiting the rate to less than 0.03 to 0.05 g/kg per hour should reduce the number of complications.

  b. **Delayed adverse reactions** include hepatomegaly, jaundice (with centrilobular cholestasis), splenomegaly, thrombocytopenia, leukopenia, and mild elevations of liver enzymes.

   (1) **The lipid overload syndrome** includes focal seizures, fever, leukocytosis, headache, abdominal pain, nausea, vomiting, sore throat, anemia, thrombocytopenia, and hepatosplenomegaly. Severe hypotension also has been described. This syndrome is very rare and does not appear to be caused by an accumulation of lipids in the blood.

   (2) **Various alterations in pulmonary function studies** have been described in patients receiving lipid emulsions. A decrease in the pulmonary diffusing capacity may be the most significant change, particularly in premature infants with hyaline membrane disease.

B. **Nonmetabolic complications**

  1. **Complications related to central catheter placement.** The complication rate should be less than 5%. Pneumothorax and hematoma are the most frequent complications. Cachectic patients are more likely to suffer one of the complications related to catheter placement.

  a. **Of the reported complications,** several may occur later in the course of TPN (47).

   (1) Undesirable direction of the catheter

   (2) Pneumothorax

   (3) Arterial puncture

   (4) Hematoma

   (5) Puncture of the thoracic duct

   (6) Subcutaneous emphysema

   (7) Air embolus

   (8) Venous thrombosis

   (9) Pulmonary embolus

   (10) Hydrothorax

   (11) Hydromediastinum

   (12) Hemothorax

   (13) Injury to the brachial plexus

   (14) Catheter fragment embolus

    b. Appropriate placement of the catheter tip in the superior vena cava always must be confirmed by chest radiography before TPN fluid is instilled. If the placement of the catheter is questionable on chest films, a radiopaque contrast material used for venography can be injected through the catheter.

    c. A prospective study suggests that central venous thrombosis may be more frequent than clinically suspected (48). Venograms from 6 of 22 patients revealed significant thrombosis, whereas venous occlusion was clinically apparent in only one patient. In another study, superior vena caval obstruction was found in 15 of 107 patients on home TPN for a total of 379 years (49).

        (1) Prevention. In one series, the incidence of detectable catheter-related thrombosis was reduced by adding 3,000 U of heparin to each liter of TPN fluid (50), and some authors advocate this practice. Others have challenged this recommendation (51).

        (2) Treatment. Methods are available to clear catheters blocked with clots, fibrin, and precipitates (52,53). Clinically significant thrombosis often requires catheter removal and systemic heparinization. The need to demonstrate, treat, or prevent clinically inapparent thrombosis remains unclear. Catheters for home TPN obstructed by thrombi have been cleared successfully by administering 250,000 U of streptokinase IV, followed by 100,000 U/h for 48 hours, with the thrombin time kept at 1.5 to 2.5 times control (54). Urokinase, either by bolus or infusion, also can be used to clear catheters obstructed by thrombi (55).

2. Allergic or sensitivity reactions. Rare hypersensitivity reactions have resulted from the infusion of amino acid solutions or lipid emulsions.

3. Infection. Catheter-related sepsis is the most common serious complication of TPN therapy. The use of strict sterile technique during catheter placement and during dressing and tubing changes probably is the most effective way to prevent this complication. The use of a protected injection port (click-lock) also significantly reduces infection rates. Large series have shown that infection rates can be very low when long Broviac or Hickman catheters are used. The data on the relative incidence of infection in single-lumen versus multiple-lumen catheters are conflicting. One prospective, randomized study found a fivefold higher incidence of sepsis in patients with triple-lumen catheters than in those with single-lumen catheters (56). However, in another study, similar complication rates were noted with single- and double-lumen catheters so long as the TPN line was absolutely dedicated to TPN (57). Severely malnourished patients may be immunocompromised and more susceptible to serious infection. Other risk factors for bacteremia include prolonged placement, distal infection, and extremes of age. Concerted efforts to reduce the infection rate should restrict this complication to fewer than 5% of patients treated with TPN.

    a. Organisms implicated in TPN catheter sepsis (58)

        (1) Relatively common organisms

            (a) *Staphylococcus aureus*

            (b) *Candida* species

            (c) *Klebsiella pneumoniae*

            (d) *Pseudomonas aeruginosa*

            (e) *Staphylococcus albus*

            (f) *Enterobacter*

        (2) Relatively rare organisms

            (a) *Serratia*

            (b) *Escherichia coli*

            (c) *Enterococcus*

> (d) *Streptococcus viridans*
> (e) *Proteus* species
> (f) *Micrococcus*
> (g) *Malassezia furfur*
> (h) *Rhodotorula rubra*

b. **Infection is detected** or suspected by new onset of glycosuria, presence of leukocytosis, and onset of spiking fever, usually to above 38°C, with chills and sweats. Fever during TPN should be systematically investigated for appropriate management according to the following protocol:

  (1) Perform a careful physical examination in search of possible sites of infection or noninfected inflammation.

  (2) For a new fever, consider discontinuing the current TPN bag and changing the system tubing with use of the usual sterile technique. In our experience, the TPN solution itself is almost never contaminated if prepared properly, and we do not routinely discontinue TPN and throw out the bag when a new fever develops in a patient.

  (3) Send a sterilely collected specimen from the bag for fungal and bacterial cultures.

  (4) Obtain a chest film, urinalysis with microscopic examination, and any appropriate cultures.

  (5) Draw blood cultures from the TPN line and a site other than the TPN line after the first definite spike above normal temperature or after the second elevation to 38°C or higher orally.

  (6) It is difficult to determine with confidence whether sepsis is catheter-related (59). Quantitative cultures with higher numbers of organisms grown from blood drawn through the catheter than from the peripheral blood suggest catheter-related sepsis. Similarly, positive cultures from the catheter and negative cultures from the peripheral blood suggest catheter-related sepsis. Finally, positive cultures with the same organism from the catheter entry site and the blood suggest catheter-related sepsis.

  (7) Make sure that vital signs, including temperature, are recorded at 4-hour intervals.

  (8) Treat possible noncatheter sources of fever appropriately. Antibiotics for diagnosed infection other than catheter-related sepsis may be initiated via a peripheral vein or another lumen of a multilumen catheter once the diagnosis has been made.

  (9) Withdraw the central catheter if no other explanation is found for the fever and if the temperature remains elevated for more than 24 to 48 hours. In a very few patients with no alternative sites for IV access, we have left the catheter in place and treated with IV antibiotics given through the catheter for a period of weeks.

  (10) Begin a peripheral IV line and infuse 5% or 10% dextrose before withdrawing the central catheter.

  (11) Draw blood for culture directly from the central catheter before it is withdrawn and label the specimens appropriately for the bacteriology laboratory.

  (12) Prepare the TPN catheter insertion site before withdrawing the catheter. Cut approximately 2 to 3 in of the catheter tip with a scalpel blade or sterile scissors, and send it for bacterial and fungal culture in a dry, sterile culture tube. Do not add anything else to the culture container. A central catheter may be exchanged over a guidewire. The exchanged catheter is used while the culture results are awaited. Use of this technique is controversial because of the risk for infection of the new catheter during the exchange.

c. **Treatment.** Noncatheter sites of inflammation should be treated appropriately. Antibiotics may be given for identified infections other than TPN catheter sepsis.

  (1) If fever persists for more than 24 to 48 hours and no other explanation for the fever is found, it must be assumed that the TPN catheter is the source of infection. Although antibiotics may temporarily suppress a fever caused by TPN catheter sepsis, the problem seldom resolves unless the catheter is withdrawn.

  (2) Fever resolves within 12 to 24 hours after removal of the catheter in most cases unless metastatic infection has occurred. In rare cases, fever persists for up to 48 hours. Although antibiotics are usually not necessary to resolve the problem, they should not be withheld from a patient who appears toxic from infection.

  (3) **Initiate a peripheral line** with 5% to 10% dextrose if the central line is to be removed abruptly.

  (4) It is recommended that at least 48 hours elapse after an infected central line is removed before central vein TPN is resumed to be certain that fever has resolved.

4. **Volume overload.** Meeting the daily calorie requirements (or exceeding them in the case of desired replacement) may require at least 4,000 mL of TPN fluid per day. This volume load may be intolerable to some patients. Weight gain of 1.0 to 1.5 kg/wk (0.5 lb/d) is the maximum expected from intensive TPN therapy. More rapid weight gain often indicates volume overload.

  a. **Detection.** Daily weights should be recorded, input and output recorded, and physical examination performed to detect edema or ascites.

  b. **Treatment** involves reduction of daily fluid delivery. If glucocorticoids are necessary, use dexamethasone or methylprednisolone to reduce mineralocorticoid effect.

IX. **Home TPN.** Patients can be discharged to their homes on TPN (60–62). Most patients requiring this therapy have either malignancies or intestinal complications related to therapy for malignancy (resection or radiation), inflammatory bowel disease, or one of a variety of intestinal disorders, including severe gastrointestinal motility disturbances (e.g., scleroderma bowel) and short-bowel syndrome following trauma or ischemic insult. Patients with malignancy are the largest and most rapidly growing group on home parenteral nutrition (63). Patients with AIDS and gastrointestinal infection are more often being discharged on TPN. The major determinant of outcome of home TPN is the patient's underlying disease. Most patients receiving home TPN for malignancy die within 6 months, whereas the 3-year survival for those with benign disease is 65% to 80%. In view of the lack of data demonstrating an improved clinical outcome, it is not clear how often home TPN is in the best interests of the patient with malignancy or AIDS. A home TPN program requires a competent team that includes all the same personnel involved in inpatient management. In addition, the patient or a personal caretaker plays an essential role in the day-to-day routine. Hospital-based programs and commercial services are sufficiently available that an interested and competent physician can provide this service in nearly any area in the United States. Comprehensive training of the patient is necessary before discharge, and the responsible physician must certify the patient's competency. The American Society for Parenteral and Enteral Nutrition has published guidelines for the use of home TPN (2).

A. **Special nutritional considerations.** Nearly all patients on home therapy receive cyclic TPN (see Section IVB9). Either SC ports or long-term catheters (e.g., Hickman) are preferred. Additional major minerals and free water may be necessary for some patients with exceptional losses; these can be added as separate infusions in the daytime. Patients must flush the catheter with heparinized saline solution after each infusion is disconnected. Uncommon deficiencies of the *trace minerals* are more likely to occur in patients on home TPN for a protracted time. These can be avoided if the comprehensive nutritional prescription outlined in Section II is followed.

B. Complications of home TPN include all the metabolic and nonmetabolic complications of inpatient TPN (see Section VIII). Although the mortality associated with home TPN is low, most patients require occasional readmission to the hospital for the management of complications if they are on home TPN for years (64). The complications for which repeated hospitalization is most often required are systemic infection, catheter-related problems (local skin infection, thrombosis, catheter breakage), and fluid and electrolyte disturbances. Although the length of time a patient is hospitalized for the management of complications may represent as much as 3% of the total time that TPM is administered, much more of the time spent in the hospital is for the management of complications of the underlying disease.

   1. Infection of the catheter is the most common reason for readmission. Risk factors for infection include Crohn's disease, jejunostomy, and poor technique in managing the catheter (65). *Fungemia* may be detected in nearly 20% of patients with documented systemic infection and should be particularly suspected in this group of patients. *Candida* species are the most frequently isolated fungal organisms. Efforts to save the infected catheter are more important in patients on home TPN, and 2- to 4-week courses of IV antibiotics may be attempted in selected patients with the usual bacterial catheter infections (see Section VIIIB1).

   2. Metabolic bone disease is more likely in patients on home TPN because this complication develops after longer courses of therapy (66) (see Section VIIIA7).

   3. Patients on home TPN should also be monitored for the development of symptomatic *cholelithiasis*.

   4. Cholestatic liver disease and complicated liver disease are likely to develop in patients on home TPN for more than a few months (52).

   5. Patients given the same formula for home TPN that they received in the hospital may be getting more calories than they need and so gain excessive weight. The calorie content of the TPN formula may need to be reduced.

C. Ethical considerations in addition to financial considerations are very important in selection of patients for nutritional "life support." Most nursing home facilities do not have the capacity to provide this form of specialized care.

Bibliography

1. Eisenberg JM, Glick HA, Buzby GP, et al. Does perioperative total parenteral nutrition reduce medical care costs? *JPEN J Parenter Enteral Nutr* 1993;17:201.
2. ASPEN. Guidelines for the use of parenteral and enteral nutrition in adult and pediatric patients. *JPEN J Parenter Enteral Nutr* 1993;17[Suppl]:1SA. Revised version *in press*, 2001.
3. Veterans Affairs TPN Cooperative Study Group. *N Engl J Med* 1991;325:573.
4. Klein S, Kinney J, Jeejeebhoy K, et al. Nutrition support in clinical practice: review of published data and recommendations for future research directions. *JPEN J Parenter Enteral Nutr* 1997;21:133.
5. Klein S. Influence of nutrition support on clinical outcome in short bowel syndrome and inflammatory bowel disease. *Nutrition* 1995;11[Suppl 2]:233.
6. Lochs H, Meryn S, Marosi L, et al. Has total bowel rest been a beneficial effect in the treatment of Crohn's disease? *Clin Nutr* 1983;2:61.
7. Jones VA. Comparison of total parenteral nutrition and elemental diet in induction of remission of Crohn's disease. *Dig Dis Sci* 1987;32[Suppl 12]:1008.
8. Greenberg GR, Fleming CR, Jeejeebhoy KN, et al. Control trial of bowel rest and nutritional support in the management of Crohn's disease. *Gut* 1988;29:1309.

9. Wright RA, Adler EC. Peripheral parenteral nutrition is no better than enteral nutrition in acute exacerbation of Crohn's disease: a prospective trial. *J Clin Gastroenterol* 1990;12:396.
10. Griffiths AM, Ohlsson A, Sherman PM, et al. Meta-analysis of enteral nutrition as a primary treatment of active Crohn's disease. *Gastroenterology* 1995;108:1056.
11. Trallori MA, D'Albasio GD, Milla M, et al. Defined-formula diets versus steroids in the treatment of active Crohn's disease. *Scand J Gastroenterol* 1996;31:267.
12. Fernandez-Banares F, Cabre E, Esteve-Comas M, et al. How effective is enteral nutrition in inducing clinical remission in active Crohn's disease? A meta-analysis of the randomized clinical trials. *JPEN J Parenter Enteral Nutr* 1995;19:356.
13. Dieleman LA, Heizer WD. Nutritional issues in inflammatory bowel disease. *Clin Gastroenterol* 1998;27:435.
14. Himal HS, Allard JR, Nadeau JE, et al. The importance of adequate nutrition in the closure of small intestinal fistulas. *Br J Surg* 1974;61:724.
15. Dickinson RJ, Ashton MG, Axon AT, et al. Controlled trial of intravenous hyperalimentation and total bowel rest as an adjunct to the routine therapy of acute colitis. *Gastroenterology* 1980;79:1199.
16. McIntyre PB, Powell-Tuck J, Wood SR, et al. Controlled trial of bowel rest in the treatment of severe acute colitis. *Gut* 1986;27:481.
17. Gonzalez-Huiz F, Fernandez-Banares F, Esteve-Comas M, et al. Enteral versus parenteral nutrition as adjunct therapy in acute ulcerative colitis. *Am J Gastroenterol* 1993;88:227.
18. Solomon SM, Kirby DF. The refeeding syndrome: a review. *JPEN J Parenter Enteral Nutr* 1990;14:90.
19. Heyman MB. General and specialized parenteral amino acid formulations for nutrition support. *J Am Diet Assoc* 1990;90:401.
20. Ziegler TR, Young LS, Benfell K, et al. Clinical and metabolic efficacy of glutamine-supplemented parenteral nutrition after bone marrow transplantation. A randomized, double-blind, controlled study. *Ann Intern Med* 1992;116:821.
21. Ardawi MSM. Effect of glutamine-supplemented total parenteral nutrition on the small bowel of septic rats. *Clin Nutr* 1992;11:207.
22. Hornsby-Lewis L, Shike M, Brown P, et al. *JPEN J Parenter Enteral Nutr* 1994; 18:268.
23. Schloerb PR, Skikne BS. Oral and parenteral glutamine in bone marrow transplantation: a randomized, double-blind study. *JPEN J Parenter Enteral Nutr* 1999;23:117.
24. Robin AP, Arain I, Phuangsab A, et al. Intravenous fat emulsion acutely suppresses neutrophil chemiluminescence. *JPEN J Parenter Enteral Nutr* 1989;13:608.
25. Gianino MS, Brunt LM, Eisenberg PG. The impact of a nutritional support team on the cost and management of multilumen central venous catheters. *J Intravenous Nurs* 1992;15:327.
26. Warshawsky KY. Intravenous fat emulsions in clinical practice. *Nutr Clin Pract* 1992;7:187.
27. Trissel LA, Gilbert DL, Martinez JF, et al. Compatibility of medications with 3-in-1 parenteral nutrition admixtures. *JPEN J Parenter Enteral Nutr* 1999; 23:67.
28. Erdman SH, McElwee CL, Kramer JM, et al. Central line occlusion with three-in-one nutrition admixtures administered at home. *JPEN J Parenter Enteral Nutr* 1994;18:177.
29. Hongsermeier T, Bistrian BR. Evaluation of a practical technique for determining insulin requirements in diabetic patients receiving total parenteral nutrition. *JPEN J Parenter Enteral Nutr* 1993;17:16.
30. Lennon C, Davidson KW, Sadowski JA, et al. The vitamin K content of intravenous lipid emulsions. *JPEN J Parenter Enteral Nutr* 1993;17:142.
31. Krzywda EA, Andris DA, Whipple JK, et al. *JPEN J Parenter Enteral Nutr* 1993;17:64.
32. Stokes MA, Hill GL. Peripheral parenteral nutrition: a preliminary report on its efficacy and safety. *JPEN J Parenter Enteral Nutr* 1993;17:145.

33. Payne-James JJ, Khawaja HT. First choice for total parenteral nutrition: the peripheral route. *JPEN J Parenter Enteral Nutr* 1993;17:468.
34. Walser M. Nutrition in renal failure. *Annu Rev Nutr* 1983;3:125.
35. Naylor CD, O'Rourke K, Detsky AS, et al. Parenteral nutrition with branched-chain amino acids in hepatic encephalopathy. A meta-analysis. *Gastroenterology* 1989;97:1033.
36. Donahoe M, Rogers RM. Nutritional assessment and support in chronic obstructive pulmonary disease. *Clin Chest Med* 1990;11:487.
37. Jimenez FJ, Leyba CO, Mendez SM. Prospective study on the efficacy of branched chain amino acids in septic patients. *JPEN J Parenter Enteral Nutr* 1991;15:252.
38. Kelts DG, Jones EG, eds. *Manual of pediatric nutrition.* Boston: Little, Brown and Company, 1984.
39. Rosmarin D, Wardlaw G, Mirtallo J. Hyperglycemia associated with high, continuous infusion rates of total parenteral nutrition dextrose. *Nutr Clin Pract* 1996;11:151.
40. Sandstrom R, Hyltander A, Korner U, et al. The effect on energy and nitrogen metabolism by continuous, bolus, or sequential infusion of a defined total parenteral nutrition formulation in patients after major surgical procedures. *JPEN J Parenter Enteral Nutr* 1995;19:333.
41. Baker AL, Rosenberg IH. Hepatic complications of total parenteral nutrition. *Am J Med* 1987;82:489.
42. Quigley Em, Marsh MN, Shaffer JL, et al. Hepatobiliary complications of total parenteral nutrition. *Gastroenterology* 1993;104:286.
43. Klein S, Nealon WH. Hepatobiliary abnormalities associated with total parenteral nutrition. *Semin Liver Dis* 1988;8:237.
44. Balistreri WF, Bove KE. Hepatobiliary consequences of parenteral alimentation. *Prog Liver Dis* 1990;9:567.
45. Lambert Jr, Thomas SM. Metronidazole prevention of serum liver enzyme abnormalities during total parenteral nutrition. *JPEN J Parenter Enteral Nutr* 1985;9:501.
46. Cavicchi M, Beau P, Crenn P, et al. Prevalence of liver disease and contributing factors in patients receiving home parenteral nutrition for permanent intestinal failure. *Ann Intern Med* 2000;132:525.
47. Pennington CR. Review article: towards safer parenteral nutrition. *Aliment Pharmacol Ther* 1990;4:427.
48. Valerio D, Hussey JK, Smith FW. Central vein thrombosis associated with intravenous feeding—a prospective study. *JPEN J Parenter Enteral Nutr* 1981;5:240.
49. Beers TR, Burnes J, Fleming CR. Superior vena caval obstruction in patients with gut failure receiving home parenteral nutrition. *JPEN J Parenter Enteral Nutr* 1990;14:474.
50. Fabri PJ, Mirtallo JM, Ruberg RL, et al. Incidence and prevention of thrombosis of the subclavian vein during total parenteral nutrition. *Surg Gynecol Obstet* 1982;155:238.
51. Macoviak JA, Melnik G, McLean G, et al. The effect of low-dose heparin on the prevention of venous thrombosis in patients receiving short-term parenteral nutrition. *Curr Surg* 1984;41:98.
52. Holcombe BJ, Forloines-Lynn S, Garmhausen LW. Restoring patency of long-term central venous access devices. *J Intravenous Nurs* 1992;15:36.
53. Holcombe BJ, Forloines-Lynn S, Garmhausen LW. Restoring patency of long-term central venous access devices: published erratum. *J Intravenous Nurs* 1993;16:55.
54. Smith NL, Ravo B, Soroff HS, et al. Successful fibrinolytic therapy for superior vena cava thrombosis secondary to long-term total parenteral nutrition. *JPEN J Parenter Enteral Nutr* 1985;9:55.
55. Haire WD, Lieberman RP. Thrombosed central venous catheters: restoring function with 6-hour urokinase infusion after failure of bolus urokinase. *JPEN J Parenter Enteral Nutr* 1992;16:129.
56. Clark-Christoff N, Watters VA, Sparks W, et al. Use of triple-lumen subclavian catheters for administration of total parenteral nutrition. *JPEN J Parenter Enteral Nutr* 1992;16:403.

57. Powell C, Fabri PJ, Kudsk KA. Risk of infection accompanying the use of single-lumen vs double-lumen subclavian catheters: a prospective randomized study. *JPEN J Parenter Enteral Nutr* 1988;12:127.
58. Howard L, Hassan N. Home parenteral nutrition. *Gastroenterol Clin North Am* 1998;27:481.
59. Kruse JA, Shah NJ. Detection and prevention of central venous catheter-related infections. *Nutr Clin Pract* 1993;8:163.
60. Ireton-Jones C, Orr M, Hennessy K. Clinical pathways in home nutrition support. *J Am Diet Assoc* 1997;97:1003.
61. Nelson JK, et al. Considerations for home nutrition support. In: *The ASPEN nutrition support practice manual*. Silver Spring, MD: American Society for Parenteral and Enteral Nutrition, 1998:35.
62. Howard L, Michalek AV. Home parenteral nutrition (HPN). *Annu Rev Nutr* 1984;4:69.
63. Howard L, Heaphey L, Fleming CR, et al. Four years of North American registry home parenteral nutrition outcome data and their implications for patient management. *JPEN J Parenter Enteral Nutr* 1991;15:384.
64. Burnes JU, O'Keefe SJ, Fleming CR, et al. Home parenteral nutrition—a 3-year analysis of clinical and laboratory monitoring. *JPEN J Parenter Enteral Nutr* 1992;16:327.
65. O'Keefe SJD, Peterson ME, Fleming CR. Octreotide as an adjunct to home parenteral nutrition in the management of permanent end-jejunostomy syndrome. *JPEN J Parenter Enteral Nutr* 1994;18:26.
66. Saitta JC, Ott SM, Sherrard DJ, et al. Metabolic bone disease in adults receiving long-term parenteral nutrition: longitudinal study with regional densitometry and bone biopsy. *JPEN J Parenter Enteral Nutr* 1993;17:214.

IV. MANAGEMENT BY USE OF DIETS

11. RESTRICTIVE DIETS

I. **General principles.** In many diets useful in managing disease, a particular element (e.g., fat or lactose) is *restricted*. In such cases, care must be taken to ensure that a balanced diet providing all the major required macronutrients and micronutrients is offered. Sometimes, supplements must be added to a restrictive diet (e.g., calcium to a low-lactose diet). In other diets, a nutrient that may be required in larger amounts than can be obtained from a usual, well-balanced diet (e.g., protein or calcium) is *added*. Finally, in some cases, either the *consistency* of a diet or the content of indigestible residue or fiber is *altered*. The availability of required nutrients is not changed in a major way, but such diets are useful in the treatment of certain intestinal disorders. This chapter begins with a review of the components of a usual, well-balanced diet because many patients do not maintain such diets, through either ignorance or a wish to avoid certain foods that seem to cause symptoms. Useful source books for information on diets are available (1,2).

A. **Normal diet**
1. **Basic food groups.** To obtain all the essential nutrients, foods from each of the four major groups—dairy products, meat (including nuts), cereals and grains, and fruits and vegetables—should be included in the diet. Macronutrients are required for different reasons.
   a. **Protein** is needed to supply essential amino acids (see Chapter 5 for a discussion of requirements). The essential amino acid content of plant proteins is lower than that of animal proteins. To obtain a mix of essential amino acids comparable with that in animal proteins, protein from various sources must be consumed (Table 11-1).
   b. **Fats** are needed to supply essential fatty acids (see Chapter 10) and vary the flavor of food. When fat is cooked, chemical changes occur that markedly affect food palatability.
   c. **Carbohydrate** is needed to provide texture and blandness, which offset the stronger flavors of protein and fats to make food pleasant-tasting. However, no carbohydrate is essential for the maintenance or growth of tissue. The distribution of macronutrients in some common foods is listed in Table 11-2.
   d. **Modification by cooking.** The values in the table refer to unprepared foods. Cooking can modify the components of food greatly (e.g., fried foods) or not at all (e.g., milk).
   e. **Distribution of micronutrients.** Micronutrients are distributed widely among the major food classes, but the distributions differ for the individual vitamins and minerals. The food sources for each micronutrient are covered in Chapters 6 and 7, but the information is summarized in Tables 11-3 and 11-4. The content of vitamins and minerals is often higher in more brightly colored fruits and vegetables. For example, vitamin A and carotenoids are more abundant in bright orange vegetables and fruits and in dark green leafy vegetables. Fortified foods are enriched with some micronutrients. Occasionally, certain foods that are sources of nutrients have special features that must be considered when the foods are used to maintain a balanced diet. For example, grapefruit juice (but not other citrus juices), a good source of vitamin C, enhances the effect of some medications by down-regulating the intestinal cytochrome P-450 system, thereby increasing their bioavailability (3). In another example, avocados provide fiber, folate, potassium, vitamin C, and vitamin B_6 in good amounts, but each ounce contains about 50 kcal and 5 g of fat (4). Both of these foods are excellent components of a balanced diet, but the special features of each should be noted.

Table 11-1. Use of vegetarian sources to provide adequate essential amino acids

Group	Major components	Limiting amino acids	Other group needed for complete proteins
A[a]	Whole grains, cereals	Lysine, threonine, tryptophan (sometimes)	B or D ± C
B	Legumes, including peanuts	Methionine, tryptophan	A
C	Nuts and seeds, except peanuts	Lysine	A + B or D
D	Vegetables, especially potato	Methionine	A

[a] Also provides iron and riboflavin
Modified from *Mayo Clinic diet manual,* 6th ed. Toronto: BC Decker, 1988.

The common macronutrients, vitamins, and minerals contained in foods are listed in Table 11-5, which provides guidelines for maintaining a balanced diet.

2. **Food guide pyramid.** An alternate method for educating consumers about a balanced diet was devised by the U. S. Department of Agriculture and introduced in 1992 as "A Guide to Daily Food Choice" (5). Fruits and vegetables are in two separate groups, so that the four basic food groups are expanded to five (Figs. 2-1 and 2-2). In the pyramid, meals are based on grains, fruits, and vegetables, which are supplemented with low-fat milk products and meat, poultry, fish, beans, and nuts. The apex of the pyramid is not a food group but rather a warning to use fats and sweets sparingly.

The placement of this warning at the top of the pyramid, whose main purpose is educational, has been controversial. In practice, the food pyramid corresponds to the basic four food groups. Depending on the desired caloric intake, the recommended servings from each group form a pyramid, although they do not decrease proportionally as in the diagram (Table 11-6). As with all diets, the difficult part is defining one serving. The definitions are generally clear in principle (Table 11-7) but often hard to follow in practice. The advantage of the food pyramid is that it can be used as a visual aid to help establish a balanced diet for patients (see Chapter 2).

The use of whole grain foods is essential to realize the distribution recommended by the food pyramid. Packaged foods with a high content of whole grains are those that list *first* among their ingredients one of the following: whole barley, cornmeal, oats, rye, wheat, brown rice, bulgur, cracked wheat, graham flour, or oatmeal. Enriched grains have for years contained added thiamine, riboflavin, niacin, and iron. Whole grain foods contain folate, but folic acid is now added to some grain products (mainly ready-to-eat cereals) to reduce the risk for certain serious birth defects.

3. **Indications.** Every adult and child should ingest a diet balanced with components from each of the major food groups. Individual items may be eliminated because of intolerance, but all macronutrients and micronutrients essential for tissue maintenance and growth should be consumed. When an entire food group is eliminated (e.g., dairy products for lactose intolerance or meat for an ovolactovegetarian diet), the nutrients supplied by that group (e.g., calcium or protein) must be obtained from other food groups (Table 11-5).

Table 11-2. Food sources of macronutrients

Food group	Serving	Protein (g)	Carbohydrate (g)	Fat (g)	kcal
Dairy					
Milk					
Whole	1 cup	8.5	12	8.5	160
2% with nonfat milk solids	1 cup	10	15	5	145
Skim	1 cup	9	12	0.2	88
Ice cream	1 cup	6	27	14	287
Butter	1 tsp	—	—	5	45
Cream, coffee	2 tbs	1	1.0	6	64
Cheese, slice	1 oz	8	0.5	8	105
Meat, fish, peanut butter					
Chicken, turkey	3 oz	21	—	15	220
Fresh fish	3 oz	21	—	15	220
Lean meats	3 oz	21	—	15	220
Egg	1	7	—	5	75
Shrimp, medium	3 oz	21	—	—	124
Tuna	3 oz	21	—	15	220
Peanut butter	1 oz	7	—	5	75
Cereals and grains					
Bread	1 slice	2	15	—	70
English muffin	1	2	15	—	70
Bagel	½	2	15	—	70
Unsweetened cereals	¾ cup	2	15	—	70
Pasta, cooked	½ cup	2	15	—	70
Rice, cooked	½ cup	2	15	—	70
Cooked hot cereal	½ cup	2	15	—	70
Fruits and vegetables					
Potato chips	1 oz	2	15	12	170
Corn	½ cup	2	15	—	70
Peas, beans, lentils (dried and cooked)	½ cup	2	15	—	70
Potatoes, baked	1	2	15	—	70
Squash, baked	½ cup	2	15	—	70
Other vegetables	½ cup	2	15	—	70
Fruit juices					
Apple, grapefruit, orange	½ cup	—	10	—	40
Apricot, cranberry, grape	¼ cup	—	10	—	40
Hi-C, prune juice					
Berries, melon	1 cup	—	10	—	40
Orange, peach, pear, apple	1 (medium)	—	10	—	40
Grapefruit, banana	½	—	10	—	40

Table 11-3. Food source of vitamins

Vitamin	Meat/ fish/eggs	Grains	Vegetables/ fruits	Dairy	Nuts/ beans	Comments
B$_1$	+	++	+	++	+	Grain products enriched
B$_2$	++	+	+	+	+	Especially organ meats
Niacin	++	+	+	—	—	Grain products enriched
B$_6$	+	++	+	+	—	Produced by bacteria
Folate	+	+	++	+	++	Especially green leafy vegetables, organ meats, eggs, whole grains, dried beans
B$_{12}$	++	—	—	++	—	Foods of animal origin only
C	—	—	++	—	—	Especially citrus fruits, green vegetables
A	++	—	++	+	—	Especially liver, pigmented vegetables, fruits
D	++	—	—	++	—	Milk enriched; made in skin; high levels in liver, fish, and eggs
E	++	—	++	+	+	Only in animal or vegetable fat
K	+	—	++	—	—	Especially green leafy vegetables; made by enteric bacteria

Estimates of content refer to raw food. Water-soluble vitamins are extracted into the cooking water.
+, present in appreciable amounts; ++, daily portion contains about 25% of RDA.

   4. **Practical aspects.** Food should be consumed as three daily meals. This
      practice avoids periods of great hunger with subsequent overeating and
      provides energy for tasks to be performed throughout the day.
      a. **Snacks** can certainly be a part of the diet and can include foods from
         any of the major groups. *Junk* or *fast foods* also can be included in a
         balanced diet. It is only when most of the daily calories are derived
         from these foods that they pose a problem. Fast foods often contain
         many calories in the form of fat and carbohydrates, with lesser
         amounts of protein. Moreover, they usually do not include fruits and
         vegetables and so do not provide all the micronutrients needed.

Table 11-4. Food source of minerals

Mineral	Meat/ fish/eggs	Grains	Vegetables/ fruits	Dairy	Nuts/ beans	Comments
Na	+	+	—	++	+	Especially processed food
K	++	+	++	+	+	Especially meat, milk, fruits
Ca	+	—	+	++	++	Especially dairy, meat, fish
P	+	+	+	+	+	Widely distributed
Mg	+	+	+	+	+	Widely distributed
Fe	++	—	+	—	++	Heme iron best
Zn	++	+	—	—	—	Complexes in grain less bioavailable
I	++	—	—	+	—	Seafood best, salt enriched
Cu	++	—	+	—	++	Shellfish, organ meats best
Mn	+	++	+	—	++	Organ, not muscle meats
F	+	+	+	+	+	Drinking water enriched
Cr	+	+	+	+	+	Widely distributed
Se	++	+	—	—	—	Especially organ meats, fish

+, present in appreciable amounts; ++, daily portion contains about 25% of RDA.

b. The term *empty calories,* which been used to describe the nutritive value of these foods, is a poor one. The caloric value of fast foods is as real as that of any other foods because all calories are equal. The foods lack many of the other nutrients, but the caloric value is the same.

c. The best way to entice a patient to follow a *balanced diet* is to review food lists, identify the perceived problems in the intake of all foods, and provide specific recommendations for foods in each major group. In addition, the health care provider must discover what behavioral patterns accompany the abnormal or irregular intake of food if an attempt to correct the diet is to be made.

d. The average *hospital house diet* is balanced so far as nutrients are concerned, although the palatability is not always good because the flavors are usually quite bland. The hospital diet provides each day between 2,000 and 2,500 kcal, 60 to 80 g of protein, 2.5 to 3.5 g of sodium, 3.5 to 4.5 g of potassium, 1.0 to 1.3 g of calcium, 1.1 to 1.5 g of phosphorus, 300 to 400 mg of magnesium, 7 to 9 mg of iron, and 13 to 14 mg of zinc. However, many teaching hospitals do not design house diets to meet nationally recognized dietary recommendations (6). Moreover, they do not always provide enough information for the patients to select appropriate and healthful choices.

Table 11-5. Distribution of nutrients among food groups for balanced meals

Food group	Major nutrients	Minimum recommended number of servings[a]					
		Child	Teenager	Adult	Pregnant woman	No meat	No milk
Dairy products	Calcium, vitamin D,[b] protein, vitamins B_1 and B_2, vitamin A[b]	3	4	2	4	4	0
Meat and meat alternates (beans, nuts, peas)	Protein, Zn, Fe, vitamins B_1, B_2, B_6, and B_{12}, folate, niacin	1–1½	2	4	3	3 (legumes)	6 (2 legumes)
Fruits and vegetables[c] Vitamin A-rich	Vitamin A, Mg, vitamins C and B_6, folate	½	1	1	1	1½	3
Vitamin C-rich	Vitamins C and A, niacin, folate, carbohydrate	½	1	1	1	3	3
Others	Vitamin B_6, folate, niacin, K, carbohydrate	2	2	2	2	0	0
Enriched or whole-grain cereals and breads	Vitamins B_1,[b] and B_2,[b] niacin,[b] protein, carbohydrate, Fe,[b] Mg	4	4	4	4	6	3
Oils and fats	Essential fatty acids, vitamins E and A[b]	Depends on caloric need					

[a] A serving equals 1 cup milk or milk products; 3 oz meat, poultry, or fish; ¾ cup cooked legumes; 1 oz nuts; ¾ cup cooked or 1 cup raw vegetables or fruit; 1 oz dry cereal; ½ cup cooked cereal or pasta; 1 slice bread; 1 tbs oil.

[b] Often fortified in the food.

[c] Representative fruits and vegetables: vitamin A—broccoli, green peppers, collards, carrots, spinach, sweet potato, cantaloupe, plums, squash; vitamin C—citrus fruits and juices, tomatoes, strawberries, green pepper, watermelon, brussels sprouts; other—banana, apple, pear, grapes, potatoes, corn, peas, green beans.

Table 11-6. How many servings are needed each day?

Daily intake	1,600 calories[a]	2,200 calories[a]	2,800 calories[a]
Appropriate groups	Children 2–6 y Women Some older adults	Older children Teenage girls Active women Most men	Teenage boys Active men
Breads, cereals, rice, and pasta	6	9	11
Vegetables	3	4	5
Fruits	2	3	4
Milk, yogurt, and cheese	2–3[b]	2–3[b]	2–3[b]
Meat, poultry, fish, dry beans, eggs, and nuts	2, for a total of 5 oz	2, for a total of 6 oz	3, for a total of 7 oz

[a] These are the calorie levels if you choose low-fat, lean foods from the five major food groups and use foods from the fats, oils, and sweets group sparingly.
[b] Women who are pregnant or breast-feeding, teenagers, and young adults to age 24 need 3 servings.
Adapted from U.S. Department of Agriculture, Center for Nutrition Policy and Promotion, *Home & Garden Bulletin 252, 1996.*

> **e. Dietary guidelines for Americans.** Many guidelines have been developed to provide a diet to minimize the risks for major chronic conditions, such as heart disease, cancer (see Chapter 14), stroke, diabetes, hypertension, dental caries, alcoholism, and obesity. With all diets, the following measures are recommended: achieving and maintaining a desirable body weight, decreasing total lipid intake

Table 11-7. What counts as one serving?

Breads, cereals, rice, and pasta
1 slice of bread
½ cup of cooked rice or pasta
½ cup of cooked cereal
1 cup of ready-to-eat cereal

Vegetables
½ cup of chopped raw or cooked vegetables
1 cup of leafy raw vegetables
¾ cup of vegetable juice

Fruits
1 piece of fruit or melon wedge
¾ cup of juice
½ cup of canned fruit
¼ cup of dried fruit

Milk, yogurt, and cheese
1 cup of milk or yogurt (or substitute)
1½ oz of natural cheese
2 oz of processed cheese

Meat, poultry, fish, dry beans, eggs, and nuts
2–3 oz of cooked lean meat, poultry, or fish
Count ½ cup of cooked beans, or 1 egg, or 2 tbs of peanut butter as 1 oz of lean meat (about ⅓ serving)

Fats, oils, and sweets
Limit calories from these, especially if you need to lose weight.

to 30% of total caloric intake, decreasing saturated fatty acid to less than 10% of total calories, decreasing cholesterol intake to less than 300 mg/d, increasing complex carbohydrate and fiber intake, and decreasing salt intake. All these recommendations are included in *Nutrition and Your Health: Dietary Guidelines for Americans, 2000* and are discussed in detail in Chapters 2 and 3 and other chapters as noted.

1. Eat a variety of foods (see Chapter 11).
2. Maintain ideal weight (see Chapter 13).
3. Avoid excess fat (total and unsaturated) and cholesterol (see Chapter 12).
4. Eat foods with adequate dietary fiber (see Chapter 11).
5. Avoid excess sugar (see Chapter 12).
6. Avoid excess salt (see Chapter 7).

The results of the National Research Council study on diet and health are available to patients in a user-friendly guide (7). Vegetarian diets achieve many of these objectives because they reduce the risks for hypertension, coronary artery disease, diabetes (type II), and gallstones (8). Diets designed to prevent cancer or heart disease are based on similar recommendations. The dietary recommendations outlined above and discussed in Chapters 2 and 3 are intended for general populations in the United States. However, some special considerations should be emphasized for African-Americans and other minority groups. The diets of middle-aged African-Americans may be lower in calcium, magnesium, iron (for women), folacin, and zinc. Obesity is more prevalent in African-American women than in white women, and it may be more difficult for them to achieve a desirable weight. Hispanic-Americans tend to consume a diet higher in fiber and with less animal fat. Overweight has been a greater problem in Hispanic-Americans than in Anglo-Americans. The diet of Asian/Pacific-Americans is generally higher in fish, shellfish, and fruits and vegetables but lower in dairy products and calcium. As these populations become more assimilated into Anglo-American societies, group differences may diminish.

II. Diets of altered consistency
A. Clear liquid diet
1. **Principles.** A clear liquid diet meets the daily requirement for water but minimally stimulates the gastrointestinal tract. This effect is achieved at the cost of minimal ingestion of protein and fat—macronutrients that are potent stimuli of gastric and pancreatic secretions and gastrointestinal motility. In addition, the diet is low in fiber. Because few unabsorbed components are provided, fecal weight and bacterial mass are decreased.
2. **Indications.** A clear liquid diet is used in the following situations:
   a. To prepare a patient for bowel surgery or colonoscopic examination.
   b. In the recovery phase of abdominal or other surgery when partial ileus is present. This restriction may not be applicable to patients after gastrointestinal surgery once bowel sounds have been heard. Early refeeding of solid food has been used successfully after colorectal surgery and perhaps should be tried more often (9).
   c. In other acute conditions associated with a serious disturbance of gastrointestinal function (e.g., acute gastroenteritis).
3. **Practical aspects.** The clear liquid diet is largely water and sugar and provides few other nutrients unless supplements are added. Without supplements, the diet provides about 1,200 kcal/d (300 g of carbohydrates) along with 1.0 g of sodium, 50 to 60 mg of calcium and magnesium, 2,000 to 2,500 mg of potassium, less than 100 mg of phosphorus, 1.2 mg of iron, and only 0.33 mg of zinc. To obtain even this supply of nutrients, one must ingest about 1,500 mL of strained fruit juice, 600 mL of gelatin or fruit ice, and 30 g of sugar added to coffee or tea. These volumes can be

achieved by healthy or younger patients. The diet of an elderly or ill patient diet may be even more restricted because intake is smaller.

Patient information on this topic is available in Appendix D.

a. **Multiple vitamin and iron supplementation** is suggested if the patient is to be on the diet for more than 3 weeks, or sooner if deficiency is present when the diet is initiated. If the diet is to be continued beyond 3 days or if fluid intake is limited, it can be supplemented with carbohydrate and a small amount of protein in addition to some micronutrients. Table 11-8 lists these modifications. The supplemented clear liquid diet provides about half the daily adult protein allowance, and it meets or exceeds allowances for vitamins E and C, folic acid, thiamine, riboflavin, niacin, vitamins B_6 and B_{12}, and iron. Vitamin A, calcium, and phosphorus are provided at about 60% of the daily allowance. Carbonated beverages can be substituted for Polycose as a source of carbohydrate, but they have many fewer calories. The use of supplements depends on the acceptability of fruit juices and gelatins as the major caloric source for the patient.

b. **Foods allowed** include coffee, tea, carbonated beverages, broth, bouillon, strained fruit juices, gelatin, sugar, and sugar candies.

c. **Caffeine.** It is generally agreed that the caffeine content of various beverages alters certain aspects of gastrointestinal function (e.g., transit time is shortened). For this reason, the inclusion of caffeinated beverages may not be desirable in other diets. However, these drinks are usually included in a clear liquid diet. Table 11-9 lists the caffeine content of some foods and drugs.

Patient information on this topic is available in Appendix D.

(1) **The caffeine content of beverages** depends on the amount of water used, method of brewing, and type of coffee or tea. Because caffeine is water-soluble, the longer the exposure to hot water, the greater the extraction of caffeine.

(2) Low doses (<50 mg/d) probably have little effect on gastrointestinal function. The actual caffeine content of cocoa is not certain because of the wide variation in reported figures and the fact that most hospitals and homes now use instant cocoa mix, a prepared product. Theobromine, not caffeine, is the major methylxanthine stimulant in cocoa (~250 mg/cup) and chocolate. Caffeine is also a component of some over-the-counter analgesics. These sources should be considered when caffeine intake seems important.

(3) **The health consequences** of caffeine ingestion are not severe (10). No consistent epidemiologic evidence has been found of an effect on birth-related outcomes, including low birth weight, pre-

Table 11-8. Nutritive value of clear liquid diets

Diet	Protein (g/d)	Fat (g/d)	Carbohydrate (g/d)	Total calories per day
No supplements (~2.5 L intake)	12	0	300	1,200
No supplements (<1 L intake)	6	0	74	320
+ Ensure (three 8-oz servings) (Ross)	32	26	167	1,040
+ Polycose (three 4-oz bottles) (Ross)	6	0	254	1,040
+ Citrotein (three 8-oz servings) (Sandoz Nutrition)	29	1	144	700

Table 11-9. Caffeine content of foods and drugs

Food	Unit	Caffeine content[a] (mg/U)
Prepared coffee	6-oz cup	
Instant, freeze-dried		61–72
Percolated		97–125
Drip		137–174
Decaffeinated coffee	6-oz cup	
Ground		2–4
Instant		0.5–1.5
Tea, bagged or loose	6-oz cup	15–75
Black, 5-min brew		40–60
Green, Japan, 5-min brew		20
Iced	12-oz cup	67–76
Cocoa beverages	6-oz cup	10–17
Chocolate		
Chocolate milk	8 oz	2–7
Milk chocolate	1 oz	1–15
Semi-sweet	1 oz	5–35
Baker's	1 oz	26
Syrup	1 oz	4
Bar	One	60–70
Carbonated drinks	12-oz can	
Colas		15–23
Diet colas		0.3
Root beer, citrus		0
Ginger ale, tonic, other nondiet		0–22
Drugs	Tablet	
Cold tablets		30–32
Alertness tablets		100–200
Weight control tablets		140–200
Pain relief OTC		32–65
Prescription pain tablets		30–100

[a] The ranges represent the range of figures from the literature because the method of preparation affects caffeine content of some beverages.
Adapted from Nagy M. Caffeine content of beverages and chocolate. *JAMA* 1974;29:337, and from Bunker ML, McWilliams M. Caffeine content of common beverages. *J Am Diet Assoc* 1979;74:28.

maturity, spontaneous abortion, and congenital anomalies. However, many studies have not been controlled for smoking, alcohol, or medication. In one case–control study, more spontaneous abortions occurred in nonsmoking women who ingested more than 100 mg of caffeine a day when the fetus had a normal karyotype (11). The risk was proportional to the dose of caffeine ingested. Considering the mixed results of earlier studies, one could cautiously recommend reducing caffeine intake during early pregnancy. The hypercalciuric effect of 300 mg of caffeine has been well established in women with a diet low in calcium (<600 mg/d), but the mechanism is not clear. However, no effects have been noted on bone health, and caffeine is not considered an important risk factor for osteoporosis, except possibly when used on a long-term basis by persons with a dietary calcium deficiency. The pharmacologic effects on the cardiovascular, renal, respiratory, gastrointestinal, and central nervous systems have been studied extensively (10). Consumption of up to 500 mg of caffeine does not cause arrhythmias, but some patients may be especially sensitive to caffeine and should limit their intake. Although data have been reported on both sides of the issue, it does not appear that caffeine causes hypertension or coronary artery disease. Nor are the data convincing that caffeine causes hyperlipidemia or fibrocystic breast disease. Although habituation to caffeine is common, it is not considered a drug of abuse, and it does not fulfill the Diagnostic and Statistical Manual-IV criteria for psychoactive substance dependence. Headache is a frequent withdrawal symptom.

4. **Side effects.** Side effects do not develop if supplements are provided.
5. **Supplements required.** Calories, protein, vitamins, and minerals are needed in the usual circumstances during long-term use.

B. Full liquid diet

1. **Principles.** The full liquid diet is designed to provide adequate nourishment in a form that requires no chewing. Such a diet can also be useful when the esophagus is narrowed and solid food cannot pass.
2. **Indications**
   a. The full liquid diet (or mechanical soft diet) is indicated for patients who cannot chew properly or who have esophageal or stomach disorders interfering with the normal digestion of solid foods.
   b. This diet can be used in conjunction with dilation in the management of esophageal stricture. Available methods for dilation include bougienage with mercury-weighted rubber catheters or with metal (olive) dilators.
   c. **Nutritional completeness.** The diets in which table foods are used can be maintained for long periods only when appropriate supplementation is provided or when all allowed food groups are included. Otherwise, this diet can be nutritionally incomplete. Alternatively, commercially available liquid diets can be used alone (see Chapter 9). However, long-term acceptability is greater when table foods are used as the major source of nutrition.
   d. Full liquid diets can be given through a gastrostomy tube to bypass esophageal obstruction. In such cases, enteral supplements that supply all nutritional needs may be preferred (see Chapter 9) because taste is no longer a factor.
   e. Full liquid diets can be helpful temporarily after many types of surgery for debilitated patients who may not have recovered sufficient strength to chew food. Usually, this phase of recovery lasts no more than a few days, except after laryngectomy, when soreness and swelling are present and a new swallowing technique must be learned. In such instances, the use of creamier foods and thicker liquids makes it easier for patients to relearn how to swallow.
3. **Practical aspects**
   a. Certain characteristics of this diet should be kept in mind, especially for successful long-term use:
      (1) Foods need not be bland.
      (2) Milk-based foods form an important part of the diet. Lactose intolerance presents a problem when this diet is used, but many milk substitutes are now available, based on either corn syrup or soy.
      (3) Flavoring is helpful for some milk-based liquids, but natural or vanilla flavor is best tolerated for long-term use.
      (4) Caloric intake should be maintained near the estimated requirement.
      (5) Medications should be given in liquid form if possible.
   b. **Table foods allowed on a full liquid diet** include all beverages, broth, bouillon, strained cream soups, poached or scrambled eggs,

cereal (e.g., cream of wheat, farina, strained oatmeal), strained fruit juices, ice cream, sherbet, gelatin, custards, puddings, tapioca, yogurt without fruit, margarine, butter, cream, and all spices.

    c. Nutrients in the full liquid diet. The full liquid diet easily provides adequate calories, protein, and essential fatty acids but not certain vitamins, notably ascorbic acid and thiamine, unless fruit juices and cereals are routinely included. The average hospital full liquid diet provides 1,900 to 2,000 kcal/d, along with 40 to 50 g of protein, 3 to 4 g of sodium, 3 to 4 g of potassium, 1.8 g of calcium, 1.3 g of phosphorus, 200 to 300 mg of magnesium, 3 mg of iron, and 8 to 9 mg of zinc.

  4. Side effects. The diet can be boring, and it is wise to include some items from the mechanical soft diet. If lactose intolerance is present, diarrhea may result, and milk substitutes can be used. If meat soups or brewer's yeast are not used, the diet will be deficient in folic acid, iron, and vitamin B_6.

  5. Supplements required. No supplements are required if all food groups are used. However, a multiple vitamin and mineral preparation, preferably liquid, is not unreasonable if this diet is to be used for a long time.

C. Mechanical soft diet

  1. Principles. The mechanical soft diet is designed to provide a greater variety of foods than the full liquid diet for patients who find it difficult to chew or have an anatomic stricture. Patients with dysphagia may require a liquid or soft solid diet. A history of coughing or choking during meals, prolonged eating time, hoarseness after eating, regurgitation of liquid or food into the nose, frequent drooling, recurrent respiratory infections, and weight loss should lead to an evaluation of oral or pharyngeal swallowing problems. The diet must be planned individually depending on the reason for the restriction. The entire range of solid and liquid foods is used so that the diet is nutritionally balanced. One attempts to provide easily masticated foods. Because texture is an important part of taste, patients must choose the foods that they tolerate best and are most acceptable to them.

  2. Indications

    a. A mechanical soft diet is indicated for patients who have difficulty chewing because of advanced age or infirmity, postoperative weakness, or dental problems.

    b. It is also indicated for patients with anatomic strictures of the esophagus, especially those caused by carcinoma.

    c. For patients with strictures in other parts of the intestinal tract, such as the duodenum in active Crohn's disease, only certain restrictions may be necessary because gastric grinding/mixing softens food.

  3. Practical aspects. Spices (except hot peppers) are allowed and are in fact desirable to make food more palatable. Food thickeners, largely gums and modified starches, are available as an aid in swallowing to avoid aspiration. Patients with oral or pharyngeal dysphagia should eat slowly, sit up as straight as possible, keep their head in an optimal position for swallowing (as determined by swallowing studies), and ingest small amounts at any one time.

    a. Foods allowed on a mechanical soft diet. All beverages and soups are allowed. Whole tender meat is permissible, as is ground or puréed meat, but not fibrous meat. Eggs and cheese are permissible. Melted cheese or nonfat dry milk can be used to increase protein content. All potatoes and starches are allowed. Breads and cereals are acceptable, except for high-fiber cereals and hard, crusty breads. Cooked or refined ready-to-eat cereals are often better. Vegetables can be included if they are well cooked or puréed, but raw vegetables must be shredded or chopped. Foods that are hard to chew must be chopped, ground, or blended. Canned or fresh fruits without skin or seeds are acceptable, but not other fresh or dried fruits. Nuts are not allowed. Desserts are acceptable if they do not contain nuts.

b. The bland diet is often combined with a mechanical soft diet and has been used for years in the treatment of ulcer disease. However, no evidence has been found of the value of a bland diet that restricts spices or coarse foods.

c. Some dietary maneuvers have been helpful in the past in the management of acid peptic disease, such as the use of small, frequent feedings to minimize acid secretion after a meal and the avoidance of snacks before bedtime to prevent acid stimulation during sleep. Other dietary modifications in peptic disease have included the elimination of alcoholic and caffeine-containing beverages and smoking. However, with the current availability of potent acid-suppressing medications, these restrictions are now usually unnecessary.

d. Certain dietary restrictions also may benefit patients with gastroesophageal reflux disease (GERD). Foods that increase lower esophageal sphincter pressure include tomatoes and tomato juice, citrus fruits, chocolate, peppermint, and very fatty foods. However, the value of restricting fatty foods in the treatment of GERD has been questioned (12).

4. Side effects have not been associated with this diet.

5. Supplements are not required.

D. Modified-fiber diets

1. Principles. Dietary fiber is not one chemical substance, nor is it completely indigestible. It is a component of the diet that either by itself or through its metabolites produces certain physiologic effects in humans, although the nature and importance of these effects are as yet poorly delineated. *Fiber* is not the same as *residue*. The latter term refers to all stool solids that result from the ingestion of any given diet. In addition to fiber, residue includes bacteria, exfoliated cells, and mucus. A full or clear liquid diet is best for minimizing fecal residue.

a. The accepted definition of dietary fiber is the following: plant cell wall components, including both polysaccharides and noncarbodydrates, that resist digestion by enzymes of the small intestine. The polysaccharide compounds in dietary fiber are both structural and matrix components of plant cell walls; they consist primarily of cellulose, hemicelluloses, pectins, fructo-oligosaccharides, and resistant starches. The compounds are branched polymers containing many uronic acids that hold water and form gels. They are highly branched in growing plants and become less branched as the support structure becomes more developed. They act as adhesives and are insoluble in the unripe fruit, becoming soluble only as the fruit matures. Nondigestible oligosaccharides, such as those associated with flatus (e.g., stachyose and raffinose), are soluble and are not included in the definition of fiber. Thus, the term *dietary fiber* includes many substances, some of which are partially fermented in the colon by bacteria and some of which escape fermentation nearly completely.

b. The **fiber content** of foods is most commonly based on the rather indirect and imprecise measurement of *crude fiber*—the residue of food that remains after sequential acid and alkali treatment. The relationship between the measurement (of the residue that escapes digestion) and the physiologic role of the residue is confusing. For an understanding of the uses of altered-fiber diets, the definition, measurement, metabolism, and possible function of dietary fiber should be considered.

c. Classes of fiber. The major chemical classes of dietary fiber are cellulose, noncellulose polysaccharides, and lignin (Table 11-10).

(1) Cellulose is a straight-chain polymer of glucose with a β-1,4 linkage. It is not digested by pancreatic or small-bowel enzymes. Cellulose is a major structural component of cell walls but rarely accounts for more than 20% of total polysaccharides.

Table 11-10. Properties of components of dietary fiber

Component	Plant function	Major food sources	Effects
Cellulose	Cell wall structure	Bran, whole wheat/other flours, legumes, root vegetables, apples	↑ Fecal bulk, ↓ transit time, ↓ micronutrient absorption (? impact)
Noncellulose polysaccharides	Cell wall stability	Bran, cereals, whole grains	Same as cellulose
Pectins	Cell wall stability	Citrus fruits, berries, apples, bananas, carrots, potatoes	Alters food consistency, ↓ cholesterol absorption, ↑ fecal water, ↓ gastric emptying
Gums and mucilages (psyllium)	Secretions	Oatmeal, dried legumes	↓ cholesterol absorption, ↑ fecal water, ↓ vitamin/mineral absorption
Lignins	Cell wall strength	Old/tough vegetables, wheat	↑ Fecal bulk, ↓ transit time
Fructo-oligosaccharides	Cell structure, secretions	Onions, bananas, tomatoes, honey, barley, garlic, wheat	Prebiotic, alters fecal flora, ↑ SCFAs, ? prevents colon cancer
Resistant starch	Storage form	Processed grains, flours	? ↓ Glycemic index, ? ↓ colon cancer

SCFA, short-chain fatty acid.

(2) **Hemicelluloses** are linear and highly branched polysaccharides of xylose, arabinose, mannose, and glucuronic acid. They act as plasticizers and intertwine with lignin between the cellulose fibers of the cell wall. *Nonstructural polysaccharides,* including pectins, gums, and mucilages, are branched polymers containing many uronic acids that hold water and form gels. They are highly branched in growing plants and become less branched as the support structure becomes more developed. They act as adhesives and are insoluble in unripe fruit, becoming soluble only as the fruit matures. Thus, the amount extracted may vary with the age of the fruit.

(3) **Polyphenols (especially flavonoids) and other cell wall-associated nonpolysaccharide substances.** Polyphenols, products of plant metabolism, range from phenols to highly polymerized compounds, such as tannins and lignins. Most of them are not currently included in the determination of dietary fiber, but lignin is the exception. *Lignin* is not a carbohydrate and constitutes about 12% of plant organic compounds. It comprises a group of phenyl propane polymers of varying sizes because polymerization continues as the plant ages. It re-

inforces the cellulose support structure and inhibits microbial cell wall digestion. Thus, lignin is resistant to all anaerobic digestion systems and is not partially metabolized in the colon, as are the cell wall polysaccharides. It represents only a small part of the human diet (~0.2%).

Phenolic acids and aldehydes, such as vanillin, are common, but the most common of the plant phenolics are the flavonoids, which consist of two aromatic rings linked through three carbons that form an oxygenated heterocyclic ring (13). Flavonoids and other polyphenols are ubiquitous in plants and beverages. They are found in tea and contribute to the bitterness of that and other beverages (14). Polyphenols usually account for less than 1% of the dry matter of plants, but they can reach concentrations of 4,000 to 7,000 mg/mL in red wines and fruit juices (13). The dietary intake of polyphenols in the United States is 1 to 1.1 g/d, with flavonoids accounting for about 4% of the total.

Like other components of fiber, polyphenols are degraded and absorbed in the colon, but the effect of these compounds on short-chain fatty acid production and microflora depends on the type of compound and the microorganisms present. Polyphenols bind proteins and precipitate in the intestinal lumen, and they can increase the fecal excretion of nitrogen and fat. They also inhibit iron absorption. Most recently, the antioxidant effects of polyphenols have been of interest, particularly as they relate to carcinogens and low-density lipoproteins (LDLs). Some evidence suggests that a moderate consumption of tea, a rich source of flavonoids, may provide protection against several forms of cancer, cardiovascular diseases, and kidney stones (14). The blacker the tea, the greater the degree of oxidation of the polyphenols and the weaker the possible effects of these compounds. Herbal teas are not true teas (*Camellia sinensis*), and their flavonoid content is much lower. Tea contributes more than 60% of dietary flavonoids and onions about 13%; grapes, apples, red wine, and dairy products provide most of the rest. The consumption of 1 to 2 cups of tea per day has been associated with health benefits in epidemiologic studies (14). Drinking tea has been as reported to decrease mortality from stroke in men by 50%, and from cancer of the mouth, pancreas, colon, esophagus, skin, lung, prostate, and bladder by 20% to 40%.

These data show only associations, not causation. Moreover, phenolics can under some conditions act as prooxidants (15). Their antioxidant effects depend on solubility and chelating potential, among other properties. Thus, it is not possible to recommend the consumption of large amounts of phenolics as foods or supplements until more data are available.

(4) **Fructo-oligosaccharides** are mixtures of β-D-fructose monomers linked by β-2,1 linkages. These molecules include inulin-type fructans (linear polymers) and levans (branched fructans). The inulin-type fructans (average molecular weight of 5,000 daltons) are present in many edible plants, such as wheat grains and members of the onion family. The daily consumption of oligofructoses by North American populations is estimated to be 1 to 12 g, and slightly more in western Europe (16). Because of the β-C2 linkage, these polymers resist hydrolysis by human digestive enzymes, and they travel to the colon, where they are fermented and metabolized to short-chain fatty acids. Only when ingested in large amounts (>80 g/d) do they produce a laxative effect. Colonic fermentation produces a change in the

microflora, enhancing bifid bacteria and decreasing *Bacteroides, Clostridium,* and other anaerobes. Fructo-oligosaccharides are the best-studied prebiotics, defined as "a nondigestible food ingredient that beneficially affects the host by selectively stimulating the growth and/or the activity of one or a limited number of bacteria in the colon and thus improves host health" (17).

(5) Resistant starches are defined as starches that enter the colon. RS1 is physically inaccessible because of its particle size or entrapment in food. RS2 and RS3 resist amylase action because of their compact (unbranched) structure; RS2 is unbranched and RS3 is retrograded (i.e., altered during processing) (18). Some starches are relatively resistant because they become available slowly in the intestinal lumen. Most resistant starches are produced during food preparation. The intake of such starches in a Western diet is estimated at 5 to 10 g/d.

2. Measurement. Four methods for measuring dietary fiber have provided enough data to be useful in assessing the fiber content of foods.

a. Crude fiber is the residue of plant food left after sequential extraction with solvent, dilute acid, and dilute alkali. Early chemists thought that residue resisting alkali and acid treatment was indigestible. The crude fiber procedure was developed in the nineteenth century and was favored because of the purity of the residue, which was low in ash and nitrogen content. Extraction and loss of hemicelluloses (>80%) and lignin (50% to 90%) are a consequence of solubility at acid and alkaline pH. All components of dietary fiber are at least partially soluble in these solutions. However, the degree of extraction varies with food preparation, particle size, and presence of other fiber components. Crude fiber is still the measure of fiber reported in some food tables and was the original basis for all altered-fiber diets. However, it provides an incomplete and inaccurate assessment of fiber because hemicellulose and lignin are extracted more than cellulose. Crude fiber is slowly being replaced by other methods. The relation of crude fiber to plant cell wall polysaccharide content depends on the proportions of pectins, cellulose, and hemicelluloses, which vary among vegetables and fruits. Monocotyledons in general are high in hemicelluloses and lignin and low in crude fiber. Legumes are higher in lignin but low in hemicelluloses and are intermediate for crude fiber. Dicotyledonous nonlegume vegetables have the highest proportion of cellulose and crude fiber.

b. Neutral detergent residues were developed by Van Soest and McQueen (19) and refined further by Englyst et al. (20) and Anderson and Bridges (21). Neutral detergent fiber or residue results from extraction with boiling sodium lauryl sulfate and ethylenediaminetetraacetate (EDTA) and is nonhydrolytic. Pectins and mucilages are removed completely, and the residue contains cellulose, lignin, and hemicelluloses (i.e., the cell wall components of fiber). This residue contains other nonlignin components that are not polysaccharides. Because neutral detergent residue includes all the major plant cell wall components, it continues to be used to assess the dietary fiber content of foods.

c. The method of Southgate (22) is the most complex but probably the most accurate because it measures both soluble polysaccharides (mucilages, gums, and pectins) and cell wall components. A series of extractions with organic solvents and acids is followed by enzymatic treatment and hydrolysis. Data derived by this method or a modification of the method are included in Table 11-11 as "total dietary fiber," which includes noncellulose polysaccharides (hemicelluloses, gums, mucilages, and pectins) and lignins.

Table 11-11. Fiber content of selected foods determined by different methods

Food	Crude fiber[a]	Total fiber (AOAC)[b]	Total fiber (Southgate)[c]	Grams per serving
		(g/100-g edible portion)		
Grains				
Flour, white	0.3	2.7	3.13	1.9/half cup
Flour, wheat	2.3	12.6	9.6	6.3/half cup
Wheat bran	9.4	35.3	43.9	13.2/half cup
Bread, white	0.2	2.3	2.7	0.8/slice
Bread, wheat	1.6	11.3	8.5	2.4/slice
Fruits				
Apples	0.6	2.2	1.5	1.3/medium
Bananas	0.5	1.6	1.8	2.4/medium
Oranges	0.5	2.4	2.9	2.0/medium
Peaches	0.6	1.6	2.3	2.1/medium
Pears	1.8	2.6	11.0	4.0/medium
Strawberries	1.3	2.6	2.1	2.1/10 large
Vegetables				
Beans, green	1.0	1.8	3.4	2.5/half cup
Broccoli	1.6	2.8	4.1	3.0/half cup
Brussels sprouts	1.6	4.3	2.9	2.0/half cup
Carrots	1.0	3.2	3.7	11.3/half cup
Cabbage, white	0.8	2.4	2.8	2.1/half cup
Cauliflower	1.0	2.2	1.8	1.1/half cup
Corn, cooked	0.8	3.7	4.7	7.4/half ear
Lettuce, romaine	0.6	1.7	1.5	1.1/cup
Pepper, green	1.4	1.6	0.9	0.8/medium
Pickle	0.5	1.1	1.5	1.0/small
Potatoes + skin	0.5	2.8	3.5	3.5/medium
Potato chips	1.6	4.8	3.2	0.96/ounce
Tomatoes	0.5	1.3	1.4	1.4/small
Turnips	0.9	2.4	2.2	1.5/half cup

AOAC, Association of Official Analytical Chemists.
[a] From U.S. Department of Agriculture Handbook No. 456.
[b] From Southgate DAT, et al. *J Hum Nutr* 1976;30:303, and Anderson JW, Bridges SR. *Am J Clin Nutr* 1988;47:440.
[c] From Paul AA, Southgate DAT. In: McNance and Widdowson's *The composition of foods.* New York: Elsevier, 1978.

d. In the **Association of Official Analytical Chemists (AOAC) method,** enzymes and gravimetry are used. After fat is extracted from food, dried samples are gelatinized and then digested with protease and amyloglucosidase to remove protein and starch. The soluble dietary fiber is precipitated with ethanol, dried, and ashed. Total dietary fiber equals ethanol-precipitated residue weight minus ashed residue weight. This is the method now used by the U.S. Department of Agriculture for its tables of food fiber content (see *www.usda.gov*).

e. **Fiber measurement techniques compared.** The variations in the actual measurements of fiber components are evident in Table 11-11. The "correct" assessment of fiber content cannot be made from these data because the physiologic importance of each component is not known. In addition, the preparation of food may alter the measurements by removing soluble and loosely bound components. Thus, fiber supplements should be offered with an understanding of the nonequivalent nature of the product sources.

3. **Fermentation of fiber**
   a. **Variations in degradation.** The proportion of cellulose digested in the colon varies widely, from 47% to 80%. Purified cellulose is handled differently from dietary cellulose and is less degraded, about 25% (23). Bran cellulose is less degraded, perhaps because of its high lignin content. Cellulose metabolism is increased by slow transit, as in the elderly. Noncellulose polysaccharides are in general more completely degraded. Wheat bran is among the most poorly digested sources of dietary fiber, for reasons not related solely to its chemical composition. The digestion of nonstarch polysaccharides is variable and unpredictable. Most freshly cooked foods and uncooked cereals contain a high percentage of readily digested starch. However, a cooled, cooked potato is less digestible than a freshly cooked one. Thus, it is not true that starch is completely digested and absorbed in the small intestine. Moreover, the fermentation products of starch and nonstarch polysaccharides differ in the large intestine. Factors that affect starch digestibility in humans include (besides the physical form) transit time, food processing, and the presence of amylase inhibitors, lectins, or phytates (24). In a Western-type diet, the amount of fermentable carbohydrate entering the colon includes, on average, 12 g of nonstarch polysaccharides and a variable amount of starch.
   b. **Volatile fatty acids** are probably the main product of fiber polysaccharides and are well absorbed by the human colon. Thus, some of the nutritive value of dietary fiber is recovered by the absorption of fermentation products. It has been estimated that from 20 g of dietary fiber, 100 mEq of volatile fatty acids is produced, of which about 20% is excreted and the rest absorbed or used by bacteria.
   c. **The overall fermentation process** as it is now understood can be defined quantitatively. Fermentation of resultant soluble hexoses is about 60%. Hydrogen produced in large amounts is converted to methane in the ruminating animal. Of humans, only 30% to 40% produce methane, so that hydrogen gas is excreted in large amounts. The gas by-products of carbohydrate fermentation are odorless but carry with them the more noticeable by-products of protein breakdown (putrefaction). The volatile fatty acids (acetate, propionate, and butyrate) are available in part as energy sources. Some of the available energy supports bacterial growth. It has been estimated that fermentation of 100 g of carbohydrate supports the growth of 30 g of bacteria. The effect of bacterial growth on other colonic functions has not been determined.

4. **Functions of dietary fiber.** A high-fiber diet increases stool bulk, produces more frequent stools, and decreases transit time through the intestine. Fecal bile acids appear to be increased when fiber is included in the diet. Table 11-10 reviews the properties of fiber components that may be responsible for the (known and postulated) effects of dietary fiber. However, the intake of fiber must be adequate if the potential benefits are to be realized. Intake in the United States remains lower than the recommended 25 g/d, averaging 17 g/d in the third National Health and Nutrition Examination (NHANES III) (25).
   a. **Factors related to increased stool weight.** Even when a function of dietary fiber has been established (water-holding capacity),

that function does not necessarily correlate with the crude fiber or total dietary fiber content of foods (Table 11-12). Moreover, the increment in stool weight is not linearly related to either the *in vitro* water-holding capacity or the water content of the food. It is possible that more than one factor (e.g., volatile fatty acid production in addition to water-holding capacity) is responsible for the observed result—an increase in stool weight. The practical aspect of this information is that not all fiber sources are alike, and the effect of a high-fiber diet may depend on the exact mixture of foods used.

b. **Possible additional clinical effects of a high-fiber diet.** The following effects are associated with increased fiber intake:

(1) **Decreased intake of food.** Obesity is rare in populations that consume a high-fiber diet, possibly because of a lower caloric intake or increased satiety (26).

(2) **Coronary heart disease** has been inversely related to fiber intake, most recently in the Nurses' Health Study, in which each increase of total daily dietary fiber of 10 g was associated with a relative risk reduction of 0.81 (27). Of the various sources of dietary fiber, only cereal fiber was strongly associated with a reduced risk for coronary heart disease (relative risk reduction of 0.63/5 g daily). However, coronary heart disease is positively associated with other dietary changes (increased animal fat and protein) that are inversely related to fiber intake.

(3) **Diabetes.** Fiber ingestion by diabetic patients leads to some delay in gastric emptying, improvement in glucose tolerance, and reduction of hyperinsulinemia and hyperlipidemia (28). The diet used for this study contained 25 g each of soluble and insoluble fiber, and the effect was greater than that seen when the American, British, and Canadian Diabetes Association recommendations were used (8 g of soluble and 16 g of insoluble fiber per day).

Table 11-12. Water-holding capacity of various foods

Food	Crude fiber content	AOAC fiber content	Capacity of fiber in 100 g of raw vegetables to absorb water (g)[b]	Moisture (g/100-g edible portion)[a]
	(g/100 g of raw food)[a]			
Potato, fresh	0.5	1.5	41	75.4
Tomato	0.5	1.3	71	94
Cucumber	0.4	1.0	77	96
Celery	0.6	1.6	97	94.7
Lettuce	0.6	1.0	99	95.7
Pear	1.4	2.6	113	83.8
Orange	0.5	2.4	122	86.8
Corn	0.7	3.7	129	69.6
Apple	0.6	2.2	177	83.9
Carrot	1.0	3.2	208	87.8
Wheat bran	9.4	35.3	447	2.9

AOAC, Association of Official Analytical Chemists.
[a] McConnell AA, Eastwood MA, Mitchell WD. A comparison of methods of measuring "fiber" in vegetable material. *J Sci Food Agric* 1974;25:1457.
[b] Human Nutrition Information Service, U.S. Department of Agriculture. *Provisional table on dietary fiber content of selected foods*, HNIS/PT-106, 1988, and updated *Appendix* Tables 8-19, 1991; and 8-20, 1989.

(4) **Mineral availability.** Binding by fiber of minerals and trace elements has been shown consistently *in vitro,* but has not been consistently reported in clinical studies. When a wide variety of food is available and ingested, it is not known whether fiber intake affects mineral availability, and micronutrient supplements are not needed when fiber intake is increased. In fact, oligofructans have been reported to improve calcium absorption and calcium balance in experimental models (16).

(5) **Colonic disorders.** The evidence for the inverse association of dietary fiber with diverticular disease, cancer of the colon, and irritable bowel syndrome is incomplete, and much of it is based on epidemiologic data. In one prospective study, a low intake of fiber (13 g/d) was associated with an increase in the relative risk for the development of symptomatic diverticular disease of 2.35 (29). Some data suggest that a fiber intake of 30 to 35 g/d is inversely related to the risk for colon cancer (see references 30 and 31 for reviews of case–control studies), but the data do not unequivocally support a protective role for fiber. The data from the Nurses' Health Study, a cohort study, do not support a protective effect against either colon cancer or adenoma (32). However, the highest quintile of fiber intake averaged only 24 g/d, not quite the recommended 25 g/d. Thus, it is possible that higher levels of fiber intake would have shown a preventive effect against colon tumors.

(6) **Lowering cholesterol levels.** Water-soluble fibers (pectins, gums, psyllium extracts) lower the cholesterol levels of hypercholesterolemic subjects. The effect may be mediated by cholesterol binding, altered gastric emptying, or both. Sources of insoluble fiber (wheat bran, cellulose) have no effect. Rice bran lowers cholesterol, but the effects appear to be produced by nonfiber components. The cholesterol-lowering effect is small but within the practical range of intake. For example, 3 g of soluble fiber from oatmeal (84 g) decreases total and LDL cholesterol by about 0.13 mmol/L (33). The addition of psyllium supplements (10.2 g/d) to a prudent American Heart Association diet can lower total cholesterol by about 5% and LDL cholesterol by 8.6% (34). Although a decreased intake of saturated fat is the most important dietary factor in lowering serum cholesterol, the effect of soluble fiber is comparable with decreasing dietary cholesterol to below 200 mg/d and with a weight loss of 5 kg (35).

(7) **Treatment of inflammatory colitis.** Some products of the fermentation of fiber (especially short-chain fatty acids, primarily butyrate) are an important energy source for colonic mucosal cells. Infusions of sodium butyrate (100 mmol/L) in the form of enemas may relieve ulcerative colitis and diversion colitis, but the data are not consistent, and a strong recommendation cannot be made with current information (36).

5. Indications for modified-fiber diets

a. **Current consumption levels.** Total dietary fiber intake has declined in recent decades in the United States, estimated as 11 to 13 g/d in NHANES II (1976–1980) (30) and as 17 g/d in NHANES III (1988–1994) (25). If these data denote a significant change, it is possible that such a decline is medically important because cereal grain fiber seems to contain the most potent of the fiber components. Fewer grain products are consumed on average than in the 1930s and 1940s, but more fresh fruits and vegetables are now consumed throughout the year than previously. The average consumption of dietary fiber in the United States in the previous decade has been estimated to be between 25 g/d (37) and 12 g/d (38).

b. **Recommended intake.** Enough fiber should be consumed to ensure normal laxation, with a wide range of bowel habits accepted as normal. For those patients with a low fiber intake, only a normal fiber intake is needed, not a high one. This same recommendation is appropriate for children. The diets of many children are low in fruits, vegetables, and cereals (39). However, it is not clear whether a higher intake of fiber need be recommended for all children because this might decrease caloric intake and possibly adversely affect the absorption of essential minerals such as calcium, iron, copper, magnesium, phosphorus, and zinc.

   Data are not yet sufficient to recommend fiber supplementation routinely for chemoprevention of colorectal cancer (30). However, because an adequate fiber intake is associated with a lower fat intake and is part of the recommendations for general health (see Chapters 2 and 3) and for cancer prevention (see Chapter 14), it is reasonable to recommend a total fiber intake of 30 to 35 g/d, the amount associated with some of the favorable results in studies. The diet should include five to seven servings of vegetables and fruits a day plus generous portions of whole grain cereals. Because the components of fiber in different foods may each play a role in the beneficial effects (if any) of fiber, single sources are not recommended for cancer chemoprevention

c. **Low-fiber diet.** This diet is indicated whenever decreased fecal bulk is desired, as during preparation for barium studies or intestinal surgery, although a clear liquid diet is often preferred in such cases. A low-fiber diet may be used in *acute diarrheal illnesses,* such as gastroenteritis and ulcerative colitis, and in *short-bowel syndrome* when the colon is still present. This diet is not indicated for the long-term treatment of diverticular disease or irritable bowel syndrome. In patients with diverticulitis presenting with a chronic partial obstruction of the colon, a low-fiber diet may be used temporarily. *Partial obstruction of any part of the intestinal tract* (e.g., pylorus, colon) may be managed either by mechanical softening of foods (more useful for upper intestinal obstructions) or by a low intake of fiber (more useful for lower intestinal obstructions).

d. **Partial low-fiber diet.** Sometimes, a diet with only a moderate restriction of fiber is indicated. When an ileal segment is very narrow in a patient with *Crohn's disease,* only the most indigestible of the fiber sources need be eliminated (bran buds, corn, nuts); the other fiber-rich foods often can be consumed in moderation. *Gastric phytobezoars* can be treated initially with a full low-fiber diet; however, to prevent recurrences, the elimination of pulpy fruits (citrus fruits, pears) and persimmons from the diet is sometimes sufficient. Alternatively, a modified low-fiber diet can be used, in which only the foods highest in fiber (Table 11-13) are avoided. Examples include fruits (oranges, grapefruits, prunes, raisins, figs, cherries, persimmons, apples, grapes, berries); vegetables (celery, pumpkin, sauerkraut, lettuce, broccoli, brussels sprouts, potato skins); and others (bran, coconut, peanut, popcorn, kidney beans).

e. **A high-fiber diet** is used in the long-term treatment of recurrent diverticulitis (not simple diverticulosis) and irritable bowel disease when altered bowel habit is a major symptom. A high-fiber diet is not essential for every healthy adult who is ingesting the recommended 25 g of dietary fiber per day. It is sometimes used nonspecifically in the treatment of chronic diarrhea to produce semiformed, less liquid stools, especially as a fiber-supplemented enteral formula (40). However, the effect is often produced at the expense of an increase in the number or volume of stools. Moreover, if a high-fiber supplement is administered to a patient through a small-bore tube, the

Table 11-13. Fiber content of commonly used foods

Total dietary fiber 5 g
Baked beans (¼ cup)
Split peas (½ cup)
Butter beans, cooled (½ cup)
Blackberries (¼ cup)
Grapes, white (12)
Raspberries (½ cup)
Bran wheat (¼ cup)
All-Bran (⅓ cup)
Shredded Wheat (2 biscuits)
Almonds (15)
Grapenuts (1 cup)
Prunes, stewed (½ cup)

Total dietary fiber ~4 g
Peas, fresh or canned (½ cup)
Turnip greens (½ cup)
Broccoli (1 cup)
Cranberries (1 cup)
Prunes, dried (3)
Pear (1 medium)
Apricots (5)
Apple (1 large)
Figs, dried (2)

Total dietary fiber ~3 g
Beets, boiled (½ cup)
Potato with skin, baked
  (one 2½-in diameter)
Rye crackers (4)
Fruit pie (9-in diameter, ⅙ of pie)
Corn flakes (1 cup)

Total dietary fiber ~2 g
Banana (1 small)
Peach (1 medium)
Potato (1 medium with skin)
Corn on cob (small ear)
Carrot (1 medium)
Cabbage, boiled (½ cup)
Tomato (1 medium)
Turnips (⅔ cup)
Cauliflower, raw (1 cup)
Rhubarb (¼ cup)
Strawberries (10 large)

Plums (2 medium)
Orange (flesh) (1 small)
Tangerine (1 large)
Cherries (15)
Puffed wheat (1 cup)
Corn flakes (1 cup)
Flour, whole-meal (3 tbs)
Peanut butter (2 tbs)
Bran, powdered (1 tbs)
Rye bread (1 slice)
Whole wheat bread (2 slices)

Total dietary fiber ~1 g
Onion (1 small)
Cauliflower, boiled (½ cup)
Celery, raw (½ cup)
Potato, boiled, no skin (1 medium)
Asparagus, boiled (4 spears)
Cucumber, raw (2 cups)
Rice Krispies (¾ cup)
Special K (¾ cup)
White bread (1 slice)
Popcorn (1 cup)
Raisins (1 tbs)
Nectarines (1 medium)
Melon, all types (¼ melon)
Pineapple, fresh (½ cup)
Grapefruit (½)
Rice, boiled white (½ cup)
Flour, white (3 tbs)
Peanuts (12)

Total dietary fiber <0.2 g
Fruit juices, strained (1 cup)
Sugar, white (1 tbs)
Mayonnaise (1 tbs)
Fruit jellies (1 tbs)
Fats (2 tbs)
Milk (1 cup)
Egg (1 medium)
Meat, fish, poultry (3 oz)
Coffee, tea, soda (1 cup)
Most seasonings

tube may become obstructed. For these reasons, a high intake of fiber must be used cautiously in most cases of diarrhea. When the diarrhea results from a motility disorder (irritable bowel syndrome), a high intake of fiber may be used more successfully in controlling symptoms.

  6. **Practical aspects.** A clear liquid diet may be substituted for a low-fiber diet, but only for a short time because caloric intake is insufficient. Alternatively, commercially prepared liquid diets can be used (see Chapter 9). Table 11-13 lists total dietary fiber per average serving. Both high-fiber and low-fiber diets can be derived from such tables. Low-

fiber diets are adequate in protein and fat. If dairy products are eliminated from the diet because of lactose intolerance, protein and calcium intake from other sources should be increased.

   a. **Commercial psyllium powders** contain about 3 g of psyllium mucilloid per teaspoon. Some plants (e.g., plantago) are very rich in psyllium, which comprises 10% to 12% of soluble fiber. The exact conversion of grams of psyllium to total dietary fiber is uncertain, but a 1:1 equivalence is practical and probably nearly correct.

   b. **Sources of fiber.** High-fiber diets can be based on foods with moderate or high amounts of fiber. Commercial psyllium seed may be used instead of, or in addition to, a high-fiber diet or a bran preparation, but this is not recommended for increasing fiber intake in healthy populations. The type of fiber is different in each source, and the effects are occasionally additive. Most often, however, a patient responds to one or another source of fiber. The psyllium seed preparations are easy to take, their effects are reproducible, and they eliminate the need to use a special diet. However, in some instances, they are ineffective, whereas other types of fiber relieve symptoms. Most dietary fiber in a Western-type diet comes from fresh fruits, vegetables, and cereals. Usual servings of fruits, vegetables, and cereals contain 2 to 4 g of dietary fiber (Table 11-13).

   c. **High-fiber diet.** *Patient information on this topic is available in Appendix D.* High-fiber diets should aim to add the equivalent of at least 10 g of total dietary fiber to the diet. This increment may be accomplished by adding a normal distribution of fiber-containing foods to the previous diet, or the use of a single, concentrated source of fiber may be required. The importance of obtaining a dietary history is obvious. Psyllium seed provides 6 to 7 g of fiber in a dosage of 2 tsp/d; All-Bran cereal contains 11.2 g of dietary fiber in each cup; wheat bran contains about 5 g of dietary fiber in each tablespoon. Table 11-14 outlines many of the available nonfood sources of fiber. In general, ingestion of two to three doses per day provides 10 g of additional dietary fiber. Keep in mind that not all sources of fiber produce the same effect (Table 11-10). Thus, it may be necessary to try different types of fiber.

   Prebiotics are an increasingly common source of fiber that are available over the counter. The major sources of prebiotics available in Europe and the United States are inulin (derived from chicory roots), fructo-oligosaccharides or oligofructose (derived from the hydrolysis of chicory inulin or synthesized from sucrose), galacto-oligosaccharides (synthesized from lactose), and soybean oligosaccharides (extracted from soybeans). The average chain lengths of most of these are quite short, with only three to four residues, except for inulin, which has an average of 10 residues. They are added as fat or sugar replacements and to add body to a variety of products, including dairy products, breakfast cereals, baked goods and breads, chocolate and confections, dietetic products, table spreads and salad dressings, and meat products. These supplements should be included on the label of the food products to which they are added, although the amount added may not be specified.

   d. **Low-fiber diet.** Allowed foods are mainly animal foods (eggs, meats, milk), fats, white bread or rice, strained juices, and low-fiber fruits and vegetables, such as peaches without skin and peeled cucumber. *Patient information on this topic is available in Appendix D.*

7. **Side effects.** An excess of fiber can increase the frequency of stools in the absence of constipation or worsen the symptoms of chronic constipation. Thus, fiber should be used cautiously to treat constipation as an isolated symptom. Excess fiber may obstruct a structural narrowing of

Table 11-14. Fiber content of commercial supplements

Product	Fiber source	Daily dose (adults)[a]	Dietary fiber
Alramucil effervescent powder	Psyllium	1 packet 1–3 times	3.6 g/packet
Bran, wheat	Wheat	1 tbs	1.6
Citrucel	Methylcellulose	1 tbs	2 g/tbs
Citrucel sugar-free	Methylcellulose	1–3 times	2 g/tbs
Correctol powder	Psyllium	1 tsp	3.5
Effer-syllium effervescent powder	Psyllium	1 tsp 1–3 times	3 g/tsp
Equalactin	Ca polycarbophil	1–2 tablet 1–2 times	0.5 g/tablet
Fiberall powder Natural Orange	Psyllium	1 rounded tsp 1–3 times	3.4 g/tsp
Fiber 10	Fiber blend	2–3 times	10 g/packet
Fiberall Wafers	Ca polycarbophil	1–2 wafers 1–3 times	3.4 g/wafer
Fiberall	Ca polycarbophil	2 tablets 2–3 times	1.0 g/tablet
FiberCon	Ca polycarbophil	1 g 1–4 times	0.5 g/tablet
Fiber-Lax	Ca polycarbophil		0.5 g/tablet
Fibermed Fruit-flavored	Corn, wheat, oats Apples, currants	1–2 biscuits 2 times	5 g 5 g
Hydrocil Instant powder	Psyllium	1 tsp 1–3 times	3.5 g/tsp
Konsyl powder	Psyllium	1 packet or rounded tsp 1–3 times	6 g/tsp or packet
Maltsupex	Barley malt extract	4 tablets 2–4 times	750 mg/tablet
Metamucil powder Regular Sugar-free Lemon-lime Orange	Psyllium	1 tsp 1–3 times daily 1 tsp 1–3 times 1 packet 1–3 times 1 tbs 1–3 times 1 packet 1–3 times	3.4 g/tsp 3.4 g/tsp 3.4 g/packet 3.4 g/tbs 3.4 g/packet
Metamucil wafers		2 wafers 1–3 times	1.7 g/wafer
Mitrolan	Ca polycarbophil	1–2 tablets 2–3 times	0.5 g/tablet
Modane bulk	Psyllium	1 tsp	3.5 g
Natural vegetable powder (many brands)	Psyllium	1 tsp 1–3 times	3.4 g/tsp
Perdiem Fiber granules	Psyllium	1–2 tsp 1–2 times	4.0 g/tsp
Phillip's Fibercaps	Ca polycarbophil	2 caplets 1–2 times	0.625 g/caplet
Serutan Toasted granules	Psyllium	1 tsp	3.4 g 2.5 g
Siblin granules	Psyllium	1 tsp 2–3 times	2.5 g/tsp
Unifiber	Cellulose	1–2 tbs	3 g/tbs

[a]All doses should be taken with 8 oz of water.

the intestinal tract. When a low-fiber diet is used inappropriately to treat diverticulitis or irritable bowel disease, symptoms may worsen.

8. **Supplements required.** A strict low-fiber diet containing 3 cups of milk per day and some meat servings is adequate for all nutrients except vitamin A (unless liver is eaten) and iron (for female patients). The caloric intake also may be inadequate, depending on the patient. In most cases, the diet is used only for a short time, and nutritional deficiency is not a problem.

III. Restrictive diets
A. Low-available-carbohydrate diet
1. **Principles.** When gastric emptying is rapid or when food enters the small intestine at an unregulated rate, the presence of small-molecular-weight foodstuffs is to be avoided.

   a. **Normal physiology.** Gastric emptying is tightly controlled by osmoreceptors in the duodenum, by vagal and hormonal regulation of intragastric pressure, and by a normally functioning pyloric sphincter. About 15 mL of liquid chyme enters the duodenum per minute after a meal. When the mechanism of gastric emptying is disturbed in such a way that emptying is more rapid, an excess of partially digested food enters the small bowel.

   b. **Pathophysiology of the dumping syndrome.** Because it is permeable in both directions, the upper small bowel rapidly corrects hypertonic or hypotonic luminal contents to isotonicity. Most meals are hypertonic, so that a net loss of fluid into the lumen of the intestine leads to a decreased plasma volume and distention of the upper intestine. The decrease in plasma volume and intestinal distention accounts for many of the symptoms associated with the dumping syndrome.

   c. **Restriction of available carbohydrates as a method to lower osmolarity.** Small-molecular-weight soluble substances exert a greater osmotic pressure than do macromolecules. The low-molecular-weight dietary components present in high concentrations are monosaccharides and disaccharides (e.g., dextrose, lactose, sucrose). Free amino acids or dipeptides are rarely encountered in the stomach. Therefore, a diet designed to decrease the osmolarity of ingested food is one low in the type of carbohydrate that is readily available for absorption. Of course, starch can be digested rapidly to maltose and glucose, and so starch also contributes to luminal osmolarity. Because milk sugar is a disaccharide, a low-available-carbohydrate diet is also a low-lactose diet.

   d. **Glycemic index.** Different starchy foods are digested at different rates. Moreover, simple sugars vary in their effect on blood glucose levels. Glucose produces a greater effect than sucrose or fructose. Some starches produce a greater effect on blood glucose than do some simple sugars. Factors that affect starch digestibility include particle size, nature of the starch, processing of the starch, presence and type of fiber, and starch–protein–fat interactions (41). Because of the difficulty in predicting the effects of starchy or sugar-containing foods on blood glucose levels, the glycemic index was developed. The glycemic index is defined as follows:

$$\frac{\text{Area under the 2-Hour Glucose Curve for Food}}{\text{Area under the 2-Hour Glucose Curve for an Equivalent Weight of Reference Sugar}} \times 100$$

The original reference sugar was glucose, but bread baked from flour of known composition has proved a better standard. A lower mean glycemic load in the diet (glycemic index of food times total daily carbohydrate intake) was associated with a twofold lower risk for the development of diabetes and cardiovascular disease in the large Nurses' Health Study (18). In the larger NHANES III sample, a lower glycemic index was a predictor of higher levels of high-density-lipoprotein (HDL) cholesterol (42). However, it is not clear what role various factors play in modifying the glycemic potency of foods, and its use in routine clinical management is still controversial.

2. Indications

a. Dumping syndrome. The low-available-carbohydrate diet is useful after vagotomy with or without a drainage procedure because many patients have symptoms of the dumping syndrome (postprandial nausea, vomiting, weakness, dizziness, cramping, diarrhea) during the early postoperative period. The rate of gastric emptying of fluids is enhanced at this time. However, the rate eventually returns to normal and the symptoms subside. Only a few patients must maintain the full diet on a long-term basis, although a large number may remain on a somewhat restricted diet. Some of the symptoms associated with dumping occur 1 to 3 hours after a meal; these may be caused by reactive hypoglycemia (see below). The diet also diminishes such symptoms by decreasing the carbohydrate load. The anatomic configuration of patients who have undergone *gastric bypass* for obesity (not gastroplasties) is associated with the dumping syndrome because the fundus of the stomach is anastomosed to the jejunum, and such patients often must remain on a low-available-carbohydrate diet.

b. Reactive hypoglycemia occurs rarely in the absence of gastric surgery, sufficient in degree to produce symptoms (dizziness, hunger, weakness, sweating, palpitations). However, these symptoms are nonspecific and often related to anxiety. The true incidence of reactive hypoglycemia is probably much lower than the frequency of the diagnosis suggests. The definitive diagnosis requires the production of typical symptoms during a 5-hour glucose tolerance test, accompanied by a low plasma glucose level (<50 mg/dL). When reactive hypoglycemia is present, the low-carbohydrate diet is helpful.

3. Practical aspects

a. General instructions. *Patient information on this topic is available in Appendix D.*

(1) Food should be taken as six dry meals per day. Because liquids leave the stomach faster than solids, it is better to allow solid foods, with a potentially high osmotic load, to liquefy slowly and be diluted with endogenous secretions.

(2) Liquids should be taken 30 to 45 minutes after solids and limited to 1 cup per meal.

(3) Milk in all forms, including ice cream and other frozen desserts, should be avoided. Even lactose substitutes contain high concentrations of monosaccharides, disaccharides, or both.

(4) Only calorie-free beverages should be consumed.

(5) Sugar, sweets, candy, syrup, chocolate, and gravies should be avoided.

(6) The stomach should not be overloaded.

(7) Foods likely to be high in sugars have the following listed as the first or second ingredient: brown or invert or table sugar, corn sweetener, corn syrup, dextrose, fructose, fruit juice concentrate, glucose, high-fructose corn syrup, honey, lactose, maltose, malt syrup, molasses, sucrose, or syrup.

b. High-fat, low-carbohydrate diet. Although it is not widely accepted that an increased intake of fat may be indicated therapeutically, a few reports suggest the possible usefulness of such a maneuver. The rationale is that fat delays gastric emptying and prolongs small-bowel transit time in a humorally mediated mechanism termed the *ileal brake* (43). A high-fat diet has been used in some cases of *short-bowel syndrome* (44). The rationale is that in a person with a short bowel and *no colon,* the importance of unabsorbed fatty acid derivatives as colonic secretagogues is limited. Thus, water secretion is regulated by the osmolarity of the diet, which is lower with a low intake of carbohydrate and a high intake of fat. Gastric emptying also is delayed by a high-fat meal. The diet used in such cases provides 60% of the total caloric intake as fat, or about 200 g of fat, and is low in carbohydrates. Lying down for 10 to 15 minutes after meals decreases the rate of gastric emptying because the factor of gravity is eliminated. Five or six glasses of suitable liquid should be ingested between meals each day, with the fluids sipped slowly.

c. **Osmolarity of foods.** Simple sugars and low-molecular-weight carbohydrates, in addition to electrolytes and amino acids, all contribute to the osmolarity of food, either as a preformed liquid or after liquefication in the intestinal lumen. Dietary fats are relatively water-insoluble and do not increase osmolarity significantly.

   (1) **Effect of reduction of available carbohydrates.** The major aim of a low-available-carbohydrate diet is to reduce the osmolarity of ingested foods. This diet eliminates foods with a sugar content likely to increase the osmolarity of the gastric contents. The osmolarity of the gastric contents is usually hypertonic after a meal, but iso-osmolar liquids are emptied most efficiently by the stomach. A diet low in available carbohydrate is used to lower the gastric and intestinal osmolarity as much as possible.

   (2) **Low-calorie iso-osmolar diet in acute illness.** In acute disorders such as gastroenteritis, in which gastric emptying is impaired, or in chronic disorders such as diabetic gastroparesis, the use of iso-osmolar foods is helpful. Unfortunately, such a diet may be low in calories because it is the calorie-containing components of food that contribute most to osmolarity. Moreover, fat decreases the rate of gastric emptying, so that low-fat liquids are needed for rapid gastric emptying. During acute illnesses, however, iso-osmolar low-calorie liquids can be used for short periods alone.

   (3) **Osmolarities of some common foods** (1)

Food	mOsmol/L	Food	mOsmol/L
Gatorade	280	Eggnog	695
Ginger ale	510	Apple juice	870
Gelatin dessert	535	Orange juice	935
Tomato juice	595	Malted milk	940
7-Up	640	Ice cream	1,150
Coca-Cola	680	Grape juice	1,170
Sherbet	1,225		

   Nearly all liquid or semisolid foods are hyperosmolar. When nausea or vomiting is among the symptoms to be treated, the use of these fluids should be modified so that appropriate dilutions decrease the osmolarity to about 280 to 300 mOsmol/L.

d. **Specific recommendations**

   (1) **Foods allowed** include those containing protein, fat, or complex polysaccharides.

      (a) Only one slice of bread, or one-half cup of rice, noodles, or cereal, or one-half cup of carbohydrate-rich vegetables (dried beans, corn, potatoes) should be eaten with any meal.

(b) **Dairy products** should be limited to margarine, butter, or small amounts of cheeses, especially harder cheeses with a lower lactose content.

(2) Sugar content of foods

(a) **Foods containing simple sugars should be avoided.** Table 11-15 lists the fructose, glucose, sucrose, and starch contents of many foods. In this table, foods are ranked in decreasing order of simple sugar content—that is, monosaccharides and disaccharides. Foods high in simple sugars should be avoided or taken in small amounts. Fructose in excess of glucose is the main determinant of fructose malabsorption and diarrhea. This excess is seen especially in honey, apples, and pears (45). However, the largest source of dietary fructose is as a sweetener in dietetic foods and soft drinks and in corn syrups (~50% fructose) (46). The mean daily intake of free fructose in the United States is 20 g. Sorbitol is ingested in fruits along with fructose, and as a sweetener in candy, mints, "sugarless" chewing gum, and dietetic foods. As much as 2 g of sorbitol can be contained in one stick of gum. The decreased carbohydrate absorption of fruit juices in young children is related to the sorbitol content of the juice (47). The lactose contents of milk products are listed in Table 11-16, and these should also be limited. In congenital sucrase–isomaltase deficiency, a rare disorder, only foods containing little sucrose can be ingested. As seen in Table 11-15, this diet eliminates many fruits and vegetables and most sweets.

(b) **Most beverages** contain available sugars and should be limited. These include beer, sodas, and iced tea or lemonade made with sugar. Canned fruits often contain extra sugar in the packing fluid; if these are used, the fluid should be drained away before the fruits are eaten.

(c) **Sweeteners.** The U.S. Food and Drug Administration has approved four sugar substitutes—*saccharine, aspartame, acesulfame-K, and sucralose.* Other sweeteners are under review (*http://vm.cfsan.fda.gov/~dms/fdsugar.html*). Despite the concerns about saccharine as a carcinogen, it remains on the market; it is 300 times sweeter than sugar and has been used safely for decades, and the dose required to see tumors in laboratory animals is huge. The Saccharine Study and Labeling Act requires the label to read "Use of this product may be hazardous to your health," but the moratorium on a final decision has been extended until 2002.

Aspartame (*NutraSweet, Equal*) is a dipeptide (phenylalanine–aspartic acid) that is 180 times sweeter than sugar. The Food and Drug Administration has reviewed more than 100 toxicologic and clinical studies that attest to its safety, although claims continue to arise regarding its possible role in causing various diseases. The very small number of patients who have phenylketonuria should not use this compound, but otherwise it appears to be safe. Urticaria has been reported with aspartame and confirmed by rechallenge (48). It is postulated that the product of degradation may form amide bonds with proteins and act as an antigen.

Acesulfame potassium (*Sunett*) is approved for use in baked goods, frozen desserts, candies, and beverages. It is 200 times sweeter than sugar and is often combined with other sweeteners. It is not degraded when cooked or baked. No evidence of toxicity has been reported.

Sucralose (*Splenda*) is 600 times sweeter than sugar and is approved for use as a table sweetener and in baked goods, nonalcoholic beverages, chewing gum, frozen dairy desserts, fruit juices, and gelatins. It is now approved as a general-purpose sweetener for all foods. It tastes like sugar because it is made from sucrose, but it cannot be digested. It is considered safe to use.

(d) **Sugar alcohols** are not technically considered artificial sweeteners, but they do not promote tooth decay or raise blood sugar, as sugar does. They include sorbitol, xylitol, lactitol, mannitol, and maltitol. Sugar alcohols are used to sweeten "sugar-free" candies, cookies, and chewing gums. Fructose is also often added to foods because, like sugar alcohols, it is less sweet than dextrose. However, these sugars are absorbed less efficiently, and ingestion of more than 10 g can produce diarrhea, gas, bloating, and cramps. Fructose is a major ingredient of soft drinks (about 40 g in a 16-oz cola). Sorbitol is added to diet gums (up to 2 g per stick) and processed apple juice (up to 0.7 g/3 oz). Labels should be read carefully for the content of these sweeteners if symptoms occur regularly after ingestion of sweetened processed foods.

(3) **For infants with sucrase–isomaltase deficiency,** glucose or fructose may be added to formulas that contain no carbohydrate (see Chapter 9). Sucrose is added to many commercial baby foods, especially puréed fruits. Labels should be read carefully. Older children with this disorder become more tolerant to sucrose, and the diet is less necessary. An unsupplemented low-sucrose diet may be limited in ascorbic acid and folic acid, and perhaps also iron, thiamine, and niacin. An oral solution is available containing sucrase from *Saccharomyces cerevisiae* (Baker's yeast), marketed as Sucraid (sacrosidase) by Orphan Medical (*www.orphan.com*). The usual dose is 1 to 2 mL per meal. About three-fourths of treated patients can be reasonably asymptomatic while ingesting sucrose. The most common side effects are abdominal pain, vomiting, and allergic reactions.

4. **Side effects.** A low-lactose diet may be low in calcium. If the diet is severely limited in fruits and vegetables, vitamin supplements, especially ascorbic acid and folic acid, may be necessary. Such severe restriction is only rarely, if ever, indicated with this diet. Because the diet is high in protein and fat, care should be taken to avoid increasing serum lipid levels in susceptible persons.

5. **Supplement required.** If the diet is used on a long-term basis, 0.5 to 1.0 g of elemental calcium should be given daily.

B. **Low-lactose diet**

1. **Principles.** Most Caucasians are lactose-tolerant, but the other peoples of the world are largely lactose-intolerant. To avoid symptoms of flatulence, bloating, cramps, and diarrhea, a low-lactose diet is indicated. However, many people who have low levels of lactase are not lactose-intolerant. This situation arises because of differences in rates of gastric emptying and intestinal transit, composition of ingested food, capture of lactose fermentation products by colonic absorption, and perhaps individual tolerance. The diagnosis is usually made either by a trial of lactose elimination or by administering a hydrogen breath test after lactose ingestion (49).

a. Lactose is commonly used as a sweetening agent in prepared foods because it is inexpensive to prepare and its taste is not excessively

Table 11-15. Carbohydrate content of selected foods

Food	Fructose[a]	Excess free fructose[b]	Glucose	Sorbitol	Reducing sugars[c]	Maltose	Sucrose	Starch	Total simple sugars[d] (g/100-g portion)
			(g/100-g edible portion)						
Fruits									
Figs, dried	30.9	—	40	—	—	—	0.1	—	73
Dates, dried	—	—	—	—	16.2	—	45.4	—	61.6
Banana, ripe	2–4	0	4.5	—	—	—	11.9	—	19.9
Grapes, white	8.0	0	8.1	0.2	—	—	0.2	—	16.1
Cherries	5–7	0	4.7	1.4–2.1	12.5	—	0.1	—	12.6
Apple juice	6–8	2–7	1–4	0.3–1.0	8.0	—	4.2	—	12.2
Plums, sweet	1–4	—	4.5	0.3–2.8	7.4	—	4.4	—	11.8
Apple	6–8	2–7	1.7	0.2–1.0	8.3	—	3.1	—	11.4
Banana, green	—	—	—	—	5.0	—	5.1	0.6	10.1
Peaches	1.6	—	1.5	—	3.1	—	6.6	—	9.7
Orange	2.7	0	2.5	—	5.0	—	4.6	—	9.6
Pears	5–9	3–8	2.5	1.2–3.5	8.0	—	1.5	—	9.5
Watermelon	—	—	—	—	3.0	—	4.9	—	7.9
Apricots	0.4	—	1.9	—	—	—	5.5	—	7.8
Orange juice, frozen	2–6	0	—	—	4.6	—	3.2	—	7.8
Melon, cantaloupe	0.9	—	1.2	—	2.3	—	4.4	—	6.7
Strawberries	2.3	0	2.6	—	—	—	1.4	—	6.3
Grapefruit	1.2	0	2.0	—	—	—	2.9	—	6.1
Prunes	15	0	30	9.4–18.8	—	—	—	—	
Vegetables									
Beets, sugar	—	0	—	—	—	—	12.9	—	12.9
Onions	1	0	2	—	—	—	0.1	—	8.3
Carrots, raw	1	0	1	—	5.8	—	1.2	—	7.9
Peas, green	<0.1	0	<0.1	—	—	—	5.5	4.1	5.5
Potatoes, sweet	0.3	—	0.4	—	0.8	1.6	4.1	16.5	4.9

Food								
Cauliflower	—	—	2.8	—	—	0.3	—	3.1
Beans, green	0–1	—	0.5–1	—	1.7	0.5	2.0	2.2
Potatoes, white	0.1	—	0.1	—	0.8	0.1	17.0	0.9
Squash, summer	0.2	—	0.1	—	—	0.4	2.6	0.7
Cucumber	—	—	0.5	—	—	0.1	—	0.6
Dry legumes								
Beans, soy	—	—	—	—	1.6	7.2	1.9	8.8
Lentils	—	—	—	—	—	2.1	28.5	2.1
Beans, navy	—	—	—	—	—	—	35.2	—
Nuts								
Peanuts	—	—	—	—	0.2	4.3	4.0	4.5
Almonds	—	—	—	—	0.2	2.3	—	2.5
Peanut butter	—	—	—	—	0.9	—	5.9	0.9
Cereals								
Wheat flour	—	—	—	—	2.0	0.2	34.7	2.2
Rice, polished	—	—	2.0	—	—	0.4	72.9	0.4
Oats	—	—	—	—	—	—	56.4	—
Sweets								
Honey	40.5	7	34.2	—	—	—	1.9	88.6
Maple syrup	—	—	—	—	1.5	62.9	—	64.4
Molasses	6.8	—	6.8	—	26.9	36.9	—	63.8
Jellies	—	—	—	—	—	—	40–65	40–65
Chocolate, sweet, dry	—	—	—	—	—	56.4	—	56.4
Corn syrup	—	—	21.2	26.4	—	—	34.7	47.6

Foods are listed with groups according to their monosaccharide and disaccharide content per 100-g edible portion. Thus, the total sugar added to the diet must take into account the size of the portion. See also *Sugar content of selected foods*, Report No. 48. Human Nutrition Information Service, U.S. Department of Agriculture.

[a] Adapted from Rumessen JJ. *Scand J Gastroenterol* 1992;27:819. Mainly monosaccharides plus maltose and lactose.

[b] Free fructose as monosaccharides in excess of free glucose.

[c] Adapted from Hardinger MG, Swarner JB, Crooks H. *J Am Diet Assoc* 1965;46:197.

[d] Total "simple" sugars equals reducing sugars plus sucrose; where total reducing sugar content is not available, the sum of the published figures for fructose, glucose, and/or maltose has been substituted.

Table 11-16. Lactose content of selected milk products

Product	Lactose content (g/unit)
Whole milk (1 cup)	11
2% Milk (1 cup)	9–13
Skim milk (1 cup)	11–14
Chocolate milk (1 cup)	10–12
Sweetened condensed milk (1 cup)	35
Reconstituted dry whole milk (1 cup)	48
Buttermilk (1 cup)	9–11
Light cream (1 tbs)	0.6
Half and half (1 tbs)	0.6
Whipped cream topping (1 tbs)	0.4
Low-fat yogurt (1 cup)	11–15
Cheeses	
Hard (Parmesan, blue, Gouda) (1 oz)	0.6–0.8
Semihard (American, Cheddar) (1 oz)	0.4–0.6
Soft (Camembert, Limburger) (1 oz)	0.1–0.2
Spread (added cream) (1 oz)	0.8–1.7
Cottage	
Regular (1 cup)	5–6
Low-fat (1 cup)	7–8
Ice creams	
Regular (1 cup)	9
Sherbet (1 cup)	4
Ice milk (1 cup)	10
Sorbets, ices (1 cup)	0
Butter (1 tbs)	0.15
Oleomargarine	0

Adapted from Welsh JD. Diet therapy in adult lactose malabsorption: present practices. *Am J Clin Nutr* 1978;31:592.

sweet. Thus, it is difficult to devise a diet completely free of lactose. In most cases, complete elimination of lactose is unnecessary because symptoms, when they occur, are dose-related. Each person has a threshold dose below which few symptoms occur.

b. Lactose, or milk sugar, is contained in human, cow's, and goat's milk and in milk products. The whey contains all the lactose; any lactose in the curds represents contamination by whey. Whey is now added to more foods than before because large amounts of whey are available as a by-product of cheese production. Milk is a remarkable food that contains more than lactose. Many nutrients are lost from the diet when lactose is restricted; however, except for calcium, most of them are readily provided by the rest of a balanced diet.

2. Indications

a. Patients with symptoms of *lactose intolerance* are candidates for the diet. Because only 50% of lactose-intolerant persons have a history of intolerance, a useful first step is to place the patient suspected of being lactose-intolerant on a low-lactose diet for 3 to 4 days. If the response is uncertain, challenge tests can help to diagnose lactose intolerance.

(1) **A positive lactose tolerance test result** is defined as a rise in blood sugar of less than 20 mg/dL after a lactose load of 50 g/m^2 in children or 50 g in adults.

(2) **The hydrogen breath test** is a better means of diagnosis. It is more sensitive than the oral lactose tolerance test and can

detect malabsorption of as little as 2 g of lactose. Thus, a lower test dose (12.5 g) can be used, an amount equal to the lactose content of one glass of milk. A rise of less than 20 ppm is consistent with lactose intolerance. Certain pitfalls are encountered in interpreting the results of a hydrogen breath test (50). A small percentage of normal persons do not produce hydrogen gas, oral antibiotics can suppress hydrogen-producing bacteria, and smoking causes an increase in breath hydrogen concentration that is unrelated to carbohydrate intake.

b. The low-lactose diet is also appropriate for *patients requiring a low-available-carbohydrate diet* after gastric surgery or during the course of an intestinal disorder. A low-lactose diet is used during the acute phase of *diarrheal illnesses,* when intestinal transit is rapid and transient lactase deficiency can develop. These illnesses include acute gastroenteritis, ulcerative colitis, and Crohn's disease. However, it is not necessary to restrict lactose from the diet in all such cases. In *sprue,* the enzyme lactase is decreased before treatment, and a low-lactose diet is helpful in the initial phase of therapy until the normal enzyme level is restored. However, restoration to normal levels may take many months.

c. Galactosemia is the only indication for very severe restriction of lactose. Virtually all dietary galactose is derived from lactose, and in galactosemia, small amounts of galactose cause symptoms. Thus, adherence to the diet must be complete.

d. Supplemental milk is offered in schools in the United States, even when the racial mixture includes a large proportion of children who would be expected to have lactase deficiency. Tolerance to a small amount of milk, such as part or even all of the cup offered with school lunches, is quite good, and the Committee on Nutrition of the American Academy of Pediatrics supports the use of milk as a good food supplement even in areas of the world where the incidence of lactose intolerance is high (51).

3. Practical aspects

   a. General instructions. *Patient information on this topic is available in Appendix D.*

   (1) Milk and liquid milk products should be avoided.

   (2) Labels should be read carefully. Products containing milk, milk products, milk solids, whey, curd, casein, lactose, galactose, skim milk powder, skim milk solids, or milk sugar contain lactose. Food that may contain "hidden" lactose include "nondairy" creamers, powdered sweeteners, breads and cakes, creamed soups, pancakes and waffles, puddings and custards, and candies. Many patients can tolerate small doses of lactose and need not be so cautious about restricting their intake of prepared foods containing small amounts of lactose. Often, however, the amount of lactose is not stated on the label. Practical information can be obtained from many Internet sites, listed on the No Milk Page *(www.panix.com/~nomilk)* along with sites for milk allergy and casein intolerance.

   (3) Milk or cream should not be used in cooking.

   (4) Small amounts of cheese and butter may be tolerated.

   (5) Commercially available fermented milk products (buttermilk, yogurt) are sometimes sweetened by adding cream or milk and are not necessarily low in lactose. The lactose content of homemade yogurt will be lower, but some lactose will remain. Nearly complete fermentation produces an inedible product. Yogurt is better tolerated by lactose-intolerant persons because the fermentation of lactose continues in the intestinal lumen (52). However, tolerance must be individualized. Frozen yogurt does not contain active bacterial cultures and is less well tolerated than fresh yogurt.

b. Specific recommendations. The average lactose-intolerant patient becomes symptomatic after ingesting 12 g of lactose, the approximate content of an 8-oz glass of milk. More lactose may be tolerated when it is ingested with other foods that delay gastric emptying. Some patients become symptomatic after ingesting as little as 3 g of lactose (53). These people must take great care to avoid foods that contain even small amounts of lactose. Patients with both lactase deficiency and irritable bowel syndrome are often extremely sensitive to small amounts of lactose.

   (1) Dairy products. Table 11-16 lists the major dietary sources of lactose in milk products.

   (2) Prepared foods that contain lactose. Not all samples of the foods listed below contain lactose, but the labels of such food groups should be read with care.

      (a) Foods with large amounts of lactose: cakes and sweet rolls, caramels, fudge, coated candies, cheese spreads, infant formulas, party dips, powdered soft drinks, puddings, sour cream, white sauces

      (b) Foods with small amounts of lactose (<1 g/100 g): canned or frozen fruits and vegetables, cookies and cookie sandwich fillings, cordials and liqueurs, dietetic and diabetic preparations, dried soups, French fries, corn cereals, instant coffee, instant potatoes, meat products prepared with fillings (e.g., frankfurters), pie crusts and fillings, salad dressings, liquid antibiotics, vitamin and mineral mixtures

      (c) Lactose-free foods: plain meat, fish, poultry, peanut butter, broth-based soups, cereals, fruits, vegetables (plain), tofu and tofu products, breads and desserts made without any milk products

   (3) Hospital diets provide lactose-containing foods with most meals. Lactose-intolerant patients may become symptomatic in the hospital, especially if they are given a modified-consistency diet with many milk products but little selection. Many commercially available protein and calorie supplements are now lactose-free (see Chapter 9).

c. Enzyme replacement. Lactose-depleted milk can be prepared by hydrolyzing the lactose with a yeast enzyme preparation (e.g., LactAid, Dairy Ease, Lactrase). Mixing five drops of LactAid liquid enzyme, which contains lactase from the yeast *Kluyveromyces lactis,* with 1 qt of milk or 12 oz of "liquid diet" or "instant breakfast" formulas at 4°C results in 70% hydrolysis of lactose in 1 day and 90% hydrolysis in 2 or 3 days. Patients with limited tolerance to lactose can use this milk, which is sweeter than regular milk but well accepted in cooking or on cereal. Dairy products other than milk cannot be treated in this way. Table 11-17 lists many of the sources of lactase, along with milk substitutes. Lactase in tablets is not always from the same source. For example, Lactrase, derived from *Aspergillus oryzae,* is stable at both acid and alkaline pH, and this stability may be advantageous in some cases. One to three capsules are ingested with milk or food, depending on the amount of lactose ingested and on individual sensitivity. Alternatively, the capsule can be opened and sprinkled on the food or liquid containing lactose.

d. Milk substitutes. Chemically defined products are now available that simulate milk; corn solids are used as the carbohydrate source (Table 11-17). These products can be used as milk substitutes if the taste is acceptable, but the sugar content is 12 g/8-oz glass and the

Table 11-17. Selected lactase replacement products and milk substitutes

Lactase products	Nondairy creamers	Milk substitutes
Lactaid (+ drops), 250 mg	Cremora	"a.m." (lactose-free)
Lactrase, 250 mg	Coffee-mate	Bordens Plus (lactose-free)
Say Yes to Dairy, 250 mg	Coffee Rich	Dairy Ease (70% ↓)
Prevail dairy enzyme, 125 mg	Vitamite	Lactaid (70% ↓)
Milk Digest-Aid, 125 mg	Creme Supreme	NutriMil (lactose-free)
Super Lactase, 125 mg	Cool Whip	Lacta-Care (99% ↓)
Swanson softgels, 150 mg	Rich Whip	
Dairy Ease (+ drops), 200 mg		

From: Steve Carper's Lactose Intolerance Clearing House/The Product Clearinghouse (*http://ourworld.compuserve.com/homepages/stevecarper*).

vegetable fat content is 5%, as in whole milk. Some of these products are cholesterol-free, and some contain micronutrient supplements.

   e. Ice cream substitutes. A wide variety of lactose-free frozen desserts are now available that provide 300 to 440 kcal/cup and contain little or no calcium. In most of the desserts, tofu is used as the base. Although they are cholesterol-free, they are high in polyunsaturated fat (10 to 26 g of fat per cup). Some widely marketed varieties are Tofree, Tofutti, and Tofulite. Frozen desserts that are both lactose-free and fat-free include fruit sorbets and ices. Low-lactose desserts can be tolerated by some patients. LactAid brand ice cream contains about 2 g of lactose per cup, compared with 9 g for regular ice cream. Frozen yogurt contains 5 g/cup but may not be tolerated because the action of the bacteria in yogurt is diminished by freezing.

  4. Side effects. A negative calcium balance may result if meat, nuts, and vegetables do not provide 0.8 to 1.0 g of calcium daily. Symptoms similar to those of lactose intolerance may develop when milk substitutes are used, which are also high in available carbohydrates.

  5. Supplement required. Calcium supplements (0.8 to 1.2 g of elemental calcium) should be given (see Chapter 7) if other sources are not ingested.

C. Low-fat diet

  1. Principles

    a. Different types of fat. Fatty acids derived from triglycerides supply energy and essential fatty acids and help absorb lipid-soluble compounds, such as fat-soluble vitamins. Saturated fats are found in high-fat dairy products, fatty fresh and processed meats, skin and fat of poultry, and lard, palm, and coconut oils. They tend to raise serum cholesterol levels. Levels of *trans* fatty acids, which also tend to raise serum cholesterol, are high in partially hydrogenated vegetable oils (margarines, shortenings) and in some commercially fried foods and bakery goods. Unsaturated fats, which tend to keep blood cholesterol levels low, are found in vegetable oils, nuts, olives, avocados, and fatty fish. These three types of fat are equivalent calorically, all produce symptoms of malabsorption, and all must be decreased in a low-fat diet designed to reduce gastrointestinal symptoms. Dietary cholesterol, found in liver and other organ meats, egg yolks, and dairy fats, is not of concern in this diet. Diets designed to lower serum cholesterol are based on an altered ratio of intake of these fats (see Chapter 12).

    Essential fatty acids (linolenic, linoleic) are found in high levels in vegetable oils (especially flaxseed, canola, and soy oils) and human milk, and dietary deficiency is rare in persons ingesting a balanced diet. Carnitine is a nonessential nutrient (synthesized from lysine and methionine) required for the entry of long-chain fatty acids into mitochondria. It is abundant in the diet, but some infant and other non–milk-based formulas are supplemented with carnitine. Sphingolipids occur widely in food (consumption ~ 0.3 to 0.4 g/d in the United States) and have some role in colon cancer prevention and lowering cholesterol in animals (54). Their role in human nutrition is not yet known.

b. **"Global" malabsorption versus predominantly fat malabsorption.** Steatorrhea of any cause is relieved when the triglyceride intake is decreased. Fat malabsorption typically predominates in disorders in which the secretion or absorption of bile acids is limited; bile acids are needed for micelle formation and the absorption of fat, but not protein or carbohydrate. Both fat malabsorption and protein malabsorption occur in pancreatic insufficiency or diffuse small-bowel mucosal disorders. When protein malabsorption accompanies fat malabsorption, it produces few symptoms except perhaps that the putrid smell of feces is increased. Severe carbohydrate malabsorption causes some of the symptoms often associated with fat malabsorption (diarrhea, bloating, gas). The demonstration of steatorrhea or carbohydrate malabsorption by itself does not always determine which factor is most important in causing symptoms in an individual patient. Response to a trial of either a low-fat or a low-carbohydrate diet is often needed to resolve this issue in patients with "global" malabsorption.

c. **Pathophysiology.** As used in this diet, the term *fat* refers to triglycerides in food, not to other lipid components, such as cholesterol. Diarrhea is relieved by a low-fat diet because the diarrhea associated with steatorrhea is partly caused by the formation of hydroxyl fatty acids that act as secretagogues in the colon (55). If fewer fatty acids reach the colon, the diarrhea is diminished and the colonic absorption of other nutrients (especially short-chain fatty acids) improves. The low-fat diet is relatively rich in other sources of calories, especially carbohydrate, and is difficult to use when carbohydrate restriction is also desired. Low-fat diets are used to control symptoms of diarrhea, bloating, and gas—not to reverse abnormal physiology. Therefore, no single level of restriction is appropriate for all patients. A low-fat diet is also relatively low in protein because most sources of protein in a Western-type diet contain triglycerides. When malabsorption is severe and strict fat restriction is required, protein supplements must sometimes be given.

2. **Indications**

a. **Patients with malabsorption.** Many disorders of digestion or absorption are characterized by steatorrhea. In general, patients with disorders in which steatorrhea is significant require a low-fat diet. These include diseases in which bile acids are poorly absorbed in the entire small bowel (e.g., sprue) or terminal ileum (e.g., Crohn's disease with or without resection, short-bowel syndrome) or in which triglyceride absorption is limited (e.g., pancreatic insufficiency). When the coefficient of fat absorption is 85% to 95% (normal, ≥95%), fat restriction need not be stringent to achieve good results. For example, in a patient with a daily intake of 80 g of triglyceride and 90% efficient absorption (mildly abnormal), the fecal output would be only 8 g/d. However, if absorption is only 60% efficient, restriction must be more severe; with an intake of 50 g, 20 g of fat would still be excreted per day.

b. **Patients with nonspecific intestinal symptoms.** Many patients complain that fatty foods cause a variety of intestinal symptoms. For such patients, it is usually enough to avoid fried foods and very fatty meats (bacon, sausage). Because the ingestion of fat is usually not specifically related to the symptoms of cholecystitis, ulcer, irritable bowel syndrome, and similar disorders, a low-fat diet is usually not indicated. Because protein is also a potent stimulus of intestinal and gastric motility, a selective restriction of fat intake serves no purpose.

  c. **Prevention of disease.** The reduced-fat diets advocated to prevent chronic diseases stipulate a reduction in fat intake of no more than 30% (56) (see Chapter 2). These diets are not the same as the low-fat diet being discussed here, and the labeling terms "light" and "lite," which mean fewer calories (see below), must be understood. However, many of the practical points relevant to a low-fat diet are also useful in a moderately reduced-fat diet. To achieve the recommended fat intake, the U.S. Department of Agriculture recommends the following upper limit of fat intake at different levels of calorie consumption:

Total kcal/d	Saturated fat (g/d)	Total fat (g/d)
1,600	≤18	53
2,200	≤24	73
2,800	≤31	93

3. **Practical aspects**
  a. **General instructions.** *Patient information on this topic is available in Appendix D.*
    (1) Broil, bake, or boil meats and fish.
    (2) Use chicken and turkey without skin as major sources of meat. The flat fish fillets usually served with sauces (flounder, sole) contain less fat than steaklike fish (salmon, halibut, tuna, trout, mackerel). Red meat trimmed of all fat or U.S. Department of Agriculture select-grade meat (8% fat content) also can be used in smaller amounts.
    (3) Use skim milk.
    (4) Avoid most desserts (cakes, cookies, pies, pastry, candy).
    (5) Avoid cream sauces and gravies.
    (6) **Label information for fat content.** As of May 1994, all manufacturers of processed foods are required by the Food and Drug Administration to use uniform definitions of claims such as "light" or "low-fat." *Light* means only that the product has one-third fewer calories or one-half the fat of its original version. Under the new law, the "% fat-free" claim appears only on low-fat products. The total grams of fat is the most important item and it is found in the middle of the label, where it may not be seen at first glance. Also, the "% daily value for calories" refers to a 2,000-calorie diet needed by "the average person." This estimate may be excessive for many people (see Appendix C for further discussion of the new food labels).
      (a) Beef, pork, and lamb products also may appear with labels indicating approval by the Nutritional Effects Foundation (NEF), a new nonprofit organization. Most producers must apply for approval and comply with limits on fat content. "NEF-1" meat contains 3.5% fat or less by weight, and "NEF-2" contains 6% fat or less. This compares with the 15% to 20% fat content in the usual meat choices.
      (b) Nearly all hard cheeses are high in fat. Part-skim cheeses are lower in fat, but most (>50%) of the calories are still derived from fat.
  b. **Specific recommendations.** To suggest a given intake of fat, the content of table foods must be known. A list of some foods with their fat content appears in Table 11-18. Based on the values for fat in this table, a general scheme of low-fat intake can be offered.

Table 11-18. Fat content of selected table foods

Food	Fat (g/unit)	Food	Fat (g/unit)
Milk products		T-bone with bone	23.9
Milk		Trimmed	3.2
Whole (1 cup)	8.6	Club steak with bone	21.2
2% (1 cup)	4.9	Trimmed	3.9
1% (1 cup)	2.5	Sirloin with bone	18.6
Skim (1 cup)	0.2	Trimmed	3
Buttermilk (1 cup)	2.4	Rib roast with bone	22.6
Ice cream		Trimmed	4.9
Regular (1 cup)	14.1	Rump roast with bone	14.5
Rich grade (1 cup)	23.8	Trimmed	3.8
Ice milk (1 cup)	6.7	Ground beef	12.4
Yogurt	8.3	Lean	7.1
Cheese and butter		Corned beef	25.9
Butter		Chicken	
Regular (tbs)	11.5	White, no skin	2.9
Whipped (tbs)	7.6	Dark, no skin	5.4
Margarine (tbs)	11.5	Fried	
Cheese		White, no skin	5.2
Blue (1 oz)	8.6	Dark, no skin	7.9
Cheddar (1 oz)	9.1	Turkey	
Cottage (1 oz)	1.2	Roasted with skin	14
Cream (1 oz)	10.7	White, no skin	3.3
Parmesan (1 oz)	8.7	Dark, no skin	7.1
Swiss (1 oz)	7.9	Lamb	
American (1 oz)	8.5	Leg	9.4
Vegetables		Chops with bone	15.8
Eggplant (½ cup)	0.6	Shoulder	13.7
Peas, green (½ cup)	0.3	Liver, fried	9.8
Spinach, cooked (1.2 cup)	0.3	Pork	
Sweet potato (½ cup)	2.8	Chop with bone	13.2
Beans, dry (½ cup)	2.0	Bacon (2 slices)	7–12
Avocado (1)	37	**Sausages**	
All others (½ cup)	<0.3	Liverwurst (1 slice)	2.7
Grains and cereals		Boiled ham (1 slice)	4.8
Bread (1 slice)	0.8	Pork sausage (1 link)	5.7
Cereal, dry (3/4 cup)	0.3	Salami (1 slice)	1.9
Rice, cooked (½ cup)	0.1	Frankfurters (1)	15.2
Roll (1)	0.6	Bologna (1 slice)	1.0
Spaghetti, cooked (½ cup)	0.4	**Fruit**	
With tomato sauce and		Apple (1)	0.6
meatballs (½ cup)	5.8	Pear (1)	0.3
Noodles (8 oz)	0.4	Watermelon (1 cup)	0.4
Meats		All others (1)	0.3
(yield from 3 oz cooked)		**Fats and oils**	
Beef		Lard (1 tbs)	13
Chuck with fat	13.5	Oils, corn, olive, peanut,	
Chuck, lean	5.6	soy, sesame (1 tbs)	13.6
Chuck steak	10.9	Salad dressing (1 tbs)	6.2–9
Trimmed	3.4	**Desserts**	
Flank steak	4.1	Cake	
Porterhouse steak with bone	23.9	Chocolate (1 slice)	6.7
Trimmed	3.4	Devil's food (1 slice)	12.3
		Pound (1 slice)	8.9
		Sponge (1 slice)	1.9

Table 11-18. (*Continued*)

Food	Fat (g/unit)	Food	Fat (g/unit)
White (1 slice)	9.7	Shrimp	
Yellow	9.5	Boiled	0.9
Candy		Fried	9.2
Chocolate, milk (1 oz)	9.2	Lobster, boiled	1.3
Fudge (1 piece)	5.3	Oysters, raw	0.5
Cookies		Sardines, canned (1 fish)	1.3
Brownie (1 piece)	5	**Nuts**	
Chocolate chip (1)	3	Almonds, roasted (1 cup)	97
Ginger snap (1)	0.6	Peanuts, roasted (10 nuts)	4.5
Oatmeal (1)	2	Pecans (10 nuts)	10
Sugar (1)	1.3	Sesame seeds (1 tbs)	4.3
Pies (⅛ of pie)	7–23	Peanut butter (1 tbs)	8.1
Fish		**Miscellaneous and**	
(yield from 3 oz cooked)		**snack foods**	
Flatfish fillets (sole, flounder)	4.8	Egg	
Steaklike fish		Boiled (1)	5–6
(swordfish, salmon)	6.5	Fried (1)	7–9
Salmon, canned	11.9	Popcorn (1 cup)	2
Tuna, canned		Potatoes	
Canned in oil	17.5	French fried (3 oz)	11.3
Solids only	7	Chips (1 oz)	11.3
Canned in water	0.7	Salad (1 cup)	7
		Olives (10)	8.3

(1) **When the fat intake must be 40 g/d,** foods allowed each day include most vegetables and fruits, breads, cereals with skim milk, two servings of lean meat (3 oz each), one egg, and 1 tsp of margarine.

(2) **When fat intake must be 60 g/d,** in addition to the preceding foods, one can add 2 cups of 2% milk or one more ounce of meat or one egg with each serving or four more teaspoons of margarine or oil.

(3) **When fat intake is 75 g/d,** in addition to foods allowed on the 60-g diet, the patient can ingest whole milk instead of 2% milk *or* two slices of bacon *or* 4 oz of ice cream *or* two larger servings of lean meat (6 oz each).

(4) **Low-fat substitutes** are available for many foods, including whole milk (skim milk), cream (evaporated skim milk), butter/oils (apple or prune sauce, no-stick sprays), eggs (egg substitute), cheese, salad dressings, coffee cream, and ice cream (ice milk, sorbet).

4. **Side effects.** The low-fat diet is a high-carbohydrate, high-osmolarity diet, and carbohydrate-induced diarrhea may occur. In such a case, the restriction of fat must be titrated to individual needs. When meats and fish must be severely restricted to control fat intake, low-fat dietary supplements may be needed to deliver adequate protein and calories (see Chapter 9). A low-fat diet is often quite bland because fat supplies much of the flavor in foods. Care must be taken to season foods so that adequate caloric intake is maintained.

5. **Fat supplements.** When steatorrhea is present, fat-soluble vitamins often must be replaced. Bile acids are necessary for the absorption of

fat-soluble vitamins; thus, the requirements are greatest in patients who have disorders associated with bile acid depletion (e.g., most cases of short-bowel syndrome). The large doses of vitamins needed to treat malabsorption are often available only as the individual vitamin, not as part of a multivitamin preparation. A discussion of vitamins A, D, E, and K is included in Chapter 6. If pancreatic insufficiency is the cause of steatorrhea, enzyme replacement is needed. When fat restriction is severe, medium-chain triglycerides or fat substitutes can be added to the diet.

a. **Medium-chain triglycerides (MCTs).** MCTs are composed of fatty acids with 6 to 12 carbon residues and are found in high concentration in kernel oils (e.g., palm oil) and coconut oil. The commercially available MCT oil is made from coconut oil; it contains mostly fatty acids with 8 to 10 carbon atoms (vs. 16 to 18 for dietary fats) and very rapidly undergoes β-oxidation. MCT oil provides 8.3 kcal/g; 1 tbs weighs 14 g and provides 116 kcal. MCTs are relatively water-soluble and can be hydrolyzed in the absence of bile salts and with minimal concentrations of pancreatic enzymes, so that they are ideal for use as a caloric supplement in fat malabsorption (57). Much interest has been shown in using MCTs as an aid to weight loss (58) and as a rapid source of energy, especially during prolonged endurance exercising, because they are metabolized more rapidly than other fats. However, little convincing evidence has been found that MCTs are useful in these roles.

   (1) **Precautions.** The rapid oxidation of MCTs leads to ketone formation. Thus, they are contraindicated in patients prone to ketosis. In cirrhosis, reduced hepatic clearance leads to increased serum MCT levels and hyperventilation, lactic acidemia, and symptoms compatible with hepatic encephalopathy. Side effects of MCT oil include nausea, vomiting, diarrhea, and abdominal cramps when the dose is excessive, either at one feeding or daily. Symptoms may be a consequence of the hyperosmolarity that develops during rapid hydrolysis of MCTs.

   (2) **Practical aspects**

      (a) Give divided doses of ½ tbs up to six times a day.

      (b) For palatability, even though the oil is tasteless, add MCT oil (1 tbs/8 oz) to fruit juice or flavored beverages.

      (c) Use MCT oil in cooking or baking if the temperature does not exceed 300° to 325°F.

      (d) Use MCT oil as a salad or vegetable dressing.

      (e) Write to Mead Johnson Nutritionals, Evansville, Indiana 47721-0001 for a copy of *Recipes Using MCT Oil and Portagen.*

b. **Fat substitutes.** The two available substitutes have been marketed as aids in weight reduction for obese patients, but they may prove useful to patients on low-fat diets. No data are currently available to evaluate this role for the compounds.

   (1) **Simplesse** is made from egg white and milk protein processed in such a way as to produce a creamy liquid with the texture of fat. It is marketed in an ice cream product (Simple Pleasures), and approval is being sought from the Food and Drug Administration to use it in other products, such as mayonnaise, salad dressings, dips, sour cream, yogurt, and cheese spreads. It cannot be used in cooking because the creamy texture is lost.

   (2) **Olestra,** a compound in which up to eight fatty acids from vegetable oil are linked to a sucrose core, is resistant to the action of pancreatic lipase. It can be used in cooking and has been approved for deep-fried snacks such as potato and corn chips. In a short-term (6-week) randomized, controlled trial of snack foods containing olestra or triglycerides, no clinically mean-

ingful gastrointestinal symptoms were caused by the ingestion of snacks that contained olestra (59). Because olestra is a nonabsorbed lipid, it can cause a false-positive reaction in measurements of stool fat (60). Public concern continues about the effects of long-term or unregulated use because unlike products made from egg and milk proteins, olestra is an entirely new compound in the food supply. Thus, the Food and Drug Administration considers that olestra must be approved as a new food additive and that studies must be performed to ensure that it is safe for each approved use.

    (3) N-3 fatty acids. Linolenic acid is found primarily in canola and soy oils, and the metabolic products, eicosapentaenoic acid (EPA) and docosahexaenoic acid (DHA), are abundant in fish and fish oils. A proposed intake of 0.65 g/d has been suggested for EPA and DHA. One gram of fish oil contains about 300 g of these substances, and commercially available sources (e.g., EPA, Max EPA, Promega, SuperEPA, Sea-Omega, Marine Lipid Concentrate) contain from 300 to 800 mg of N-3 fatty acids per capsule. However, the commercial products are not the same mixture as fish oil, and the optimal dose has not been established. Doses of 10 to 20 g/d may be needed to produce a biochemical effect on LDL and HDL cholesterol. It is still uncertain whether these nutrients should be added to commercial supplements, such as infant formulas (61). Food enrichment with N-3 fatty acids has not been successful thus far because it causes a fishy taste, and oxidation occurs during processing. These fatty acids are not required for patients on a low-fat diet who are ingesting vegetable oils or fish. It has been proposed that N-3 fatty acids play a role in preventing or treating many diseases, including coronary artery disease, Crohn's disease, autoimmune disorders, and various cancers, but it is premature to recommend their routine use (61).

D. Low-protein diet
1. Principles
    a. Pathophysiology. In chronic hepatic disease with cirrhosis and portal–systemic shunting, exogenous protein bypasses the liver, and the products of protein degradation induce hepatic encephalopathy. Protein restriction is most effective when liver disease is stable and the episodes of encephalopathy are related to exogenous sources. When encephalopathy is caused by active hepatic disease and an inability to utilize endogenous amino acids, the diet is less effective. The cause of encephalopathy is uncertain. The "false-neurotransmitter" theory suggests that biogenic amines derived from tyrosine and phenylalanine may be involved in the development of hepatic encephalopathy. In cirrhosis, the ratio of branched-chain amino acids (BCAAs) (leucine, valine, and isoleucine) to tyrosine and phenylalanine is decreased from between 3 and 3.5 to less than 1.0. Because BCAAs compete with aromatic and sulfur amino acids for transport into the brain, it is rational to use either a low intake of protein or a relative increase in BCAAs in the diet to prevent this effect.

    Nutritional support enriched with BCAAs increases the recovery rate in patients with acute hepatic encephalopathy in comparison with dextrose solutions without amino acids (62). However, it is not known whether BCAA mixtures are superior to standard amino acid mixtures. Protein-sparing nutritional support produces some improvement in liver function, but it is not clear that such support alters mortality or morbidity (63).

    b. In chronic renal failure, a low-protein diet is used to decrease the production of nitrogenous waste products that must be excreted (e.g., urea, uric acid). This diet stresses the essential amino acids because they tend to be used preferentially for protein synthesis and are not deaminated with subsequent production of urea. Restriction of dietary protein to about 0.6 g/kg of body weight reduces the relative risk for renal failure by about 33% (64). The details of this special use of the low-protein diet are discussed in Chapter 12.

    c. Hospitalized patients. Many elderly hospitalized patients meet less than 50% of their recommended protein and energy requirements, so that the risk for a poor outcome is increased (65). This unintended low-protein diet is a consequence of many factors, including a decreased appetite and the administration of medications. Supplementing the hospital diet with 20 g of milk protein per day (up to about 1.0 g of total protein per kilogram per day) slowed the rate of bone loss, increased levels of insulin-like growth factor 1, and shortened hospital stay in patients after hip fracture (66). Whether supplementation with specific growth factors is needed or whether protein replacement alone is enough is still a matter of considerable debate (67).

2. Indications

    a. In patients with chronic liver disease and hepatic encephalopathy, a low-protein diet can be useful. However, the diet must still supply protein at the required rate of 0.5 to 0.8 g/kg per day. For this reason, restricted diets that provide less than 40 g/d for an adult or 1.0 to 2.5 g of protein per kilogram daily for a growing child may be associated with a negative nitrogen balance.

    b. In hyperammonemia of any cause, such as certain *inborn errors of metabolism* (e.g., isovaleric acidemia), this diet decreases available substrate.

    c. Renal failure, whether acute or chronic, must be treated with a low-protein diet (see Chapter 12).

3. Practical aspects

    a. General instructions

        (1) The caloric intake as carbohydrate should be sufficient to prevent the use of protein in muscle for energy (25 to 40 kcal/g of protein). For patients too ill to eat, parenteral administration is appropriate.

        (2) For patients with renal disease, 80% of the daily protein allotment should be protein of high biologic value—eggs, meat, fish, poultry, milk.

        (3) For patients with hepatic encephalopathy, the intestinal absorption of protein by-products should be reduced by concomitant treatment with lactulose (30 mL three or four times daily to produce loose stools) or neomycin (1 g two to four times daily).

        (4) An intake of 40 g of protein barely maintains nitrogen balance. Lesser amounts of protein can be used acutely but should not be prescribed on a long-term basis. Vegetable protein may be better tolerated than animal protein because it contains less tryptophan and sulfur amino acids, which are thought to contribute to hepatic encephalopathy.

        (5) The use of BCAA supplements is still not established, and no convincing data are available to indicate that such supplements are more effective in relieving acute or chronic encephalopathy than are standard amino acid mixtures (63). The guidelines for patient selection and the endpoint of therapy are unclear, as is the demonstration of clear long-term benefit to the patient. Recommended doses of the oral products (e.g., Hepatic-Aid) are 15 to 60 g/d; for IV use (e.g., HepatAmine), they are 80 to 120 g/d (see Chapters 9 and 10 for the composition of these products). HepatAmine contains three amino acids (methionine, phenylalanine, and tryptophan) thought to contribute to hepatic encephalopathy. The doses mentioned above are recommended by the manufacturer and may be too high. Because efficacy is not proven, these products should be used with caution, especially at the recommended high doses.

(6) For patients with renal disease, sodium and potassium must also be restricted.

b. **Specific instructions.** Each ounce of meat, fish, poultry, or cheese contains about 7 g of protein, an egg contains 6 g, and 1 cup of milk contains 8 g. One-half cup of cereal, bread, pasta, or a vegetable contains 2 g of protein, whereas the same amount of dried beans, peas, or nuts contains 5 g or more. Table 11-19 lists the protein content of various foods. The National Kidney Foundation (116 East 27th Street, New York, New York 10016) provides further information useful for patients. See Chapter 12 for details of the use of protein restriction in renal disease.

Table 11-19. Protein content of selected foods

Food	Protein (g/unit)	Food	Protein (g/unit)
Egg, 1 large (100)[a]	6.5	**Breads and cereals** (65)	
Milk products (93)		Bread (1 slice)	2.2
Milk		Cereal, dry (¾ cup)	1.1–2.1
Whole (1 cup)	8.5	Rice, cooked (½ cup)	2.0
Skim (1 cup)	8.8	Roll (1)	2.6
Buttermilk (1 cup)	8.1	Spaghetti, cooked (½ cup)	3.4
Ice cream (1 cup)	9.6	**Vegetables** (72)	
Cheese (1 oz)	6.6–7.5	Asparagus, cooked (⅔ cup)	2.2
Yogurt, low-fat, fruit (1 cup)	9.8	Broccoli, cooked (⅔ cup)	1.7
Meat, fish, poultry (75)		Cabbage, raw (½ cup)	1.3
Hamburger (3 oz)	21.9	Cauliflower, cooked (⅔ cup)	2.3
Sirloin steak (3 oz)	22.2	Cucumber, raw (½ cup)	0.3
Lamb chop (3 oz)	19.2	Eggplant, cooked (½ cup)	2.0
Lamb leg (3 oz)	23.4	Lettuce (4 leaves)	1.7
Pork chop (3 oz)	22.2	Green pepper, raw (1)	1.2
Liver, beef (3 oz)	23.7	Spinach, cooked (½ cup)	3.0
Chicken, white meat (3 oz)	21.6	Green beans (½ cup)	0.8
Chicken, dark meat (3 oz)	18.6	Tomato (1)	1.1
Frankfurter (3 oz)	18.6	Green peas, cooked (½ cup)	4.3
Fish		Legumes, dried (1 oz)	6.7
Cod (3 oz)	25.5	**Fruits**	
Halibut (3 oz)	22.8	Apple (1)	0.2
Salmon, canned (3 oz)	17.7	Apricots (1)	0.5
Tuna, canned (3 oz)	26.1	Bananas (1)	1.2
Shellfish		Cantaloupe (quarter)	1.0
Crabmeat (3 oz)	12.9	Orange (1)	1.0
Lobster (3 oz)	12.6	Orange juice (½ cup)	0.7
Shrimp (3 oz)	14.4	Pear, peach (1)	0.6
Bacon (2 slices)	6.0	Watermelon (1 cup)	0.9
Nuts (55)			
Peanuts (6 nuts)	2.6		
Peanut butter (1 tbs)	4.2		

[a] Biologic value is based on the ability of the protein to produce positive nitrogen balance. The numbers in parentheses correspond to an average value for that food group versus 100% for egg.

4. **Side effects.** When protein restriction is too severe, catabolized muscle mass provides the amino acids needed for daily use (see Chapter 5). It is not wise to restrict protein to less than 0.4 g/kg of body weight (~ 30 g of protein for the average 70-kg patient). If the symptoms of hepatic encephalopathy or uremia do not respond to this degree of restriction, it is unlikely that more stringent restriction will help. When the intake of meat and milk is restricted, it is possible that calcium, iron, and B vitamins (thiamine, riboflavin, niacin) will be needed.

5. **Supplements required.** In renal failure, calcium is often needed to compensate for hypocalcemia and a decreased calcium intake. Iron deficiency resulting from bleeding gastrointestinal lesions often complicates renal failure, but iron is sometimes needed even in the absence of overt gastrointestinal bleeding.

E. Gluten-restricted diet

1. **Principles**

   a. **Toxic grain products.** Nontropical sprue (celiac sprue, gluten-sensitive enteropathy) is a disorder characterized by sensitivity to certain glutens. Glutens are a family of proteins found in many grains, including corn and rice, which are safe for patients with celiac disease. The glutens that produce symptoms in this disorder are those in wheat, rye, barley, and buckwheat. The data implicating oats are not so certain as those implicating other grains, and oats have been well tolerated in patients with dermatitis herpetiformis, a related disorder (68). Nonetheless, oats are usually omitted from the gluten-free diet.

      (1) **Substitutions.** Glutens from corn and rice, in addition to those from wheat starch, potato flour, soybean flour, and tapioca, may be used as substitutes for the omitted cereal grains.

      (2) **Wheat products are used as fillers in many processed foods.** It is helpful for the patient with sprue to develop an extensive list of acceptable products.

   b. **Duration of diet.** Although a gluten-free diet was formerly thought to be needed only until remission occurred in some patients, it is now clear that use of the diet should be lifelong (69). No convincing evidence indicates that the diet is useful for the nonspecific therapy of other diarrheal illness. However, acute intestinal damage resulting from conditions other than sprue may cause temporary gluten intolerance, especially in children. The long-term use of this diet should be limited to patients with gluten-induced enteropathy.

   c. **Relationship to traditional allergy.** The abnormal response to wheat and other glutens in sprue differs from other food allergies in that the process is not mediated by immunoglobulin E. However, abnormalities of the intestinal immune system are involved in some way. In some cases, treatment with glucocorticosteroids can supplement dietary management of the disease (55).

2. **Indications.** A gluten-restricted diet is necessary for patients with biopsy-proven *nontropical sprue* or the related disorder *dermatitis herpetiformis.*

3. **Practical aspects**

   a. **General instructions**

      (1) Eliminate foods containing wheat, rye, barley, and probably oats (Table 11-20). These glutens are the components that give form to dough. The flours allowed on a gluten-restricted diet produce flat or crumbly baked products. Any commercial product with a crown contains a forbidden gluten.

      (2) Read labels carefully. Avoid products that contain wheat, rye, barley, oats, unspecified flour or starch, emulsifiers, stabilizers, hydrolyzed plant/vegetable protein, vegetable monoacylglycerols or diacylglycerols, and natural flavorings. Some of

these products may in fact be gluten-free, but the absence of gluten should be verified with an up-to-date gluten-free product list, or the company should be contacted.

(3) The foods most likely to contain glutens include cereal beverages (beer, Ovaltine), some commercial ice creams, commercial cakes and cookies, salad dressings, canned or processed meats, soups, candy bars, catsups, mustards, frozen foods with sauces, processed cheeses, chocolate milk, cream soups, and breaded, creamed, or scalloped vegetables.

(4) Products made from cornmeal, cornstarch, corn flour, rice, rice flour, tapioca, soybean, potato starch, or arrowroot may be used. For baking, 1 cup of wheat flour may be replaced by 1 cup of corn flour, 1 cup of fine cornmeal, $\frac{3}{4}$ cup of coarse cornmeal, 10 tbs of potato flour, or 14 tbs of rice flour. For thickening, 1 tbs of wheat flour can be substituted with $\frac{1}{2}$ tbs of cornstarch, potato flour, rice, or arrowroot starch or 2 tbs of quick-cooking tapioca.

(5) Fresh meats, milk, fish, eggs, fresh vegetables, and fruits are all acceptable.

(6) A low-lactose diet may be needed in the early stages of treatment if lactose intolerance is present.

Patient information on this topic is available in Appendix D.

b. **Specific recommendations**

(1) **Patient support groups.** Each of these groups can provide recipes, lists of gluten-free commercial products, and information on gluten content in medications.

(a) CSA/USA (Celiac Sprue Association) (*http://www. csaceliacs.org*). The website contains useful information on grains and flours, gluten-free diets, and lactose intolerance.

(b) Gluten Intolerance Group of North America (*gig@accessone.com*).

(c) Celiac Disease Foundation (*http://www.celiac.org*).

(d) Coeliac Society of the United Kingdom (*http://www. coeliac.co.uk*).

(2) **Gluten-free cookbooks** are available in many of the large retail bookstores.

(3) **Safe commercial products.** Among the many foods that often contain offending glutens, it is possible to select products that are safe. Therefore, another brand name should not be substituted for one known to be gluten-free unless it, too, is known to be gluten-free. The Celiac UPC database (*http://www.brandbeach.com/celiac/upc/index.html*) has been created to help patients with celiac disease determine whether a product is gluten-free according to the product's UPC code. The database can be used on line or on a hand-held personal computer. For a "complete" list of products, one of the patient support groups can also be contacted.

(4) **Gluten in drug products.** Gluten is often added as an "inert" filler in tablets, capsules, and suspensions. Most major manufacturers do not use gluten. The CSA/USA has a listing of relevant pharmaceuticals.

4. **Side effects.** The gluten-restricted diet can be well balanced for all nutrients and so no side effects are associated.

5. **Supplements required.** No supplements are needed unless the malabsorption has caused specific deficiencies or unless the lactose intolerance is permanent and calcium supplements are required. Celiac disease is an important cause of osteoporosis, and adequate calcium (1,200 mg/d) and vitamin D (400 IU) must be provided to restore bone density in patients whose axial bone density is decreased.

(*text continues on page 444*)

Table 11-20. Sources of gluten[a]

Food groups	Foods that contain gluten	Foods that contain malt	Foods that may contain gluten	Foods that do *not* contain gluten
Beverage	Cereal beverages (e.g., Postum), malt Ovaltine, beer, and ale		Commercial chocolate milk; cocoa mixes; other beverage mixes; dietary supplements; commercial rice and corn cereals[b]	Coffee; tea; decaffeinated coffee, carbonated beverages; chocolate drinks made with pure cocoa powder; wine; distilled liquor
Meat and meat substitutes			Meat loaf and patties; cold cuts and prepared meats; sausage; stuffing; breaded meats; cheese foods and spreads; commercial soufflés, omelets, and fondues; soy protein meat substitutes	Pure meat, fish, fowl, egg, cottage cheese, cheeses, and peanut butter
Fat and oil			Commercial salad dressing and mayonnaise, gravy, white and cream sauces, nondairy creamer	Butter, margarine, vegetable oil
Milk		Milk beverages that contain malt	Commercial chocolate milk	Whole, low-fat, and skim milk; buttermilk
Grains and grain products	Bread, crackers, cereal, and pasta that contain wheat; oats; rye; malt and, malt flavoring; graham flour, durum flour, pastry flour; bran or wheat germ; barley; millet; pretzels; communion wafers		Commercial seasoned rice and potato mixes, commercial corn, rice, and potato snacks	Specially prepared breads made with wheat starch,[c] rice, potato, or soybean flour, or cornmeal; pure corn or rice cereals; hominy grits; white, brown, and wild rice; popcorn; low-protein pasta made from wheat starch
Vegetable			Commercial seasoned vegetable mixes; commercial vegetables with cream or cheese sauce; canned baked beans	All fresh vegetables; plain commercially frozen or canned vegetables

Fruit		Commercial pie fillings	All plain or sweetened fruits; fruit thickened with tapioca or cornstarch
Soup	Soup that contains wheat pasta; soup thickened with wheat flour or other gluten-containing grains	Commercial soup, broth, and soup mixes	Soup thickened with cornstarch, wheat starch, or potato, rice, or soybean flour; pure broth
Desserts	Commercial cakes, cookies, and pastries; commercial dessert mixes	Commercial ice cream and sherbet	Gelatin; custard; fruit ice; specially prepared cakes, cookies, and pastries made with gluten-free flour or starch; pudding and fruit filling thickened with tapioca, cornstarch, or arrowroot flour; some commercial ice creams
Sweets		Commercial candies, especially chocolates	
Miscellaneous		Catsup; prepared mustard; soy sauce; commercially prepared meat sauces and pickles; vinegar; flavoring syrups (syrups for pancakes or ice cream)	Monosodium glutamate; salt; pepper; pure spices and herbs; yeast; pure baking chocolate or cocoa powder; flavoring extracts; artificial flavoring

[a] The terms *commercially prepared* and *commercial* are used to refer to partially prepared foods purchased from a grocery or food market and to prepared foods purchased from a restaurant.
[b] Check up-to-date lists of gluten-free commercial products.
[c] Wheat starch may contain trace amounts of gluten. Avoid if not tolerated.
Modified from *Mayo Clinic diet manual*, 6th ed. Toronto: BC Decker, 1988.

F. Low-oxalate diet

1. **Principles.** Hyperoxaluria resulting from an increased absorption of dietary oxalate occurs in disorders in which bile acids are poorly absorbed, enter the colon, and increase its permeability (55). The degree of oxaluria in such cases is inversely correlated with the degree of fat absorption. The excessive free fatty acids in the lumen of the small bowel that result from fat malabsorption bind calcium, which is then not available to form the insoluble calcium oxalate salt. Consequently, the more soluble sodium oxalate forms and is absorbed in the colon. However, only about 10% of the body oxalate is normally derived from the diet. Therefore, a low-oxalate diet is not always effective in reducing hyperoxaluria.

2. **Indications.** This diet is used in cases of *hyperoxaluria* (>40 mg/d). Hyperoxaluria develops in a subset of patients with renal stones (idiopathic hyperoxaluria) and in patients with *steatorrhea* resulting from *bile acid malabsorption* (e.g., short-bowel syndrome). The diet can begin before calcium oxalate stones have formed. After the diet has been started, urinary excretion should be remeasured to ascertain that the diet is effective.

   Calcium supplements often must be added in cases of short-bowel syndrome because poor calcium absorption and a negative calcium balance can lead to osteopenia. When luminal calcium is increased, the calcium oxalate salt may re-form and the hyperoxaluria decrease without use of the diet. In some instances, both treatments are given together.

3. **Practical aspects**

   a. The low-oxalate diet is often part of the regimen of patients requiring a *low-fat diet.* In evaluating the progress of a patient on a restrictive diet, one should determine the patient's compliance. A full listing of oxalate content of selected foods is available from the General Clinical Research Center, University of California, San Diego Medical Center (Brzezinski E, Durning AM, Grasse B, et al. Oxalate content of selected foods. 1998).

   b. **Foods high in oxalate.** Certain snack foods are high in oxalates, such as cola beverages, nuts, potatoes, tea, and foods containing chocolate. Cereals, meats, and dairy products are generally low in oxalate. Foods with a very high content (>10 mg per serving) should be avoided completely. A detailed listing of the oxalate content of foods can be found in standard diet manuals and nutrition textbooks (1,2,70). The following paragraphs indicate the oxalate content of selected foods:

      Patient information on this topic is available in Appendix D.

      (1) **Foods very high in oxalate** (>10 mg per serving): spinach, rhubarb, cocoa, chocolate, tea, Ovaltine, beer, peanut butter, green beans, beets, Swiss chard, collards, kale, eggplant, sweet potatoes, blueberries, Concord grapes, strawberries, raspberries, fruit cocktail, wheat germ, pepper (>1 tsp/d), turmeric, tomato soup, nuts (especially peanuts, pecans, walnuts, almonds). Indian or Chinese teas made from *Camellia sinensis* are rich in oxalate; herbal teas, which are not true teas but derived from other plant sources, contain much less oxalate (70).

      (2) **Foods moderately high in oxalate** (2 to 20 mg per serving): parsley, turnip greens, brussels sprouts, tomatoes, lima beans, lettuce, corn, broccoli, figs, oranges, cola beverages, juices (orange, tomato, grape), apple, pear, pineapple, sardines.

4. **Side effects.** None.

5. **Supplements required.** None.

G. Elimination diets for allergy or intolerance to foods

1. **Principles**

   a. **Food allergy and intolerance.** The Committee on Adverse Reactions to Foods of the American Academy of Immunology defines *food allergy* as a reaction to a specific food that is mediated by classic immune mechanisms (71,72). In the absence of evidence of classic immune mechanisms, it is better to refer to such a reaction as *food intolerance* (Table 11-21). Even in the latter case, the food should provoke a clear reaction that recurs each time the food is eaten. This sequence is lacking in many cases of so-called food intolerance.

   b. **True allergic reactions to food,** which occur infrequently in adults, are most often caused by fruit juices, nuts, chocolate, milk, and shellfish (73). The organs usually affected are the skin (~45%), respiratory tract (~25%), and gastrointestinal tract (~20%). In the oral allergy syndrome, the most common form, early symptoms develop within minutes of ingestion and include swelling of the lips, tingling in the throat, and rhinorrhea. Later symptoms (developing within 2 hours of ingestion) may include asthma, urticaria, eczema, vomiting, diarrhea, abdominal pain, headache, and general malaise. Allergens can be inhaled as well as ingested (e.g., flour, spices, egg white, steam produced when legumes or crustaceans are cooked), and inhalation leads to respiratory symptoms. Tests that identify immunoglobulin G antibodies (e.g., radioallergosorbent test, enzyme-linked immunosorbent assay) do not prove the presence of an immunoglobulin E immune complex. Allergies are more common in children because their immunoglobulin E levels are much higher than those of adults. Most reactions to fruits/juices disappear by age 3. Allergy to pollen-related food is the most common food allergy in adults in countries where tree pollen allergy is common. Primary pulmonary sensitization to pollen from trees, grasses, or herbs can give rise to food allergies when epitopes are shared. For example, natural latex dermatitis can be associated with food allergies to banana or avocado, and birch pollen allergy can be associated with hazelnut or kiwi food allergy (71). The value of an elimination diet is that an offending food is identified by adding a single food at a time. This maneuver is necessary when the history does not provide the clue, and it can be used to identify allergies to both food additives and natural food components. The history remains the best means of identifying symptom complexes caused by true allergies.

Table 11-21. Classification of food-induced reactions

IgE-mediated	Not IgE-mediated	Food intolerance	Food aversion
Urticaria/ angioedema	Dermatitis herpetiformis	Lactose/sucrose	Chronic fatigue
Atopic dermatitis	Contact dermatitis	Fructose/sorbitol	Irritable bowel
Rhinoconjunctivitis	Celiac disease	Histamine (scombroid)	Depression
Oral allergy syndrome	Eosinophilic enteritis	Bacterial enterotoxins	Phobias
Anaphylaxis	Heiner's syndrome[a]	Plant/phytotoxins	ADHD
Food protein enteropathies	Migraine headaches	Food additives	IBD, flatus

ADHD, attention-deficit hyperactivity disorder; IBD, inflammatory bowel disease.
[a] Heiner's syndrome is milk-induced alveolitis and hemorrhagic gastroenteritis in infants.

2. Diagnosis

a. Foods most commonly implicated include milk, eggs, nuts, and shellfish. Less commonly involved are wheat, chocolate, cheese, soft fruits, and meat. Artificial coloring agents in addition to virtually all foods have been implicated in nonimmunologic adverse food reactions. One should remember the rules for food labeling when trying to determine the presence of a food additive. The Codex General Standard on Labeling states that "all ingredients shall be listed in descending order of ingoing weight at the time of the manufacture of the food." When a compound ingredient constitutes less than 25% of a food, ingredients other than food additives need not be declared (71). In other words, a substance that is present as only a minor ingredient of a food must be declared, but a substance that is more abundant but part of a compound ingredient may not be listed. In addition, food additives with no technologic function in the finished product (e.g., egg whites or milk used as clarifying agents in juices or wine) may not be declared on the label. New labeling laws may change these rules, but currently one must realize that not all substances that might cause a food allergy must be listed on the label.

b. Tests. If anaphylaxis occurs, no challenge should be given. If the response is mild, skin tests and food challenge may be used. If the response is sporadic, a food diary may help. Double-blinded challenge may be needed because many patients are placebo reactors, and food intolerance is demonstrated in only a few of the adults in whom it is suspected (74). Both skin tests and radioallergosorbent tests give many false-positive results, and cross-reactions between allergens occur. In fact, results of skin testing for immediate hypersensitivity have not been shown to be reliable (71,75). In most patients presenting with possible food allergy, psychiatric disease may be a major cause of symptoms (76). Other tests have been suggested for diagnosis (71). These include radioallergosorbent tests for total serum immunoglobulin E and allergen-specific immunoglobulin E, neither of which adds much if the results of oral testing (elimination and provocation) are positive. If tests are performed, the results should match the clinical history. The problem with oral testing is that it is time-consuming.

c. Double-blinded oral control challenge is the "gold standard" but is difficult to carry out in clinical practice and can be dangerous if anaphylaxis is suspected. It is usually more convenient to use an open or single-blinded food challenge. Both negative and positive results are highly predictive of the correct answer. When a positive allergic history is present or a food allergy is strongly suspected, an *elimination diet* can be tried. This diet is usually reserved for patients having daily or almost daily symptoms.

3. Practical aspects

a. True food allergies (adults)

(1) **The strictest diet,** which is rarely needed, consists of lamb, rice, dry puffed rice, salt, and water for 5 to 7 days. One new food is then added each day, with relatively nonallergenic foods usually added first. Allergenic foods such as milk, eggs, wheat, and corn are finally added. No fat can be added to any prepared food. Salt or baking soda must be used to brush the teeth (77).

(2) **A less strict initial diet** (modified from Golbert TM. In: Patterson R, ed. *Allergic Diseases*. Philadelphia: JB Lippincott Co, 1972:362) allows the following foods and beverages (all fruits and vegetables *must be cooked*): lamb, poi, rice, rice cereals, water, pineapple, apricot, cherries, blueberries, lettuce, artichokes, beets, spinach, celery, sweet potatoes, salt, sugar, and tapioca. Any vegetable oil is allowed except oleomargarine

and soy oil. Mazola margarine contains no milk and is acceptable. Specific foods to be avoided include pork, beef, fish and seafood, eggs, milk and milk products, and baked goods made with wheat, oats, corn, or rye flour. Also to be avoided are butter, margarine, tea, coffee, cola, soft drinks, chewing gum, alcohol, and chocolate. This diet may be more useful for outpatient use. Egg is often hidden in such foods as pastries, ice creams, marshmallows, sausages, salad dressings, instant coffee, and root beer.

   (3) **Addition of other foods.** The patient is instructed to continue the basic diet for 5 to 7 days. On each successive day, a single cooked food is added. The patient keeps a diet diary and records the time foods are ingested, with any untold reactions. For those unable to begin with such a strict diet, same basic diet can be used, with the following foods added: chicken, turkey, beef, boiled ham, bacon, potatoes, potato chips, carrots, soybeans, asparagus, maple syrup, ginger ale, plums, prunes, lentils, navy beans, and kidney beans. These are poorly allergenic foods that can be added in the early stages of an elimination diet. When foods must be added in double-blinded fashion, dried foods can be placed into gelatin capsules. A dose of 8 g of each food is commonly used.

   (4) **Foods should be cooked** in the strictest diets because heating can denature proteins and render them less allergenic.

   (5) **Patients with a history of severe (anaphylactic) reactions** to eggs or chicken should be tested with intradermal extracts before receiving egg-derived vaccines.

b. **Milk allergy (infants).** In infants with suspected milk allergy, formulas containing casein hydrolysates (e.g., Pregestimil, Nutramigen, Alimentum) work well. Because 20% of milk-allergic patients react to soy protein, soy-based formulas are not suggested.

c. **Elimination diet for intolerance to foods.** A low-lactose diet for lactose intolerance is discussed in separately in this chapter. The other intolerance most commonly encountered is to gas-producing foods (primarily flatus). Although it is not clear that gas production or the perception of gas production is related to the intake of specific foods, some foods undoubtedly contain oligosaccharides (e.g., stachyose, raffinose) or components of dietary fiber that escape digestion in the small bowel and are fermented in part in the colon. For the occasional patient with intolerance to gas-producing foods, an elimination diet can be suggested (78).

   (1) **Foods to be avoided in diet for gassy food intolerance** (elimination on a trial basis):

Class	Examples
High-lactose foods	Dairy products
Vegetables	Legumes (beans, peas, lentils)
	Cruciferous vegetables (broccoli, cauliflower, brussels sprouts)
	Root vegetables (radishes, onion, rutabaga), cabbage, kohlrabi, cucumber, sweet peppers
Fruits	Prunes, apples, raisins, bananas
Grains	Whole wheat bread, bran cereals
Fatty foods	Fried foods, cream sauces, gravies
Artificial sweeteners	Fructose (soft drinks), sorbitol

   (2) **The enzyme α-galactosidase (Beano),** derived from a mold, is marketed with the claim that it prevents gas from occurring with a high fiber intake. The manufacturer recommends that three to eight drops of Beano be added to a food after it has

cooled below 130°F. Some evidence indicates that the treatment may be effective (79).

  d. **Adverse reactions to food additives.** The same range of symptoms seen in food allergy can be caused by food additives. However, food allergies are much less common, and it may not be necessary to eliminate foods with troublesome additives from the diet completely. The mechanisms for many of the reactions are unknown but may be pharmacologic, toxic, or truly allergic. These reactions are most often to salicylates, tyramine, sulfites, and monosodium glutamate.

  (1) **Pharmacologic reactions:** caffeine (see earlier section in this chapter), monosodium glutamate (headache, asthma), tyramine, phenylethylamine in chocolate (headache), nitrite and nitrates (headache), histamine-releasing foods such as egg white, strawberry, shellfish (anaphylactoid reaction), histamine poisoning from tuna, mackerel, Swiss cheese (anaphylactoid reaction), sodium metabisulfite (asthma), salicylates in candies

  (2) **Toxic reactions:** ethanol, acid juices (heartburn), toxins from infectious agents

  (3) **Allergic reactions to common food chemicals:** tartrazine, menthol in breakfast cereals, candy, gum (urticaria), EDTA in mayonnaise and salad dressings (dermatitis), erythrosine in maraschino cherries and fruit cocktail, breakfast cereals (photosensitivity), sodium benzoate in catsup (purpura), quinine in tonic water, bitter lemon (purpura), sulfites

  4. **Side effects.** Care must be taken to provide a well-balanced diet, including foods from all basic groups.

  5. **Supplements required.** None.

H. **Restricted diets for allergy or intolerance to food additives**

  1. **Salicylates/tartrazine.** The most common drug allergy for which an altered diet is important is salicylate hypersensitivity. Salicylates and tartrazine, a salicylate-related compound, can produce chronic urticaria in the sensitive patient. Most patients sensitive to aspirin also react to tartrazine.

  a. **Food sources.** Many colas, Dr. Pepper, root beer, most carbonated soft drinks, many cereals and baked goods mixes, many fruits (apples, oranges, peaches, plums, cherries, grapefruit, berries), prepared meats, nondairy creamers, yogurt, ice cream, sherbet, most commercial dessert mixes, prepared pies and cakes, frostings, puddings, rolls, and candies contain salicylates. Methyl salicylate is commonly used as a flavoring agent under the name *wintergreen.* Candies containing wintergreen include gums, mints, and jelly beans. Cereals containing salicylate include breakfast squares and fruit turnover pastries. Tartrazine is included in many yellow and green candies, fruit crushes, and many antibiotic capsules and vitamin preparations.

  b. **Salicylate or tartrazine-free foods** include milk and milk products, most vegetables (except cucumbers, peppers, broccoli, asparagus, okra, spinach, squash, sweet potato, zucchini, and tomatoes), all fish, red meat, cheese, eggs, poultry, pasta, rice, white potatoes, most breads, all fats, sugar, syrup, and molasses. A more complete list of foods allowed has been published (80).

  c. **Supplements required.** A salicylate-free diet is adequate for all nutrients except vitamin C. Supplements (60 mg/d) can be provided for such patients.

  2. **Tyramine**

  a. **Population at risk.** Patients taking monoamine oxidase inhibitors are at risk for the development of headache, palpitations, nausea, vomiting, and in some cases hypertensive crises if they ingest sympathomimetic drugs (methyl dopa, L-dopa, dopamine, epinephrine, ephedrine) or foods with a high concentration of tyramine. Tyramine is a biogenic amine derived from tyrosine metabolism. Inhibition of tyramine metabolism can cause hypertensive crises, which begin 30 to 60 minutes after the offending food is ingested, with headache, palpitations, nausea, and vomiting. At high doses (60 mg/kg of body weight), tyramine can cause cardiac arrhythmias, with a loss of P waves, atrial ectopies, ventricular and atrial premature beats, junctional rhythm, bigeminy, and Wenckebach phenomenon (81). It is not known whether the intake of tyramine-rich foods should be decreased in patients with arrhythmias.

b. **Drugs that inhibit monoamine oxidase,** a widely distributed complex enzyme system, include furazolidone (Furoxone), isocarboxazid (Marplan), phenelzine sulfate (Nardil), procarbazine (Matulane), selegiline HCl (Eldepryl), and tranylcypromine (Parnate). Patients taking these drugs should also refrain from taking medication containing sympathomimetic drugs, especially nose drops and cold capsules, and most antidepressant medications.

c. **A restricted-tyramine diet** should be followed by patients taking these drugs, as they may be intolerant of ingested tyramine. The details of this diet, which provides less than 2 mg of tyramine per day, are listed in Table 11-22. Usually, more than 6 mg of tyramine must be ingested to cause symptoms when it cannot be metabolized. Cheeses with the highest content of tyramine (>200 mg/g in some cheeses) are cheddar, Camembert, and Stilton.

3. **Sulfites**
   a. **Uses and abundance.** Six sulfiting agents have been declared safe by the Food and Drug Administration. These chemicals are listed on labels as sulfur dioxide, sodium sulfite, sodium and potassium bisulfite, and sodium and potassium metabisulfite. Sulfites are widely used in the processing of wine and beer and in restaurants to maintain the crispness and freshness of salads, fruits, and potatoes. They are also used for bleaching food starches and in producing cellophane for food packaging. The Food and Drug Administration prohibits the use of sulfites in foods that are important sources of thiamine because they destroy the vitamin. In 1986, the Food and Drug Administration also banned the use of sulfites in fruits and vegetables meant to be eaten raw. Sulfite sensitivity can develop even in persons without an allergic history, and it is not certain that all reactions are mediated by allergy. Symptoms include wheezing, hives, nausea, and diarrhea. Rarely, anaphylaxis may occur. With increased awareness and restricted use, adverse reactions to sulfites are now relatively uncommon. Updated information can be obtained from the Food and Drug Administration website (*http://vm.cfsan.fda.gov/~dms*).

   b. **Foods containing sulfites** are so common that the average person ingests 2 to 3 mg/d, and when beer or wine is included in the diet, this figure can reach 5 to 10 mg/d. Foods frequently preserved with sulfites include instant tea, beer, wine, wine coolers and spirits, dried citrus fruit beverage mixes, condiments and relishes, confections and frostings, canned soups, dried mixes, seafood (especially shrimp), baked goods, processed and dried fruits, gelatin, puddings and fillings, jams and jellies, corn and maple syrup, molasses, breading, batters, noodle mixes, and processed vegetables (vegetable juices; canned, pickled, dried vegetables; potato chips).

   c. **Treatment** is complicated by the widespread presence of the chemical, which makes the problem difficult to diagnose before the episode is complete. Moreover, several treatments for acute allergic response may contain potassium metabisulfite as a preservative, especially epinephrine and some IV solutions and medications. Terbutaline can be used safely in such a situation.

Table 11-22. Restricted-tyramine diet

Food group	Unrestricted foods (<5 µg/g)	Foods allowed in moderation (5–20 µg/g)	Foods to avoid (>20 µg/g)
Cheese	Cottage cheese, ricotta, cream cheese	Processed American cheese, Gouda	Aged cheeses—brick, blue, cheddar, Camembert, Swiss, Romano, Roquefort, Stilton, mozzarella, Parmesan, provolone, Emmentaler, boursin, sour cream, Brie
Beverages	Milk	Coffee, hot chocolate, cola drinks (1–3 cups per day)	Ale, beer, sherry, red and white wines,[a] yogurt, bouillon
Meats	Fresh or fresh frozen meat, poultry		Canned meats, chicken liver, beef liver, fermented (hard) sausage or salami, pepperoni, summer sausage, bologna, Genoa salami
Fish	Fresh or fresh frozen fish or shellfish		Salt herring, dried fish, caviar, pickled herring
Vegetables	Most		Italian flat beans, Chinese pea pods, broad (fava) beans, mixed Chinese vegetables, eggplant
Fruit	Most		Figs, avocados
Miscellaneous			Chocolate, soy sauce, protein extracts, yeast concentrates or products made with them

[a] Fermentation of wine and beer does not ordinarily involve processes that result in the production of tyramine. Despite this, levels in beer are variable. The production of appreciable amounts of tyramine in red wines results from contamination with other than the usual fermenting organisms and from the inclusion of grape pulp and seeds in the process. These potential sources of amino acids are not used in making white wines. Because of the unpredictable variability in tyramine levels, all the beverages listed are generally excluded (*Med Lett Drugs Ther* 1976;18:32).

4. Monosodium glutamate (MSG)
   a. Use in foods. MSG is the sodium salt of glutamic acid. It is made by fermenting starch, sugar beets, sugar cane, or molasses and is used to enhance flavor, perhaps by stimulating glutamate receptors on the tongue. Foods labeled "no MSG" may in fact contain hydrolyzed protein, a source of free glutamate. Some products containing protein hydrolysates with substantial amounts of glutamate are labeled "contains glutamate."
   b. Safety. MSG has been classified as GRAS (generally recognized as safe), but because of its presumed role in "MSG syndrome" and asthma attacks, its use is subject to repeated review by the Food and Drug Administration, American Medical Association, European Communities, and World Health Organization. All have found the additive to be safe. The most recent Food and Drug Administration/Federation of Associated Societies of Experimental Biology (FASEB) review (1995) concluded that a symptom complex may develop in an unknown percentage of people after the ingestion of 3 g or more of MSG without other food (*http://vm.cfspan. fda.gov/~lrd*). Most food servings contain no more than 0.5 g of MSG. The syndrome includes burning and numbness in the neck and arms, chest pain, facial pressure, headache, nausea, tachycardia, weakness, and bronchospasm in patients with asthma. However, no evidence for causation of other medical illnesses has been documented.

I. Low-sodium diet
   1. Principles. Disorders in which sodium retention or hypertension is a prominent feature are treated with a low-sodium diet. The usual intake of sodium on a Western-style diet is greatly in excess of daily needs. Moreover, many processed foods contain sodium (see Chapter 7). Therefore, the diet seems quite restrictive. When sodium is retained, the ability to excrete excess ingested sodium is limited. The less sodium that is ingested, the easier is the task of removing excess sodium from the body. Potassium salts are often used to replace sodium. A high-sodium diet alone will not cause hypertension in an otherwise normotensive person. Thus, the diet is probably not needed to prevent hypertension.
   2. Indications. A low-sodium diet is used in the management of *acute and chronic congestive heart failure, chronic hepatic failure with ascites, acute and chronic renal failure,* and *hypertension.* Less often, it may be indicated when the administration of exogenous corticosteroids causes salt retention in women with premenstrual edema. A low-sodium diet is often used together with diuretic agents. In certain cases, only one or the other of these therapies is necessary. In disorders associated with sodium retention and low levels of urinary sodium, the diet may be very important. In many cases of hypertension, drug therapy, perhaps in conjunction with mild sodium restriction, may be more useful, with better patient compliance.
   3. Practical aspects
      a. General instructions. *Patient information on this topic is available in Appendix D.*
         (1) The degree of sodium restriction required differs greatly among patients; a no-added-salt diet may suffice, or one that strictly limits salt-containing foods may be necessary.
         (2) Sodium is present in table salt, drinking water (depending on the source), medicines, and baked goods in which regular baking powder or soda is used. It is also present in foods seasoned with monosodium glutamate; preserved with brine, sodium benzoate, or sodium sulfite; or processed with sodium hydroxide, sodium alginate, or sodium propionate.
         (3) Many products used in food preparation contain sodium. Products that should not be used in food preparation unless their sodium content is known include baking powder, baking soda,

barbecue sauce, beverages (fruit-flavored mixes, many car-bonated sodas), bouillon cubes, canned broth, catsup, celery salt, celery flakes, celery seed, chili sauce, consommé, garlic salt, horseradish (prepared), instant cocoa mixes, olives, onion salt, commercial gelatin (Jell-O), monosodium glutamate, mustard (prepared), meat extract and sauces, meat tenderizers, molasses, parsley flakes, pickles, relishes, soy sauce, salad dressing, sodium saccharine, Worcestershire sauce, rennet tablets, some salt substitutes, mayonnaise, bacon bits, maraschino cherries, and salted nuts.

(4) **The sodium content** given for foods is approximate but much larger than usually appreciated. It is helpful to consider which foods are equivalent to a given amount of sodium. For example:

(a) **50 mg of sodium:** 1 tsp salted butter or margarine, $\frac{1}{2}$ cup raw carrots, $1\frac{1}{2}$ tsp mayonnaise, 1 small egg, $\frac{1}{2}$ cup ice cream or sherbet

(b) **250 mg of sodium:** 1 oz canned tuna, $\frac{2}{3}$ cup buttermilk, $\frac{1}{2}$ cup canned vegetables, 5 salted crackers, $1\frac{1}{2}$ tbs salad dressing, 1 large strip of bacon, $\frac{1}{2}$ cup cold cereal, $\frac{1}{4}$ cup cottage cheese, $\frac{1}{8}$ of a 9-in pie, 2 slices of bacon

(c) **500 mg of sodium:** $\frac{1}{4}$ scant tsp salt, $\frac{3}{4}$ tsp monosodium glutamate, $\frac{1}{2}$ bouillon cube, $\frac{2}{3}$ cup canned tomato juice, 1 average-sized frankfurter, 7 or 8 green olives (small), 2 tsp regular soy sauce

(d) **800 to 1,000 mg of sodium:** 1 dill pickle, 1 cup canned vegetable soup (preparations vary)

(5) **Sodium labeling.** The daily value for sodium is 2,400 mg in the United States.

Sodium-free: <5 mg per serving

Very low in sodium: ≤35 mg per serving

Low in sodium: ≤140 mg per serving

Light in sodium/lightly salted: ≤50% reduction in sodium per serving versus reference food

Reduced in sodium or less sodium: ≤25% reduction in sodium per serving versus reference food

(6) Cooking "from scratch" is usually the best way to prepare foods. Salt should not be added in cooking unless the patient can tolerate the added sodium. Patients should cook with oil or with unsalted butter or margarine.

(7) Lemon juice, onion, red pepper, Tabasco sauce, and garlic are excellent substitute seasonings for meats and fish. See Table 7-10 for a list of other natural seasonings that can be substituted for salt to flavor foods.

(8) Low-sodium baking powder is available in many stores that sell dietetic foods. If it is not available, the pharmacist can make it up with the following formula:

Potassium bicarbonate	39.8 g
Cornstarch	28.0 g
Tartaric acid	7.5 g
Potassium bitartrate	56.1 g

If the patient is on a diet that limits potassium, excessive amounts of potassium-containing baking powder should not be ingested.

(9) **A large number of cookbooks for low-sodium diets** are available in most retail bookstores. One suggested title is Franey P. *Low-Calorie Gourmet* (New York: Times Books, 1984). The recipes use small amounts of salt that can be replaced with a salt substitute. Many spices are included in the recipes, so that the replacement is relatively easy.

b. Specific recommendations

    (1) Diets are ordered as salt (sodium chloride) or as sodium, which is about 40% of the weight of salt. Ordering *dietary prescriptions* by sodium content is more sensible because the "salt" content cannot actually be measured. The usual restrictions ordered are listed in Table 11-23.

    (2) Decrease the use of table salt and seasonings high in sodium (e.g., soy sauce, garlic salt, onion salt), and substitute herbs and other spices. If salt substitutes are used, make certain that the patient is not on medication that causes hyperkalemia (e.g., triamterene).

    (3) Limit intake of foods known to be high in sodium.

    (4) Avoid less obvious sources of sodium, including foods that contain MSG, sodium saccharine, sodium nitrate (curing agent), and sodium benzoate (preservative). Some over-the-counter medications, such as antacids, laxatives, and sleeping pills, contain large quantities of sodium. For example, Alka-Seltzer effervescent antacid tablets contain 276 mg of sodium per tablet. Labels of over-the-counter products should be read carefully.

    (5) Modify recipes to include low-sodium ingredients—either prepared products labeled as such or fresh fruits, vegetables, meats, and fish. Particularly avoid canned products. Low-sodium cheese and peanut butter are available, as are unsalted crackers, low-sodium canned soups, and unsalted chips and popcorn.

    (6) When dining out, choose foods without sauces or gravies, use oil/vinegar dressing for salads, choose fresh fruit for dessert, and ask that no salt be added to individually prepared dishes (e.g., steak or fish). Avoid fast foods.

4. Side effects. The low-sodium diet is not easy for some patients to follow because the intake of sodium in most Western diets is large. Care must be taken to maintain good protein intake. Because large amounts of fruits and vegetables are allowed, the intake of most vitamins and minerals is adequate.

    a. When a patient on a low-sodium diet also takes a diuretic, *hypokalemia* often develops. Potassium can be replaced by table foods or by medication (see Chapter 7).

    b. Sodium depletion can develop in a patient on a low-sodium diet when urinary sodium losses are continuously high, as in chronic renal disease. Patients with obligatory sodium losses from ileostomies are also at risk for the development of sodium depletion if dietary sodium is restricted.

5. Supplements required. Potassium may be needed if diuretics are used, but no other supplements are required.

J. Restriction of serotonin-rich foods. When a urinary collection for 5-hydroxyindoleacetic acid (5-HIAA) is ordered, the patient should not consume foods rich in serotonin or medications that react with the reagents used in the test. Foods to be avoided include avocado, bananas, butternut squash, eggplant, kiwi fruit, pecans, plantains, pineapple, plums, tomatoes, walnuts, and alcohol (82). Alcohol presumably stimulates the production of serotonin. Medications to be avoided are glyceryl guaiacolate, acetaminophen, and phenacetin; they interfere with the urinary and serum determinations.

K. Diet for occult blood screening (low-peroxidase diet)

1. Principle. Screening for occult blood in stool is of proven efficacy. When standard low-sensitivity, peroxidase-based tests (e.g., Hemoccult) are used, the ingestion of red meat and uncooked peroxidase-rich plants (radish, turnip, broccoli) can produce false-positive results, although the effect is small. The low-meat diet and six mail-in stool sample cards are

Table 11-23. Salt-restricted diets

Daily intake (g)		Restrictions					Practicality
Sodium	Salt	Added salt	Visibly salted items[a]	Processed foods[b]	Milk, bread[c]	Meat, eggs	
5–6	12.5–15	Yes	Yes	Yes	Yes	Yes	Average U.S. diet
4	10	No	Yes	Yes	Yes	Yes	Home use
3	7.5	No	No	Many	Yes	Yes	Home use
2	5.0	No	No	Few	Yes	Yes	Home use; needs cooperation
1	2.5	No	No	No	Salt-free bread	Yes	Needs great cooperation for home use
0.5	1.25	No	No	No	1 pt milk	4 oz meat, 1 egg	Hospital use

[a]Includes potato chips, pretzels, crackers or snacks, pickles, olives, and bacon.
[b]Includes most canned foods, dry cereals, prepared meats, ham, cheese, and prepared desserts.
[c]One hundred twenty milligrams of sodium per 8 oz of milk or 1 slice of bread.

generally used, especially if the level of meat intake is high. The specificity of the available tests for routine fecal blood testing is affected by peroxidase-containing foods. The use of rehydrated Hemoccult or similar guaiac-impregnated cards increases the false-positive rate, and a low-peroxidase diet has been shown to reduce the false-positive rate from above 6% to 0.6% (55). Many clinicians have abandoned rehydrated guaiac techniques and ignore diet in their screening programs (83). However, a small increase in specificity can have a major impact on clinical decisions, so that when outpatient screening for occult blood is performed, it seems prudent at the present time to recommend a meat-free, low-peroxidase diet (84).

2. **A low-peroxidase diet is indicated** when guaiac-containing cards are used to screen for colorectal neoplasms.

3. **Practical aspects**
   a. **General instructions.** The low-peroxidase diet avoids red meat, raw or cooked. Although the peroxidase activity of most fruits and vegetables is destroyed completely by cooking at 100°C for 20 minutes, well-cooked red meat retains some activity. Because of the high level of peroxidase activity in red meat and uncertainty regarding how thoroughly cooked meat may be, all red meat is proscribed. Peroxidase-rich fruits and vegetables (categories 1 through 5, Table 11-24) are also eliminated.
   b. **Specific recommendations.** Foods in categories 1 to 5 (Table 11-24) are eliminated for 1 to 2 days before stool sampling begins and for 3 days consecutively, during which time one sample is collected per day. Aspirin-containing medications are not permitted, but it is not clear whether aspirin in modest doses increases fecal blood loss.
   Patient information on this topic is available in Appendix D.

L. **Vitamin K-restricted diet**
   1. **Principle.** Foods with a high content of vitamin K may interfere with the smooth control of anticoagulation. The dietary intake of vitamin K is only one of many factors influencing blood clotting in patients on long-term

Table 11-24. Peroxidase levels in foods

Category	Peroxidase activity[a] (mL of blood equivalent)	Food items
1	>20	Broccoli, turnip[b]
2	10–20	Rare red meat, cantaloupe, cauliflower, red radish, parsnips
3	5–10	Bean sprouts, cucumber, green beans, mushrooms, parsley, zucchini, lemon rind
4	2–5	Grapefruit, carrot, cabbage, potato, pumpkin, fig
5	1–2	Peach, celery, lettuce, spinach, pickles
6	0.2–1.0	Blackberries, pineapple, watermelon, walnuts, sweet peppers
7	0.1–0.2	Banana, black grapes, pear, plum
8	<0.1	Well-cooked meat, apples, apricot, olives, raspberries
9	Peroxidase undetectable	Roast chicken, turkey, cooked fish, organ meats, pork, ham and bacon, white grapes, lemon, nectarine, orange, strawberries, tomato, raisins

[a] The peroxidase activity in 100 g of food is reported as the equivalent of "x" milliliters of blood.
[b] The data refer to uncooked vegetables. Adequate cooking destroys peroxidase activity.
Adapted from Caligore P, et al. *Am J Clin Nutr* 1982;35:1487.

warfarin therapy. It is not clear whether the dietary intake of vitamin K is a significant factor because fecal flora produce the vitamin, and it can be absorbed in the colon.

2. **Indication.** This diet is used for patients receiving anticoagulant therapy when the regulation of anticoagulation is difficult or the patient is more resistant to warfarin therapy than expected.

3. **Practical aspects.** All foods are allowed except those containing more than 100 mg of vitamin K per 100 g. These include broccoli, brussels sprouts, green or white cabbage, cauliflower, kale, lettuce, soybeans, spinach, turnip greens, beef liver or kidney, and pork liver.

M. Copper-restricted diet

1. **Principle.** Wilson's disease is characterized by an increase in total body and hepatic copper. Treatment consists of a low copper intake plus chelating therapy. Other cholestatic liver diseases (e.g., primary biliary cirrhosis) are characterized by elevated levels of hepatic copper, but it is not clear that removal of copper alters the clinical course.

2. **Indication.** For patients with Wilson's disease.

3. **Practical aspects.** Milk, coffee, lemonade, carbonated beverages, and vanilla ice cream may be consumed freely. Regular table salt should be avoided. Analytic reagent-grade salt, available through the pharmacist, may be used as desired. Almost no foods are copper-free, so the more caloric and protein needs can be met by low-copper foods, the better. A list of foods low in copper has been published (85). As Wilson's disease is diagnosed earlier and effective drug therapy is used to create a negative copper balance, the strict use of low-copper diets becomes unnecessary. Obviously, the less copper ingested, the less drug theoretically needed to produce a negative copper balance, although this effect has not been quantified.

N. Dietary supplements. Products are marketed as supplements, functional foods, "dietetic" foods, "neutriceuticals," and phytochemicals. Their purpose is to improve function not only in healthy people but also in patients with restricted diets. Such use has been spurred by the passage of the Dietary Supplement Health and Education Act of 1994, which formally defined dietary supplements. Because these supplements were regulated as foods and not as drugs, manufacturers did not have to prove efficacy. As of March 1999, all vitamin, mineral, herbal, and supplement products must include "nutrition facts" in their label. Nutrients are listed as percentage of daily value, although the dose is called a "serving." Nutrients labeled "high potency" must supply at least 100% of the daily value, and multivitamins must supply 100% of the daily value of two-thirds of the contents. "Antioxidants" must prevent chemical damage *in vitro*. However, neither label means that the product is effective. For any health claims, the label must carry the following disclaimer: "This statement has not been evaluated by the Food and Drug Administration." The National Institutes of Health Office of Dietary Supplements views a supplement as any substance consumed in addition to the regular diet—that is, in addition to meals, snacks, and beverages (86). The American Dietetic Association has published a useful guide to many of these supplements (87).

Table 11-25 lists many of the supplements that are specific nutrients. Those that are micronutrients (vitamins and minerals) are discussed in Chapters 6 and 7. Some of the others are discussed in Chapter 15, "Alternative Nutritional Therapy." The National Institutes of Health Office of Dietary Supplements and the Consumer Healthcare Products Association have initiated a bibliography to highlight scientifically sound research on dietary supplements and their role in health maintenance. Copies of the document are posted on the Internet (*http://ods.od.nih.gov/publications/publications.html*) and are available from the Office of Dietary Supplements at *ods@nih.gov* or 301-435-2920.

O. "Functional" foods. This term is used to describe physiologically active foods and is often used synonymously with the terms *neutriceutical, de-*

Table 11-25. Selected dietary supplements

Supplement	Marketing claims	Efficacy	Adverse effects
Alanine	Spares muscle	Not proven	None
	Stabilizes blood sugar	Equivocal	
Arginine	Helps CV disease, immune Fx	Possibly Equivocal	None
	Builds muscle mass	Not proven	
Boron	Prevents osteoporosis	Not proven	Toxic >50 mg/d
	Improves memory, libido		
BCAA	↑ Muscle mass, exercising	Not proven	↑ NH_3 if >20 g/d
Calcium	Prevents osteoporosis	Proven	U.L. 2,500 mg/d
	↓ Blood pressure	Possibly	↑ Absorption of Fe,
	↓ Colon cancer risk	Equivocal	other drugs
L-Carnitine	Helps heart, immune function	Not proven	Diarrhea >6 g/d
β-Carotene	↓ Cancer prevalence	Probably not	May ↑ lung cancer in
	↑ Immunity, helps CV disease	No	male smokers
Chromium	Helps control diabetes	Possibly	Safe daily intake
	Lowers cholesterol	Equivocal	50–200 µg
	↓ Body fat	No	
Creatine	↑ Muscle strength, ↑ muscle mass	Equivocal Not proven	Water retention
Folate	Prevents birth defects	Yes	Masks B_{12} deficiency
	Prevents colon cancer	Not proven	at >400 µg/d, impairs
	Prevents depression	Not proven	Anticonvulsants >5 mg/d
Fructo-oligosaccharides	Supports GI tract health	Equivocal	Bloating, cramps, diarrhea at >50 g/d
	Controls blood sugar, cholesterol	Not proven	
Glucosamine	Relieves arthritis pain	Possibly	None
Glutamine	Enhances immune system	Equivocal	None
Lecithin	Helps Alzheimer's, memory	No	Diarrhea >20 g/d
Lysine	↓ Herpesvirus effect	Equivocal	↓ Arginine absorption
	↓ Angina	Not proven	
Magnesium	↓ CV disease, BP	Equivocal	U.L. 350 mg/d
	↓ Migraine, PMS	Equivocal	
Pantothenate	Blocks stress, ↓ cholesterol	Not proven	None
Phosphatidylserine (source, bovine brain extract)	Improves memory in elderly, raises IQ	Equivocal Not proven	? Contains B_{12}
Potassium	↓ Blood pressure	Possibly	GI ulcer, bleeding >6 g/d
			↑ [K], inhibits ACE
Pyruvate	↓ Cholesterol, weight	Not proven	Flatus, diarrhea
Selenium	↓ Cancer risk	Possibly	Toxic >750 µg/d
	Helps heart, immune function	Not proven	

continued

Table 11-25. (Continued)

Supplement	Marketing claims	Efficacy	Adverse effects
Vitamin A	Improves immunity	Possibly	Toxic >50,000 IU/d
	Improves skin disease	Yes	Teratogenic
	Reverses skin aging	Not proven	>3,000 IU/d
Vitamin B_1	↑ Energy	No	None
B_2	↑ Energy, helps migraine	No	None
B_3	↓ Cholesterol	Yes	Flushing, diarrhea
B_6	Improves PMS, autism	Equivocal	Nerve damage
	Improves heart Fx	Possibly	>500 mg/d
B_{12}	Improves dementia, energy	No	None
	↑ Function in elderly deficient	Yes	
Vitamin C	Improve cold Sx, ↓ heart disease	Equivocal	Diarrhea >3 g/d
	Protects vs. cancer, cataracts	Possibly	↑ Fe absorption in hemochromatosis ↑ Oxalate excretion
Vitamin D	↑ Ca^{++} absorption, bone health	Yes	U.L. 1,000 IU (50 μg)
	↓ Cancer risk	Equivocal	
Vitamin E	Improve diabetes, immunity	Possibly	↑ Bleeding if on Anticoagulants
	↓ Heart attack, cataracts	Possibly	
	Improve lung Fx, psychiatric illness	Possibly	
Zinc	Improve cold Sx, taste	Not proven	↓ Cu absorption >100 mg/d
	↑ immunity, fertility, skin	No	↑ Cholesterol, nausea at high dose

Explanation of efficacy: Yes, several controlled trials in humans; possibly, preliminary data from controlled trials; equivocal, conflicting controlled data in humans; not proven, not enough data in humans or data are poor; no, human data not supportive.
U.L., upper limit recommended by Food and Nutrition Board, National Academy of Science; PMS, premenstrual syndrome; ACE, angiotensin-converting enzyme; BCAA, branched-chain amino acid.

signer food, and *medical food.* The orphan drugs amendment to the Food, Drug, and Cosmetic Act (1988) defines *medical food* as "a food which is formulated to be consumed or administered enterally under the supervision of a physician and which is intended for the specific management of a disease or condition for which distinctive nutritional requirements, based on recognized scientific principles, are established by medical evaluation." However, medical foods are not subject to regulation by the Food and Drug Administration, and in 1990, the National Labeling Education Act exempted medical foods from its labeling requirements (88). "Functional" foods were defined in the Food, Drug, and Cosmetic Act of 1938 as "articles intended for the diagnosis, cure, mitigation, treatment, or prevention of disease." More recently, they have been defined as "any food or food ingredient that may provide a health benefit beyond that conferred by the nutrients the food contains" (86).

The European definition is by consensus the following: "A food can be regarded as functional if it is satisfactorily demonstrated to affect beneficially one or more target functions in the body, beyond adequate nutritional effects, in a way which is relevant to either the state of well-being and health or the reduction of the risk of a disease" (89).

Currently, the Food and Drug Administration has approved health claims for the following foods in the prevention of chronic disease: fiber-containing products for cancer and cardiovascular disease, fruits and vegetables for cancer, and calcium for osteoporosis. It also recognizes the relationship between saturated fat and cholesterol and the risk for cardiovascular disease, dietary fat and cancer, sodium and hypertension, and sugar alcohols and dental caries (86,88). The Dietary Supplement Health and Education Act of 1994, which exempts dietary supplements from regulation as drugs and food additives, also allows structure/function claims to be made and literature about functional foods to be distributed. Claims can be made that functional foods are modifiers of oxidative damage, anticarcinogens, enhancers of gastrointestinal function (including probiotics and prebiotics), and agents of immunomodulation, neuroregulation, cholesterol metabolism, blood pressure control, and allergic responses. Prebiotics and probiotics are considered "functional" foods by some because they contain or produce components similar to those in some functional foods (90). Probiotics, such as yogurt, are viable microbial dietary supplements that benefit the host by altering the milieu in the intestinal lumen. The number of organisms studied is small but growing, and their use must be confirmed by double-blinded, placebo-controlled trials. Indications that appear promising include rotavirus- and antibiotic-associated diarrhea in children, *Clostridium difficile*-associated diarrhea, traveler's diarrhea (91), and chronic pouchitis after ileoanal anastomosis for ulcerative

Table 11-26. Physiologically active compounds in functional foods

Compound	Food source	Potential health benefit
Isothiocyanates	Cruciferous vegetables	Chemoprevention of cancer by altering drug-metabolizing enzymes
Epigallocatechin	Green tea	↓ Cancer/heart disease by antioxidation
Carotenoids	Tomatoes, carrots, citrus fruits, yams	↓ Cancer/heart disease by antioxidation
Lactoferrin	Milk	Stimulate immune system, antimicrobial
Conjugated linoleic acid	Dairy products	Prevention of cancer/ atherosclerosis
Genestein and other isoflavones	Soybeans, soy foods	↓ Menopausal symptoms, osteoporosis, cancer, heart disease
Diallyl disulfide	Garlic, onions	Prevention of cancer, ↑ immune function, ↓ serum cholesterol, triglyceride
Limonene	Citrus fruits	Prevention of cancer
Nondigestible oligosaccharides	Garlic, asparagus, chicory	↑ Immune function, ↓ serum cholesterol
ω-3 Fatty acids	Algae, fish	↓ Serum cholesterol/heart disease, suppress immune function
Coumarins	Vegetables, citrus fruits	↓ Blood clotting, anticarcinogenic

colitis (92). However, current commercial probiotic preparations often contain nonviable organisms or bacterial counts well below those on the label. Prebiotics are food ingredients that are not digested in the small intestine, such as fiber components or fructo-oligosaccharides, and that selectively stimulate the growth or activity of some colonic bacteria. The numbers of many of these products (supplements, functional foods, prebiotics, probiotics) on the market have been increasing, so that they now account for a significant proportion of the total food market in Western countries. It will take years to discover and evaluate their potential therapeutic value, and so only some of the better-defined substances, such as vitamins and minerals, can be covered any detail in this manual. Table 11-26 lists some of the compounds included in functional foods and the claims that may be made for them (87).

Bibliography

1. American Dietetic Association. *Handbook of clinical dietetics*. New Haven: Yale University Press, 1981.
2. Nelson JK, Moxness KE, Gastineau CF. Mayo Clinic diet manual, 7th ed. Mosby—Year Book, 1994.
3. Feldman EB. How grapefruit juice potentiates drug bioavailability. *Nutr Rev* 1997;55:398.
4. Rainey C, Affleck M, Bretschger K, et al. The California avocado. *Nutrition Today* 1994;29:23.
5. The Dietary Guidelines 2000 Committee to Build a Healthy Base. *http://www.ars. usda.gov/dgac.*
6. Singer AJ, Werther K, Nestle M. The nutritional value of university-hospital diets. *N Engl J Med* 1996;335:1466.
7. Wotecki CE, Thomas PR. *Eat for life*. Washington, DC: National Academy Press, 1992.
8. Dwyer JT. Health aspects of vegetarian diets. *Am J Clin Nutr* 1988;48:712.
9. Eagon JC, Alpers D. Gut rest versus early feeding after elective abdominal surgery. *Nutrition* 1997;13:155.
10. Emerson JL, Chappel CI. Health effects of coffee, tea, mate, cocoa, and their major methylxanthine components. In: Van der Heijden K, Younes M, Fishbein L, et al., eds. *International food safety handbook*. New York: Marcel Dekker, 1999:141.
11. Cnattingius S, Signorello LB, Anneren G, et al. Caffeine intake and the risk of first-trimester spontaneous abortion. *N Engl J Med* 2000;343:1839.
12. Pehl C, Waizenhoefer A, Wendl B, et al. Effect of low and high fat meals on lower esophageal sphincter motility and gastroesophageal reflux in healthy subjects. *Am J Gastroenterol* 1999;94:1192.
13. Bravo L. Polyphenols: chemistry, dietary sources, metabolism, and nutritional significance. *Nutr Rev* 1998;56:317.
14. Trevisanato SI, Kim Y-I. Tea and health. *Nutr Rev* 2000;58:1.
15. Decker EA. Phenolics: prooxidants or antioxidants. *Nutr Rev* 1997;55:396.
16. Roberfroid MB. Fructo-oligosaccharide malabsorption: benefit for gastrointestinal functions. *Curr Opin Gastroenterol* 2000;16:173.
17. Gibson GR, Roberfroid MB. Dietary modulation of the human colonic microbiota: introducing the concept of prebiotics. *J Nutr* 1995;125:1401.
18. Jenkins DJA, Kendall CWC. Resistant starches. *Curr Opin Gastroenterol* 2000;16:178.
19. Van Soest PJ, McQueen RW. The chemistry and estimation of fibre. *Proc Nutr Soc* 1973;32:123.
20. Englyst HN, Quigley ME, Hudson GJ. Determination of dietary fibre as non-starch polysaccharides with gas-liquid chromatographic, high-performance liquid chromatographic or spectrophotometric measurement of constituent sugars. *Analyst* 1994;119:1497.
21. Anderson JW, Bridges SR. Dietary fiber content of selected foods. *Am J Clin Nutr* 1988;47:440.
22. Southgate, DAT, Waldron K, Johnson LT, Fenwick GR. *Dietary fiber: chemical and biological aspects*. Boca Raton, FL: CRC Press, 1991.
23. Cummings JH. Cellulose and the human gut. *Gut* 1984;25:805.

24. Cummings JH, Englyst HN. Fermentation in the human large intestine and the available substrates. *Am J Clin Nutr* 1987;45:1243.
25. *National Health and Nutrition Examination Survey III, 1988–94.* NCHS CD-ROM series 11, No. 2A. ASCII version. Hyattsville, MD: National Center for Health Statistics, April 1998.
26. Kritchevsky D, et al., eds. *Dietary fiber.* New York: Plenum Publishing, 1990.
27. Wolk A, Manson JE, Stampfer MJ, et al. Long-term intake of dietary fiber and decreased risk of coronary heart disease among women. *JAMA* 1999;281:1998.
28. Chandalia M, Garg A, Jutjohann D, et al. Beneficial effects of high dietary fiber intake in patients with type 2 diabetes mellitus. *N Engl J Med* 2000;342:1392.
29. Aldoori WH, Giovannucci EL, Rimm EB, et al. A prospective study of diet and the risk of symptomatic diverticular disease in men. *Am J Clin Nutr* 1994;60:757.
30. AGA Clinical Practice and Practice Economics Committee. AGA technical review: impact of dietary fiber on colon cancer occurrence. *Gastroenterology* 2000;118:1235.
31. Hill MJ. Cereals, cereal fibre and colorectal cancer risk: a review of the epidemiological literature. *Eur J Cancer Prev* 1998;7[Suppl 2]:S5.
32. Fuchs CS, Giovannucci, Colditz GA, et al. Dietary fiber and the risk of colorectal cancer and adenoma in women. *N Engl J Med* 1999;340:169.
33. Brown L, Rosner B, Willett WW, et al. Cholesterol-lowering effects of dietary fiber: a meta-analysis. *Am J Clin Nutr* 1999;69:30.
34. Levin EG, Miller VT, Muesing RA, et al. Comparison of psyllium hydrophilic mucilloid and cellulose as adjuncts to a prudent diet in the treatment of mild to moderate hypercholesterolemia. *Arch Intern Med* 1990;150:1822.
35. Jenkins DJA, Kendall CWC, Vuksan V. Viscous fibers, health claims, and strategies to reduce cardiovascular risk. *Am J Clin Nutr* 2000;71:401.
36. Kim Y-I. Short-chain fatty acids in ulcerative colitis. *Nutr Rev* 1998;56:17.
37. Bright-See E, McKeown-Eyssen GE. Estimation of per capita crude and dietary fiber supply in 38 countries. *Am J Clin Nutr* 1984;39:821.
38. Lanza E, Jones DY, Block G, et al. Dietary fiber intake in the U.S. population. *Am J Clin Nutr* 1987;46:790.
39. Committee on Nutrition, American Academy of Pediatrics. *Pediatrics* 1981;67:572.
40. Lin HC, Zhao XT, Chu AW, et al. Fiber-supplemented enteral formula slows intestinal transit by intensifying inhibitory feedback from the distal gut. *Am J Clin Nutr* 1997;65:1840.
41. Jenkins DJA, Jenkins AL, Wolever TM, et al. Simple and complex carbohydrates. *Nutr Rev* 1986;44:44.
42. Frost G, Leeds A, Dore C, et al. Glycaemic index as a determinant of serum HDL-cholesterol concentration. *Lancet* 1999;353:1045.
43. Lin HC, Zhao T, Wang L. Intestinal transit is more potently inhibited by fat in the distal (ileal brake) than in the proximal (jejunal brake) gut. *Dig Dis Sci* 1997;42:19.
44. Simko V, McCarroll AM, Goodman S, et al. High-fat diet in a short bowel syndrome. Intestinal absorption and gastroenteropancreatic hormone responses. *Dig Dis Sci* 1980;25:333.
45. Ladas SD, Haritos DN, Raptis SA. Honey may have a laxative effect on normal subjects because of incomplete fructose absorption. *Am J Clin Nutr* 1995;62:1212.
46. Riby JE, Fujisawa T, Kretchmer N. Fructose absorption. *Am J Clin Nutr* 1993;58[Suppl 5]:748S.
47. Nobigrot T, Chasalow FI, Lifshitz F. Carbohydrate absorption from one serving of fruit juice in young children: age and carbohydrate composition effects. *J Am Coll Nutr* 1997;16:152.
48. Kulczycki A. Aspartame-induced urticaria. *Ann Intern Med* 1986;104:207.
49. Shaw AD, Davies GJ. Lactose intolerance: problems in diagnosis and treatment. *J Clin Gastroenterol* 1999;28:208.
50. Paige DM, Bayless TM, eds. *Lactose digestion.* Baltimore: Johns Hopkins University, 1981.
51. Committee on Nutrition, American Academy of Pediatrics. The practical significance of lactose intolerance in children. *Pediatrics* 1990;86:643.

52. Kolars JC, Levitt MD, Aouji M, et al. Yogurt—an autodigesting source of lactose. *N Engl J Med* 1984;310:1.
53. Martini MC, Savaiano DA. Reduced intolerance symptoms from lactose consumed during a meal. *Am J Clin Nutr* 1988;47:57.
54. Vesper H, Schmelz E-M, Nikolova-Karakashian MN, et al. Sphingolipids in food and the emerging importance of sphingolipids to nutrition. *J Nutr* 1999;129:1239.
55. Yamada T, Alpers DH, Laine L, et al., eds. *Textbook of gastroenterology,* 3rd ed. Philadelphia: Lippincott–Raven Publishers, 1999.
56. American Dietetic Association. *Nutrition trends survey 1997.* Chicago: The American Dietetic Association, 1997.
57. Bach A, Babayan VK. Medium-chain triglycerides—an update. *Am J Clin Nutr* 1982;36:950.
58. Bach AC, Ingenbleek Y, Frey A. The usefulness of dietary medium-chain triglycerides in body weight control: fact or fancy? *J Lipid Res* 1996;37:708.
59. Sandler RS, Zorich NL, Filloon TG, et al. Gastrointestinal symptoms in 3,181 volunteers ingesting snack food containing olestra or triglycerides. *Ann Intern Med* 1999;130:253.
60. Balasekaran R, Porter JL, Santa Ana CA, et al. Positive results on tests for steatorrhea in persons consuming olestra potato chips. *Ann Intern Med* 2000;132:279.
61. Connor WE, Bendich A. Highly unsaturated fatty acids in nutrition and disease prevention. *Am J Clin Nutr* 71[Suppl 1]:169S.
62. Naylor CD, O'Rourke K, Detsky AS, et al. Parenteral nutrition with branched-chain amino acids in hepatic encephalopathy. A meta-analysis. *Gastroenterology* 1989;97:1033.
63. Klein S, Kinney J, Jeejeebhoy K, et al. Nutrition support in clinical practice: review of published data and recommendations for future research directions. *JPEN J Parenter Enteral Nutr* 1997;21:133.
64. Pedrini MT, Levey AS, Lau J, et al. The effect of dietary protein restriction on the progression of diabetic and nondiabetic renal diseases: a meta-analysis. *Ann Intern Med* 1996;124:627.
65. Sullivan DH, Sun S, Walls RC. Protein-energy undernutrition among elderly hospitalized patients: a prospective study. *JAMA* 1999;281:2013.
66. Schurch M-E, Rizzoli R, Slosman D, et al. Protein supplements increase serum insulin-like growth factor-I levels and attenuate proximal femur bone loss in patients with recent hip fracture. A randomized, double-blind, placebo-controlled trial. *Ann Intern Med* 1998;128:801.
67. Ziegler TR, Mulligan K, eds. ASPEN research workshop: anabolic hormones in nutrition support. *JPEN J Parenter Enteral Nutr* 1999;23[Suppl 6]:S173.
68. Hardman CM, Garioch JJ, Leonard JN, et al. Absence of toxicity of oats in patients with dermatitis herpetiformis. *N Engl J Med* 1997;337:1884.
69. Murray JA. The widening spectrum of celiac disease. *Am J Clin Nutr* 1999;69:354.
70. Bloch AS, Shils ME. *Appendix.* In: Shils ME, Olson JA, Shike M, et al., eds. *Modern nutrition in health and disease,* 9th ed. Baltimore: Williams & Wilkins, 1999:A198.
71. Madsen C, Wuthrich B. Food sensitivities, allergic reactions, and food intolerances. In: van der HeijdenK, Younes M, Fishbein L, et al., eds. *International food safety handbook.* New York: Marcel Dekker, 1999:447.
72. Frieri M, Kettelhut BV. *Food hypersensitivity and adverse reactions: a practical guide for diagnosis and management.* New York: Marcel Dekker, 1999.
73. Sampson HA. Food allergy. *JAMA* 1997;278:1888.
74. Sampson HA, Sicherer SH, Birnbaum AH. AGA technical review on the evaluation of food allergy in gastrointestinal disorders. *Gastroenterology* 2001;120:1026.
75. Bengtsson U, Hanson LA, Ahlstedt S. Survey of gastrointestinal reactions to foods in adults in relation to atopy, presence of mucus in the stools, swelling of joints and arthralgia in patients with gastrointestinal reactions to foods. *Clin Exp Allergy* 1996;26:1387.
76. Rix KJ, Pearson DJ, Bentley SJ. A psychiatric study of patients with supposed food allergy. *Br J Psychiatry* 1984;145:121.
77. Atkins FM, Metcalf DD. The diagnosis and treatment of food allergy. *Annu Rev Nutr* 1984;4:253.

78. Levitt MD, Bond JH. Flatulence. *Annu Rev Med* 1980;31:127.
79. Alpha-galactosidase to prevent gas. *Med Lett Drugs Ther* 1993;35:29.
80. Swain AR, Dutton P, Truswell AS. Salicylates in foods. *J Am Diet Assoc* 1985; 85:950.
81. Tiller JW, Dowling JT, Tung LH, et al. Tyramine-induced cardiac arrhythmias. *N Engl J Med* 1985;313:266.
82. Feldman JM, Lee EM, Castleberry CA. Catecholamine and serotonin content of foods: effect on urinary excretion of homovanillic and 5-hydroxyindoleactetic acid. *J Am Diet Assoc* 1987;87:1031.
83. Simon JB. Occult blood screening for colorectal carcinoma: a critical review. *Gastroenterology* 1985;88:820.
84. Markowitz AJ, Winawer SJ. Screening and surveillance for colorectal cancer. *Semin Oncol* 1999;26:485.
85. Pennington TH, Calloway DH. Copper content of foods. Factors affecting reported values. *J Am Diet Assoc* 1993;63:143.
86. Marriott BM. Functional foods: an ecologic perspective. *Am J Clin Nutr* 2000; 71[Suppl]:1728S.
87. DHHS/FDA. Food labeling: general requirements for health claims for food. *Federal Register* 1993;58:2478.
88. Ross S. Functional foods: the Food and Drug Administration perspective. *Am J Clin Nutr* 2000;71[Suppl]:1735S.
89. Bidlack WR, Wang W. Designing functional foods. In: Shils ME, Olson JA, Shike M, et al., eds. *Modern nutrition in health and disease,* 9th ed. Baltimore: Williams & Wilkins, 1999:1823.
90. Diplock AT, Aggott PJ, Ashwell M, et al. Scientific concepts of functional foods in Europe: consensus document. *Br J Nutr* 1999;8[Suppl]:S1.
91. Vanderhof JA, Young RJ. The role of probiotics in the treatment of intestinal infections and inflammation. *Curr Opin Gastroenterol* 2001;17:58.
92. Gionchetti P, Rizzello F, Venturi A, et al. Oral bacteriotherapy as maintenance treatment in patients with chronic pouchitis: a double-blind, placebo-controlled trial. *Gastroenterology* 2000;119:305.

12. DIETARY MANAGEMENT OF DIABETES, RENAL DISEASE, AND HYPERLIPIDEMIA

I. Diabetes

A. Goals and strategies. More than 10 million Americans have diagnosed diabetes, and another 5 to 6 million persons are estimated to have undiagnosed diabetes. Together, they constitute nearly 6% of the population. Diabetes is the seventh leading cause of death in the United States and the sixth leading cause of death by disease. It is the leading cause of blindness in people between the ages of 20 and 74, the leading cause of end-stage renal disease, and a principal cause of neuropathy and peripheral vascular disease. The relative risk for stroke and heart disease is increased twofold to fourfold in patients with diabetes, and heart disease kills nearly 80,000 Americans annually. The overall costs of diabetes treatment and the associated loss of productivity amount to nearly $100 billion annually.

The chronicity of the disease and its myriad complications make diabetes one of the most common problems encountered by physicians.

The National Institutes of Health Diabetes Control and Complications Trial (DCCT) demonstrated unequivocally that prolonged near-normalization of blood glucose in persons with type I diabetes significantly reduces the development and progression of retinopathy, clinical neuropathy, abnormalities of the autonomic nervous system, albuminuria, and microalbuminuria (1–10). On the other hand, at this point in the ongoing 10-year follow up of the original cohort, intensive treatment does not appear to influence the signs of atherosclerosis, which is more influenced by traditional risk factors such as smoking, obesity, and low-density-lipoprotein (LDL) cholesterol (8). Control of dietary intake is one of the key elements of any diabetic treatment regimen aimed at normalizing blood glucose; it is also crucial in the management of obesity and hypercholesterolemia.

1. **Role of dietary management.** Diet plays a major role in regulating carbohydrate, fat, and protein homeostasis in patients with diabetes. Furthermore, proper dietary management is required for the safe and effective use of insulin.

   a. **Successful dietary management of the obese diabetic** leads to weight loss, improves the control of blood sugar, and almost certainly slows the progression of complications. Because the subjects enrolled in the DCCT were nonobese persons with type I diabetes, we do not yet know whether the results can be extrapolated directly to obese persons with type II diabetes, although it is likely that the fundamental conclusions of the DCCT also apply to the latter group. These issues are currently under study in the 27-center, randomized Diabetes Prevention Program Trial, which is attempting to determine whether interventions can delay or prevent the development of type II diabetes in persons at risk, most of whom have a body mass index of 30 or more and approximately half of whom have abnormal lipid profiles (11). Because of poor patient compliance, dietary management in diabetes is usually only partially successful and is frequently totally unsuccessful.

   The obese diabetic usually does not achieve and maintain significant weight loss. The likelihood of compliance is increased by adequate patient education and by attempts to tailor diets according to the needs of individual patients. If a patient is offered no personal dietary instruction other than a preprinted guide to the diabetic diet, the chances of successful compliance are nil.

   b. Most physicians have neither the time nor the knowledge to develop an individualized diet plan for each patient, educate each patient adequately, and follow the patient's dietary progress. *Dietitians, certified diabetes educators,* and other properly trained physician's assistants, who are based in the hospital or physician's office or are in private practice in the community, can formulate plans in cooperation with the physician and instruct patients. Local chapters of the American Diabetes Association and the Juvenile Diabetes Foundation can provide educational support.

2. **Types of diabetes**
   a. **Insulin-dependent (type I) diabetes mellitus** usually begins in childhood or at puberty. Characteristic features are a diminished capacity for insulin secretion at presentation and an absence or virtual absence of insulin secretion within 5 years of onset. The initial diagnosis is usually heralded by the sudden appearance of hyperglycemia, polyuria, polydipsia, polyphagia, weight loss, ketosis, and often coma. However, the pathogenesis of type I diabetes begins long (often years) before the presenting episode with a complex autoimmune response to various pancreatic beta-cell autoantigens that eventually leads to diminished insulin secretion and ultimately beta-cell destruction. Patients with type I diabetes are usually of normal weight. Insulin-dependent diabetics account for approximately 5% to 10% of the diabetic population.
   b. **Non–insulin-dependent (type II) diabetes** usually develops in adulthood, frequently in middle age. However, with an approximate doubling of the prevalence of childhood obesity during the last two decades, the incidence of type II diabetes in children and adolescents has increased dramatically. In type II diabetes, the ability of tissues to respond to insulin action is impaired (insulin resistance). Secondarily, the ability of the pancreas to maintain a compensatory augmented insulin secretory response fails, so that relative insulinopenia (i.e., relative to the degree of hyperglycemia) results. Persons with type II diabetes are usually obese; generally, ketoacidosis does not develop, and they can be managed with diet, oral hypoglycemic agents, or both. Many are best managed by means of exogenous insulin supplementation together with diet therapy. Obesity *per se* contributes to insulin resistance, and insulin secretion must keep up with the demands of increased caloric intake. Thus, the insulin secretion of type II diabetic subjects is frequently adequate to meet the demands of a regular diet in a person whose body weight is not excessive but inadequate to meet the same demands if the subject is overweight and consumes a high-calorie diet. A significant number of adult Americans and, of concern, an increasing number of children and adolescents have type II diabetes. In even more, glucose tolerance is impaired. Strong genetic determinants of type II diabetes have been identified. Defects of single genes cause only a minority of the cases of type II diabetes. A unique form of type II diabetes, maturity-onset diabetes of youth, is sometimes caused by mutations in the glucokinase gene, the hepatic nuclear factor 1α, 1β, and 4α genes, and the pancreatic insulin promoter factor genes, and maternally inherited diabetes with deafness is caused by a mitochondrial DNA gene defect. However, the vast majority of cases of type II diabetes are the result of polygenetic interactions that are as yet unknown.
   c. **Other forms of diabetes.** Clinically significant hyperglycemia is the result of a wide variety of disorders, of which insulin-dependent and non–insulin-dependent diabetes are the most common. Even these two conditions are heterogeneous. In addition, the diabetic phenotype is known to result from genetic defects in the insulin receptor or in insulin processing, and it may also be caused by autoantibodies to the insulin receptor. The diabetic syndrome can be a

secondary finding in various conditions, including pancreatectomy, pancreatitis, hemochromatosis, a wide variety of endocrinopathies, and assorted genetic syndromes (e.g., cystic fibrosis and the chromosomal defects of Down's, Turner's, and Klinefelter's syndromes), and it can be a complication of the use of a variety of drugs.

3. **Diet therapy**

a. For practical purposes, the major divisions of type I (insulin-requiring) and type II (often non–insulin-requiring) diabetes provide a means of classifying dietary management issues (12), although the *goals of diet therapy* in these two groups are similar in most respects (13).

(1) Maintain a nearly normal blood glucose level by balancing food intake, physical activity, and appropriate medical therapy with insulin or oral hypoglycemic agents.

(2) Normalize serum lipid levels.

(3) Provide adequate calories to achieve and maintain a reasonable body weight in adults and to achieve normal growth and development in children and adolescents.

(4) Prevent or delay the progression of the acute and long-term complications of diabetes, including retinopathy, nephropathy, neuropathy, and vascular disease, including hypertension.

(5) Improve overall health through optimal nutrition, as outlined in *Nutrition and Your Health: Dietary Guideline for Americans, 2000* (14) (see Chapter 2).

b. **Strategy of diet therapy for obese, non–insulin-dependent (type II) diabetics.** Although the major goals of dietary therapy for the two types of diabetes are similar, the strategies for reaching these goals differ in some important ways (Table 12-1). Recent extensive and detailed reviews are available (15–18).

(1) The primary therapeutic goal for patients with non–insulin-dependent diabetes is to maintain normal glucose, lipid, and blood pressure levels. Achieving this goal is facilitated by *weight loss,* which is a major focus of diet therapy in obese patients with type II diabetes. However, current strategies for achieving *significant and sustained weight loss* are often ineffective. For this reason, practical therapeutic approaches emphasize pharmacologic and other supportive approaches to control serum glucose, serum lipids, and blood pressure and use moderate caloric restriction paradigms to achieve and sustain at least a modest reduction of weight, in the range of 10 to 20 lb (see Chapter 13).

Regular clinical and biochemical monitoring is essential to evaluate the effects of various treatment regimens aimed at accomplishing the stated goals. For obese diabetics who are not taking insulin or oral hypoglycemic agents, the timing of meals, precise distribution of macronutrients, and day-to-day consistency in dietary patterns are in general somewhat less important than they are in insulin-dependent subjects. However, consistency of meal content and timing may be an adjunct to therapy in selected patients with type II diabetes, as it is in patients with type I diabetes. Management should follow certain principles (13):

(a) Food choices should be guided by the standards of a healthy diet as outlined in the *Nutrition and Your Health: Dietary Guidelines for Americans, 2000* with the food guide pyramid used as a tool (see Chapter 2). These expert recommendations aim for a modest total intake of fat, with a reduction in intake of saturated fat to less than 10% of energy intake, and they often produce a corresponding reduction in total calorie intake because excessive energy

Table 12-1. Dietary strategies for patients with diabetes

Strategy	Obese diabetics who do not require insulin (type II)	Nonobese, insulin-dependent diabetics (type I)
Decrease caloric intake	Yes	No
Protect or improve pancreatic beta-cell function	Priority	Seldom important because beta cells are usually extinct
Increase frequency and number of feedings	Helpful	Yes
Maintain day-to-day consistency of intake of kilocalories, carbohydrate, protein, and fat	Not as crucial as dietary total energy and fat content	Very important
Maintain day-to-day consistency of ratios of carbohydrate, protein, and fat for each of the feedings	Helpful	Desirable
Time meals consistently	Not crucial	Very important
Allow extra food for unusual exercise	Not usually appropriate	Usually appropriate
Use food to treat, abort, or prevent hypoglycemia	Not necessary	Important
During complicating illness, provide small frequent feedings, or give carbohydrate IV to prevent starvation ketosis	Often not necessary because of resistance to ketosis	Important

Adapted from West KM. Diet and diabetes. *Postgrad Med* 1976;60:209.

consumption is linked to dietary intake of fat. Thus, some weight loss is often achieved. *Any* sustained weight loss is a beneficial goal in the management of type II diabetes. A sustained weight loss in the range of 10 to 20 lb can significantly improve the metabolic control of a type II diabetic patient. If for other pressing medical reasons weight loss is a primary therapeutic concern, a more aggressive reduction of dietary fat intake should be recommended. Similarly, if LDL cholesterol is not normalized with a saturated fat intake of less than 10% of total energy intake, a further reduction in saturated fats to less than 7% of energy intake may be advisable (19,20). Compelling data are now available indicating that modest reductions in total fat intake, in which dietary unsaturated fats replace dietary saturated fats, improve serum lipid profiles (21–23).

(b) Long-term compliance with a weight loss diet is more likely if the *caloric restriction is not too stringent.* Moderate caloric reductions to 250 to 500 kcal less than the subject's usual intake are appropriate. An overall calorie allowance of 20 to 25 kcal/kg of ideal body weight allows gradual weight loss (1 to 3 lb/wk) without being so restrictive that compliance is unlikely.

(c) Adjuncts to dietary therapy often can improve both compliance and efficacy. Some patients are able to maintain a reduced dietary intake of energy if their caloric intake is spread throughout the day in the form of meals and snacks rather than three meals alone. Similarly, in addition to improving glycemic control, maintaining lean body mass, and enhancing a general feeling of well being, regular exercise augments energy expenditure. A diabetic patient who exercises can accelerate weight loss on a fixed intake of energy; conversely, the patient can maintain the same rate of weight loss on a smaller reduction in dietary energy intake.

(2) **Supplementation.** Except for diabetic patients on reducing regimens that entail substantial dietary restriction (<1,500 kcal), those with uncontrolled glycosuria, or those who are pregnant, lactating, elderly, or strict vegetarians, routine dietary vitamin and mineral supplementation is not necessary. The primary exceptions are the two that apply to nondiabetic as well as diabetic persons. First, folic acid supplementation or the consumption of foods fortified with folic acid may be necessary for all diabetic women of childbearing age to achieve the CDCP recommendations for a daily folic acid intake of 400 μg. Secondly, elderly persons with diabetes are advised to take supplemental vitamin B_{12} or foods fortified with vitamin B_{12} to achieve an adequate daily intake of that vitamin. Although no consensus recommendation has been made, diabetic women should consider taking a calcium supplement if their dietary calcium intake does not meet current recommended levels.

Dietary deficits of chromium and zinc have been reported in diabetic persons, but little systematic evidence is available to indicate that dietary zinc or chromium supplementation is of clinical benefit. Magnesium deficiency may follow sustained polyuria secondary to hyperglycemia or the use of diuretics, but this also is not a common problem or one that requires routine supplementation. Similarly, iron replacement should be reserved for patients with demonstrable iron deficiency.

(3) **Exchange list.** In many hospitals and outpatient facilities, obese patients with type II diabetes are placed on the same dietary regimen as patients with insulin-dependent type I diabetes and are taught the American Diabetes Association exchange list system. The exchange system is the most extensively used tool for the nutritional instruction of diabetics but is merely a guide to understanding intelligent food choices within the context of a balanced diabetic diet. Alternative approaches are available, and selected patients with type II diabetes may be better served by flexible diet plans if they facilitate compliance and help the patients achieve the goals outlined above. Nonetheless, the American Diabetes Association exchange system remains one of the best ways to provide dietary choice and flexibility and at the same time maintain reasonably consistent energy and macronutrient intake from day to day.

(4) **Prudent diet.** To maintain normal blood lipid profiles, diabetic patients should aim for a prudent diet with a modest intake of total fat (approximately 30% of dietary energy intake), a reduction of saturated fatty acid intake to less than 10% of energy intake, a substitution of monounsaturated and polyunsaturated fats for saturated fats to increase the dietary ratio of polyunsaturated to saturated fats (P:S ratio), and a limited cholesterol intake (although cholesterol-rich foods without high levels of saturated fat, such as egg yolks, have a relatively small effect on plasma cholesterol levels).

(5) **Simple sugars.** In some diabetics, restriction of the intake of simple sugars can be a helpful adjunct to dietary treatment. Little evidence is available to indicate that simple sugars enhance the hyperglycemic response in the context of a complete meal. However, the caloric content of the sugars consumed should be included in the total daily carbohydrate intake and its relationship to energy balance.

c. **Strategy of diet therapy for insulin-dependent (type I) diabetics**

(1) **Insulin secretion in nondiabetics.** In nondiabetics, insulin secretion changes in response to blood sugar. After a meal, insulin secretion increases as blood sugar starts to rise. Nondiabetics can increase or decrease their caloric intake by several times from day to day without becoming hyperglycemic or hypoglycemic because their insulin secretion is tightly regulated.

(2) **Insulin requirements in patients with type I diabetes.** Insulin-requiring, type I diabetics are unable to secrete insulin in response to a rise in blood sugar. Most diabetics who take insulin inject a combination of rapid-, short-, intermediate-, and long-acting insulin on a set schedule more than once a day. The amount and proportions of the insulin dose are determined by preceding glycemia and anticipated glycemic response. Serum insulin levels are determined largely by the types of insulin injected and by the size and timing of the injected insulin dose.

(3) **Timing of food intake.** *None of the currently available insulins, even the so-called rapid-acting insulins, can provide a serum insulin profile to match the immediate release of insulin that occurs in nondiabetic subjects following the ingestion of food.* Thus, the timing of a meal following an injection of insulin is critical. Depending on the type of insulin used, meals are delayed for 15 to 60 minutes after an SC injection of insulin because this period of time is required to achieve an effect of circulating insulin. Furthermore, it is imperative that the composition and distribution of meals be consistent with the composition and expected actions of the insulins injected. Because most patients with type I diabetes inject insulin on a relatively consistent schedule, they also consume meals on a relatively consistent schedule. Insulin doses should be adapted to the patient's lifestyle, schedule, eating preferences, and level of activity. Tailored regimens of this type are the rule for patients who monitor their blood glucose adequately. However, adjustment of the insulin dose is effective only if the caloric content is regular and the temporal distribution of food is consistent with the insulin regimen employed.

(4) **Consistency of composition of meals.** Some *regularity* in the ratio of carbohydrates, proteins, and fats is necessary in each meal. The amount of insulin needed to "cover" a meal can be determined empirically, whatever the composition of the meal, and will remain fairly constant if the total number of ingested calories and ratio of macronutrients remain constant. The purpose of the dietary exchange list system is to provide consistency yet allow flexible food choices.

(5) **The degree of flexibility in the diet** that is consistent with good metabolic control varies from patient to patient. Some patients can vary their caloric intake and dietary composition from day to day and still tightly regulate their blood sugar level by paying careful attention to blood sugar monitoring and insulin dose adjustment. Others require a fixed regimen to control hyperglycemia. The DCCT demonstrated an unequivocal

reduction in diabetic complications following prolonged control of blood sugar, and good control should not be sacrificed for a more liberal diet.

    (6) **Adverse consequences** of rigid glycemic control include (a) the risk for obesity because of diminished urinary loss of glucose calories and the antilipolytic effects of insulin and (b) excessive, significant hypoglycemia. Because we are unable to match plasma insulin and glucose profiles adequately, consistently, and precisely, diabetics who aim for normoglycemia are at a significantly increased risk for episodes of serious hypoglycemia requiring the assistance of another person for resolution. Such episodes can lead to permanent detrimental consequences, both to the diabetic patient and others (e.g., auto accidents). Careful and regular monitoring for adverse effects is required, and the insulin dose and calorie intake must be adjusted as necessary.

B. The dietary prescription must be individualized to accommodate the diabetic patient's lifestyle, eating habits, age, and concurrent disease. The following list can be used to establish such a prescription (12):

1. In order of priority, what are the main general purposes (not strategies or methods) of this patient's prescription?
2. How much does the patient weigh? How much do the doctor, dietitian, and patient think the patient should weigh? How much would the patient like to weigh?
3. What is the appropriate level of caloric consumption for the patient?
4. Does the patient require insulin? If so, is the blood glucose level relatively stable, moderately labile, or severely labile? What kind of insulin is to be given? At what time? In what amount?
5. What, when, and how much would the patient like to eat if he or she did not have diabetes? Are there any special considerations relating to economic factors or to family or cultural dietary propensities?
6. Is the level of carbohydrate to be limited? To what level or range? To what extent and under what conditions, if any, are concentrated carbohydrates to be used?
7. Are there any special requirements concerning levels of protein?
8. Are there any specific or general requirements with respect to levels of dietary fat, either saturated or unsaturated?
9. How much alcohol is to be permitted? Under what conditions? Should alcohol be exchanged for food? If so, what kind and in what amount?
10. If the temporal distribution of food is of any importance, are there specific requirements concerning the following:
    a. The relative size and timing of each of the three main meals?
    b. The timing, size, and characteristics of any extra feedings?
11. To what degree is day-to-day consistency required in
    a. Total kilocalories?
    b. Size and characteristics of specific feedings, such as lunch?
12. Are dietary adjustments to be made for exercise or marked glycosuria? Of what nature?
13. Are there any special conditions unrelated to diabetes that require a special diet (e.g., gout, hyperlipidemia, renal or cardiac failure)?
14. Can all elements of the prescription be reconciled, and how should this be done? (For example, it is usually not feasible to construct a palatable diet for a lean diabetic if the prescription restricts both carbohydrate and fat.)
15. What kind and degree of changes are to be made subsequently by the dietitian without consulting the physician?
16. What should the patient do if it becomes necessary to postpone or modify a meal (e.g., when attending a dinner meeting or social affair)?
17. Tactical questions:

a. How much precision is required in the various elements of this prescription?
b. What foods can be freely allowed?
c. What foods, if any, are to be weighed or measured?
d. Are any modifications of the standard exchange system appropriate, such as simplification?
e. In general, is food to be unmeasured, estimated, measured, or weighed?
f. Is it necessary or desirable to instruct the patient about the carbohydrate, protein, and fat contents of the common foods?
g. Under what circumstances are artificial sweeteners and diet drinks to be used?

18. Has the patient's understanding of dietary principles and methods been systematically evaluated?

C. **Setting up the diabetic diet**
1. **Calculating caloric needs.** The first step in formulating the diabetic diet is to calculate the number of calories the patient requires to achieve or maintain ideal body weight. This is no easy task because no simple approach to the accurate and precise estimation of a specific patient's energy requirements in a clinical setting is available. Caloric requirements are related to the patient's age, level of activity, and desired weight. Basal metabolic rates (BMRs) are in the range of 21 to 29 kcal/kg daily for adults below the age of 60, with women, on average, having BMRs slightly lower than those for men. Above the age of 60, the daily BMR is in the range of 19 to 23 kcal/kg. It is most appropriate to start at the low end of these ranges to estimate energy expenditure (see Chapter 5, Section IA for the World Health Organization/FAO equations used to estimate BMR according to age).

An additional caloric allowance must then be added for the patient's level of physical activity (Tables 5-5 and 5-6). For sedentary persons who engage in only light activity (defined as sitting or standing 75% of the time), the BMR is multiplied by 1.2 to 1.4. For persons who are moderately active, the BMR is multiplied by 1.5 to 1.7. For persons engaged in heavy work, the BMR is multiplied by approximately a factor of 2. Most patients with type II diabetes fall into the sedentary category. Moderately active people are those who engage in regular exercise (e.g., an hour of singles tennis a day). Only those engaged in the most arduous work fall into the marked activity group. As with the initial BMR estimation, it is most appropriate to assume initially that the patient is reasonably sedentary unless clear evidence to the contrary is noted. Thus, for most patients with type II diabetes, the initial estimation of daily caloric requirements will be in the range of about 25 kcal/kg.

2. **Determining the dietary distribution of protein, carbohydrate, and fat.** The various consensus guidelines (13–24) provide for a diet consisting of 12% to 15% of calories as protein, 50% to 60% as carbohydrate (5% to 20% as monosaccharides and disaccharides and 35% to 40% as complex carbohydrates), and approximately 30% as fat, with an emphasis on restriction of saturated fat (<10% of energy) and enhanced provision of monounsaturated and polyunsaturated fatty acids. In all ways, this diet is the same as that recommended for all healthy adults in the *Nutrition and Your Health: Dietary Guidelines for Americans, 2000* (14).

a. **The relaxed restriction on carbohydrates** in current diabetic diets is a result of a better understanding of glucose homeostasis. Previous recommendations restricted carbohydrate intake because high-carbohydrate diets were thought to raise blood levels of sugar. High-starch (complex carbohydrate) diets are well tolerated by diabetics as long as the total caloric intake is controlled. A high-complex carbohydrate diet with an optimal caloric intake is better tolerated than a low-carbohydrate diet with excess calories. Furthermore, a high-complex carbohydrate diet provides the additional known nutritional benefits of a diet rich in fruits and vegetables.

   b. **The reason for the more recent moderation of total fat intake** is the realization that a reduction in intake of saturated fat and the substitution of monounsaturated and polyunsaturated fatty acids for saturated fatty acids provide the most appropriate dietary pattern for normalizing blood lipid profiles, a critical endpoint because the leading cause of death among diabetics is coronary artery disease.

   c. **The glycemic index (GI)** represents an attempt to classify foods according to the extent to which they raise the blood sugar level (17). Different foods with the same caloric value can produce markedly different elevations in the blood sugar. The GI has been defined as the area under the 2-hour blood glucose response curve for a food expressed as a percentage of the area after ingestion of the same number of calories as glucose. In general, the GIs of complex carbohydrates, especially in fiber-rich foods, are low. However, no simple algorithm can predict the GI *a priori*. Soybeans and peanuts have very low GIs, but the GIs of lentils, chick-peas, green peas, kidney beans, and pinto beans are two to fourfold higher. The GI of fructose is equivalent to that of soybeans, the GI of honey is nearly equivalent to that of glucose, and the GI of table sugar (sucrose) is less than that of a baked potato. The blood glucose response after ingestion of a baked potato is essentially the same as that after oral glucose, but rice and pasta evoke a much lower blood glucose response.

   The reason for the differences in the glycemic response is not completely understood. The GI is influenced by the rate at which foods are digested and absorbed and the degree to which they raise the blood glucose level. The rate of gastric emptying and the presence of fat and protein affect the glycemic response. The glycemic response in patients with type II diabetes is similar to that seen in normal persons, but the glycemic response in patients with type I diabetes is more variable. These individual variations limit the usefulness of the GI as a teaching tool for patients with diabetes. Also, in the context of mixed meals, the GI tends to lose its practical usefulness because the distinctions between individual foods are blurred. For this reason, many experts do not consider the GI to be a valuable adjunct to diabetes management but prefer to regulate total carbohydrate intake. However, for selected, well-monitored patients, the realization that modifying carbohydrate food choices may help to "fine tune" diabetic control is important. It is also important to keep in mind that the long-term glycemic load, reflected by an estimate of the dietary GI (25–29), may play a role in the development of coronary heart disease and type II diabetes, although these hypotheses are currently the subject of vigorous debate.

3. **Dividing the daily prescription into meals.** The distribution of calories during the day must be adjusted to the patient's lifestyle and insulin program.

   a. **A typical diet** provides 20% to 30% of calories at breakfast, 20% to 35% at lunch, 25% to 40% at supper, and none to 15% as snacks.

   b. **Snacks** are usually taken at midmorning, at midafternoon, and near bedtime. Tight control of blood sugar is easier if snacks are part of the diet regimen. Midmorning and midafternoon snacks may prevent hypoglycemia by providing calories at times when levels of regular and intermediate-acting insulin reach their peak. Similarly, a bedtime snack may prevent nighttime hypoglycemia. Snacks also reduce the number of calories that are taken at meals and thus help prevent episodes of postprandial hyperglycemia.

4. **Formulation of the meal plan.** After the patient's calorie requirement has been calculated, the next step is to formulate a specific meal

plan. The standard exchange system is the method used to formulate diabetic meal plans in almost all U.S. hospitals. The exchange lists most commonly used are those developed jointly by the American Dietetic Association and the American Diabetic Association and most recently revised in 1995 (30).

a. The purpose of the exchange system is to allow a patient to vary the foods eaten from day to day and still consume a constant number of calories with a relatively fixed distribution of calories among carbohydrates, proteins, and fat and a fixed distribution of calories among the meals. The macronutrient contents of the various exchange groups are shown in Table 12-2, and detailed exchange lists can be found in reference 17 (Appendix Section V, Tables A-25-a through A-25-k).

b. Application of the exchange system. A thorough explanation of the exchange system is beyond the scope of this manual and the interests of most health care providers who are not dietitians, but it is useful to understand how it works. For example, an 1,800-cal diet in which the calories are distributed as 50% carbohydrate, 30% fat, and 20% protein would contain 224 g of carbohydrate, 92 g of protein, and 59 g of fat. One slice of white bread contains 15 g of carbohydrate, 3 g of protein, and no fat. This is one bread exchange with a caloric content of 80 cal. An 1,800-kcal diet might include eight bread exchanges (120 g of carbohydrate, 24 g of protein), with two of those exchanges assigned to breakfast. Thus, every breakfast would include two slices of white bread or their equivalent. Foods equivalent to two slices of bread include one cup of bran flakes or one bagel. On three successive mornings, a diabetic patient could have a breakfast that included three different items (bread, bran flakes, and

Table 12-2. Nutritional values of the exchange lists

	CHO	Protein	Fat	Calories
Carbohydrate group				
Starch	15	3	≤1	80
Fruit	15	—	—	60
Vegetables	5	2	—	25
Milk				
Skim	12	8	≤1	90
Low-fat	12	8	5	120
Whole	15	Varies	Varies	Varies
Meat and meat substitutes group				
Very lean	—	7	≤1	35
Lean	—	7	3	55
Medium-fat	—	7	5	75
High-fat	—	7	8	100
Fat group	—	—	5	45
Free foods group	<5	—	—	<20
Combination foods group	Varies	Varies	Varies	Varies
Fast foods group	Varies	Varies	Varies	Varies

CHO, carbohydrate.
From the American Dietetic Association and the American Diabetes Association. *Exchange lists for meal planning.* New York: American Diabetes Association, 1995, with permission.

bagel) while still consuming the same number of calories with the same distribution of macronutrients.

D. Modifying the diet

1. Use of dietetic foods and sweeteners

a. A widespread misconception is that by spending more money for *dietetic foods,* persons with diabetes can eat what they like and still control their disease. Most dietetic foods contain a significant number of calories; some dietetic candies and cookies contain as many calories as the comparable nondietetic foods.

b. Nonsucrose sweeteners come in two varieties—nutritive and non-nutritive (see discussion of low-available-carbohydrate diets in Chapter 11).

(1) Saccharine, aspartame, acesulfame-K, and sucralose are four non-nutritive sweeteners commonly used in diet soft drinks and other "diet" products. On a gram-for-gram basis, they are many times sweeter than sucrose and do not contribute to the caloric content of foods. Saccharine has been implicated as a carcinogen in rats. The incidence of bladder cancer was increased in male rats fed a large amount of saccharine. The role of saccharine as a carcinogen in humans is not established. Studies in human users and nonusers of saccharine reveal no differences in the incidence of cancer.

(2) Partially in response to the saccharine–cancer controversy, interest in *nutritive sweeteners—fructose, sorbitol, mannitol, and xylitol*—has increased. These compounds are all carbohydrates and, like sucrose, contain 4 kcal/g. Fructose is somewhat sweeter than sucrose, and less is required for sweetening.

(a) Metabolism. Sorbitol is metabolized to fructose but is less sweet than sucrose.

(b) Sorbitol (and xylitol) may not be well absorbed and can cause *osmotic diarrhea.*

(c) One of the reasons for using fructose and sorbitol is that insulin is not required for the early steps in their metabolism, and they do not produce such a steep rise in blood sugar. However, the liver converts fructose to glucose, so that fructose does eventually contribute to the blood sugar. Also, diets with a very high fructose content can have an adverse effect on the secretion of very-low-density lipoproteins (VLDLs) in some persons, so that levels of serum VLDL triglycerides and LDL cholesterol are increased.

(d) Caloric content. The chief disadvantage of these compounds and the reason that they are unlikely to have major roles in the dietary management of diabetes is their high caloric content. The obese diabetic should be warned that fructose, xylitol, and sorbitol are not like saccharine; they cannot be viewed as "calorie-free sweeteners." The use of nutritive sweeteners should be reserved for the diabetic who is at ideal body weight and whose blood sugar and serum lipids are under good control.

2. Modifying the diet for illness

a. Illness in diabetics who are not dependent on insulin. Acute illnesses are frequently accompanied by nausea, vomiting, and anorexia. In patients with type II diabetes, acute illness usually does not have a markedly adverse effect on diabetic control. For these patients, the major concern is avoiding dehydration by ensuring adequate fluid intake, usually by frequently ingesting small volumes of liquids and soft foods. Occasionally, during an intercurrent illness such as influenza, insulin dependence develops in a patient with non–insulin-dependent diabetes; all diabetic patients should carefully monitor their blood sugar and their urine for the appearance of ketonuria during acute illness.

   b. **In the patient with insulin-dependent diabetes, acute illness** may result in profound hypoglycemia or hyperglycemia and ketosis. Usually, the acute illness tends to increase insulin requirements. The only way to assess the insulin need is by frequent monitoring of blood glucose and urine ketones. The diabetic patient must take in enough carbohydrate (200 g/d) to prevent starvation ketosis. To prevent hypoglycemia during bouts of illness when appetite is depressed, adequate carbohydrate can be obtained by the frequent ingestion of sweetened fluids and soft, easily digested foods such as ice cream, juices, sweetened Jell-O, and soups. The ingestion of small amounts of fluid on a 15- to 30-minute basis helps to prevent dehydration (see Table 7-10 for selected oral rehydration solutions).

3. **Modifying the diet for activity**
   a. **Changes in activity level in diabetic patients who are not insulin-dependent.** Patients with non–insulin-dependent diabetes do not have to alter their diet to accommodate changes in exercise patterns. Exercise is a useful adjunct to caloric restriction in the attempt to lose weight. The overweight diabetic who begins an exercise program should gradually lose weight if the caloric intake is constant. However, it should be emphasized that daily regular physical activity of all kinds is beneficial to persons with type II diabetes. The diabetic patient should not be led to interpret "physical activity" as traditional "exercise" (e.g., running, tennis) but made to understand that all forms of nonsedentary behavior are valuable. Brisk walking is one of the most beneficial activities for obese diabetics and has been shown to be an effective adjunct in reducing the risk for coronary heart disease (31,32).
   b. **Changes in exercise patterns in patients with insulin-dependent diabetes,** however, must be accompanied by adjustments in the diet and insulin doses.
      (1) **Regular exercise** every day at a set time, at a set level of activity, for a set length of time is easily fitted into the diabetic dietary regimen.
      (2) **Irregular exercise** is a more difficult problem. An hour of vigorous exercise (e.g., cycling, basketball) may require two extra bread exchanges or one bread and one fruit exchange. An hour of moderate exercise (walking) may require the addition of half as much carbohydrate. If the exercise is to last for less than 2 hours, the consumption of extra food can be delayed until the exercise is complete and the patient determines whether any food is necessary by measuring the blood glucose. Often, however, depending on the subject's prior history of hypoglycemia with moderate exercise for this length of time, a snack of 10 to 15 g of carbohydrate may be consumed before exercise. Among the foods that may be eaten before exercise are low-fat cottage cheese, fruit, yogurt, bread, and crackers. These should be eaten about 30 minutes before exercise. If the exercise is vigorous or of long duration, a carbohydrate-rich snack may have to be consumed every 30 minutes. The amount of food required to cover exercise depends on body size and the duration and intensity of activity.

4. **Alcohol.** Alcohol is a component of the diet of many Americans. Most diabetics can consume limited amounts of alcohol, but several considerations peculiar to diabetes must be kept in mind.
   a. **Caloric content.** Because alcohol contains a significant number of calories (7 kcal/g), it is difficult to fit much alcohol into a weight loss diet and still obtain adequate protein, vitamins, and minerals. In

the obese diabetic, alcohol consumption should be minimized or eliminated until the excess weight is lost.

b. Carbohydrate content. Some alcoholic beverages, especially beer and sweet wines, contain a substantial number of calories in the form of carbohydrate in addition to those in alcohol. These may contribute to hyperglycemia and must be considered in the diet.

c. The effect of alcohol on blood glucose depends on such factors as time, consumption of other foods, and type of beverage. In fasting, insulin-dependent diabetics, the ingestion of a large amount of alcohol can induce profound hypoglycemia by inhibiting the release of glucose from the liver. Alcohol can also impair counterregulation in insulin-induced hypoglycemia. This effect may be most pronounced in tightly controlled patients with an increased incidence of hypoglycemia. Because the symptoms of hypoglycemia closely resemble those of alcohol intoxication, the hypoglycemia may go unrecognized. Alcoholism and insulin-dependent diabetes are an unfortunate combination of diseases.

d. Effect on triglyceride levels. Diabetes is frequently accompanied by hyperlipidemia, especially hypertriglyceridemia, and alcohol consumption can cause an abrupt rise in triglycerides. Fortunately, control of the blood sugar and achievement of ideal body weight may return the triglycerides levels to normal, so that moderate alcohol consumption can be allowed.

e. Some patients taking sulfonylureas experience flushing, nausea, dyspnea, and palpitations when they drink alcohol. This reaction, which resembles the effect of disulfiram (Antabuse), can be prevented by taking antihistamines before alcohol, although the preferred solution is abstinence.

f. On the whole, the clearly positive reasons for diabetics to consume alcohol are few. Nonetheless, despite all these reservations, most diabetics can consume limited amounts of alcohol (generally no more than one drink daily) as long as their diabetes is under control and they are at ideal body weight. *Alcohol is substituted for fat exchanges* (1-oz of whiskey is the equivalent of two to three fat exchanges; 12 oz of low-calorie beer is the equivalent of two fat exchanges).

E. Diabetes in special groups

1. Diabetes in pregnant women. Insulin-requiring diabetes is frequently more difficult to control during pregnancy, and pregnancy may cause glucose intolerance in a woman with previously normal glucose control.

a. Special modifications of the diabetic diet are not needed to accommodate the additional requirements of pregnancy other than those recommended for pregnant women in general, as described in detail in Chapter 4.

b. Weight gain during pregnancy is frequently excessive in diabetic patients. Because obese women often have heavier babies, they are advised to limit their weight gain during pregnancy (see Chapter 4).

c. Insulin requirements

(1) During the second and third trimesters, insulin requirements usually increase, and dietary manipulation may be necessary to accommodate the changing levels of blood sugar and insulin.

(2) During the first trimester and immediately after delivery, insulin requirements are usually reduced, and hypoglycemia may develop.

2. Diabetes in children. Diabetes is one of the most common serious chronic diseases of childhood. Whereas most adults with diabetes do not require insulin and are obese, 98% of children with diabetes require insulin, and few are obese.

a. **The goals of dietary therapy** in children with diabetes are the same as in adults with diabetes, but in addition, dietary therapy must promote normal growth and development. The calorie requirements for children are based on sex, age, size, growth rate, and physical activity. Although the recommended daily allowances (RDAs) are a general guideline (see Appendix B), each child's caloric requirement must be determined individually.

b. **During adolescence,** the caloric requirements increase with the rate of growth. The energy cost of growth is about 120 kcal/d at peak growth during adolescence, although this still represents only 3% to 4% of the total energy requirement. The energy requirements of individual adolescents vary markedly. The total daily expenditure of energy in adolescent boys ranges from about 50 to 75 kcal/kg daily, depending on the BMR and habitual level of physical activity. In adolescent girls, the corresponding range of total daily expenditure of energy is between about 50 to 65 kcal/kg.

c. **Underweight children.** The calorie allotments for children should be modified according to their progress on the weight and height charts. Many juvenile diabetics at the time of diagnosis are underweight. A common error is to place underweight children on a diet calculated to meet the needs of children of normal weight of the same age. Underweight children may require an additional several hundred calories per day to regain lost weight and maintain growth.

3. **Diabetes in patients with hypertension, hyperlipidemia, or renal failure.** Diabetes is frequently associated with other chronic illnesses for which the management includes diet therapy. Chronic renal failure is a common complication of diabetes. Familial dysbetalipoproteinemia, familial endogenous hypertriglyceridemia, and mixed hypertriglyceridemias are common among diabetics. Finally, hypertension, although not directly related to diabetes, is common among the obese, middle-aged patients who comprise the majority of the diabetic population. Because each of these illnesses is treated in part by dietary measures, the formulation of a diet for patients with more than one of these illnesses requires additional planning. Fortunately, the diets used in the management of these several illnesses do not conflict with, but frequently complement, each other.

a. **Patients with chronic renal failure** treated without dialysis require a protein-restricted diet that favors protein of high biologic value, as described later in this chapter. In addition, their intake of phosphorus, potassium, and sodium must be restricted. None of these requirements should interfere with the recommended diabetic diet. Since the recent recommendations for a higher content of complex carbohydrates in the diabetic diet, a combined renal–diabetic diet is easier to devise.

b. **Hypertriglyceridemia** occurs in about 20% of patients with type II diabetes. Management regimens, including appropriate blood glucose control with insulin or oral agents, reduction of alcohol intake, and caloric restriction to attain ideal body weight, should result in reduced blood levels of both lipids and sugar.

c. **Hypertension.** The major dietary manipulations in the treatment of hypertension are caloric restriction, to help obese patients lose weight, and sodium restriction. Although sodium restriction is largely independent of the diabetic diet, certain foods have a high content of both calories and sodium. Examples of these are TV dinners, cold cuts, sausage, French fries, salted nuts, and snack chips. Eliminating these items helps control both diabetes and hypertension (see Chapter 11 for a discussion of the low-sodium diet). Regular exercise and a reduced alcohol intake are also useful adjuncts in the treatment of hypertensive diabetics.

II. Renal disease

A. General principles. Diet therapy is an important component of the management of renal disease, although whether these regimens slow the progression of renal disease remains controversial (33–37).

1. **The goals of diet therapy** are to (a) provide adequate nutrition, (b) minimize uremia and other metabolic derangements, and (c) delay the progression of renal failure. Improvement in the patient's metabolic status reduces the symptoms associated with uremia, including fatigue, nausea, pruritus, and anorexia.

2. **A wasting syndrome in uremic patients** is secondary to inadequate dietary intake of protein and energy, altered protein metabolism, and the endocrine abnormalities associated with renal failure (hyperparathyroidism, insulin resistance). In addition, patients on dialysis lose nutrients into the dialysate, which further contributes to wasting.

3. A major factor contributing to malnutrition in chronic renal failure is the *anorexia* caused by uremia. Uremia also diminishes taste acuity, so that food seems bland and unappealing. Proper nutrition may help reverse the wasting syndrome. For example, the correct manipulation of dietary protein can reduce the degree of uremia; if the patient's appetite improves, the caloric intake increases and wasting is reversed.

4. **Total parenteral nutrition (TPN)** can be used in patients with chronic renal failure, whether they are managed conservatively or on dialysis. The use of TPN in the renal patient is covered in Chapter 10.

B. The dietary management of chronic renal disease depends on the degree of renal failure and the need for dialysis.

1. **Phases of management**

   a. **Conservative (predialysis) management.** In the *predialysis phase,* chronic renal disease has not yet progressed to the point at which dialysis is indicated, but conservative dietary therapy is critically important.

      (1) **Patients at this stage** include those with a glomerular filtration rate (GFR) between 25 mL/min and 5 to 10 mL/min. For patients who are managed conservatively, proper dietary management may delay the need for dialysis. As noted above, the latter issue has remained controversial since the Modification of Diet in Renal Disease (MDRD) study produced ambiguous results (38,39); Maroni and Mitch (33) discussed at length potential reasons for the lack of conclusive evidence of benefit, including the fact that the MDRD study lasted only 2.2 years. The corresponding DCCT, discussed earlier in this chapter, was a much longer study in which beneficial outcomes did not become apparent until after 3 to 4 years of therapy. Two large metaanalyses have supported the effectiveness of a low intake of protein in slowing the progression of renal disease (40,41).

      (2) **The goals of therapy** at the predialysis stage are those listed above (maintain good nutritional status, relieve symptoms, and if possible slow disease progression), in addition to minimizing the secondary effects of renal failure (e.g., renal osteodystrophy).

   b. **Management during long-term dialysis.** When the GFR falls to approximately 5 mL/min, dietary manipulation alone can no longer control the metabolic abnormalities associated with renal failure, and transplantation or dialysis is required. *The goals of diet therapy for patients on dialysis* are to minimize metabolic abnormalities, correct for nutrients lost during dialysis, and provide sufficient nutritional support to prevent the protein–energy malnutrition that is commonly seen in patients undergoing maintenance dialysis (36,42,43,44).

2. **Protein requirements.** As renal disease progresses, the ability of the kidneys to excrete urea diminishes. The load of urea presented to the kidneys is usually proportional to the amount of protein in the diet; however,

even patients on a zero-protein diet produce some urea as a result of the breakdown of tissue proteins. If too much protein is included in the diet, the level of blood urea nitrogen (BUN) rises and symptoms of uremia develop. If dietary protein is inadequate, the supply of amino acids required for the synthesis of necessary proteins is inadequate (36,43) (Table 12-3).

   a. Type of protein. Not only is it important for a patient to consume an adequate amount of protein; it is also important that the protein be of the right type. Amino acids are either nonessential or essential. Because the body cannot synthesize essential amino acids, they must come from the diet. Nonessential amino acids can be ingested or synthesized. In chronic renal failure, endogenous synthesis of the nonessential amino acids is preferable to ingestion for two reasons:

Table 12-3. Nutritional requirements for patients with chronic renal failure

	Chronic renal failure	Maintenance dialysis
Dietary nutrients		
Protein	0.55–0.6 g/kg/d (≥0.35 g/kg/d of high biologic value)	Hemodialysis: 1.0–1.2 g/kg/d (≥50% high biologic value) Peritoneal dialysis: 1.2–1.3 g/kg/d
Calories	>35 kcal/kg/d[a]	>35 kcal/kg/d[a]
Fat	30–40% Energy	30–40% Energy
P:S fat ratio	1:1	1:1
Carbohydrate	Rest of nonprotein calories	Rest of nonprotein calories
Fiber	20–25 g	20–25 g
Fluids	Up to 3 L/d[b]	Usually 750–1,500 mL/d[b]
Sodium	1–3 g/d[b]	0.75–1.0 g/d[b]
Potassium	40–70 mEq/d	40–70 mEq/d
Phosphorus	5–10 mg/kg/d	8–17 mg/kg/d
Calcium	1.4–1.6 g/d	1.4–1.6 g/d
Magnesium	200–300 mg/d	200–300 mg/d
Iron	≥10–18 mg/d[c]	≥10–18 mg/d[c]
Zinc	15 mg/d	15 mg/d
Vitamin supplements		
Thiamine	1.5 mg/d	1.5 mg/d
Riboflavin	1.8 mg/d	1.8 mg/d
Pantothenic acid	5 mg/d	5 mg/d
Niacin	20 mg/d	20 mg/d
Pyridoxine HCl	5 mg/d	10 mg/d
Vitamin A	0	0
Folic acid	1 mg/d	1 mg/d
Vitamin B_{12}	3 μg/d	3 μg/d
Vitamin C	60 mg/d	60 mg/d
Vitamin D	See text	See text
Vitamin E	8 mg/d[d]	8 mg/d[d]
Vitamin K	0	0

[a] Unless patient is >120% ideal body weight or is gaining unwanted weight.
[b] Can be higher in patients with greater urinary or dialysis losses.
[c] Ten milligrams for men and nonmenstruating women; 18 mg for menstruating women.
[d] As α-tocopherol (includes *RRR*-α-tocopherol and the 2*R*-stereoisomeric forms).
Adapted from Kopple JD. Renal disorders and nutrition. In: Shils ME, Olson JA, Shike M, et al., eds. *Modern nutrition in health and disease*, 9th ed. Baltimore: Williams & Wilkins, 1999:1439.

(1) The synthesis of an amino acid uses up an amino group that would otherwise go into urea.

(2) The synthesis of an amino acid reduces the amount of dietary protein required and thus diminishes the substrate for urea production. An adjunct to this approach is the use of dietary α-ketoacid analogues of essential amino acids. Via transamination, these ketoacids are converted into the respective essential amino acids, so that an amino acid group is salvaged while simultaneously an essential amino acid is provided.

b. **Biologic value of protein.** Essential amino acids should be present in the diet in quantities adequate to allow required protein synthesis.

    (1) Proteins are said to be of *high biologic value* if they meet the following criteria:

        (a) Most of the nitrogen is in the form of essential amino acids.

        (b) All essential amino acids are present.

        (c) The essential amino acids are present in concentrations proportional to the minimum daily requirements.

    (2) **Eggs are the food with proteins of the highest biologic value.** Other foods with proteins of high biologic value include fish, poultry, lean meat, and dairy products.

    (3) **Protein of low biologic value** is found in some grains, nuts, seeds, and legumes.

c. **Certain abnormalities of amino acid homeostasis are peculiar to uremia.** Plasma concentrations of valine, leucine, isoleucine, lysine, and tryptophan are reduced, whereas the concentrations of many nonessential amino acids are elevated. The conversion of phenylalanine to tyrosine is impaired, so that the requirement for phenylalanine is decreased and the requirement for tyrosine is increased. Histidine may be considered an essential amino acid because patients in renal failure are unable to synthesize enough histidine to meet their needs.

d. **Protein requirements during conservative management**

    (1) **The recommended daily protein intake for a healthy adult** is 0.8 g/kg per day, or 56 g/d for a 70-kg man. Most Americans consume more than 100 g/d.

    (2) **GFR.** In individuals with a GFR of 25 to 70 mL/min, despite the controversy generated by the results of the previously mentioned MDRD study, the support for dietary protein restriction is substantial (33,34,36). Therefore, the recommended dietary protein intake is reduced to 0.55 to 0.6 g/kg per day, of which at least 35 g/kg per day is protein of high biologic value. When the GFR falls below 25 mL/min, the argument for dietary protein restriction become far more powerful. In this circumstance, a reduction in dietary protein intake not only reduces the generation of deleterious nitrogenous metabolic products but also leads to a concomitant reduction in the intake of both phosphorus and potassium, which generate additional deleterious metabolites. The recommended protein intake remains at the level stated above (36). Although some evidence indicates that ketoacid and amino acid supplementation of a low-protein or very-low-protein diet may further retard the progression of renal disease, the data are insufficient to recommend such supplementation outside a research setting at this time.

    (3) When the GFR falls below 5 mL/min, patients do better if they undergo dialysis and consume a regular diet with a higher daily intake of protein (in the range of 1.0 to 1.3 g/kg per day), at least half of which is of high biologic value. This regimen avoids protein–energy malnutrition; the capacity of these patients to conserve body protein and amino acids is reduced, and

other biologically important nitrogenous compounds are lost in the dialysate (43). In hemodialysis, losses are estimated to be as high as 1 g of free amino acids per hour and 3 g of total (free plus protein-bound) amino acids per hour. Thus, a standard 4-hour session of hemodialysis results in losses equivalent to 5 to 10 g of protein. Because a large proportion (30% to 40%) of the amino acids lost in the dialysate are essential amino acids, it is important that at least half of the dietary protein be of high biologic value, as noted above.

(4) **Patients undergoing long-term peritoneal dialysis** may require even a greater intake of protein than patients on hemodialysis. The "pores" of the peritoneum are larger than those of dialysis tubing and so allow larger proteins to be lost into the dialysate. On average, these patients lose 10 to 14 g of protein, peptides, and amino acids daily into the dialysate. The recommended protein intake for patients on long-term peritoneal dialysis may be increased to the range of 1.2 to 1.5 g/kg of body weight (36).

(5) **Patients with nephrotic syndrome** require approximately 0.7 g of protein per kilogram per day plus an additional gram per day of high-biologic-value protein for each gram of protein lost in the urine daily.

(6) **Potassium and phosphorus.** Foods high in protein are usually also high in potassium and phosphorus, and if they are given to patients with a low GFR, hyperkalemia and hyperphosphatemia may develop. Thus, a diet restricted in protein is usually also restricted in potassium and phosphorus. This is just as well because patients with chronic renal failure require a diet restricted in all three. Specific diets for phosphorus and potassium restriction are available (45).

3. **Energy requirements.** The caloric requirements are similar for conservatively managed patients with chronic renal failure and for patients undergoing dialysis (Table 12-3). Patients with chronic renal failure are frequently calorie-deficient, the deficiency being manifested as weight loss, diminished adipose tissue, and loss of muscle mass. Because these patients tend to be volume-expanded, their muscle mass and fat stores may be even lower than their weight would suggest. The average calorie intake of dialysis patients is usually lower than 30 kcal/kg per day, and they have a better clinical course if dietary energy intakes above this level can be achieved.

a. **Prevention of protein catabolism.** An adequate intake of calories in the form of carbohydrates and fats is required to prevent the use of dietary or tissue protein as a source of energy. The catabolism of proteins results in increased urea production. The ideal calorie intake is whatever is required to achieve and maintain an ideal body weight. Patients who are below their ideal body weight need more calories.

b. **Dietary instructions** for renal patients must be complete, given by professionals, and reinforced regularly. Patients who are told to restrict their protein intake and handed a preprinted diet sheet without further instructions may inadvertently reduce an already inadequate caloric intake. Achieving an adequate caloric intake is a major problem in the management of patients with chronic renal failure. In some cases, compliance with other dietary restrictions must be sacrificed to attain an adequate caloric intake. The vigorous pursuit of perfect metabolic balance may result in a diet that is totally unpalatable and a patient with an inadequate calorie intake.

c. **Nutritional supplements.** Because they are frequently anorectic and have difficulty in maintaining an adequate calorie intake, patients with chronic renal failure may require *nutritional supplements.*

Many commercial nutritional supplements are now available that are especially appropriate for patients with renal failure. In some supplements, the calories are all carbohydrate (e.g., Polycose) (Table 9-1). Other supplements are more specific to renal failure; they contain a mixture of fat and carbohydrate and are designed to be low in protein, phosphorus, sodium, and potassium for readily apparent reasons (e.g., Nepro). Table 9-7 lists the supplements specifically intended for patients with renal disease, and Table 9-5 provides the detailed nutritional content of some of them.

4. **Sodium requirements** are outlined in Table 12-3, and sodium-restricted diets are readily available (45). As chronic renal disease progresses, the ability of the kidneys to respond to variations in sodium intake diminishes. The normal kidney responds to a low-sodium diet by reabsorbing virtually all the filtered sodium and responds to a high-sodium diet by reabsorbing less. The failing kidney progressively filters and reabsorbs less sodium and cannot adapt to changes in sodium intake. The goal is to have the daily sodium intake equal the fixed daily loss.

   a. **Urinary sodium measurements.** One approach to determining the sodium requirement is to put the patient on moderate sodium restriction (3 to 6 g of salt per day; 1 g of salt equals 410 mg of sodium) and measure the 24-hour urinary sodium. The dietary intake can be adjusted on the basis of the urinary sodium. The patient's sodium status is also roughly reflected by changes in weight. Weight gain reflects sodium intake in excess of sodium excretion, and weight loss reflects net sodium loss.

   b. Most patients with renal disease require 2 to 8 g of salt (1 to 3 g of sodium) per day, although *variation among individual patients is significant.* As renal function deteriorates, the requirement may diminish. The risks attached to inappropriate sodium intake are considerable. Too much dietary sodium can cause edema, hypertension, and congestive heart failure. Too little sodium intake can result in dehydration, a reduced GFR, and acceleration of the deterioration in renal function. Patients with renal disease are often placed on diets in which the sodium restrictions are excessively stringent. A rising BUN may reflect dehydration instead of excessive protein intake.

   c. Not all forms of chronic renal failure affect sodium homeostasis in the same way.

      (1) **Pyelonephritis and polycystic kidney disease** tend to be salt-wasting conditions requiring increased dietary sodium.

      (2) **Glomerulonephritis** is associated with hypertension and may require a lower salt intake.

   d. In any case, dietary sodium requirements change with *nonurinary salt losses* (e.g., in sweat). Sodium restrictions must be liberalized in warm climates whose homes are not air-conditioned. Some patients require sodium bicarbonate for the treatment of acidosis. In such cases, dietary sodium must be reduced to compensate for the sodium in the sodium bicarbonate. Two grams of sodium bicarbonate contain the same amount of sodium as 1.5 g of salt.

5. **Water requirements** are not usually a major problem for patients with chronic renal failure who are not on dialysis. Fluid intake should equal insensible loss (water lost from skin and lungs, which is usually 400 to 600 mL/d) plus urine volume. Most conservatively managed patients do well on 1.5 to 3.0 L/d (36).

   The goal of salt and fluid management in the patient on dialysis is to limit the rate of weight gain between dialysis treatments to 1 lb/d. This can be achieved with a diet containing 750 to 1,000 mg of sodium plus a water intake in the range of 750 to 1,000 mL daily. These values may be increased in patients undergoing long-term peritoneal dialysis and in those on hemodialysis who have greater urinary losses. Thus, in the absence of anuria, urinary salt and water losses can be added to these allowances.

  a. **Stringent salt restrictions** may improve metabolic control but make the diet unpalatable. Nonetheless, patients with hypertension and congestive heart failure may have to reduce their salt intake.

  b. **The daily fluid allotment** of 1,000 mL includes 500 mL for insensible losses and 500 mL for a 1-lb weight gain. Fluid in food must be subtracted from the fluid allotment. Any food that is liquid at room temperature (e.g., gelatin, ice cream) is counted as fluid. Fruits and vegetables are 85% to 90% water, cooked cereals are 70% to 85% water, and meat is 45% to 60% water. It should be readily apparent that 1,000 mL/d is a severe fluid restriction; compliance is difficult for many patients.

6. **Potassium requirements.** Guidelines for the management of potassium are similar for both conservatively managed and dialysis patients (Table 12-3), and dietary prescriptions are available (45). The standard American diet contains 50 to 100 mEq of potassium per day. Patients with a GFR of less than 15 mL/min usually require potassium restriction to 40 to 70 mEq/d. Hyperkalemia is less likely in those with a urine output of 1,000 mL or more per day.

  a. **Sources of potassium.** A 40-g protein diet provides 50 to 60 mEq of potassium per day. Excessive dietary potassium can lead to hyperkalemia and the danger of cardiac arrhythmias. Patients with renal failure should not use salt substitutes that contain large amounts of potassium (Table 7-15). Similarly, they should not be given potassium supplements when treated with thiazides or furosemide.

  b. **Hyperkalemia is exacerbated by acidosis and catabolic stress with muscle protein breakdown.** These conditions should be prevented by proper medical management and corrected expeditiously when they occur.

  c. **Potassium restriction is often unnecessary.** Despite nearly normal serum potassium levels, the total body potassium pool and intramuscular potassium concentration are frequently low in chronic renal failure. This may reflect acidosis or impaired transport into cells. Because total body potassium is usually low, dietary potassium should not be appreciably restricted unless hyperkalemia is a problem and the urine output is below about 1,000 mL/d.

7. **Phosphorus, calcium, and vitamin D requirements**

  a. **Renal osteodystrophy,** a major problem in chronic renal disease, results from the abnormalities in calcium, phosphorus, parathyroid hormone (PTH), and vitamin D homeostasis brought on by renal failure. As the kidney fails, its ability to clear phosphate diminishes, and the serum phosphate level rises. Hyperphosphatemia is accompanied by hypocalcemia, which causes the release of PTH. Elevated levels of PTH result in increased renal phosphate clearance and bone resorption.

    (1) **The goals of therapy in renal osteodystrophy** are the following:

      (a) Suppression of secondary hyperparathyroidism

      (b) Normalization of osteoid mineralization

    (2) These goals are achieved by the following means:

      (a) Reducing phosphate absorption by reducing dietary phosphate and using phosphate-binding gels

      (b) Supplementing the diet with calcium and vitamin D

  b. **Phosphate absorption.** PTH levels rise with the loss of as little as 25% of renal function. Thus, one of the earliest interventions required in renal failure is the reduction of phosphate absorption. Phosphate absorption is reduced by lowering the dietary intake of phosphate and administering phosphate-binding gels.

(1) Dietary phosphate. The usual American diet contains 1.0 to 1.8 g of phosphorus per day. The elimination of milk, milk products, cheese, colas, and instant powdered beverages combined with protein restriction (40 g/d) will reduce intake to 600 mg/d (45). Nonetheless, when the GFR falls below about 25 mL/min per day, this level of dietary phosphorus restriction is still not adequate to prevent hyperphosphatemia. The diet of patients on dialysis is higher in protein than that of conservatively managed patients, so that their dietary intake of phosphorus is also usually higher.

(2) The need for phosphate binders is just as great for dialysis patients as for nondialysis patients, and several commercial phosphate binders are available. The goal in using phosphate binders is to keep the serum phosphorus level in the range of 4 to 5 mg/dL. Most clinicians use phosphate-binding gels early in the course of renal disease before imposing any dietary restrictions.

c. Calcium balance. Although chronic renal failure causes a positive phosphorus balance, it results in a negative *calcium balance*. Several factors contribute to the negative calcium balance—hyperparathyroidism, calcium malabsorption secondary to vitamin D deficiency, and a diet low in calcium because phosphorus-rich dairy products are restricted.

(1) Oral calcium supplements are recommended for the reasons that have been outlined; approximately 1.5 g of elemental calcium per day should be given to patients with a GFR below 25 mL/min. Because a diet with 40 g of protein provides about 300 to 400 mg of calcium daily, these subjects require approximately 1.0 to 1.2 g of calcium supplements daily.

(a) Before calcium supplementation is started, it is important that the *serum phosphorus* be under control. If calcium supplements are given in the face of hyperphosphatemia, calcium phosphate is deposited in the soft tissues.

(b) For dialysis patients, the goal is to keep the serum calcium in the range of 10.5 to 11.0 mg/dL to suppress PTH secretion.

(c) If patients on dialysis ingest 1.2 g of protein per kilogram per day, the weekly phosphorus intake averages 8,400 mg. If 5,000 mg of this is absorbed and dialysis can remove only 900 mg at a time (average of three sessions per week), 2,300 mg of phosphorus is retained each week. When the amount of calcium supplement needed to normalize the serum phosphorus level in patients on dialysis (often in the range of 10 to 16 g of calcium carbonate per day) is given, calcium is deposited ectopically in arterial walls and other tissues, and this process may contribute to an increase in mortality from heart disease. It may be advisable to give the phosphate binder Renagel (sevelamer hydrochloride), which does not contain calcium, to such patients to avoid a serum calcium phosphate product above 66.

(2) Vitamin D supplements. The reduction in functioning renal mass in chronic renal failure is accompanied by a decreased conversion of 25-hydroxycholecalciferol to 1,25-dihydroxycholecalciferol. The decreased levels of 1,25-dihydoxycholecalciferol result in a decreased absorption of dietary calcium. Rocaltrol, which is a trade name for 1,25-dihydroxyvitamin D$_3$, is useful in managing the hypocalcemia and osteodystrophy of chronic renal disease, but it is very expensive. The starting dose is 0.25 µg/d, which can be increased to 0.50 µg/d after a period of 4 to 6 weeks. It is possible to induce hypercalcemia by giving calcium and vitamin D supplements. Therefore, the serum calcium level should be monitored carefully. Vitamin D increases the absorption of both phosphate and calcium; thus, serum phosphorus levels also must be monitored during vitamin D therapy.

8. **Iron requirements.** Twenty-five percent of nontransfused patients on long-term hemodialysis are deficient in iron. Iron intake (especially heme iron intake) is frequently low. A major cause of iron deficiency in these patients is the loss of 5 to 20 mL of blood left in the dialyzer after each treatment, which can amount to a loss of anywhere from a few hundred milligrams to a gram of iron per year. In addition, the heparin used as an anticoagulant may increase gastrointestinal and uterine blood loss. For these reasons, many dialysis patients receive supplementation with ferrous sulfate.

9. **Vitamin requirements.** Patients with chronic renal failure are frequently vitamin-deficient because of their poor dietary intake. However, the alterations in vitamin requirements caused by chronic renal failure are poorly defined, and the systematic data are insufficient to set new dietary reference intakes (DRIs) for vitamins. Supplementation with *vitamin A* should be avoided because chronic renal disease is associated with elevated levels of vitamin A. *Vitamin K* supplementation is not routinely required but may be necessary in patients who are receiving TPN and antibiotics. The loss of *water-soluble vitamins* into the dialysate in hemodialysis creates an additional demand. Nonetheless, although no consensus recommendations regarding the increased needs have been made, many experts advise prudent supplementation of water-soluble vitamins (Table 12-3). One standard multivitamin plus 1 mg of folic acid per day should meet the requirements. The recommended vitamin supplementation is the same for both conservatively managed patients and those on dialysis.

10. **Dietary management of concomitant hypertriglyceridemia** (type IV hyperlipoproteinemia). The relationship of hypertriglyceridemia to coronary heart disease is complex, and the status of elevated plasma triglycerides *per se* as a risk factor is still debated. Nonetheless, elevated triglycerides are generally accepted as a risk factor in many parts of the world, and a large metaanalysis found elevated triglycerides to be associated with a significantly increased risk for cardiovascular incidents (46). Many clinicians recommend a prudent National Cholesterol Education Program step 1 diet (described previously for diabetes) for patients with renal failure.

   a. **Dietary management of type IV hyperlipoproteinemia.** The mainstays of diet therapy for hypertriglyceridemia are caloric intake to maintain reasonable body weight, limitation of sugars and alcohol, moderation of dietary fat intake to about 30% of total calories, restriction of saturated fat to less than 10% of total calories, restriction of cholesterol intake to less than 300 mg/d, and a high ratio of polyunsaturated to saturated fats.

   b. **Dietary management in patients with chronic renal failure.** In chronic renal failure, the caloric intake is more likely to be inadequate than excessive; thus, caloric restriction is usually not appropriate. On the other hand, the proper dietary management of chronic renal failure is quite compatible with a diet low in sugars and alcohol and high in polyunsaturated fats.

   c. **Monitoring diet therapy in the patient with chronic renal failure.** A brief physical examination in addition to standard blood chemistry studies should make it possible to determine patient compliance and any needed changes in the diet. Various laboratory tests and other criteria assist in monitoring the adequacy of specific nutrients.

   (1) **Protein.** In patients who undergo dialysis three times a week, a reasonable goal is a BUN of 60 to 80 mg/dL after the longest interval between dialysis sessions (3 days). A higher BUN suggests excessive protein intake if weight is maintained or gained. It suggests protein catabolism if associated with recent weight loss.

   (2) **Calories.** Inability to achieve or maintain ideal body weight is a sign of poor caloric intake. A rising BUN may reflect protein catabolism in a patient with inadequate caloric intake.

   (3) **Salt and water.** Excessive weight gain between dialysis sessions with a normal serum sodium level reflects excess salt and water ingestion. Excessive weight gain with a low serum sodium level suggests excessive ingestion of fluids but not salt. Edema, congestive heart failure, and increasing blood pressure may be signs of excess sodium intake. Weight loss, diminished urine output, and a rising BUN all point to inadequate salt ingestion.

   (4) **An elevated potassium level** reflects increased potassium ingestion or acidosis.

   (5) **An elevated phosphorus level** may reflect either failure to take phosphate binders or excessive dietary phosphorus intake, usually in the form of dairy products.

  d. **Practical dietary aids.** Many commercial products are now available to facilitate the dietary management of uremia (see reference 37 and Table 9-7).

  e. **Dietary management of acute renal failure.** The goals of diet in acute renal failure are to provide adequate calories to maintain body weight and minimize catabolism of tissue proteins. The major difficulty in managing patients without dialysis is providing adequate calories without fluid overload. Whenever possible, the patient should receive nutrition via the enteral route. The following are suggested guidelines (36):

   (1) **Fluids** should be given at a rate of 400 mL/d plus urinary and all other fluid losses. The goal is a normal serum sodium level and no weight gain.

   (2) **The ideal caloric intake** is whatever it takes to maintain body weight. The minimum is at least 200 g of carbohydrate (usually as a 50% to 70% solution) to minimize protein breakdown. Desirable energy intake is 30 to 40 kcal/kg per day, of which 10% to 30% is given as liquid emulsions.

   (3) **Protein intake** in acute renal failure is a highly debated topic (36). If patients are otherwise adequately nourished and expected to regain renal function within a few weeks, 0.3 to 0.5 g of high-biologic-value protein or essential amino acids per kilogram per day is used. For patients who are highly catabolic, who have high levels of urinary nitrogen, or who are not expected to recover for more than 2 weeks, additional protein intake is advisable, up to 1.2 g/kg per day.

   (4) **Salt intake** should equal salt losses (urine, stool, gastric aspirate).

   (5) **Potassium.** Because acute renal failure may be accompanied by substantial tissue destruction and acidosis, the possibility of rapidly developing hyperkalemia is greater than in chronic renal failure. Serum potassium should be monitored carefully and dietary potassium minimized (see Tables 7-12 and 7-13 for sources of dietary potassium).

   (6) **Dialysis.** In acute renal failure, dialysis makes it possible to control hyperkalemia, fluid overload, acidosis, and uremia. After

the initiation of dialysis, less stringent restriction of protein, fluids, and potassium may be possible.

III. **Hyperlipoproteinemia.** According to recent estimates, nearly 60 million Americans have one or more forms of cardiovascular disease. In 1997, it was estimated that 12 million persons had coronary heart disease, which caused nearly 500,000 deaths. Coronary heart disease is the number one cause of death in America today, and more than 1 million Americans will have a new or recurrent coronary event this year. More than 200 risk factors for cardiovascular disease have been identified, but the major factors are far fewer in number. Some, like male sex, increasing age, and genotype, cannot be modified. Others, such as increased plasma LDL cholesterol, increased circulating triglycerides, low plasma high-density-lipoprotein (HDL) cholesterol, cigarette smoking, hypertension, obesity, and reduced physical activity, are potentially reversible. Reductions in LDL cholesterol, hypertension, and cigarette smoking have been shown clearly to lower risk. Increases in HDL cholesterol and physical activity are highly likely to lower risk. Because many of these risks are related to diet and lifestyle, a highly significant reduction in the risks for cardiovascular disease can be achieved through the nutritional practices outlined in this volume and presented in detail elsewhere (24,47–50).

A. **Definitions**

1. **Hyperlipidemias.** The population distributions (fifth through ninety-fifth percentiles) of cholesterol and triglyceride levels are given in Table 12-4.

   a. **Hypercholesterolemia,** the elevation of serum LDL cholesterol, is one of the major risk factors for the development of coronary artery disease. A progressive curvilinear or logarithmic–linear relationship exists between increases in the incidence of coronary artery disease and increases in serum total or LDL cholesterol concentrations (49–53). Similarly, extensive evidence indicates that interventions to lower serum LDL cholesterol in secondary prevention trials are highly beneficial (53–56). Serum cholesterol appears to be the most significant determinant of geographic variations in the incidence of coronary heart disease.

      (1) **Normal cholesterol levels.** The relationship between cholesterol level and heart disease extends even into the range of cholesterol levels that most would consider "normal"—that is, the incidence of coronary artery disease is lower among persons with a cholesterol level of 180 mg/dL than it is among those with a level of 220 mg/dL.

         (a) If the upper limit of normal for the cholesterol level among American adults is set to exclude the upper 5% of each age group, then many persons with an increased risk for coronary artery disease are included in the normal group.

         (b) Because the risk for coronary artery disease decreases with serum cholesterol over the entire range of cholesterol levels found in the American population, it is difficult to define a "normal" cholesterol level.

      (2) **Reduction of cholesterol level.** Based on extensive worldwide and U.S. epidemiologic data, a persuasive argument can be made that the desirable range of plasma total cholesterol is below 200 mg/dL (49). Given this argument, approximately half the U.S. population has a cholesterol level above the desirable range. The National Cholesterol Education Program has categorized the risk levels for coronary heart disease on the basis of plasma total and LDL cholesterol levels (57–59) (Table 12-5). According to this classification, about one-fourth of Americans are at high risk. Based on a modification of this scheme, Grundy (49) has classified hypercholesterolemia as mild, moderate, or severe based on total and LDL cholesterol

(*text continues on page 490*)

Table 12-4. Population distributions for plasma total cholesterol and plasma triglycerides

Age (ys)	White males (percentiles)							White females (percentiles)						
	5	10	25	50	75	90	95	5	10	25	50	75	90	95
Plasma total cholesterol (mg/dL)														
0–4	—	—	—	—	—	—	—	—	—	—	—	—	—	—
5–9	125	131	141	153	168	183	189	131	136	151	164	176	190	197
10–14	124	131	144	160	173	188	202	125	131	142	159	171	191	205
15–19	118	123	136	152	168	183	191	118	126	140	157	176	198	207
20–24	118	126	142	159	179	197	212	121	132	147	165	186	220	237
25–29	130	137	154	176	199	223	234	130	142	158	178	198	217	231
30–34	142	152	171	190	213	237	258	133	141	158	178	199	215	228
35–39	147	157	176	195	222	248	267	139	149	165	186	209	233	249
40–44	150	160	179	204	229	251	260	146	156	172	193	220	241	259
45–49	163	171	188	210	235	258	275	148	162	182	204	231	256	268
50–54	157	168	189	211	237	263	274	163	171	188	214	240	267	281
55–59	161	172	188	214	236	260	280	167	182	201	229	251	278	294
60–74	163	170	191	215	237	262	287	172	186	207	226	251	282	300
65–69	166	174	192	213	250	275	288	167	179	212	233	259	282	291
70+	144	160	185	214	236	253	265	173	181	196	226	249	268	280

Plasma triglycerides (mg/dL)

	—	—	—	—	—	—	—	—	—	—	—	—	—	—
0–4	—	—	—	—	—	—	—	—	—	—	—	—	—	—
5–9	28	34	39	48	58	70	85	32	37	45	57	74	103	126
10–14	33	37	46	58	74	94	111	39	44	53	68	85	104	120
15–19	38	43	53	68	88	125	143	36	40	52	64	85	112	126
20–24	44	50	61	78	107	146	165	37	42	60	80	104	135	168
25–29	45	51	67	88	120	171	204	42	45	57	76	104	137	159
30–34	46	57	76	102	142	214	253	40	45	55	73	104	140	163
35–39	52	58	80	109	167	250	316	40	47	61	83	115	170	205
40–44	56	69	89	123	174	252	318	45	51	66	68	116	161	191
45–49	56	65	88	119	165	218	279	44	55	71	94	139	180	223
50–59	63	75	94	128	178	244	313	53	58	75	103	144	190	223
55–59	60	70	85	117	167	210	261	59	65	80	111	163	229	279
60–64	56	65	84	111	150	193	240	57	66	78	105	143	210	256
65–69	54	61	78	108	164	227	256	56	64	86	118	158	221	260
70+	63	71	87	115	152	202	239	60	68	83	110	141	189	289

Adapted from Lipid Metabolism Branch, National Heart, Lung, and Blood Institute, U.S. Department of Health and Human Services. *Lipid research clinics population studies data book.* NIH Publication No. 80-1527, 1980.

Table 12-5. Classification of coronary heart disease risk for adults

Classification	Total cholesterol (mg/dL)	LDL cholesterol (mg/dL)
"Optimal"	<150	<100
Desirable	150–199	100–129
Borderline high	200–239	130–159[a]
High	≥240	≥160[b]

LDL, low-density-lipoprotein.
[a] Properly called "borderline high-risk."
[b] Properly called "high-risk."
From Report of the National Cholesterol Education Program Expert Panel on detection, evaluation, and treatment of high blood cholesterol in adults. *Arch Intern Med* 1988;148:36, and Expert Panel on detection, evaluation, and treatment of high blood cholesterol in adults. *JAMA* 1993;269:3015, with permission.

levels (Table 12-6). If these definitions are used, about 25% of Americans have mild hypercholesterolemia and about 20% have moderate hypercholesterolemia.

To reduce the risk for coronary heart disease, the National Cholesterol Education Program further recommended almost a decade ago that "step 2" dietary intervention be initiated for all persons in the high-risk group (Table 12-7). The Program also recommended a "step 1" diet for all persons, regardless of their plasma total cholesterol level (Table 12-7). Today, the "step 1" diet, with the modification that total fat intake be set at about 30%, is virtually identical to the dietary recommendations for Americans found in *Nutrition and Your Health: Dietary Guidelines for Americans, 2000* (14) and the American Heart Association guidelines (24).

A host of additional factors affect both plasma cholesterol levels and the specific risk for coronary heart disease in any given person. For example, approximately half the variations in plasma lipid levels between individuals are genetically determined, and some people have genotypes that increase susceptibility to coronary heart disease, even though their plasma lipid levels are normal by population standards. Also, a wide degree of variability is observed between individuals in regard to the cholesterol-lowering effects of dietary intervention. However, the diet recommended by all expert committees (14,24,57,58) is both wholesome and health-promoting according to the information available at this time, so it is reasonable to accept these recommendations for the general population.

Table 12-6. Classification of hypercholesterolemia

Classification	Total cholesterol (mg/dL)	LDL cholesterol (mg/dL)
Mild	220–239	130–159
Moderate	240–299	160–219
Severe	≥300	≥220

LDL, low-density-lipoprotein.
From Grundy SM. Nutrition and diet in the management of hyperlipidemia and atherosclerosis. In: Shils ME, Olson JA, Shike M, et al., eds. *Modern nutrition in health and disease,* 9th ed. Baltimore: Williams & Wilkins, 1999:1199.

Table 12-7. Dietary recommendations

Nutrient[a]	Current intakes	Recommended intakes	
		Step 1	Step 2
Total fat	35	<30%	<30%
Saturated + *trans*	12	<10%	<7%
Monounsaturated	14	10–15%	
Polyunsaturated	6	<10%	
Carbohydrate	50	50–60%	
Protein	15	10–20%	
Cholesterol (mg/d)	300–400	<300	<200
Calories		To achieve/maintain desirable weight	

[a] As percentage of total dietary energy.
Adapted from references 49, 57, and 58.

(3) Cholesterol-carrying lipoproteins. Plasma total cholesterol is a discriminating risk factor for heart disease. However, the relationship between plasma total cholesterol and coronary heart disease can be assessed confidently only after the total cholesterol is further fractionated into the components carried by the two principal cholesterol-containing lipoproteins, LDLs and HDLs (Table 12-8). Most plasma cholesterol is carried by LDLs, and increases in plasma LDL cholesterol are highly associated with an increased incidence of coronary heart disease. For this reason, LDL cholesterol is popularly referred to as "bad cholesterol." LDL cholesterol is a better predictor of risk than plasma total cholesterol. Desirable levels of LDL cholesterol are below 130 mg/dL (Table 12-5).

An average of 45 to 55 mg of cholesterol per deciliter of plasma is carried by HDLs. HDL cholesterol and coronary heart disease are inversely related. A fourfold increase in the incidence of coronary heart disease is noted as HDL cholesterol levels decline from a range of 65 to 74 mg/dL to a range of 25 to 44 mg/dL, and an additional threefold increase is noted with HDL cholesterol values below 25 mg/dL. For these reasons, HDL cholesterol is referred to as "good cholesterol." The fifth

Table 12-8. Plasma lipoproteins

Class	Size (Å)	Composition (%)			
		Protein	Cholesterol	Triglycerides	Phospholipids
Chylomicrons	750–10,000	2	5	90	3
VLDLs	300–800	10	12	60	18
IDLs	250–400	10	30	40	20
LDLs	200–220	25	50	10	15
HDLs	75–100	50	20	5	25

VLDL, very-low-density lipoprotein; IDL, intermediate-density lipoprotein; LDL, low-density lipoprotein; HDL, high-density lipoprotein.
From Kuo PT. Prevention and treatment of hyperlipidemia. In: Halpern SL, ed. *Quick reference to clinical nutrition.* Philadelphia: JB Lippincott Co, 1979:137.

percentile population value for HDL cholesterol in adult men is approximately 30 mg/dL, and the corresponding value for adult women is approximately 35 mg/dL. Desirable levels, however, are above the twenty-fifth percentile, which correspond to values of approximately 38 mg/dL in adult men and about 48 mg/dL in adult women.

b. Hypertriglyceridemia. It is not entirely clear whether elevations in plasma triglyceride levels alone augment the risk for coronary heart disease. A metaanalysis lends support to the arguments of those who support hypertriglyceridemia as a risk factor (46). The issue is confounded by the fact that circulating triglycerides carried in very-low-density lipoproteins (VLDLs) are of two principal types: those recently secreted by the liver and those that have been partially metabolized (remnant particles). Because they have been metabolized, the remnants have less triglyceride and more cholesteryl esters, and these modifications probably promote atherogenicity, whereas the newly secreted VLDLs are probably not associated with an increased risk for coronary artery disease (49). The issue is further confounded by the fact that many persons with hypertriglyceridemia have additional risk factors, such as obesity and diabetes. Estrogen treatment and alcohol consumption also may elevate plasma triglycerides. Because triglycerides and HDLs are related inversely, it is not clear whether elevated triglyceride levels carry a risk truly independent of the association with lower HDL levels.

Some agreement has been reached that persons with pronounced hypertriglyceridemia (>1,000 mg/dL) require treatment to prevent pancreatitis, and that persons with combined elevations of triglycerides and cholesterol (mixed hyperlipoproteinemia or atherogenic dyslipoproteinemia) require treatment according to the guidelines of the National Cholesterol Education Program. Patients with modestly elevated plasma triglycerides (>200 mg/dL) should be evaluated for associated risk factors, educated about prudent dietary habits (including the maintenance of reasonable body weight), and given individualized treatment recommendations as necessary.

c. Treatment of hyperlipidemia. Firm evidence is available to implicate elevated LDL cholesterol as a risk factor for coronary heart disease (49–53). Also, extensive data from epidemiologic studies, clinical treatment trials, primary prevention trials, and secondary prevention trials show that lowering plasma cholesterol levels reduces coronary heart disease risk (53–56). These data drive consensus recommendations to treat elevated plasma cholesterol levels by diet and supplemental pharmacologic intervention to achieve desirable plasma cholesterol levels.

2. Lipoproteins. By definition, lipids are insoluble in water. So that they can be transported in blood, triglycerides and cholesterol are complexed with apoproteins and phospholipids to form the soluble particles called *lipoproteins*. The major lipoprotein classes are outlined in Table 12-8 (48–50,60).

a. Chylomicrons. The major function of chylomicrons is to carry exogenous dietary fat from the intestine to peripheral tissues. Chylomicrons are formed in the endoplasmic reticulum of enterocytes. During transit through the Golgi apparatus, they acquire apoproteins (apo) A-I, A-II, A-IV, and B-48 (an edited product of the same gene that produces apo B-100 in the liver) (60). After passing through the lacteals of the intestinal villi, the chylomicrons are transported through the thoracic duct into the bloodstream, where they acquire the additional apoproteins apo C-II and apo E via transfer from HDLs. Thereafter, the chylomicrons interact with the enzyme lipoprotein lipase, located on the endothelial surface of blood capillaries in many

organs (60). Apo C-II is a required cofactor in the activation of lipoprotein lipase. Lipoprotein lipase hydrolyzes the chylomicron triglycerides into unesterified fatty acids and glycerol. At the same time,
the apo A peptides are transferred to HDLs. The remaining, much
smaller chylomicron particle, still containing apo B-48 and now called
a *chylomicron remnant,* is taken up by a specific hepatic receptor that
recognizes the apo E peptide on its surface.

b. VLDLs are synthesized by the liver. Their principal role is the transport between organs of endogenously synthesized triglycerides of
hepatic origin. VLDLs resemble chylomicrons in that they are rich in
triglycerides (albeit somewhat smaller in size), receive small amounts
of apo E and apo C-II from HDL, and lose their triglycerides via
lipoprotein lipase-catalyzed hydrolysis. VLDLs are unique in that
they acquire apo B-100 during intrahepatic assembly. VLDL hydrolysis proceeds more slowly than that of chylomicrons and results in
two lesser VLDL particles, the larger of which is called a *VLDL remnant* (removed by the hepatic LDL receptor) and the smaller of which
is called an *intermediate-density lipoprotein* (IDL). In humans, about
half of IDLs are also taken up by hepatic receptors, but the remaining half are further converted to LDL, with apo B-100 as the predominant remaining peptide.

c. LDLs are the principal carrier of plasma cholesterol, accounting for
approximately 60% of the total in normal persons. Half of the LDL
particle is cholesterol; only 10% is triglyceride, and most of it is apo
B-100 (Table 12-8). LDLs are the vehicles whereby cholesterol synthesized in the liver is delivered to peripheral tissues. LDLs are metabolized slowly over several days. LDLs are taken up by cells
principally through interaction with a specific LDL receptor (60).

d. HDLs are secreted in an immature, disklike, nascent form largely by
the liver but also by the intestine. Through the action of a circulating cholesteryl ester transfer complex containing lecithin-cholesterol
acyltransferase (LCAT, a plasma enzyme that esterifies cholesterol
by transferring acyl groups from phosphatidylcholine to the free cholesterol being carried back to the liver from various cells and tissues)
and cholesteryl ester transfer protein (CETP, which is essential to
the clearance of HDL and transfers cholesteryl esters from HDL to
apo B-100 containing other lipoproteins), the mature, spherical HDL
particle is produced. In the process, cholesterol is transported from
the peripheral tissues to lipoproteins (so-called reverse cholesterol
transport) and eventually removed by the liver. The liver, in turn, ultimately disposes of the cholesterol by excreting it in bile.

The principal apoprotein of HDL is apo A-I, deficiency of which
leads to HDL deficiency and an increased risk for coronary heart disease (60). However, a genetic variant of apo A-I, apo A-I$_{Milano}$, causes
an HDL deficiency that is not associated with an increased susceptibility to cardiovascular disease; this effect may be secondary to its
ability to reduce damage to the vascular wall (60).

3. Hyperlipoproteinemias. The term *hyperlipoproteinemia* describes a
group of disorders in which serum lipoproteins are elevated. Because
the concentrations of plasma lipids are continuous variables, any definition of hyperlipoproteinemia is somewhat arbitrary. These disorders
are traditionally classified into six clinically useful types according to
which lipoproteins are elevated (Table 12-9).

Each type of hyperlipoproteinemia is not a single disease, but rather a
group of "genotypic" disorders marked by a similar "phenotypic" abnormality in circulating lipoproteins. Each type includes primary genetic defects and some secondary disorders. When the latter occur because of a
specific primary disease, such as uncontrolled diabetes, treatment of the
underlying disorder frequently corrects the lipid abnormality. Similarly,

Table 12-9. Lipid levels in hyperlipoproteinemia

Type	Cholesterol	Triglycerides	Atherogenicity
I Chylomicronemia	Normal or slightly elevated	Very high	Uncertain
IIa Hypercholesterolemia	Elevated LDL cholesterol	Normal	+++
IIb Familial combined hyperlipemia	Elevated LDL cholesterol	Elevated	+++
III[a] Dsybetalipoprotinemia	Elevated	Elevated	+++
IV Hypertriglyceridemia	Normal or slightly elevated	Elevated	? to +
V Mixed hypertriglyceridemia	Moderately elevated	Markedly elevated	+

[a] Increased intermediate-density lipoproteins. Also called *remnant hyperlipoproteinemia*. Definitive diagnosis of type III requires lipoprotein ultracentrifugation and characterization of Apo E isoforms.

when the primary disorder is aggravated by obesity, alcohol consumption, or estrogen or glucocorticoid treatment, elimination of the aggravating factor facilitates diet therapy. Because obesity and excessive consumption of cholesterol, total fat, and saturated fat increase plasma lipoprotein concentrations in many people, diet is an important component of the management of hyperlipidemia.

a. **Type I** hyperlipoproteinemia is an uncommon pattern marked by substantial chylomicronemia. Plasma cholesterol is usually normal and plasma triglycerides are markedly elevated, generally to a level above 1,000 mg/dL. Because chylomicrons contain a small amount of cholesterol, when the chylomicron concentration is very high, a slight secondary elevation of plasma cholesterol may develop. The classic form of this disease is an autosomal recessive disorder caused by more than 60 identified mutations in the gene for the enzyme lipoprotein lipase (48,49,60). It is usually identified in childhood by symptoms of eruptive xanthomata and pancreatitis. Chylomicronemia is less frequently caused by autosomal recessive defects in the gene for the apo C-II peptide activator of lipoprotein lipase. At least 10 distinct mutations of this gene have been described to date.

b. **Type IIa** hyperlipoproteinemia is marked by high LDL levels and normal VLDL levels. Thus, plasma cholesterol is elevated but triglycerides are normal. The principal genetic disorder associated with this phenotype is familial hypercholesterolemia, an autosomal dominant condition. The carrier frequency for this disorder is approximately 1/500. Familial hypercholesterolemia results from a defect in the LDL cell surface receptor that controls the plasma removal of LDLs. More than 40 mutations of the gene for the LDL receptor have been characterized at the DNA level, and many more potential receptor mutants remain to be characterized.

c. **Type IIb** hyperlipoproteinemia is the most common pattern found in families with premature coronary heart disease, with a population prevalence of 0.5% to 1.0%. It is characterized by increases in both circulating VLDLs and LDLs; thus, plasma cholesterol and triglycerides are both elevated. Additionally, HDL levels tend to be reduced. The genetic defects that result in this phenotype, called *familial combined* *hyperlipidemia,* are as yet unidentified. The type IIb phenotype is aggravated by obesity or glucocorticoid treatment and also can be seen as a secondary consequence of the nephrotic syndrome.

d. **Type III** hyperlipoproteinemia is characterized by an accumulation of IDLs, which results in combined cholesterolemia and triglyceridemia, usually to about the same level. This condition is also called *remnant hyperlipoproteinemia, dysbetalipoproteinemia,* or *broad-beta disease* because the accumulated IDLs are remnants of incompletely metabolized triglyceride-containing lipoproteins with a relatively high cholesterol content that migrate beyond the usual "beta" or LDL cholesterol band during electrophoresis.

Type III hyperlipoproteinemia is relatively uncommon, with an incidence of between 1/5,000 and 1/10,000 (48,60). Clinically, it is characterized by unusual xanthomata, called *planar xanthomata,* in the creases of the palms of the hand and by tuberous xanthomata over the elbows and knees. Diagnosis of this disorder requires identification of IDLs by ultracentrifugation. The apo E phenotype of the patient should be determined because more than 90% of people with type III hyperlipoproteinemia are homozygous for two apo E-II isoforms that cannot bind effectively with the hepatic receptor responsible for removing apo E-containing lipoprotein remnant particles, including IDLs. The pathogenesis of dyslipidemia in type III hyperlipoproteinemia is not completely understood (61).

e. **Type IV** hyperlipoproteinemia is a common pattern occurring in about 1/300 individuals and characterized principally by an increase in plasma triglycerides secondary to elevated VLDLs. The pathogenic mechanisms of type IV hyperlipoproteinemia are not entirely elucidated; hepatic overproduction of VLDL appears to be the primary mechanism, although some evidence for diminished removal has also been found. Elevated VLDL levels are seen commonly secondary to diabetes, uremia, nephrotic syndrome, alcohol ingestion, and glucocorticoid or estrogen treatment. Obesity may aggravate VLDL elevations in subjects with primary hyperlipidemia, but obesity usually does not cause significant hypertriglyceridemia in persons with normal lipoprotein metabolism. As discussed, the role of triglycerides *per se* as a cardiovascular risk factor is still unsettled, although current evidence supports the position that it is a factor (46,62)

f. **Type V** hyperlipoproteinemia is a rare pattern marked by elevations in both chylomicrons and VLDLs. Thus, triglycerides are significantly elevated, and the phenotype is often called *mixed hypertriglyceridemia* because the triglycerides are contained in both VLDL and chylomicrons. Mild elevations in cholesterol may be secondary to the cholesterol content of VLDLs and chylomicrons. The underlying mechanisms and genetics of this phenotype are unknown, but it does not generally appear until later in life. Most patients have diabetes, renal failure, or other disorders, abuse alcohol, or are on various medication regimens. The common feature in this disorder appears to be an inherent or acquired defect in the capacity to metabolize triglyceride-rich lipoproteins that have been produced in excess quantity by the liver in response to excessive fatty acid release by adipose tissue (49).

4. **Atherogenic dyslipidemia** is a newly named entity (49). A particularly important constellation of lipoprotein abnormalities of great clinical significance appear to result from the coexistence of several defects, lipoprotein or otherwise, of lipid metabolism. The specific findings are (a) mild hypercholesterolemia, (b) mild to moderate hypertriglyceridemia, (c) the presence of circulating small, dense LDL particles, and (d) a low serum concentration of HDL cholesterol. Although genotype and aging are strong contributors, three additional lifestyle factors are also apparently

contributory or causative. These include obesity, physical inactivity, and diets high in fatty acids that increase serum cholesterol. Naturally, the latter three factors are clinically relevant because they are potentially modifiable.

B. Diagnosis

1. **Measurement of cholesterol and triglycerides.** Because of the association of hyperlipidemia with coronary heart disease, it is generally recommended that plasma cholesterol and triglycerides be measured periodically during adult life. If a family has a history of hyperlipidemia or premature coronary heart disease, children should also be tested.

   a. **Timing of measurement.** The serum cholesterol level is relatively unaffected by eating, but a recent meal can cause a marked elevation of plasma triglycerides. Triglycerides should be measured only after a 12- to 14-hour fast. Plasma lipid values are best determined while patients are maintaining a steady weight and have been on their usual diet for several weeks.

   b. **Repeated measurements.** Before a firm diagnosis is made, fasting lipid levels should be measured on two or three occasions separated by 2- to 3-week intervals.

2. **The presence of chylomicrons** can be detected by refrigerating the plasma overnight at 4°C. If chylomicrons are present, they will form a creamy layer on top of the plasma. The presence of chylomicrons in plasma drawn after a 12-hour fast is abnormal and indicative of type I or type V hyperlipoproteinemia. Fasting chylomicronemia is usually seen only when plasma triglyceride levels are above 1,000 mg/dL.

3. **Effect of elevation of different lipoproteins.** The implications of elevated plasma cholesterol depend on the lipoprotein class with which the cholesterol is associated. As noted earlier, a risk for coronary heart disease is associated with an elevated level of LDL cholesterol. A marked increase in VLDL may result in some increase in plasma cholesterol because VLDL contains about 1 mg of cholesterol for every 4 mg of triglyceride. After ultracentrifugation to separate VLDL, HDL cholesterol can be determined easily by precipitating lipoproteins containing apo B; the nonprecipitated cholesterol that remains is HDL cholesterol. Then, by simultaneous measurement of total and HDL cholesterol, LDL cholesterol can be calculated as follows:

$$\text{LDL Cholesterol} = \text{Total Cholesterol} - \text{HDL Cholesterol} - (\text{Triglycerides}/5)$$

   If the LDL cholesterol level by this clinical screening method is abnormal, more specific LDL cholesterol measurements must be made because this approach also precipitates IDL cholesterol and apolipoprotein[a] cholesterol. The former is a particular problem if the patient has the homozygous apo E-II phenotype and type III dyslipoproteinemia.

4. **Diagnosis.** Most patients can be assigned to a specific diagnostic category on the basis of total and LDL cholesterol, triglycerides, and the presence or absence of chylomicronemia. To establish the diagnoses of type III hyperlipoproteinemia or apo C-II deficiency, appropriate apoprotein quantification is necessary. Confirmation of the specific genetic defects in lipoprotein lipase deficiency, apo C-II deficiency, and familial hypercholesterolemia require appropriate studies at the DNA level.

C. Dietary therapy

1. **General principles.** Dietary therapy is the mainstay of lifestyle-altering treatment of all the hyperlipoproteinemias. However, dietary therapy alone is most often today reserved for persons without coronary heart disease, with LDL cholesterol values in the range of 160 to 189 mg/dL, and with fewer than two major cardiovascular risk factors, including hypertension, diabetes, obesity, smoking, decreased physical

activity, male sex, advanced age, and decreased HDL cholesterol. Even these patients may require drug therapy if the target goal for LDL cholesterol reduction is not met. Persons with LDL cholesterol values of 190 mg/dL or higher require drug therapy in addition to dietary intervention (48,49,53,63).

The manipulation of serum lipids by changes in diet has been an area of active research for several decades. Although the responses of serum lipids to dietary manipulations are known, the biochemical mechanisms for the responses are not completely clear. The following statements summarize the response of serum lipids to dietary manipulation:

a. Despite the fact that most (two-thirds to three-fourths) of the serum cholesterol is endogenous rather than of dietary origin, *alterations in diet* can change serum cholesterol levels. However, the effect of dietary alterations on serum cholesterol varies greatly from person to person. Dietary changes that cause a marked fall in cholesterol in one person may have little or no effect in another.

b. The reduction in serum cholesterol is most marked when dietary cholesterol is reduced to a very low level (<100 mg/d). In *severe cholesterol restriction*, the diet consists largely of cereals, legumes, fruits, and vegetables, with only small allowances of meat and dairy products.

c. The fall in serum cholesterol is not directly proportional to the degree of dietary restriction. A substantial reduction in dietary cholesterol (e.g., from 600 to <300 mg/d) usually results in only a modest reduction in serum cholesterol.

d. An increased dietary P:S ratio reduces serum cholesterol levels. Reducing the dietary cholesterol in addition to increasing the P:S ratio reduces serum cholesterol more than does reducing dietary cholesterol alone. The mechanism by which an increased P:S ratio decreases serum cholesterol is not established, but a decrease in the synthesis of endogenous cholesterol has been postulated. Monounsaturated fatty acids, such as are found in olive and peanut oils, have cholesterol-lowering effects similar to those of polyunsaturated oils (64).

e. The major determinant of chylomicron production and VLDL production is the rate of synthesis of triglycerides in the enterocytes and hepatocytes, respectively. The rate of triglyceride synthesis in enterocytes is determined by the intake of fat. The rate of triglyceride synthesis in hepatocytes is determined by total caloric intake and fat intake. Thus, caloric restriction reduces both chylomicron and VLDL production by reducing the synthesis of triglycerides.

f. Elevated triglycerides are associated with obesity. Weight loss usually reduces the hypertriglyceridemia associated with obesity. In many patients with hypertriglyceridemia, a pronounced rise in triglyceride levels occurs after alcohol ingestion. Elimination or marked curtailment of alcohol results in decreased triglycerides.

g. As discussed above, a trial of *dietary therapy alone* is indicated for persons with modestly elevated LDL cholesterol and fewer than two cardiovascular risk factors *before drugs are used* to alter serum lipids.

h. Repeated measurements of serum lipids. Because the individual response to diet therapy is variable, and because dietary compliance is frequently less than perfect, it is important to follow the patient and measure serum lipids again after 4 to 6 weeks of dietary therapy.

2. Specific recommendations for dietary therapy. For dietary purposes, it is useful to think of the hyperlipoproteinemias according to the previously described, practical clinical classification that divides the various disorders into those with elevated cholesterol, those with elevated triglycerides, and those with both (Table 12-9).

a. **Hypercholesterolemia.** For patients with hypercholesterolemia, the National Cholesterol Education Program recommends a decrease in the intake of total fat, saturated fat, and cholesterol. Two progressive steps are described (Table 12-7). Individuals on the step 2 diet for therapeutic purposes (as opposed to voluntary lifestyle preferences) will almost certainly be receiving cholesterol-lowering drugs. As mentioned previously, the step 1 diet is essentially the same diet recommended by the American Heart Association (24) and in *Nutrition and Your Health: Dietary Guidelines for Americans, 2000* (14,21):

Step 1: In this diet, no more than 30% of total calories is provided by fat and less than 10% of total calories is provided by saturated fat. Monounsaturated fats should contribute 10% to 15% and polyunsaturated fats should contribute 10% or less of the total daily energy intake. Cholesterol intake should be less than 300 mg/d.

Step 2: In this diet, less than 30% of the total calories (preferably <25%) should be from fat, with less than 7% of dietary energy from saturated fat. Cholesterol intake should be less than 200 mg/d. In selected patients with severe hypercholesterolemia, even further reductions in total fat intake to less than 20% of calories and in cholesterol intake to 100 to 150 mg/d may be required. Step 2 diets contain little meat and may be deficient in iron. Even though certain vegetables may contain considerable amounts of iron, it is not readily absorbed as heme iron. The risk for iron deficiency is particularly high in women consuming less than 1,500 cal and in those with increased iron requirements, as in pregnancy. The patient's iron status should be measured and supplements given as necessary.

   (1) An important component of dietary therapy for patients with hypercholesterolemia is an attempt to achieve *desirable weight.* Any overweight patient should be put on a weight-reduction diet low in both fat and cholesterol. This is especially important in persons exhibiting the characteristics of atherogenic dyslipoproteinemia, described earlier.

   (2) **Other medical conditions** must be considered when a cholesterol-lowering diet is designed. If renal disease is present, it may be necessary to lower the protein intake, and if the patient has hypertension, further limitation of the salt intake may be required, as described earlier in this chapter.

b. **Hypertriglyceridemia**

   (1) **Eliminating precipitating factors.** Obesity and alcohol consumption both commonly precipitate hypertriglyceridemia. Weight-reduction diets and elimination of alcohol should be applied as indicated. Weight loss reduces VLDL production and thus lowers triglycerides. When high plasma levels of triglycerides are secondary to other diseases, therapy should be directed first toward the underlying disorder. Non–insulin-dependent diabetes, when poorly controlled, is a common cause of hypertriglyceridemia; treatment with caloric restriction, exercise, or insulin often normalizes triglyceride concentrations. When hypothyroidism is associated with hypertriglyceridemia, patients usually are obese and may have a familial form of hyperlipidemia; with this combination of disorders, thyroid hormone therapy alone may not correct the hypertriglyceridemia completely.

   (2) **Diet.** As noted, the first goal of diet therapy is to achieve ideal body weight. The second goal is to moderate total fat intake to about 30% of dietary energy intake and to reduce saturated fat intake to below 10% of energy intake, aims achieved by the step 1 diet and related recommendations (14,21,24). For patients at

ideal body weight, calories from saturated fat can be replaced with calories from carbohydrates; for those who are overweight, the calories are best eliminated. Patients whose hyperlipoproteinemias do not respond adequately to diet therapy probably require drug intervention, as discussed (48,49,53,61).

3. Practical dietary management

    a. Decreasing cholesterol intake. The average American consumes between 300 to 400 mg of cholesterol daily.

        (1) Cholesterol intake can be reduced to about 300 mg by *eliminating foods very high in cholesterol and in saturated and* trans *fatty acids* (organ meats, butter fat, lard, certain margarines), and by substituting skim milk for whole milk (Table 12-10). The cholesterol contents of some common foods are as follows: a large egg, 240 mg; 1 tbs of butter, 30 mg; a hamburger made with a quarter of a pound of beef, 85 mg; one

Table 12-10. Lipid content of selected foods

Specific food (100 g)	Total fat (g)	P:S ratio[a]	Cholesterol (g)
Beef, lean, cooked	14.9	0.1	80
Beef, fatty, cooked	29.8	0.1	85
Chicken and turkey (light meat, no skin)	3.9	0.8	77
Frankfurter, all beef, cooked	28.5	0.1	61
Bologna, salami, cold cuts	30.0	0.1	85
Bacon, regular, cooked	49.0	0.3	85
Fish (cod)	1.5	1.7	68
Shrimp	1.1	1.54	195
Clams, mussels, cooked	1.9	2.9	67
Tuna, canned, water-packed	0.8	1.5	30
Eggs (equivalent to 2 whole)	10.5	0.4	425
Egg, yolk	30.9	0.4	1,281
Egg, white	0	—	0
Milk, whole	3.5	0.1	13.6
Milk, 1% fat	1.1	0.1	4
Milk, skim	0.2	0.1	2
Cheese, cheddar, American	33.1	0.1	105
Cheese, cottage, low-fat	1.9	0.1	8
Ice cream, regular (11% fat)	11	0.1	44
Butter	81.0	0.1	219
Oils			
Corn	100.0	4.6	0
Cottonseed	100.0	2.0	0
Safflower	100.0	8.2	0
Sesame	100.0	2.9	0
Soybean, partially hydrogenated	100.0	2.5	0
Olive	100.0	0.6	0
Peanut	100.0	1.9	0
Coconut	100.0	0.1	0
Peanut butter	50.6	1.6	0

[a] P:S ratio is the ratio of polyunsaturated fatty acids to saturated fatty acids; values less than 0.1 have been rounded to 0.1. For dairy products, the values average closer to 0.05, and for coconut oil, the P:S ratio is closer to 0.02.

Adapted from Grundy SM. Nutrition and diet in the management of hyperlipidemia and atherosclerosis. In: Shils ME, Olson JA, Shike M, et al., eds. *Modern nutrition in health and disease,* 9th ed. Baltimore: Williams & Wilkins, 1999:1199.

strip of bacon, 16 mg; and 1 cup of whole milk, 34 mg. Although eggs contain a significant amount of cholesterol, they are relatively "poor" in saturated fatty acids. Evidence indicates that they raise LDL cholesterol considerably less than might be anticipated (65–68).

(2) A further reduction to about 200 mg of cholesterol per day can be achieved by *reducing the amount of animal fats* consumed.

(a) **Meat and fish.** Up to 9 oz of fish, shellfish, poultry, or veal is allowed per day. Beef, lamb, ham, and pork are limited to a 3-oz serving three times per week. Although the cholesterol content of shrimp is high, they contain many noncholesterol sterols (e.g., sitosterol) that compete for absorption. Thus, like eggs, shrimp do not appear to raise cholesterol levels substantially (69). Also, shrimp are not usually consumed daily or in as large quantities as animal products containing cholesterol.

(b) **Most whole milk cheeses,** except for cottage cheese and farmer's cheese, are high in cholesterol and should be limited. Some whole milk substitutes, made for lactose-intolerant patients, are composed entirely of vegetable products and oils (often soy) and are acceptable for patients with hypercholesterolemia (e.g., Vita Rich, Vitamite). However, they contain as many calories as whole milk.

(c) **Many homemade and commercially prepared baked goods** contain significant amounts of saturated fat in the form of butter, lard, and whole milk in addition to the cholesterol of egg yolks. These products include waffles, pancakes, muffins, pastries, French toast, potato chips, cakes, and pies. Low-cholesterol baked goods can be made at home, with either egg whites or egg substitutes used instead of whole eggs, skim milk instead of whole milk, and soft margarine instead of butter and lard. A variety of low-fat, low-cholesterol bakery products is now available commercially.

(3) **Commercially prepared low-cholesterol egg substitutes** may be useful in a low-cholesterol diet. They are made principally from egg whites but, unfortunately, are considerably more expensive than fresh whole eggs.

(4) **Fat-modified cheeses** are now commonly available in supermarkets. The calorie content of *low-fat or nonfat cheeses* is reduced in comparison with that of regular cheese, and *cheeses made from vegetable fats* rather than animal fats have no cholesterol and a high P:S ratio, although their calorie content is about the same as that of natural cheese.

(5) **Meat analogues** made from a variety of vegetable sources are now available in virtually every supermarket and in almost every meat product configuration, including "bacon," "sausage," "ground beef," and "turkey." Surimi, a form of processed pollock that is low in fat and cholesterol, is sold as imitation crab meat and is a reasonably priced substitute for meat protein.

b. For a few patients with hypercholesterolemia, an even *more stringent restriction of dietary cholesterol* (in the range of 100 mg/d) is required. These are patients whose cholesterol levels do not fall into the acceptable range with a dietary restriction of 200 mg/d. Restriction of dietary cholesterol to 100 mg/d requires that meat consumption be limited to about 3 oz/d and that low-cholesterol cheese be used. When meat consumption is reduced to this level, meat cannot be used as the main course of a meal. Instead, it is used as a supplement or side dish. The current availability of cholesterol- and triglyceride-lowering drugs has helped persons with severe hypercholesterolemia significantly because it is now possible to liberalize to some extent severely restricted and relatively unpalatable dietary regimens that preclude compliance.

c. **Modifying the P:S ratio.** The P:S ratio in the standard American diet is less than 1.0. Most polyunsaturated fats come from vegetable oils, whereas most saturated fat comes from meat and dairy products.

   (1) **Margarines** are all made by partially hydrogenating vegetable oils.

   (a) **Hydrogenation** increases saturation and therefore reduces the P:S ratio. Generally, tub margarines are less hydrogenated than stick margarines and have a higher P:S ratio. This is not always true, however, and each margarine must be evaluated individually by reading the label. During the hydrogenation process, some fatty acids are converted to *trans* fatty acids. Substantial evidence now indicates that *trans* fatty acids may raise LDL cholesterol and reduce HDL cholesterol as much as saturated fatty acids do (21,70,71). When buying margarine, it is very important to read the label. Some margarine labels now indicate that they are low in, or free of, *trans* fatty acids. Further, given the listing of grams of saturated and unsaturated fats on the label, one can calculate the P:S ratio, which is best when above 2.0.

   (b) A label stating "vegetable fat" or "containing no animal fat" or "nondairy" does not always mean "unsaturated fat." "Vegetable fat" may refer to coconut oil or other relatively saturated vegetable oils. Always read the label.

   (2) **Vegetable oils.** Of all the vegetable oils, safflower oil has the highest P:S ratio. Other vegetable oils with a high P:S ratio are corn, soybean, and sunflower oils. The P:S ratio for olive oil (0.6) is lower than that for most other vegetable oils because olive oil is predominantly a monounsaturated oil; however, monounsaturated oils lower cholesterol as effectively as polyunsaturated oils. The P:S ratios for palm oil (0.2) and coconut oil (0.2) are even lower, and these are not effective cholesterol-lowering oils. Vegetable oils can be used for baking, in salad dressings, and in preparing meat (e.g., frying, marinating).

   (3) **Most regular commercially prepared baked goods,** including crackers for snacks, cookies, cakes, and pies, have low P:S ratios because they are made with animal fats or hydrogenated vegetable fats. Commercial cake mixes have low P:S ratios for the same reason.

   (4) Although the P:S ratios for vegetable products are generally high, those for *animal products* are very low. Fish and poultry have higher P:S ratios than do other animal products. To raise the P:S ratio of the diet, one must reduce the consumption of meat, eggs, butter, and whole milk and increase the consumption of foods and oils with a high P:S ratio. The dietary changes that decrease cholesterol intake also generally lower the intake of saturated fat because, in the American diet, the foods that are high in cholesterol are also high in saturated fat (e.g., meat, butter, and dairy products made from whole milk).

   (5) It is relatively easy to think in terms of the P:S ratio of a single food but more difficult to calculate the *P:S ratio of an entire diet.*

   (a) For example, in a meal including 1 egg (50 g) and 1 tbs of butter (14 g), the egg contains 5.5 g of fat with a P:S ratio

Table 12-11. Polyunsaturated substitutes for saturated fats useful in changing a recipe that may be high in saturated fat to one that is high in polyunsatured fat

Saturated fat	Polyunsaturated fat
1 oz chocolate	= 2 tbs cocoa + 2 tsp margarine
1 egg	= 1 tbs flour for thickening
1 egg	= 2 egg whites
1 cup butter	= 1 cup margarine
1 cup sour cream	= 1 cup yogurt
1 cup whole milk	= 1 cup skim milk + 2 tsp margarine
1 tbs butter	= ¾ tbs oil
1¼ cup butter	= 1 cup oil

From the Washington University Lipid Research Center.

of 0.4 and the butter contains 11.3 g of fat with a P:S ratio of 0.1. Thus, the meal contains a total of 16.8 g of fat with a P:S ratio of 0.2. If 1 tbs (14 g) of margarine with a high P:S ratio (14 g of fat with a P:S ratio of 2.4) is substituted for the butter, the meal then contains 19.5 g of fat with a P:S ratio of 1.9.

   (b) Many recipes call for saturated fats; Table 12-11 provides a list of polyunsaturated substitutes for these saturated fats.

4. **Fish oils.** Marine fish oils, often given as supplements containing the long-chain φ-3 fatty acids eicosapentaenoic acid (EPA) and docosahexaenoic acid (DHA), have received considerable attention for their potential role in the prevention of coronary artery disease (24). Epidemiologic studies indicate that populations that consume large amounts of marine fish oils (Greenland Eskimos and Japanese fishermen) have low plasma levels of cholesterol and triglyceride and a low incidence of coronary artery disease. The EPA- and DHA-containing triglycerides of marine fish are not found in significant quantities in other foods. These fatty acids are found in much larger amounts in oily fish (mackerel, menhaden, herring) than in nonoily fish (sole, flounder, turbot). The highly unsaturated fatty acids of fish oil may retard the development of coronary artery disease by two mechanisms: effects on platelet aggregation by decreasing production of thromboxane A_2, and effects on reducing plasma triglycerides by decreasing hepatic secretion of VLDL and increasing VLDL turnover and catabolism (48). Fish oil has little effect on LDL cholesterol levels.

   The appropriate role of fish oil in the *prevention* of coronary artery disease and the *management* of hyperlipidemia is not yet established, and appropriate doses of fish oil and DHA and EPA to prevent coronary heart disease have not been determined. Nonetheless, the accumulated evidence suggests that some persons may benefit from the consumption of one meal of fatty marine fish per day or a fish oil supplement yielding approximately 900 mg of DHA and EPA, the amount shown to be beneficial in some studies (24).

Bibliography

1. The Diabetes Control and Complications Trial Research Group. The effect of intensive treatment of diabetes on the development and progression of long-term complications in insulin-dependent diabetes mellitus. *N Engl J Med* 1993;329: 977.

2. The Diabetes Control and Complications Trial Research Group. Progression of retinopathy with intensive versus conventional treatment in the diabetes control and complications trial. *Ophthalmology* 1995;102:647.
3. The Diabetes Control and Complications Trial Research Group. Effect of intensive therapy on the development and progression of diabetic nephropathy in the diabetes control and complications trial. *Kidney Int* 1995;47:1703.
4. The Diabetes Control and Complications Trial Research Group. Influence of intensive diabetes treatment on quality-of-life outcomes in the diabetes control and complications trial. *Diabetes Care* 1996;19:195.
5. The Diabetes Control and Complications Trial Research Group. Lifetime benefits and costs of intensive treatment as practiced in the diabetes control and complications trial. *JAMA* 1996;276:1409.
6. The Diabetes Control and Complications Trial Research Group. Hypoglycemia in the diabetes control and complications trial. *Diabetes* 1997;46:271.
7. The Diabetes Control and Complications Trial Research Group. The effect of intensive diabetes therapy on measures of autonomic nervous system function in the diabetes control and complications trial. *Diabetologia* 1998;41:416.
8. The Epidemiology of Diabetes Interventions and Complications Research Group. Effect of intensive diabetes treatment on carotid artery wall thickness in the epidemiology of diabetes interventions and complications. *Diabetes* 1999;48:383.
9. The Diabetes Control and Complications Trial/Epidemiology of Diabetes Interventions and Complications Research Group. Retinopathy and nephropathy in patients with type 1 diabetes four years after a trial of intensive therapy. *N Engl J Med* 2000;342:381.
10. The Diabetes Control and Complications Trial Research Group. Effect of pregnancy on microvascular complications in the diabetes control and complications trial. *Diabetes Care* 2000;23:1084.
11. The Diabetes Prevention Program. Baseline characteristics of the randomized cohort. *Diabetes Care* 2000;23:1619.
12. West KM. Diet and diabetes. *Postgrad Med* 1976;60:209.
13. American Diabetes Association. Nutrition recommendations and principles for people with diabetes mellitus. *Diabetes Care* 2000;23[Suppl 1]:S43.
14. U.S. Department of Health and Human Services, U.S. Department of Agriculture. Nutrition and your health: dietary guidelines for Americans, 2000, 5th ed. Washington, DC: U.S. Government Printing Office, 2000. Booklet available on line at *http://www.usda.gov/cnpp/DietGd.pdf* via the Internet. Accessed December 11, 2000.
15. Beebe CA. Kilocalorie- and nutrient-controlled diet for diabetes. In: *The American Dietetic Association handbook of clinical dietetics,* 2nd ed. New Haven: Yale University Press, 1992:405.
16. Crapo PA. Dietary management. In: Kahn CR, Weir GC, eds. *Joslin's diabetes mellitus,* 13th ed. Philadelphia: Lea & Febiger, 1994:415.
17. Anderson JW. Nutritional management of diabetes mellitus. In: Shils ME, Olson JA, Shike M, et al., eds. *Modern nutrition in health and disease,* 9th ed. Baltimore: Williams & Wilkins, 1999:1365.
18. Lean MEJ, Ha TKK. Nutrition and dietary advice for diabetics. In: Garrow JS, James WPT, Ralph A, eds. *Human nutrition and dietetics,* 10th ed. Edinburgh: Churchill Livingstone, 2000:605.
19. Adult Treatment Panel II. Expert panel on detection, evaluation, and treatment of high blood cholesterol in adults: summary of the second report of the National Cholesterol Education Program (NCEP) expert panel on detection, evaluation, and treatment of high blood cholesterol in adults. *JAMA* 1993;269:3015.
20. Expert Panel on Blood Cholesterol Levels in Children and Adolescents. Treatment recommendations of the National Cholesterol Education Program report of the expert panel on blood cholesterol levels in children and adolescents. *Pediatrics* 1992; 89[Suppl]:525.
21. U.S. Department of Health and Human Services, U.S. Department of Agriculture, Dietary Guidelines Advisory Committee. Report of the Dietary Guidelines Advisory

Committee on the dietary guidelines for Americans, 2000, 5th ed. Washington, DC: U.S. Government Printing Office, 2000. Report available on line at *http://www. usda.gov/cnpp/Pubs/DG2000/Full%20Report.pdf* via the Internet. Accessed December 11, 2000.

22. Gumbiner B. Treating obesity in type II diabetes: calories, composition, and control. *Diabetes Care* 1999;22:886.

23. Heilbronn LK, Noakes M, Clifton PM. Effect of energy restriction, weight loss, and diet composition on plasma lipids and glucose in patients with type II diabetes. *Diabetes Care* 1999;22:889.

24. Krauss RM, Eckel RH, Howard B, et al. AHA dietary guidelines revision 2000: a statement for healthcare professionals from the nutrition committee of the American Heart Association. *Circulation* 2000;102:2284.

25. Salmeron J, Manson JE, Stampfer MJ, et al. Dietary fiber, glycemic load, and risk of non–insulin-dependent diabetes mellitus in women. *JAMA* 1997;277:472.

26. Salmeron J, Ascherio A, Rimm EB, et al. Dietary fiber, glycemic load, and risk of NIDDM in men. *Diabetes Care* 1997;20:545.

27. Liu S, Willett WC, Stampfer MJ, et al. A prospective study of dietary glycemic load, carbohydrate intake, and risk of coronary heart disease in US women. *Am J Clin Nutr* 2000;71:1455.

28. Stampfer MJ, Hu FB, Manson JE, et al. Primary prevention of coronary heart disease in women through diet and lifestyle. *N Engl J Med* 2000;343:16.

29. Liu S, Manson JE, Stampfer MJ, et al. A prospective study of whole-grain intake and risk of type 2 diabetes mellitus in US women. *Am J Public Health* 2000; 90:1409.

30. The American Dietetic Association and The American Diabetes Association. *Exchange lists for meal planning.* New York: American Diabetes Association, 1995.

31. Yamanouchi K, Shinozaki T, Chikada K, et al. Daily walking combined with diet therapy is a useful means for obese NIDDM patients not only to reduce body weight but also to improve insulin sensitivity. *Diabetes Care* 1995;18:775.

32. Manson JE, Hu FB, Rich-Edwards JW, et al. A prospective study of walking as compared with vigorous exercise in the prevention of coronary heart disease in women. *N Engl J Med* 1999;341:650.

33. Maroni BJ, Mitch WE. Role of nutrition in prevention of the progression of renal disease. *Annu Rev Nutr* 1997;17:435.

34. Walser M, Mitch WE, Maroini BJ, et al. Should protein intake be restricted in predialysis patients? *Kidney Int* 1999;55:771.

35. Mitch WE. Dietary therapy in uremia: the impact of nutrition on progressive renal failure. *Kidney Int* 2000;57[Suppl 75]:S38.

36. Kopple JD. Renal disorders and nutrition. In: Shils ME, Olson JA, Shike M, et al., eds. *Modern nutrition in health and disease,* 9th ed. Baltimore: Williams & Wilkins, 1999:1439.

37. Mitch WE, Klahr S. *Nutrition and the kidney.* Boston: Little, Brown and Company, 1993.

38. Klahr S, Levey AS, Beck GJ, et al. The effects of dietary protein restriction and blood pressure control on the progression of chronic renal disease. *N Engl J Med* 1994;330:877.

39. Levey AS, Adler S, Caggiula AW, et al. Effects of dietary protein restriction on the progression of advanced renal disease in the modification of diet and renal disease study. *Am J Kidney Dis* 1996;27:652.

40. Fouque D, Laville M, Boissel JP, et al. Controlled low-protein diets in chronic renal insufficiency: meta-analysis. *Br Med J* 1992;304:216.

41. Pedrini MT, Levey AS, Lau J, et al. The effect of dietary protein restriction on the progression of diabetic and nondiabetic renal diseases: a meta-analysis. *Ann Intern Med* 1996;124:627.

42. Kopple JD. Therapeutic approaches to malnutrition in chronic dialysis patients: the different modalities of nutritional support. *Am J Kidney Dis* 1999;33:180.

43. Lim VS, Kopple JD. Protein metabolism in patients with chronic renal failure: role of uremia and dialysis. *Kidney Int* 2000;58:1.

44. Kopple JD. Dietary protein and energy requirements in ESRD patients. *Am J Kidney Dis* 1998;32[Suppl 4]:S97.
45. American Dietetic Association. Diets to control protein, sodium, potassium, phosphorus, and fluids (renal diets). In: *The American Dietetic Association handbook of clinical dietetics,* 2nd ed. New Haven: Yale University Press, 1992:187.
46. Austin MA, Hokanson JE, Edwards KL. Hypertriglyceridemia as a cardiovascular risk factor. *Am J Cardiol* 1998;81:7B.
47. Grundy SM, Pasternak R, Greenland P, et al. Assessment of cardiovascular risk by use of multiple-risk-factor assessment equations: a statement for healthcare professionals from the American Heart Association and the American College of Cardiology. *Circulation* 1999;100:1481.
48. Gotto A, Pownall H. *Manual of lipid disorders,* 2nd ed. Baltimore: Williams & Wilkins, 1999.
49. Grundy SM. Nutrition and diet in the management of hyperlipidemia and atherosclerosis. In: Shils ME, Olson JA, Shike M, et al., eds. *Modern nutrition in health and disease,* 9th ed. Baltimore: Williams & Wilkins, 1999:1199.
50. Mann J. Diseases of the heart and circulation: the role of dietary factors in aetiology and management. In: Garrow JS, James WPT, Ralph A, eds. *Human nutrition and dietetics,* 10th ed. Edinburgh: Churchill Livingstone, 2000.
51. Kannel WB, Castelli WP, Gordon T, et al. Serum cholesterol, lipoproteins, and the risk of coronary heart disease. The Framingham study. *N Engl J Med* 1971;74:1.
52. Kannel WB. Range of serum cholesterol values in the population developing coronary artery disease. *Am J Cardiol* 1995;76[9 Suppl]:69C.
53. Jacobson TA. "The lower the better" in hypercholesterolemia therapy: a reliable clinical guideline? *Ann Intern Med* 2000;133:549.
54. Randomized trial of cholesterol lowering in 4,444 patients with coronary heart disease: the Scandinavian simvastatin survival study. *Lancet* 1994;344:1383.
55. Sacks FM, Pfeiffer MA, Moyle LA, et al. The effect of pravastatin on coronary events after myocardial infarction in patients with average cholesterol levels. *N Engl J Med* 1996;335:1001.
56. The Long-term Intervention with Pravastatin in Ischemic Disease (LIPID) Study Group. Prevention of cardiovascular events and death with pravastatin in patients with coronary heart disease and a broad range of initial cholesterol levels. *N Engl J Med* 1998;339:1349.
57. Report of the National Cholesterol Education Program expert panel on detection, evaluation, and treatment of high blood cholesterol in adults. *Arch Intern Med* 1988;148:36.
58. Summary of the second report of the National Cholesterol Program (NCEP) Expert panel on detection, evaluation, and treatment of high blood cholesterol in adults (Adult Treatment Panel II). *JAMA* 1993;269:3015.
59. Kuo PT. Prevention and treatment of hyperlipidemia. In: Halpern SL, ed. *Quick reference to clinical nutrition.* Philadelphia: JB Lippincott Co, 1979:137.
60. Semenkovich CF. Nutrient and genetic regulation of lipoprotein metabolism. In: Shils ME, Olson JA, Shike M, et al., eds. *Modern nutrition in health and disease,* 9th ed. Baltimore: Williams & Wilkins, 1999:1199.
61. Mahley RW, Huang Y, Rall SC. Pathogenesis of type III hyperlipoproteinemia (dysbetalipoproteinemia): questions, quandries, and paradoxes. *J Lipid Res* 1999; 40:1933.
62. Triglycerides and heart disease. *Harvard Health Lett* 2000;11:1.
63. Gould AL, Rossouw JE, Santanello NC, et al. Cholesterol reduction yields clinical benefit: impact of statin trials. *Circulation* 1998;97:946.
64. Kris-Etherton P (for the American Heart Association Nutrition Committee). Monounsaturated fatty acids and risk of cardiovascular disease. *Circulation* 1999;100:1253.
65. Vorster HH, Benade AJ, Bernard HC, et al. Egg intake does not change plasma lipoprotein and coagulation profiles. *Am J Clin Nutr* 1992;55:400.
66. McNamara DJ. The impact of egg limitations on coronary heart disease risk: do the numbers add up? *J Am Coll Nutr* 2000;19[5 Suppl]:540S.
67. McNamara DJ. Dietary cholesterol and atherosclerosis. *Biochim Biophys Acta* 2000;15:1529.

68. Howell WH, McNamara DJ, Tosca MA, et al. Plasma lipid and lipoprotein responses to dietary fat and cholesterol: a meta-analysis. *Am J Clin Nutr* 1997; 65:1747.
69. De Oliveira E, Silva ER, Seidman CE, et al. Effects of shrimp consumption on plasma lipoproteins. *Am J Clin Nutr* 1996;64:712.
70. Judd JT, Clevidence BA, Muesing RA, et al. Dietary *trans* fatty acids: effects on plasma lipids and lipoproteins of healthy men and women. *Am J Clin Nutr* 1994;59:861.
71. Lichtenstein AH, Ausman LM, Jalbert SM, et al. Effects of different forms of dietary hydrogenated fats on serum lipoprotein cholesterol levels. *N Engl J Med* 1999;340:1933. [Published erratum appears in *N Engl J Med* 1999;341:856.]

13. OBESITY

I. **Definition of obesity.** *Obesity* is an excess amount of body fat. Although a variety of methods have been used to estimate body fat for decades, *no definition of normal quantities of body fat is uniformly accepted, and therefore no single definition of obesity based on excessive accretion of body fat exists.* This confusion results from the fact that the presence of abnormal amounts of body fat associated with medical complications is caused by many factors, including gender, age, distribution of fat, weight (fat) gain since early adulthood, level of fitness, genetic factors, and other disease risk factors. In recent years, guidelines for assigning risk have been proposed by classifying weight status according to body mass index (BMI) (Table 5-20). Thus, the World Health Organization has defined the preobese state as a BMI between 25 and 29.9, class I obesity as a BMI between 30.0 and 34.9, class II obesity as a BMI between 35.0 and 39.9, and class III obesity as a BMI above 40 (1,2). The U.S. National Center for Health Statistics classifies the BMI range of 25.0 to 29.9 as overweight, and obesity as a BMI of 30.0 or more (3). Based on these definitions, the prevalence of overweight in American adults in the 1999 National Health and Nutrition Examination Survey (NHANES) was 35% (an increase of 2% from NHANES III, conducted between 1988 and 1994), and the prevalence of obesity in adult Americans in 1999 was 26% (an increase of 3% from NHANES III, and an approximate doubling of the prevalence of obesity in NHANES II, conducted between 1976 and 1980). The BMI has been accepted as the guideline for classifying weight status by the National Institutes of Health (4), the U.S. Department of Health and Human Services (5), and the committee developing *Nutrition and Your Health: Dietary Guidelines for Americans, 2000* (6). These empirically derived ranges based on the BMI (as calculated in the equation shown below) have now become a global tool for evaluating healthy and unhealthy body sizes, and as a practical field surrogate for body fatness.

The *BMI* is a useful and very practical way of estimating relative body mass and assigning a relative associated disease risk. As a result, it has become the *de facto* standard for characterizing overweight and underweight for size (7). It is important to emphasize that the BMI does not measure body fat, although it is highly correlated with fat mass in a curvilinear fashion (8). For example, at the same BMI, women and elderly persons have more body fat than young men. Thus, persons with an elevated BMI are properly referred to as *overweight,* not *obese.* However, in general practice, once the BMI becomes elevated significantly, it is far more likely that the incremental changes represent accumulated body fat rather than accretion of lean tissue.

The BMI is calculated by dividing the weight (in kilograms) by the square of the height (in meters), or by multiplying the weight (in pounds) by 704 and dividing the product by the square of the height (in inches). Thus, for an 80-kg man who is 180 cm tall,

$$BMI = \frac{80}{(1.80)^2} = 24.7$$

In adults, a BMI between 18.5 and 24.9 is healthful, based on the relationships between the BMI and diseases that are a consequence of obesity (7). A BMI above 25 or 26 correlates with a Metropolitan relative weight of more than 120%, and a BMI above 30 corresponds to Metropolitan relative weight of more than 130%. A BMI table for adults (Table 13-1), which can be downloaded, and an English and metric unit calculator are available at the Centers for Disease Control web site *(www.cdc.gov/nccdphp/dnpa/bmi/bmi-adult.htm).* In children, the range of normal BMIs changes with age, and therefore no single range is healthful. BMI tables for children between the ages of 2 and 20 years, which can be downloaded,

Table 13-1. Adult body mass index (BMI)

BMI	19	20	21	22	23	24	25	26	27	28	29	30	31	32	33	34	35
Height									Weight (lb)								
4'10" (58")	91	96	100	105	110	115	119	124	129	134	138	143	148	153	158	162	167
4'11" (59")	94	99	104	109	114	119	124	128	133	138	143	148	153	158	163	168	173
5' (60")	97	102	107	112	118	123	128	133	138	143	148	153	158	163	168	174	179
5'1" (61")	100	106	111	116	122	127	132	137	143	148	153	158	164	169	174	180	185
5'2" (62")	104	109	115	120	126	131	136	142	147	153	158	164	169	175	180	186	191
5'3" (63")	107	113	118	124	130	135	141	146	152	158	163	169	175	180	186	191	197
5'4" (64")	110	116	122	128	134	140	145	151	157	163	169	174	180	186	192	197	204
5'5" (65")	114	120	126	132	138	144	150	156	162	168	174	180	186	192	198	204	210
5'6" (66")	118	124	130	136	142	148	155	161	167	173	179	186	192	198	204	210	216
5'7" (67")	121	127	134	140	146	153	159	166	172	178	185	191	198	204	211	217	223
5'8" (68")	125	131	138	144	151	158	164	171	177	184	190	197	203	210	216	223	230
5'9" (69")	128	135	142	149	155	162	169	176	182	189	196	203	209	216	223	230	236
5'10" (70")	132	139	146	153	160	167	174	181	188	195	202	209	216	222	229	236	243
5'11" (71")	136	143	150	157	165	172	179	186	193	200	208	215	222	229	236	243	250
6' (72")	140	147	154	162	169	177	184	191	199	206	213	221	228	235	242	250	258
6'1" (73")	144	151	159	166	174	182	189	197	204	212	219	227	235	242	250	257	265
6'2" (74")	148	155	163	171	179	186	194	202	210	218	225	233	241	249	256	264	272
6'3" (75")	152	160	168	176	184	192	200	208	216	224	232	240	248	256	264	272	279

From NIH/National Heart, Lung, and Blood Institute (NHLBI). *Evidence report of clinical guidelines on the identification, evaluation, and treatment of overweight and obesity in adults, 1998,* and Centers for Disease Control and Prevention, U.S. Department of Health and Human Services *(www.cdc.gov/nccdphp/dnpa/bmi/bmi-adult.htm).*

and a BMI calculator are available at *www.cdc.gov/nccdphp/dnpa/bmi/bmi-for-age.htm.*

From the recommended range of BMIs (between 19 and 25), it is possible to "back-calculate" combinations of height and weight that yield healthful BMI values. Based on this calculation, Table 13-2 shows healthful weight ranges for adults that are offered as guidelines for persons of given heights.

II. **Relative disease risks in obesity.** The BMI cutoff values are based on large epidemiologic studies correlating BMIs and mortality rates (9–11). Men and women with a BMI of 30 kg/m$_2$ or more are considered to be obese and at higher risk for adverse health events (Table 5-20). It has been argued that this cutoff value is too high because it is based on associations with mortality; the incidence of the diseases that are associated with obesity and lead to mortality (i.e., diabetes, hypertension, coronary artery disease) begins to increase at lower BMI values. Classifying disease risk according to BMI values tends to efface this continuum; the same problem arises in the evaluation of risk in hypertensive patients. Thus, the BMI should be considered as only one component of risk assessment in patients of various heights and weights. In general, the higher the BMI, the greater the risk for obesity-related disease and accompanying mortality. Other risk factors include the following:

A. **Age.** The relative rates of death associated with increasing BMI values decrease with advancing age (12), but the absolute mortality risk increases up to age 75 because of the marked effect of age on overall mortality.

B. **Fat distribution.** Morbidity is greater in persons with excess intraabdominal or subcutaneous truncal fat (android or "apple-shaped" distribution) than in those with excess gluteofemoral fat (gynoid or "pear-shaped" distribution), and the risk for diabetes, hypertension, dyslipidemia, and ischemic

Table 13-2. U.S. weight guidelines for adult men and women[a]

Height[b]	Weight[c] (lb)
4'10"	91–119
4'11"	94–124
5'0"	97–128
5'1"	101–132
5'2"	104–137
5'3"	107–141
5'4"	111–146
5'5"	114–150
5'6"	118–155
5'7"	121–160
5'8"	125–164
5'9"	129–169
5'10"	132–174
5'11"	136–179
6'0"	140–184
6'1"	144–189
6'2"	148–195
6'3"	152–200
6'4"	156–205
6'5"	160–211
6'6"	164–216

[a] Calculated from the "low-risk" BMI range: 19–25 kg/m^2.
[b] Without shoes.
[c] Without clothes.
From Willett WC, Dietz WH, Colditz GA. Guidelines for healthy weight. *N Engl J Med* 1999;341:427, with permission.

heart disease is greater in the former group (13–15). Waist circumference is often used as a surrogate marker because it correlates with abdominal fat mass (16). The National Institutes of Health Expert Panel on the Identification, Evaluation, and Treatment of Overweight and Obesity in Adults has proposed the following values for weight circumference that are associated with an increased risk for disease: more than 102 cm (40 in) in men, and more than 88 cm (35 in) in women (4).

C. **Weight gain during adulthood.** Weight gain of more than 5 kg after ages 18 to 20 increases obesity-related disease risk in both men and women (17). Unfortunately, this risk factor applies even in lean adults.

D. **State of fitness.** Subjects with better oxygen consumption during exercise had lower rates of diabetes and cardiovascular mortality across a range of body weight values (18).

E. **Ethnic background.** At the same BMI values as Caucasians, Asian-Pacific populations are at increased risk for the development of diabetes and cardiovascular disease (19).

III. **Recommended weight.** To interpret energy balance or weight change, other measurements of recommended body size have been used. For the application or interpretation of such tables, it is important to emphasize the following:

1. The use of terms such as *recommended* or *desirable weight* implies that we know what the criteria for *normal* or *optimal weight* should be. We do not, and no uniform agreement has been reached on otherwise arbitrary definitions.

2. The so-called normal range of adult weights gradually increases with age. A reasonable consensus exists that this increment is not a "normal," healthful effect of aging but rather the potentially detrimental consequence of inactivity and loss of lean body mass with aging.

3. Total weight alone does not permit an estimate of body composition (i.e., how much fat and how much lean tissue are present). A person can be overweight but not overly fat. No convenient "field" method is available for reliably determining a person's body composition.

A. **Weight tables for children.** Population reference values for the weights of American infants and children, recently revised by the National Center for Health Statistics, can be downloaded from the Centers for Disease Control and Prevention web site (20). *It is very important to realize that these weight charts are not the true current weight distributions of American children 6 years of age or older.* The height data at all ages and the weight data for infants and children below the age of 6 years are the most currently available. However, because of the increasing prevalence of overweight children, the advisory group chose to exclude weight data from NHANES III and use earlier, age-normalized weight values for children 6 years of age or older (21).

B. **Weight tables for adults.** Standard values for adult weights have been compiled by the Society of Actuaries and Association of Life Insurance Medical Directors (22) (Table 13-3). It is important to realize that the life insurance figures in Table 13-3 refer to *weights at ages 25 to 29 associated with minimal mortality rates* at a later age and are not necessarily related to average nutritional status. Moreover, the subjects for this study were self-selected from persons eligible to be insured; they were predominantly middle or upper class and largely Caucasian (they could afford insurance), tended to be healthier and weigh less than the general population, and were weighed in their clothes and shoes. Finally, no widely accepted standard algorithm is available for determining frame size. For these reasons, *these statistics cannot be relied on completely to provide advice about the ideal weight of all adults.*

IV. **Pathogenesis of obesity.** Genetic, endocrine, neurologic, psychological, and environmental factors are all involved in the pathogenesis of obesity to differing degrees in different persons. The factors contributing to obesity in a given individual may be difficult to define, but it is clear that obesity is not a single disease but rather a heterogeneous group of disorders, each of which is manifested by excess body fat.

Table 13-3. Weights of men and women ages 25 to 59 correlated
with the lowest mortality

Height[a]		Weight (lb)[b]		
Feet	Inches	Small frame	Medium frame	Large frame
Men				
5	2	128–134	131–141	138–150
5	3	130–136	133–143	140–153
5	4	132–138	135–145	142–156
5	5	134–140	137–148	144–160
5	6	136–142	139–151	146–164
5	7	138–145	142–154	149–168
5	8	140–148	145–157	152–172
5	9	142–151	148–160	155–176
5	10	144–154	151–163	158–180
5	11	146–157	154–166	161–184
6	0	149–160	157–170	164–188
6	1	152–164	160–174	168–192
6	2	155–168	164–178	172–197
6	3	158–172	167–182	176–202
6	4	162–176	171–187	181–207
Women				
4	10	102–111	109–121	118–131
4	11	103–113	111–123	120–134
5	0	104–115	113–126	122–137
5	1	106–118	115–129	125–140
5	2	108–121	118–132	128–143
5	3	111–124	121–135	131–147
5	4	114–127	124–138	134–151
5	5	117–130	127–141	137–155
5	6	120–133	130–144	140–159
5	7	123–136	133–147	143–163
5	8	126–139	136–150	146–167
5	9	129–142	139–153	149–170
5	10	132–145	142–156	152–173
5	11	135–148	145–159	155–176
6	0	138–151	148–162	158–179

[a] In shoes with 1-in heels.
[b] Men: in indoor clothing weighing 5 lb; women: in indoor clothing weighing 3 lb.
From Society of Actuaries and Association of Life Insurance Medical Directors of America. *Build study, 1979.* Chicago: Society of Actuaries, 1980, with permission.

A. **Genetics.** Genes clearly influence the development of body size, and *heredity* plays a definite role in human obesity (23–30). If neither parent is obese, the offspring have a 10% chance of becoming obese. Having one obese parent increases the risk for obesity to 40%. If both parents are obese, the risk rises to 80%. The roles of heredity and childhood environment have been separated by studies of adopted children with obese biologic parents. The incidence of obesity is higher in children with obese biologic parents and normal-weight adoptive parents than in children with normal-weight biologic parents and normal-weight adoptive parents, so that a role for heredity in human obesity is indicated. Furthermore, convincing evidence of the importance of genetic factors in the pathogenesis of obesity comes from multiple studies of monozygotic twins reared together or apart, which show that variability in BMI is largely independent of shared environment. The data in these and other studies suggest that genes account for as much as 60% to 80% of variations in BMI and body fat mass (25–28,31–33). However, familial studies that do not involve twins suggest a somewhat lower contribution (~ 40%) of genetics to variability in body weight (34).

Nonetheless, although more than 200 genes are now linked with the human obesity phenotype and 20 mendelian disorders with obesity as a prominent part of the phenotype, defects in only five genes, affecting a very small number of persons, have been shown to cause obesity in humans (23). These are the genes for leptin, the leptin receptor, proopiomelanocortin (POMC), the melanocortin-4 receptor, and prohormone convertase-1 (23,25). Only one of these defects, a deficiency of melanocortin-4 receptor, has been shown to account for more than sporadic cases of severe obesity (35–37). The genes and polygenetic interactions underlying the common forms of human obesity are unknown. Furthermore, it is critical to emphasize that the prevalence of obesity in the United States has approximately doubled in the last two decades, a period inconsequential in the context of genetic changes. Individual genotypes have not been the principal reason for the dramatic increase in obesity.

B. **Studies of the central nervous system control of food intake** have produced the most dramatic advances in obesity research in the past 5 years (38,39). Leptin, which is released from fat cells and circulates in the plasma in proportion to body fat mass, interacts within the arcuate nucleus of the hypothalamus with two principal neuronal cell types, one in which neuropeptide Y (NPY) and agouti-related (AGRP) proteins co-localize, and a second that contains POMC. Leptin signaling in the former neurons inhibits *NPY* and *AGRP* gene expression and leads to a decrease in the release of NPY and AGRP. Because these peptides normally cause an increase in food intake, inhibition of their secretion by leptin causes a decrease in food intake. In the second family of neurons, leptin signaling causes an increase in *POMC* gene expression and, consequently, increased generation of the peptide α-MSH, a melanocortin produced from the cleavage of POMC by prohormone convertase-1. Released MSH, in turn, binds to the melanocortin-4 receptor and inhibits food intake (38,39). Other hypothalamic neuropeptides have been identified as additional mediators of the effects of leptin on appetite and satiety. These include the appetite-stimulating (orexigenic) peptides hypocretin-1 and -2, orexin A and B, and galanin, which are down-regulated by leptin or insulin, and the anorexigenic (appetite-suppressing) peptides corticotropin-releasing hormone, thyrotropin-releasing hormone, and cocaine- and amphetamine-regulated transcript (CART), which are up-regulated by leptin or insulin (38).

C. **Energy metabolism** varies considerably from person to person. In fact, the resting metabolic rate varies more between families than within families, presumably on the basis of genetic determinants of energy expenditure. Some evidence has been found that low rates of resting energy expenditure (REE) may predispose both children and adults to the development of obesity (40). However, these findings do not necessarily describe the primary mechanism for the development of obesity; if appetite, satiety, and the other mechanisms that maintain energy balance by affecting food intake all functioned normally, the person with a low expenditure of energy would eat less.

The relationships between altered energy metabolism and obesity were carefully examined in cross-sectional studies. The REE was greater in obese than in lean persons of the same height because of their greater lean tissue cell mass (41). The small reduction in the thermic effect of food (TEF) may be related to insulin resistance and the depressed sympathetic nervous system activity seen in obesity (42). The same amount of energy was needed for the same amount of work in both obese and lean persons (43). The metabolic rates during sleep, rest, exercise, and eating were the same in lean and obese children when the rates were adjusted for differences in body composition (44). Moreover, defects in REE or TEF were not found in patients who failed to lose weight despite apparent adherence to a low-calorie diet (45). Thus, it seems unlikely that significant alterations in the components of energy metabolism account for the wide variation in body weights found among free-living persons.

Because these data were obtained at only one time, significant energy changes may have been missed during development or at other times of life. Although in some studies persons with lower daily REE or TEF values gained more weight in later years, larger (46) and longer (47) studies did not find a relationship between initial REE or TEF and subsequent weight changes. Some data suggested that the amount of weight gained after overfeeding might be genetically determined, but when the components of energy metabolism were examined before and after 8 weeks of overfeeding, the gain in body fat was found to be inversely related to changes in nonvolitional energy expenditure (48). Thus, it is possible that differences in weight gain are determined by genetic differences in the ability to dissipate excess ingested energy.

Weight loss during dieting decreased the REE 15% to 30%, and the decrease did not appear to be explained entirely by the loss of lean body mass. This phenomenon led to the "set-point" theory, which states that body weight is predetermined because changes in weight alter the metabolic rate to return the body weight to a preset value. One difficulty with this theory is that the decline in REE below predicted values occurs only during negative energy balance and does not persist when the lower weight is maintained (49). In a metaanalysis of 15 studies, the REE, when adjusted for body composition, was similar in formerly obese and never-obese subjects (50). Thus, the fall in REE during dieting probably accounts for some failures to continue dieting, but the decrease seems appropriate to the changes that occur in body composition and might be interpreted as part of the metabolic adaptation to energy restriction.

Although we do not yet understand the full significance of intersubject variations in energy expenditure or energy intake in the generation of obesity, the role of energy intake in the *maintenance* of obesity is now absolutely clear. Energy expenditure can be measured very accurately and precisely, both under controlled conditions on a metabolic ward with a room calorimeter and under free-living conditions with isotopic methods. In each case, all such studies have shown unequivocally *that the total daily energy expenditure of obese adults is greater than that of lean adults*. Therefore, the energy intake of obese adults must be greater (i.e., they must eat more) than that of lean adults for them to maintain their body weight.

D. **Energy intake.** On the other hand, no method reliably measures energy intake in free-living subjects. The best approaches entail uncertainties greater than the precision required to answer basic questions of energy balance in humans. Studies have shown repeatedly that adults tend to underestimate their energy intake, and that overweight persons tend to underestimate their dietary intake more than subjects of normal body weight. Nonetheless, for all persons, no matter how energy-efficient their metabolism, a level of calorie consumption exists below which they lose weight. Despite the many different mechanisms underlying obesity, *calorie restriction and increased energy expenditure through exercise are always effective in achieving weight loss.*

As discussed above, the degree of calorie restriction or energy expenditure increase required for weight loss varies from person to person. Energy efficiency varies among individuals and also varies for a given individual over time. The basal metabolic rate declines when an obese person loses weight on a calorie-restricted diet. This adaptation contributes to the difficulty in maintaining weight loss. On most conventional weight-loss programs, the obese person loses weight fairly rapidly for a few weeks, and then the rate of weight loss declines markedly or even stops although the person adheres to the weight-loss program. Several factors contribute to this pattern. First, the initial weight loss may involve a significant loss of tissue glycogen and protein, which is associated with loss of water. Later, most of the weight loss involves fat, and fat loss is not associated with water loss. Second, as weight declines, the basal metabolic rate also declines because less lean tissue must be supported. These factors combine to reduce the rate of weight loss, so that discouragement and diminished compliance ensue. Although earlier studies suggested that the body attempts to maintain weight by reducing the metabolic rate, most studies suggest this is not so (49).

Dieters should be warned that the rate of weight loss will decrease. Moreover, when the rate of weight loss declines, the dieter should not necessarily be accused of backsliding. A major unfortunate issue that plagues all dieters is that they regain lost weight. One possible explanation for this response is that the reduction in energy expenditure associated with successful dietary therapy predisposes one to regain lost weight. Available energy expenditure data are conflicting on this issue (51–53).

E. **The macronutrient composition of foods** may play an important role in the development of obesity. Gene–diet interactions and epidemiologic evidence support a role for a high intake of fat in promoting obesity (54,55). Although some disagree with the proposition that a high intake of fat contributes significantly to obesity (56), data on energy expenditure collected during controlled feeding experiments support the contention that it is more difficult to reestablish energy balance during periods of a high intake of fat. Consequently, the fat is stored in adipose tissue (57,58).

V. **Morbidity and mortality.** A BMI above 30 is clearly associated with an increase in morbidity and mortality (2,7,59–61). Figure 13-1 shows how the risk for mortality from obesity is estimated as a function of the BMI. Obese persons have an increased risk for diabetes, hypertension, coronary artery disease, hyperlipidemia, arthritis, gout, and gallstones. In older adults (>75 years old), the difference between the mortality rates of obese and nonobese persons is less striking than in the young. The development of obesity in middle age appears to

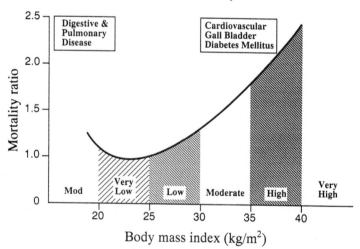

All Cause Mortality

FIG. 13.1. Use of body mass index to estimate excess mortality risk from obesity in persons ages 20 to 29 years and 30 to 39 years. (Based on data from Les EA, Garfunkel L. Variation in mortality by weight among 750,000 men and women. *J Chron Dis* 1987;32:563, as adapted by Bray GA. Obesity: basic considerations and clinical approaches. *Dis Mon* 1989;18:449.)

increase mortality less than the presence of obesity from childhood. In the past, it was debated whether obesity itself is a risk factor for coronary artery disease independently of other risk factors because almost all severely obese persons have at least one other risk factor (smoking, diabetes, hypertension, or hypercholesterolemia). However, data have now confirmed that obesity is an independent risk factor for the development of coronary heart disease (2,59–61).

VI. **Management of obesity.** The management of obesity is difficult, and the rate of success, defined as adequate weight loss followed by a prolonged period in which the lost weight is not regained, is low. Obesity can be managed by diet, exercise, surgery, drugs, behavior modification, or combinations of these modalities. Here, we focus primarily on diet, with the recognition that the long-term results of obesity treatment by diet alone have been disappointing on the whole (2,59,62,63). Although epidemiologic data have failed to demonstrate conclusively that weight reduction is associated with a reduction in mortality (64), the data in this area are scarce. Weight loss decreases the risk for some obesity-related diseases, such as diabetes and hypertension, independently of the effect on obesity itself. Thus, there is every reason to offer therapy to overweight persons.

A. **Dietary management.** A realistic goal in the dietary management of obesity is to have the patient lose 5% to 10% of body weight and then maintain this reduced weight. Ideally, one should lose weight down to one's ideal body weight, but this goal is unrealistic for most patients. Many more dieters achieve an initial significant weight loss than maintain such weight loss. In fact, 80% to 90% of dieters regain some or all lost weight. In prescribing a diet, it is important to choose one that the patient will comply with long enough to lose the necessary amount of weight. The more weight that must be lost, the longer the diet will have to be maintained and the more carefully the diet should be designed. For patients with a BMI above 35 who have demonstrated an ability to lose weight and maintain a lower weight and for whom further weight loss is advisable for medical or social reasons, treatment with pharmacologic agents should be considered (65).

The patient must understand that the process is long (Fig. 13-2). To lose a modest amount of weight within a short period of time, patients will comply with almost any diet. However, when a large amount of weight must be

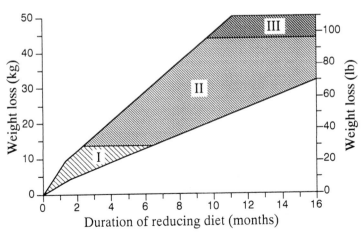

FIG. 13.2. Duration of reducing diets calculated to achieve weight losses of approximately 75% fat and 25% fat-free tissue at acceptable rates of weight reduction. *Shaded areas* show length of treatment required for patients with grade I, II, or III obesity according to body mass index. (From Garrow JS. *Obesity and related diseases.* Edinburgh: Churchill-Livingstone, 1988.)

lost over a long period, compliance is better when the diet is nutritionally balanced and palatable. The longer an unbalanced weight loss diet is continued, the greater the risk for the development of nutritional deficiency. Thus, it is important that markedly obese patients be placed on diets that fulfill the requirements for vitamins and minerals. Properly constructed diets in the 1,200-kcal range are nutritionally adequate without supplements. Equally important is the need for patients to establish new eating habits so that they will be able to maintain a lower weight after the desired weight loss has been achieved. This is one goal of behavior modification, discussed below. A major problem with many weight loss programs is that they are designed to help patients lose weight but not to make permanent changes in their eating habits. In fact, many weight loss diets are so monotonous or unpalatable that it is impossible to continue them for many months. As a result, after losing weight, patients discontinue the hypocaloric diet and resume the diet that led to obesity. This is one reason for the low success rate in keeping off lost weight.

1. **Low-calorie, nutritionally balanced diets.** The most direct and reasonable approach to weight loss is a nutritionally balanced diet that is low enough in calories to result in weight loss, developed according to the principles outlined in *Nutrition and Your Health: Dietary Guidelines for Americans, 2000* (66,67) and the *American Heart Association Dietary Guidelines Revision 2000* (68). The lower the number of calories, the more rapid the weight loss. The most reasonable and conservative recommendation for adults is a caloric intake of 1,200 to 1,400 kcal/d. It is not particularly useful to attempt to calculate a specific caloric deficit from the subject's diet history because obese (and most other) persons invariably underreport their true energy intake. A representative 1,200-kcal nutritionally balanced diet is given in Table 13-4. A balanced diet with this caloric content should supply the required amounts of proteins, vitamins, and minerals, although even balanced diets in the range of 1,000 kcal may provide inadequate amounts of niacin, thiamine, folate, pyridoxine, iron, zinc, and calcium. Diets of less than 1,000 kcal must be supplemented with essential vitamins and minerals, but it is almost never necessary to prescribe a diet of less than about 1,000 kcal/d *if the patient complies* with the 1,000-kcal program. Caloric restrictions in the range of 1,200 to 1,400 kcal can be achieved by following several principles.

   a. **Eliminate or markedly limit concentrated sources of calories.** Certain foods are energy-dense (high in caloric content per volume) but contribute little to the daily nutrient needs. These include potato chips, cream sauces, pastries, and doughnuts. Alcoholic beverages also have a high caloric content (168 kcal for a 12-oz beer, 172 kcal for 2 oz of whiskey). Many people consume 10% to 20% of their calories as alcoholic beverages. Eliminating alcoholic beverages without making other dietary changes leads to significant weight loss in such persons.

   b. **Reduce the portions of foods with significant caloric content.** Fats have a higher caloric content (9 kcal/g) than carbohydrates (4 kcal/g) or protein (4 kcal/g). Thus, reducing the portions of foods high in fat (meat, butter, margarine, salad oil) has a greater effect on caloric intake than reducing the portions of foods high in carbohydrates (fruits and vegetables, breads, potatoes, pasta). It is difficult to design a successful low-calorie diet if the proportion of calories coming from fat is in the range of the typical U.S. diet (35% to 45%). It is also important to recognize that the portions of foods eaten in America have become absurdly large. In fact, "small" portions have virtually disappeared from restaurants, fast-food and otherwise. Even when portions are small, they are invariably larger than the portions recommended in the U.S. Department of Agriculture (USDA) food guide pyramid (67).

Table 13-4. Sample meal plan for a 1,200-kcal diet

Kilocalories	Exchanges	Carbohydrate (g)	Protein (g)	Fat (g)
Breakfast				
1 cup skim milk 90	1 nonfat milk	12	8	0
½ cup orange juice 60	1 fruit	15	0	0
¾ cup corn flakes 80	1 bread	15	3	0
1 slice white toast 80	1 bread	15	3	0
Coffee 0	—	0	0	0
Lunch				
2 oz chicken 110	2 lean meat	0	14	6
2 slices white bread 160	2 bread	30	6	0
½ cup tomato 25	1 vegetable	5	2	0
1 tsp mayonnaise 45	1 fat	0	0	5
1 apple 60	1 fruit	15	0	0
Diet soda 0	—	0	0	0
Dinner				
2 oz broiled beef 150	2 medium-fat meat	0	14	10
½ cup carrots 25	1 vegetable	5	2	0
½ cup asparagus 25	1 vegetable	5	2	0
Lettuce 0	—	0	0	0
1 tbs French dressing 45	1 fat	0	0	5
¼ cup strawberries 60	1 fruit	15	0	0
1 plain dinner roll 80	1 bread	15	3	0
1 cup skim milk 90	1 nonfat milk	12	8	0
Snack				
2 graham crackers 80	1 bread	15	3	0
Totals 1,265		174	68	26

c. Change the methods of food preparation. The caloric content of food can be greatly affected by the method of preparation. The caloric content of fried chicken is greater than that of baked chicken. Significant calorie (and fat) reduction can be achieved simply by removing the skin from chicken. Similarly, the caloric content of French fries is much greater than the energy content of an equivalent weight of baked potato. The way food is treated at the table also affects its caloric content. The salad dressing has more calories than the salad, the gravy may have more calories than the biscuit, and the sour cream may have more calories than the potato.

d. Add high-fiber, low-calorie foods to the diet. High-fiber foods frequently take longer to chew and can contribute to a sense of satiety (presumably by increasing gastric distension) without contributing much to caloric intake. High-fiber, low-calorie foods include bran, most nonstarchy vegetables (carrots, celery, green beans, asparagus, cabbage), and many fruits. Recommended fiber intakes in adults are in the range of 20 to 40 g/d. Most Americans consume far less, and people can easily tolerate a modest increase (10 g) in their daily intake of dietary fiber. However, very large quantities of fiber can make a diet unpalatable and enhance caloric fermentation, which causes considerable discomfort in the form of bloating, gas, and abdominal cramps.

e. Be aware of calories. If weight is to be lost with a low-calorie, nutritionally balanced diet, the dieter must be aware of the caloric content of food. The dieter should be encouraged to buy and use one of the pocket calorie counters that are available at all major bookstores. Table 13-4 provides a representative 1-day meal plan for a 1,200-calorie diet, and Table 13-5 is a partial list of portion sizes that contain 100 calories. Table 13-4 also shows how the caloric content and macronutrient composition of a meal plan can be calculated by using the exchange lists described for the diabetic diet. The diet shown contains two nonfat milk exchanges, six bread exchanges, three fruit exchanges, three vegetable exchanges, two fat exchanges, two lean meat exchanges, and two medium-fat meat exchanges. Knowing that carbohydrates and proteins contain 4 cal/g and that fats contain 9 cal/g, we can calculate the caloric distribution for this meal plan as 55% carbohydrate, 22% protein, and 18% fat.

By using the same number and distribution of exchanges, a large number of meal plans can be developed, each with the same number of calories and macronutrient distribution. These simple dietary modifications are safe and reasonable and, if followed for a long enough period of time, should lead to significant weight loss. The rate of weight loss is a function of the caloric deficit (the difference between the number of calories in the new diet and the number in the patient's original diet). Thus, a 1,200-kcal diet results in more rapid weight loss in a person who previously consumed 3,000 kcal/d (caloric deficit of 1,800 kcal/d) than in someone who previously consumed 2,000 kcal/d (caloric deficit of 800 kcal/d). For each pound of weight lost, a caloric deficit of 3,400 kcal is required, rounded off to 3,500 kcal for ease of calculation (see Chapter 5, Section VIB). A woman on a 1,700-kcal diet whose weight was constant on a diet of 2,200 kcal/d has a caloric deficit of 500 kcal/d or 3,500 kcal/wk. On this diet, she should lose a pound a week (Table 13-6). This rule of thumb must be modified for some circumstances. At the beginning of a period of dieting, a mild diuresis frequently develops that results in a more rapid weight loss than what is projected by the caloric deficit. After a few weeks, the rate of weight loss becomes slower. The reason for this change in the rate of weight loss is that

(text continues on page 522)

Table 13-5. One hundred-kilocalorie portions

Food (oz)	Portion	Wt/vol
Apple		
Fresh	1 (3-in diameter)	8
Juice	¾ cup	6
Pie	½ part (9-in pie)	2
Sauce	½ cup	4
Bacon, broiled	2 slices	⅔
Banana, fresh	1 medium	3½
Beans		
Baked with pork	⅓ cup	3
Lima, green, canned	¾ cup	5
String	3½ cups	14
Beef		
Consommé	10 cups	80
Corned	1 slice	1
Loin (lean)	1 slice	1½
Rib (lean)	1 slice	1⅓
Roast	1 slice	2
Sirloin steak (lean)	1 small slice	2
Tongue	2 slices	1½
Beer	½ can	6
Biscuits, baking powder	1 (2-in diameter)	1
Bran, wheat	1 cup	2
Bread	1½ slices	1
Broccoli	3 stalks	10
Butter	2 small squares	½
Cabbage, fresh, cooked	2½ cups	12
Cake		
Angel	1 slice (2 in)	1⅓
Fruit	1 small slice	1
Sponge	1 slice (2 in)	1
Candy bar, chocolate	1 piece	⅔
Cantaloupe	½ melon (5-in diameter)	15
Carrots, fresh, cooked	2 cups	10
Cauliflower, raw	3 cups	12
Celery, raw, diced	6 cups	18
Cheese		
American	Small cube	1
Cheddar	1-in cube	1
Cottage	4 tbs	3½
Sandwich, American	⅓ sandwich	4
Soufflé	½ cup	2
Chicken		
Broiled	1 slice	2
Roast	1 slice	2
Club sandwich	¼ sandwich	—
Cookies		
Plain	1 medium (3-in diameter)	1
Lady fingers	3	1
Oatmeal raisin	1	1½

continued

Table 13-5. (*Continued*)

Food (oz)	Portion	Wt/vol
Corn		
Canned	½ cup (creamed)	4
Flakes	1¼ cups	1
Corned beef sandwich	⅓ sandwich	—
Crackers		
Cheese or oyster	20	1
Normal-sized	3	1
Saltines	7	1
Cream, heavy	2 tbs	—
Cream cheese	2 tbs	1
Cucumbers	3 whole (large)	24
Doughnuts	½	1
Eggs		
Raw	1⅓	2
Boiled	1⅓	2
Whites only	7	7½
Yolk only	2	1
Flounder	1 slice	3
Frankfurter	1	1½
French dressing	1½ tbs	¾
Fruit salad	1 cup	8
Grapefruit		
Fresh	½ fruit (4-in diameter)	8
Juice, canned	1 cup	8
Grapes	1 large bunch (40)	5
Griddle cake	1 (4-in diameter)	2
Haddock, cooked	⅔ fillet	5
Ham, fresh, lean	1 slice	1
Hamburger, lean	Very small patty	2
Hash, corned beef	¼ cup	1½
Ice cream	⅓ cup	2
Jam, marmalade, jellies	1½ tbs	1½
Lettuce	2 heads	20
Luncheon meat	1 slice	1¼
Macaroni, elbow, cooked	½ cup	2½
Manhattan cocktail	½ glass	1½
Mayonnaise	1 tbs	½
Milk		
Skim	1¼ cups	10
Whole	⅔ cup	5
Muffins	1	2
Nonfat solids	3½ tbs	—
Noodles		
Soup	1 cup	8
Uncooked	¼ cup	1
Oatmeal, cooked	¾ cup	5
Oil, cooking or salad	⅘ tbs	½

Table 13-5. (*Continued*)

Food (oz)	Portion	Wt/vol
Olives		
Green	16 (extra large)	—
Ripe	12	—
Onions	2 medium (2½-in diameter)	7
Oranges		
Fresh	1 large	7
Juice, fresh	1 cup	8
Marmalade	1 tbs	1
Oysters	8–12 medium	5
Peanuts, roasted	20	½
Peanut butter	1 tbs	½
Pears		
Fresh	1 large (3-in diameter)	6
Canned	2½ halves	5
Peas		
Canned	¾ cup	3½
Dried, split	2 tbs	1
Green, fresh	¾ cup	4
Soup	½ cup	4
Peppers, green	5	12
Pickles		
Dill	6 large (1¾ × 4 in)	—
Sweet	3 small (¾ × 2¾ in)	—
Pineapple		
Canned or fresh	2 slices	6
Juice	¾ cup	6
Pizza (tomato and cheese pie)	3-in section (14-in pie)	1½
Plums, canned or fresh	4 fruits	6½
Pork		
Chops, broiled	½ lean chop	2
Tenderloin, broiled	½ slice	2½
Potato		
Boiled or baked	1 medium	3
Chips	8 large	½
Mashed, white	½ cup	3½
Salad	¼ cup	2
Soup	½ cup	4
Pretzels	2 large or 8 small	1
Prune		
Dried or fresh	4 medium	1½
Juice	½ cup	4
Whip	½ cup	2½
Raisins	2 tbs	1
Red wine (dry)	1⅓ glasses	4
Rice, boiled	¾ cup	4
Rice Krispies	¾ cup	1
Rye bread	1 slice	1½
Salami	⅔ slice	¾

continued

Table 13-5. (*Continued*)

Food (oz)	Portion	Wt/vol
Salmon		
Fresh or canned	½ cup	2½
Smoked	½ small slice	2
Shrimp	15 medium	3
Soft drinks, carbonated	1 cup	8
Spaghetti, cooked	¾ cup	4
Spinach, cooked	2 cups	12
Split pea soup	¾ cup	6
Squash		
Summer, boiled	3 cups	21
Winter, boiled	1⅓ cups	9
Strawberries, fresh, no sugar	2 cups	9
Sugar		
Cubes	4 lumps	—
Granular	6½ tbs	—
Powdered	2½ tbs	—
Syrup, maple or corn	1½ tbs	1
Tomatoes		
Fresh	3	16
Canned	2⅙ cups	—
Juice	2 cups	16
Soup	1 cup	8
Triscuit	5 wafers	1⅔
Turkey	1 slice	2
Veal		
Breast	½ slice	2
Cutlet	½	1½
Steak	⅓	1½
Vegetable soup	1 cup	8
Waffles	1	1½
Watermelon	1 medium slice	12
Wheat bread	1⅓ slices	1
Whitefish	⅓ portion	2
White wine (dry)	1½ glasses	5
Yogurt	⅔ cup	6

the basal metabolic rate and caloric cost of exercise both diminish as weight decreases. A 70-kg man jogging a mile in 9 minutes expends 18 fewer calories than an 80-kg man.

f. Some nutritionally sound weight loss programs are listed in Table 13-7. These programs offer diets that are nutritionally balanced, and they encourage eating habits that can be maintained after the desired amount of weight has been lost. One major appeal of the balanced diet with a moderate caloric deficit is that it forms a basis for dietary habits that can be continued indefinitely and help to maintain weight at a desirable level. The balanced diet with a modest caloric deficit is perfectly reasonable, but the success rate is low. Many people fail to lose weight with a conservative approach

Table 13-6. Calorie intake calculator

Present weight (lb)	Present daily intake (total number of calories to maintain present body weight)[a]	Daily calorie intake to lose 1 lb/wk (500 kcal less per day than present daily intake)	Daily calorie intake to lose 2 lb/wk (1,000 kcal less per day than present daily intake)
295	4,425	3,925	3,425
290	4,350	3,850	3,350
285	4,275	3,775	3,275
280	4,200	3,700	3,200
275	4,125	3,625	3,125
270	4,050	3,550	3,050
265	3,975	3,475	2,975
260	3,900	3,400	2,900
255	3,825	3,325	2,825
250	3,750	3,250	2,750
245	3,675	3,175	2,675
240	3,600	3,100	2,600
235	3,525	3,025	2,525
230	3,450	2,950	2,450
225	3,375	2,875	2,375
220	3,300	2,800	2,300
215	3,225	2,725	2,225
210	3,150	2,650	2,150
205	3,075	2,575	2,075
200	3,000	2,500	2,000
195	2,925	2,425	1,925
190	2,850	2,350	1,850
185	2,775	2,275	1,775
180	2,700	2,200	1,700
175	2,625	2,125	1,625
170	2,550	2,050	1,550
165	2,475	1,975	1,475
160	2,400	1,900	1,400
155	2,325	1,825	1,325
150	2,250	1,750	1,250
145	2,175	1,675	1,175
140	2,100	1,600	1,100
135	2,050	1,525	1,025
130	1,950	1,450	950
125	1,875	1,375	875

[a] Daily calorie intake to maintain present weight equals weight times 15.

because they do not comply with the diet for a sufficiently long period of time. Weight loss with this program is slow, averaging a pound a week. The rate is not slow if one considers the caloric deficit necessary to lose 1 pound, but it is slow compared with the dieter's expectations and with the claims of commercial diet programs. If the dieter's expectations are realistic, the likelihood of discouragement will be lessened. Another factor contributing to poor compliance with this kind of program is the palatability of the food. On a balanced diet with a modest caloric deficit, the patient consumes many of the foods that were eaten before the diet was started, but in smaller portions. The foods are palatable and familiar, and the like-

Table 13-7. Nutritionally sound weight-loss programs

Weight Watchers International
175 Crossways Park Dr.
Woodbury, NY 11799
516-677-3755
www.weightwatchers.com

Take Off Pounds Sensibly (TOPS) Club
4575 South 5th St.
P.O. Box 07360
Milwaukee, WI 53207-0360
414-482-4620
www.tops.org

Overeaters Anonymous
World Service Office
6075 Zenith Ct. NE
Rio Rancho, NM 87124
505-891-2664
www.overeaters.com/home.htm

lihood that the dieter will eat more than the diet allows is high. The issue of palatability is a two-edged sword. If the food is too palatable, the dieter will eat too much; if the food is not palatable enough, the dieter will lose enthusiasm and abandon the diet.

2. **Other dietary approaches.** Because of the low success rate of the balanced diet with a modest caloric deficit, a wide variety of other dietary approaches to weight loss have been developed. Almost every type of dietary manipulation conceivable has been put forth as a weight loss program. Most of these approaches are based on misinformed concepts of nutrition, and a few of them are dangerous. Some diets manipulate the major sources of calories (high-carbohydrate, low-fat; high-protein, low-carbohydrate; high-fat, low-carbohydrate). The American Heart Association has identified the features of a fad diet: (a) magic or miracle foods that burn fat, (b) bizarre quantities of only one food or type of food, (c) rigid menus, (d) specific food combinations, (e) promises of rapid weight loss, (f) no recommendations for increasing physical activity, and (g) no warnings for persons with medical conditions.

Table 13-8 lists some popular and fad diets according to macronutrient distribution. When the distribution of calories becomes highly skewed in favor of a single macronutrient, the diet tends to become monotonous and unpalatable. As a result, the dieter's caloric intake decreases and weight is lost. Another dietary approach to weight loss is a nutritionally unbalanced diet that focuses on the consumption of large amounts of a single food (e.g., the "grapefruit" diet). These diets are also unpalatable and monotonous and so lead to short-term weight loss. A third approach is to limit food intake to a single product sold by the promoters of the diet. These products are usually liquids, which may be nutritionally balanced or unbalanced. Weight loss with these regimens may be based in part on the fact that monotony leads to a diminished consumption of energy. Nonetheless, some of the commercially available prepared food supplements, used in conjunction with an overall dietary plan, have been shown to lead to sustained, long-term weight reduction (69). All these approaches have an advantage over the nutritionally balanced low-calorie diet in that the dieter is not tempted by exposure to familiar and palatable foods. Overweight persons seem to

Table 13-8. Selected fad diets and other popular weight-loss programs

Low-carbohydrate diets: These diets are based on the misconception that carbohydrates *per se* promote weight gain. The diets induce ketosis and diuresis and can lead to dehydration. In addition, some of them, the Atkins diet in particular, are unbalanced and high in fat and cholesterol.
Dr. Atkins' New Diet Revolution. From Atkins RC, *Dr. Atkins' New Diet Revolution* (New York: Avon Books, 1998).
The Stillman Diet. From Stillman IM, Baker S, *Doctor's Quick Weight Loss Diet* (New York: Dell, 1977, out of print). This is a severely restricted form of a ketogenic diet that is not likely to be kept for long periods of time.

High-carbohydrate, low-fat diets:
Pritikin Diet. From Pritikin R, Rubenstein J (ed), *The New Pritikin Program* (New York: Pocket Books, 1991) and Pritikin R, *The Pritikin Principle* (New York: Time Life, 2000). This diet is fundamentally a nutritionally adequate vegetarian diet and thus is not strictly a fad diet. For many people, however, the low-fat content makes it unpalatable and reduces the likelihood of compliance.
Ornish Diet. From Ornish D, *Dr. Dean Ornish's Programs for Reversing Heart Disease: the Only System Scientifically Proven to Reverse Heart Disease without Drugs or Surgery* (New York: Ivy Books, 1996). Severe fat-restriction diet designed for people with heart disease. Fat restriction to <10% energy is significantly more restrictive than the American Heart Association diets for similar persons, and the very high carbohydrate content may increase triglyceride levels and lower HDL cholesterol concentrations.
T-Factor Diet. From Katahn M, The T-Factor Diet (New York: Bantam Books, 1994). This diet is adequate by itself but offers no advantages over the nutritional advice contained in *Nutrition and Your Health: Dietary Guidelines for Americans, 2000* (U.S. Department of Agriculture). Moreover, it is suggested that the diet contains a special component for efficacy, but this rationalization is without scientific validation, for which reason we have classified this diet as a fad diet.
Rice Diet Report. From Moscovitz J, *The Rice Diet Report* (New York: Putnam, 1986, out of print). This diet is deficient in protein, calcium, iron, and zinc.

Diets with severe caloric restrictions: Most conservative weight-loss regimens include a caloric deficit of from 500 to 1,000 kcal/d. This level of caloric deficit results in a daily calorie intake of 1,200 to 1,500 kcal for most adults. A diet containing less than 1,200 kcal is frequently deficient in essential nutrients, including protein, iron, and calcium. Several fad diets provide 500 to 750 kcal/d. Like the low-carbohydrate diets, these diets are ketogenic and may result in dehydration if fluid intake is inadequate. Prolonged use of these diets may result in deficiencies of vitamin A, riboflavin, iron, calcium, protein, niacin, and thiamine.
Scarsdale Diet. From Tarnhower H, Baker SB, *The Complete Scarsdale Medical Diet plus Dr. Tarnhower's Lifetime Keep-Slim Program* (New York: Bantam Books, 1995). One thousand calories per day, low in carbohydrate.
Richard Simmons Diet. From Toews J, *Never Say Diet Book and Program Planner Package* (Toronto: Key Porter Books, 1998). Nine hundred calories per day.

Protein-supplemented or protein-modified fasts: No data support the concept that a high intake of protein augments weight loss. Severe caloric restriction diets with liquid protein supplements to replace obligatory body protein losses were popularized in the mid-1970s. These fell from favor after nearly 60 deaths occurred, largely from refractory cardiac arrhythmias. The protein supplements then available were of poor quality and also deficient in many minerals normally present in food protein sources. The use of protein-sparing modified fast diets has regained some popularity because high-biologic-value protein supplements are now commercially available.
The Last Chance Diet. From Linn R, *The Last Chance Diet* (New York: Bantam Books, 1977, out of print).

continued

Table 13-8. (*Continued*)

Diets of highly dubious rationale: These diet regimens are based on biochemical, physiologic, or nutritional "principles" as yet unknown to the evidence-based scientific community. Although some plans contain supportable facts, the derived fundamental weight loss rationales are nonsensical and the consequent rules have no scientific bases. If weight loss is achieved, it is on the basis of the hypocalorie menu plans (as in the case of the Fitonics, 5-Day Miracle, and Zone plans).

The Beverly Hills Diet. From Mazel J, *The New Beverly Hills Diet* (Deerfield Beach: Health Communications, 1996). This diet is deficient in protein, vitamins (e.g., B_{12}), and the minerals iron, calcium, and zinc.

The Carbohydrate Addict's Diet Program. From Heller RF, Heller RF, *The Carbohydrate Addict's Lifespan Program* (New York: Dutton, 1998). Menus are often high in fat and not necessarily low in calories. Some of the optional supplements, such as chromium, are of dubious value.

Fitonics. From Diamond M, Schnell DB, *Fitonics for Life* (New York: Avon Books, 1998). The proposition that we are enzyme-deficient from eating predominantly cooked foods has no scientific basis. The proposition that correcting the "deficiency" by eating predominantly uncooked and unprocessed foods has even less basis.

Five-Day Miracle Diet. From Puhn A, *The 5-Day Miracle Diet* (New York: Ballantine Books, 1997). Very-low-calorie menus with energy intakes in the range of the severely calorie-restricted diet plans listed above. Timing of food combinations for good blood sugar maintenance is of little known value in persons with normal carbohydrate tolerance.

Somersizing. From Somers S, *Suzanne Somers' Eat Great, Lose Weight Diet* (New York: Three Rivers Press, 1999). Elimination of all sugar sources and certain starches, specified bad food combinations, and protein and carbohydrate combinations have no basis in fact.

Eat Right for Your Type. From D'Adamo PJ, *Eat Right 4 Your Type* (Chicago: Putnam Publishing Group, 1997). The selection of diet composition based on the nature of one's distant ancestors is a highly dubious hypothesis with no direct experimental support.

The Zone Diet. From Sears B, *Mastering the Zone* (New York: Regan Books, 1997). This complex zone system has no proven advantage over the simpler balanced, sensible macronutrient intake "zone system" offered in *Dietary Guidelines for Americans, 2000.*

prefer unusual diets to diets that simply reduce the portion of foods they normally eat.

Many fad diets separate dieting from ordinary life—that is, they do not promote long-term lifestyle changes. Most are based on a gimmick (e.g., eating just one food or eating different foods on an unusual schedule), and many dieters find the gimmicks useful. They lose weight on unusual diets because the gimmicks provide a focus for the weight loss program. Even though the nutritional basis for these diets is incorrect, weight is lost because the caloric intake is decreased. However, the same "strangeness" that makes unbalanced regimens successful for short periods of time makes them unsuccessful as programs to maintain weight loss. They do not modify the dieter's eating habits or bring about other lifestyle changes that are necessary to maintain the desired reduced weight after it has been reached.

    a. Some forms of nutritionally unbalanced diets have special characteristics that are worth pointing out. Low-calorie, low-carbohydrate diets are associated with rapid weight loss early in the diet period. With low-calorie, low-carbohydrate diets, the body initially breaks down glycogen and protein to glucose to maintain the blood glucose level. The water associated with both glycogen and protein is lost from the body when they are broken down. Diuresis contributes to the large weight loss seen early in the course of low-calorie, low-carbohydrate diets. These diets also cause ketosis, which may induce anorexia and hence enhance compliance. Ketosis and the accompanying acidosis can result in bone demineralization and osteoporosis. Other possible effects of these diets include menstrual dysfunction, increases in serum cholesterol levels, formation of kidney stones, and exacerbation of gout. A potentially dangerous form of weight loss is protein-modified fasting or protein-supplemented fasting. In these programs, a diet very low in calories is supplemented with 1.0 to 1.4 g of high-quality protein per kilogram of body weight. The programs claim to allow weight loss without protein breakdown. In reality, when protein is ingested without sufficient caloric intake, much of the ingested protein is used as a source of energy rather than for protein synthesis. Ketosis and significant diuresis develop early in the program, and as a consequence, significant weight is lost. The early versions of these diets were associated with hypokalemia and cardiac arrhythmias, and nearly 60 fatalities occurred. The newer protein-sparing, modified fasting regimens use high-biologic-value protein and require supplementation with vitamins, minerals, and potassium. After the initial, relatively rapid weight loss, a steady weight loss of 2 to 3 lb/wk can be expected with protein-modified fasting. These programs should be used only under close medical supervision and only in patients at high risk for disease (BMI >30) who have no existing serious diseases, particularly cardiovascular disease.

b. **A modest increase in the consumption of high-fiber foods,** as noted above, may be a reasonable part of a balanced, low-calorie diet. High-fiber food increases the effort of eating because more chewing is required, and it contributes to satiety without adding many calories. Some diet promoters have made high-fiber foods the centerpiece of their programs. These diets eliminate all products made with refined flour and sugar. They include high-fiber foods (whole grain bread, bran, fruits, and vegetables) and moderate amounts of low-fat meat and fish. For those who can tolerate the plans, they are reasonable diets, based in large part on the foundation layers of the USDA food guide pyramid (67). Moreover, these diets promote eating habits that can be maintained after the desired amount of weight has been lost. High-fiber diets are usually adequate in nutrients and do not lead to ketosis. The major disadvantage of diets very high in fiber is their frequent association with gas, cramps, bloating, and flatulence. Weight loss with high-fiber diets tends to be slow because the caloric deficit is usually small. No good evidence has been found that dietary fiber significantly decreases the absorption of calories. Fiber does diminish the absorption of selected micronutrients, but this effect does not seem clinically significant.

c. **Exercise.** Energy economy is a balance between intake and expenditure. Increasing the expenditure of energy through physical activity is a cornerstone of maintaining a healthful weight and an important adjunct in losing weight (4,66,67,70). The health benefits of regular physical activity of all kinds are extensive and extend beyond those afforded to persons who want to lose weight. Unfortunately, though, when it comes to the arithmetic of energy expenditure, the number of calories burned during exercise is not as great as some might hope. A 70-kg man jogging a mile in 9 minutes expends only 126 additional calories (Table 13-9). However, recent studies suggest that exercise may influence energy balance through more mechanisms than the direct expenditure of calories, although it must be understood that exercise enhances weight maintenance much more than it increases weight loss. Exercise has a small and

Table 13-9. Energy expenditure resulting from exercise

Activity	kcal/min/kg	kcal per half-hour	
		Reference female (5 ft 5 in, 128 lb)	Reference male (5 ft 9 in, 154 lb)
Badminton	0.097	170	205
Basketball	0.138	240	290
Canoeing	0.044	75	90
Cycling			
5.5 mph	0.064	110	135
9.4 mph	0.100	175	210
Dancing, ballroom	0.051	90	90
Field hockey	0.134	235	280
Golf	0.085	150	180
Gymnastics	0.066	115	140
Horseback riding	0.110	190	230
Jogging (9 min/mile)	0.193	335	405
Judo, karate	0.195	340	410
Running (6 min/mile)	0.252	460	535
Skiing			
Cross-country	0.143	250	300
Downhill	0.098	190	230
Squash	0.212	370	445
Swimming, slow crawl	0.128	225	270
Tennis	0.109	190	230
Volleyball	0.050	90	105
Walking (normal pace, 15 min/mile)	0.080	140	165

Adapted from Katch F, McArdle W. *Nutrition, weight control and exercise.* Boston: Houghton-Mifflin, 1983.

probably clinically insignificant effect on preserving lean body mass. Exercise may also affect appetite; engaging in exercise shortly before a meal reduces food intake. Increased physical activity, including traditional exercise activities if possible, is thus an important adjunct to dietary therapy in the management of obesity. If incorporated into a healthful lifestyle and sustained over the long term, a combination of increased exercise and decreased caloric intake will surely promote negative energy balance more effectively than either modality alone and can also contribute to weight maintenance when hypocaloric diets are discontinued (71–74).

d. Behavior modification. In persons of normal weight, eating is prompted by hunger. However, in many obese persons, eating is triggered by factors such as environment and mood rather than hunger. Some eat because they are angry or depressed, and some eat because "it is time to eat," irrespective of their own hunger or satiety signals. Many people will eat when presented with especially attractive food, even if they are not hungry. Such eating habits have led some therapists to use behavior modification as the cornerstone of obesity management. The goal of behavior modification is to make changes in the daily patterns of eating and achieve permanent alterations in lifestyle behavior that will be continued far beyond the period of weight reduction. Through behavior modification techniques, obese persons gain insights into why they start eating, how they choose what to eat, and why they stop eating. Patients then learn a method for controlling their eating behavior. Some sample techniques for altering the environment to reduce stimuli to eating are applicable to most people.

1. Eat in only one place.
2. Eat only while sitting down at a table.
3. Do not eat while watching television.
4. Eat slowly and pause between bites.
5. Make food inconspicuous when not eating.

Many obese people benefit from initial self-monitoring—that is, keeping a record of eating behavior: where and when they eat, what mood they are in, what they choose to eat and how much, and activities during eating. A review of this material provides insight into the events that trigger eating and how they can be modified. The self-monitoring period is followed by a period of goal setting in regard to caloric intake and physical activity and the introduction of behavioral modification strategies, including stimulus control, problem solving, cognitive restructuring, and relapse prevention (73.) Although many of the principles underlying behavioral modification therapy have come under criticism, behavioral modification in practice has proved more effective than other weight loss regimens or has enhanced their effects (59,62,73).

e. **Prominent international weight loss programs** (Table 13-7). *Weight Watchers,* founded in 1963, is a well-established self-help program in which diet, exercise, behavior modification, and group support are used to promote weight loss. The food program meets national nutritional recommendations. Dieters are assigned to a group that meets weekly. At these meetings, with the accompanying weigh-ins, peer pressure and group solidarity help dieters stay with the program. The success of the program is tied to a certain degree to the group leader, who provides support for the dieters. The Weight Watchers program is well designed and professionally backed. The diets are nutritionally balanced and encourage eating habits that are useful after a desirable weight has been achieved. *Take Off Pounds Sensibly (TOPS),* founded in 1948, is another well-established program based on a group support approach to weight control. It does not supply a specific diet, as Weight Watchers does, but maintains that participants should receive a dietary program from a medical professional. Group support is provided through weekly meetings. Like Weight Watchers, TOPS is a reasonable weight loss program that has been successful for a large number of persons. *Overeaters Anonymous,* founded in 1960, is a cost-free program with minimal group organization in the structured sense. Their 12-step recovery program is modeled after the successful Alcoholics Anonymous program.

3. **Drug therapy.** The use of drug therapy depends on many factors, such as the patient's willingness to attempt lifestyle changes and ability to maintain a modest reduction in weight without drugs. Although most obese persons are not candidates for drug therapy (mostly because of a lack of willingness to make them part of a total treatment approach), candidates for drug treatment are usually those with a BMI above 35. Patients with a BMI above 30 and additional risk factors may also be considered potential candidates (65,75). Drugs that can lead to weight loss include the following:

a. **Drugs that reduce food intake by decreasing appetite or increasing satiety.** These include the currently approved sympathomimetic agent phentermine, and the serotonin–norepinephrine reuptake inhibitors mazindol and sibutramine (which also blocks serotonin reuptake). However, phentermine and mazindol are not currently recommended for use in obesity. Sibutramine is the only drug in this category that has been evaluated extensively; it has been effective in clinical trials and is reasonably safe (65,75). About 40% of patients lose weight on sibutramine, and the overall weight loss of treated patients is 9% at 1 year. It should be used cautiously in combination with drugs that increase blood pressure and is contraindicated in persons with cardiovascular disease and stroke.

Ephedrine and caffeine are commonly given to obese patients, but neither has been approved by the Food and Drug Administration for the treatment of obesity. These drugs cause an increase in energy and a reduction in food intake. In fact, the latter mechanism seemed to predominate over the former in two studies from the same research group that demonstrated an augmented weight loss during combined therapy (75). Interestingly, ephedrine and caffeine in combination also act as "nutrient-partitioning" agents by enhancing fatty acid oxidation and reducing the loss of lean body mass. Many other agents (e.g., growth hormone, testosterone, corticosteroids) are also known to alter macronutrient partitioning, but each has significant side effects and none has been approved for the treatment of obesity.

- **b. Drugs that block nutrient absorption.** The absorption of dietary fat is diminished by the use of orlistat, a pancreatic lipase inhibitor. This agent has been shown to augment weight loss in several clinical trials, producing a loss of 9% to 10% in 1 year, in comparison with a loss of 4% to 5% in controls (75). Gastrointestinal side effects are those expected as a consequence of fat malabsorption. Daily fat-soluble vitamin supplements are recommended with use of this compound.
- **c. Drugs that modulate central nervous system control of body weight.** Potential agents in this class include newly recognized peptides and their receptors that may, depending on the mode of action, be blocked or enhanced to reduce food intake. Although this is one of the most exciting developmental areas in the clinical pharmacology of agents to treat obesity, no such compounds are yet commercially available. Leptin has been shown to produce modest weight loss (~ 8%) at 24 weeks in a single clinical trial involving only six to eight patients per treatment arm (76), and it has also been clinically effective in leptin-deficient persons (77).

B. Surgical management. Three surgical approaches to weight reduction have been popularized. These should be used only in patients with documented failure on medical weight loss programs. Practically, these procedures have generally been made available to patients with a BMI above 40 kg/m^2, those with serious obesity-related comorbidities and a BMI above 35 kg/m^2, and those who are more than 100 lb over ideal body weight and offer a personal history of failure in weight reduction programs (78).

- **1. Gastric bypass and gastroplasty.** Three procedures have produced the best results to date: adjustable silicone gastric banding, vertical gastric banding, and gastric bypass. These operations are designed to induce satiety by creating a small gastric pouch, so that the stomach becomes distended quickly. In gastroplasty or gastric stapling, a small gastric pouch in continuity with the esophagus is segregated from the rest of the stomach. In gastric bypass, a small pouch is connected with a loop of jejunum; this procedure also produces some degree of malabsorption. The mechanical procedures increase dietary compliance by inducing satiety after the ingestion of a small volume of food, but they also decrease hunger for unknown reasons. They produce a loss of about 50% of excess weight, but patients who cannot maintain a diet regain the weight. Weight loss with these procedures depends on the patient's adhering to a low-calorie, nutritionally balanced diet. After these procedures, a patient can maintain weight, or even gain weight, by consuming significant amounts of concentrated calories, particularly as liquids.
- **2. Gastric bypass with partial/selective malabsorption.** Many variants of this approach have been described previously, in which nutrient

malabsorption was produced by bypassing varying lengths of the small intestine (jejunal–ileal bypass). Although weight loss is achieved, this approach is associated with many complications, including electrolyte abnormalities and vitamin deficiencies, so that its use has been discontinued. Currently offered variants aim to establish selective malabsorption and at the same time decrease gastric capacitance. These procedures include partial biliopancreatic bypass and duodenal switch with partial biliopancreatic bypass (79). Experience with these procedures is much less than with the more standard gastric bypass or gastroplasty procedures.

3. **Liposuction.** In this procedure, subcutaneous fat is aspirated under local anesthesia. Only limited quantities of fat can be removed, and the procedure is more cosmetically than medically beneficial for anyone with significant obesity.

References

1. World Health Organization. *Obesity: preventing and managing the global epidemic. Report of a WHO consultation on obesity.* Geneva: World Health Organization, 1998.
2. Garrow JS. Obesity. In: Garrow JS, James WPT, Ralph A, eds. *Human nutrition and dietetics,* 10th ed. New York: Churchill Livingstone, 2000:527.
3. National Center for Health Statistics. Prevalence of overweight and obesity among adults: United States, 1999. Available on line at *www.cdc.gov/nchs/products/pubs/pubd/hestats/obese/obese99tab2.htm* via the Internet. Accessed December 23, 2000.
4. National Institutes of Health, National Heart, Lung and Blood Institute. *Clinical guidelines on the identification, evaluation, and treatment of overweight and obesity in adults.* U.S. Department of Health and Human Services, Public Health Service, 1998. Abstracted in *Obes Res* 1998;6[Suppl 2]:53S.
5. U.S. Department of Health and Human Services. Nutrition and overweight. In: *Healthy people 2010.* Washington, DC: U.S. Government Printing Office, 2000:19-1.
6. U.S. Department of Agriculture and U.S. Department of Health and Human Services. *Nutrition and your health: dietary guidelines for Americans, 2000* 5th ed. Washington, DC: U.S. Government Printing Office, 2000 (Home and Garden Bulletin No. 232). Booklet available on line at *http://www.usda.gov/cnpp.* Accessed December 11, 2000.
7. Willett WC, Dietz WH, Colditz GA. Guidelines for healthy weight. *N Engl J Med* 1999;341:427.
8. Gallagher D, Heymsfield SB, Heo M, et al. Health percentage body fat ranges: an approach for developing guidelines based on body mass index. *Am J Clin Nutr* 2000;72:694.
9. Troiano RP, Frongillo Jr EA, Sobal J, et al. The relationship between body weight and mortality: a quantitative analysis of combined information from existing studies. *Int J Obes* 1996;20:63.
10. Calle EE, Thun MJ, Petrelli JM, et al. Body-mass index and mortality in a prospective cohort of U.S. adults. *N Engl J Med* 1999;341:1097.
11. Manson JE, Willett WC, Stampfer MJ, et al. Body weight and mortality among women. *N Engl J Med* 1995;333:677.
12. Stevens J, Cai J, Pamuk ER, et al. The effect of age on the association between body mass-index and mortality. *N Engl J Med* 1998;338:1.
13. Han TS, van Leer EM, Seidell JC, et al. Waist circumference action levels in the identification of cardiovascular risk factors: prevalence study in a random sample. *Br Med J* 1995;311:1401.
14. Lemieux S, Prud'homme D, Bouchard C, et. al. A single threshold value of waist girth identifies normal-weight and overweight subjects with excess visceral adipose tissue. *Am J Clin Nutr* 1996;64:685.
15. Rexrode KM, Carey VJ, Hennekens CH, et al. Abdominal adiposity and coronary heart disease in women. *JAMA* 1998:280;1843.
16. Pouliot MC, Despres JP, Lemieux S, et al. Waist circumference and abdominal sagittal diameter: best simple anthropometric indices of abdominal visceral adipose

tissue accumulation and reduced cardiovascular risk in men and women. *Am J Cardiol* 1994;73:460.

17. Rimm EB, Stampfer MJ, Giovannucci E, et al. Body size and fat distribution as predictors of coronary heart disease among middle-aged and older U.S. men. *Am J Epidemiol* 1995;141:1117.

18. Lee CD, Blair SN, Jackson AS. Cardiorespiratory fitness, body composition, and all-cause and cardiovascular disease mortality in men. *Am J Clin Nutr* 1999; 69:373.

19. International Diabetes Institute, World Health Organization. *The Asia-Pacific perspective: redefining obesity and its treatment.* Geneva: World Health Organization, 2000:1. Available on line at *http://www.idi.org.au/obesity_report.htm.* Accessed December 23, 2000.

20. National Center for Health Statistics, National Health and Nutrition Examination Survey. Clinical growth charts. Available on line at *http://www.cdc.gov/nchs/about/major/nhanes/growthcharts/clinical_charts.htm* via the Internet. Accessed December 23, 2000.

21. Kuczmarski RJ, Ogden CL, Grummer-Strawn LM, et al. CDC growth charts: United States. *Advance Data* 2000;314:1 [DHHS Publication No. (PHS) 2000-1250 0-0431 (5/00)]. Available, with listing of errata, on line at *http://www.cdc.gov/nchs/data/ad314.pdf* via the Internet. Accessed December 23, 2000.

22. Society of Actuaries and Association of Life Insurance Medical Directors of America. *Build study, 1979.* Chicago: Society of Actuaries, 1980.

23. Chagnon YC, Perusse L, Weisnagel SJ, et. al. The human obesity gene map: the 1999 update. *Obes Res* 2000;8:89.

24. Comuzzie AG, Allison DB. The search for human obesity genes. *Science* 1998;280: 1363.

25. Barsch GS, Farooqi IS, O'Rahilly S. Genetics of body-weight regulation. *Nature* 2000;404:644.

26. Bouchard C, Perusse L, Rice T, et al. The genetics of human obesity. In: Bray GA, Bouchard C, James WPT, eds. *Handbook of obesity.* New York: Marcel Dekker Inc, 1998:157.

27. Rosenbaum M, Leibel RH, Hirsch J. Obesity. *N Engl J Med* 1997;337:396.

28. Maes HHM, Neale MC, Eaves LJ. Genetic and environmental factors in relative body weight and human adiposity. *Behav Genet* 1997;27:325.

29. Hewett JK. The genetics of obesity: what have genetic studies told us about the environment? *Behav Genet* 1997;27:353.

30. Allison DB, Faith, MS. A proposed heuristic for communicating heritability estimates to the general public, with obesity as an example. *Behav Genet* 1997;27:441.

31. Allison DB, Heshka S, Neale MC, et. al. A genetic analysis of relative weight among 4,020 twin pairs, with an emphasis on sex effects. *Health Psychol* 1994;4:362.

32. Allison DB, Kaprio J, Korkeila M, et. al. The heritability of body mass index among an international sample of monozygotic twins reared apart. *Int J Obes Res Relat Metab Disord* 1996;6:501.

33. Faith MS, Pietrobelli A, Nunez, et. al. Evidence for independent genetic influences on fat mass and body mass index in a pediatric twin sample. *Pediatrics* 1999;104:61.

34. Bouchard C, Perusse L. Genetics of obesity. *Annu Rev Nutr* 1993;3:337.

35. Cone RD. Haploinsufficiency of the melanocortin-4 receptor: part of a thrifty genotype? *J Clin Invest* 2000;106:185.

36. Vaisse C, Clement K, Durand E. Melanocortin-4-receptor mutations are a frequent and heterogeneous cause of morbid obesity. *J Clin Invest* 2000;106:253.

37. Farooqi, IS, Yeo GSH, Keogh JM. Dominant and recessive inheritance of morbid obesity associated with melanocortin-4-receptor deficiency. *J Clin Invest* 2000; 106:271.

38. Schwartz, MW, Woods SC, Porte D Jr, et. al. Central nervous system control of food intake. *Nature* 2000;404:661.

39. Woods SC, Seeley RJ, Porte D Jr, et al. Signals that regulate food intake and energy homeostasis. *Science* 1998;280:1378.

40. Ravussin E. Metabolic differences and the development of obesity. *Metabolism* 1995;44:12.

41. Ravussin E, Burnand B, Schutz Y, et al. Twenty-four-hour energy expenditure and resting metabolic rate in obese, moderately obese, and control subjects. *Am J Clin Nutr* 1982;35:566.
42. de Jonge L, Bray GA. The thermic effect of food and obesity: a critical review. *Obes Res* 1997;5:622.
43. Segal KR, Presta E, Gutin B. Thermic effect of food during graded exercise in normal-weight and obese men. *Am J Clin Nutr* 1984;40:95.
44. Trueth MS, Figueroa-Colon R, Hunter GR, et al. Energy expenditure and physical fitness in overweight vs non-overweight prepubertal girls. *Int J Obes Relat Metab Disord* 1998;22:440.
45. Lichtman SW, Pisarka K, Berman ER, et al. Discrepancy between self-reported and actual caloric intake and exercise in obese subjects. *N Engl J Med* 1992;327:1893.
46. Stunkard AJ, Berkowitz RI, Stallings VA, et al. Energy intake, not energy output, is the determinant of body size in infants. *Am J Clin Nutr* 1999;69:524.
47. Seidell JC, Muller DC, Sorkin JD, et al. Fasting respiratory exchange ratio and resting metabolic rate as predictors of weight gain: the Baltimore Longitudinal Study on Aging. *Int J Obes* 1992;16:667.
48. Levine JA, Eberhardt NL, Jensen MD. Role of nonexercise activity thermogenesis in resistance to fat gain in humans. *Science* 1999;282:212.
49. Weinsier RL, Nagy TR, Hunter GR, et al. Do adaptive changes in metabolic rate favor weight regain in weight-reduced individuals? An examination of the set-point theory. *Am J Clin Nutr* 2000;72:1088.
50. Astrup A, Gotzsche PC, van de Werken K, et al. Meta-analysis of resting metabolic rate in formerly obese subjects. *Am J Clin Nutr* 1999;69:1117.
51. Amatruda JM, Statt MC, Welle SL. Total and resting energy expenditure in obese women reduced to ideal body weight. *J Clin Invest* 1993;92:1236.
52. Larson DE, Ferraro RT, Robertson DS, et al. Energy metabolism in weight-stable postobese individuals. *Am J Clin Nutr* 1995;62:735.
53. Weyer C, Walford RL, Harper IT, et al. Energy metabolism after 2 years of energy restriction: the biosphere experiment. *Am J Clin Nutr* 2000;72:946.
54. Perusse L, Bouchard C. Gene–diet interactions in obesity. *Am J Clin Nutr* 2000; 72[Suppl]:1285S.
55. Bray G, Popkin BM. Dietary fat intake does affect obesity! *Am J Clin Nutr* 1998; 68:1157.
56. Willett WC. Dietary fat and obesity: an unconvincing relation. *Am J Clin Nutr* 1998;68:1149.
57. Flatt J-P. Energy expenditure and substrate oxidation. In: Bray GA, Bouchard C, James WPT, eds. *Handbook of obesity.* New York: Marcel Dekker Inc, 1998:513.
58. Schutz Y. Macronutrients and energy balance in obesity. *Metabolism* 1995; 44[Suppl 3]:7.
59. Pi-Sunyer FX Obesity. In: Shils ME, Olson JA, Shike M, et al., eds. *Modern nutrition in health and disease,* 9th ed. Baltimore: Williams & Wilkins, 1999:1395.
60. Kopelman PG. Obesity as a medical problem. *Nature* 2000;404:635.
61. Solomon CG, Manson JE. Obesity and mortality: a review of the epidemiologic data. *Am J Clin Nutr* 1977;66[Suppl]:1044S.
62. Ayyad C, Andersen T. Long-term efficacy of dietary treatment of obesity: a systematic review of studies published between 1931 and 1999. *Obes Rev* 2000;1:113.
63. Jealian E, Saelens BE. Empirically supported treatments in pediatric psychology: pediatric obesity. *J Pediatr Psychol* 1999;24:223.
64. Blair SA, Lee I-M. Weight loss and risk of mortality. In: Bray GA, Bouchard C, James WPT, eds. *Handbook of obesity.* New York: Marcel Dekker Inc, 1998:805.
65. Bray GA. A concise review of the therapeutics of obesity. *Nutrition* 2000;16:953.
66. U.S. Department of Health and Human Services, U.S. Department of Agriculture. *Nutrition and your health: dietary guidelines for Americans, 2000,* 5th ed. Washington, DC: U.S. Government Printing Office, 2000. Booklet available on line at *http://www.usda.gov/cnpp/DietGd.pdf* via the Internet. Accessed December 11, 2000.
67. U.S. Department of Health and Human Services, U.S. Department of Agriculture. Dietary Guidelines Advisory Committee. Report of the Dietary Guidelines Advisory

Committee on *Dietary guidelines for Americans, 2000,* 5th ed. Washington, DC: U.S. Government Printing Office, 2000. Report available on line at *http://www. usda.gov/cnpp/Pubs/DG2000/Full%20Report.pdf* via the Internet. Accessed December 11, 2000.

68. Krauss RM, Eckel RH, Howard B, et al. AHA dietary guidelines revision 2000: a statement for health care professionals from the nutrition committee of the American Heart Association. *Circulation* 2000;102:2284.

69. Ditschuneit HH, Flechtner-Mors M, Johnson TD, et al. Metabolic and weight-loss effects of a long-term dietary intervention in obese patients. *Am J Clin Nutr* 1999; 69:198.

70. Rippe JM, Hess S. The role of physical activity in the prevention and management of obesity. *J Am Diet Assoc* 1998;98:S31.

71. Fogelholm M, Kukkonen-Harjula K. Does physical activity prevent weight gain— a systematic review. *Obes Rev* 2000;1:95.

72. Wing RR, Venditti E, Jakicic JM, et al. Lifestyle intervention in overweight individuals with a family history of diabetes. *Diabetes Care* 1998;21:350.

73. Wing RR. Behavioral approaches to the treatment of obesity. In: Bray GA, Bouchard C, James WPT, eds. *Handbook of obesity.* New York: Marcel Dekker Inc, 1998:855.

74. Ballor DL, Poehlman EP, Toth MJ. Exercise as a treatment for obesity. In: Bray GA, Bouchard C, James WPT, eds. *Handbook of obesity.* New York: Marcel Dekker Inc, 1998:891.

75. Bray GA, Tartaglia LA. Medicinal strategies in the treatment of obesity. *Nature* 2000;404:672.

76. Heymsfield SB, Greenberg AS, Fujioka K, et al. Recombinant leptin for weight loss in obese and lean adults: a randomized, controlled, dose-escalation study. *JAMA* 1999;282:1568.

77. Farooqi IS, Jebb SA, Langmack G, et al. Effects of recombinant leptin therapy in a child with congenital leptin deficiency. *N Engl J Med* 1999;341:879.

78. Albrecht RJ, Pories WJ. Surgical intervention for the severely obese. *Baillieres Clin Endocrinol Metab* 1999;13:149.

79. Balsiger BM, Murr MM, Poggio JL, et al. Bariatric surgery. Surgery for weight control in patients with morbid obesity. *Med Clin North Am* 2000;84:477.

14. NUTRITIONAL CONSIDERATIONS IN WASTING DISEASES (CANCER, AIDS)

I. Cancer

A. Dietary guidelines to minimize cancer risk. Much epidemiologic evidence is available to suggest that environmental/dietary factors play a role in the development of carcinomas in a variety of organs (1–3). Individual dietary components have been examined as part of an effort to compile recommendations for reducing the risk for cancer (Table 14-1). All reports suggest increasing one's intake of fruits, vegetables, and grains/cereals; decreasing one's intake of fatty meats, fats/oils, saturated fats, and refined sugars; and avoiding excessive salt. All recent reports also suggest maintaining a healthful body weight, engaging in physical activity, and limiting one's intake of alcohol to less than two drinks a day for men, or one for women.

The National Research Council of the National Academy of Sciences concluded that the human diet contains anticarcinogens and protective factors, most of which have not been identified. It also contains carcinogens. The precise role of diet in reducing cancer risk is poorly defined, but 30% of cancers may be affected. The recommendations for a prudent diet are included in the reports of the Council (1,2). The recommendations are not novel, and their effectiveness has never been prospectively demonstrated. However, they are sensible guidelines for sound nutrition, and their use can certainly be encouraged for that reason alone. Although the consumption of some micronutrients, such as vitamins A and C, has been correlated with a lower incidence of cancer, no evidence has been found that consuming excessive amounts of these nutrients (beyond what is obtained from a balanced diet) is helpful (see the sections on folate and vitamins C, A, and E in Chapter 6). In the Lyon Diet Heart Study, prospective use of a Mediterranean-type diet (more bread and cereals, more fresh fruit and vegetables, more legumes and fish, less beef and pork, no butter and cream, and replacement with an experimental canola oil margarine) was associated with a reduced cancer death rate in comparison with the step 1 American Heart Association prudent diet (4). The numbers are quite small, and the protective effect of such a diet has not yet been proved, but similar prospective studies should be forthcoming in the future.

1. **Reduce intake of dietary fat (saturated and unsaturated) from 40% to 30% of total calories.** The evidence for this recommendation is twofold. First, an increased intake of fat is correlated with an increased incidence of cancer of the breast, colon, and prostate. However, a low-cholesterol diet is not the same thing as a low-fat diet because the total intake of fat is not usually decreased unless a low-cholesterol diet is combined with a weight-reducing diet. Second, in animal studies, caloric restriction appears to decrease cancer risk. In humans, obesity is connected with cancer of the breast, endometrium, colon, and prostate. However, case–control and cohort studies have not provided conclusive evidence for an association between total dietary fat and breast, colorectal, or prostate cancer, but this may be related to the difficulty of measuring dietary fat and the genetic variability of populations. To carry out the recommendation for a reduced intake of fat, the guidelines for a low-fat diet should be followed.

   a. Bake, broil, or boil foods instead of frying them.

   b. Trim excess fat off meat or buy low-fat meats.

   c. Use less cooking oil, butter, margarine, salad dressing, and cream.

   d. Use fat substitutes when possible (e.g., nondairy creamer).

2. **Increase intake of fruits and vegetables.** The best evidence at present involves foods containing β-carotenes, vitamin A, and vitamin C. It is possible that cruciferous vegetables contain other, undefined inhibitors of carcinogens. Most of the data in humans are from case–control and cohort studies showing an inverse correlation between cancer rates and

Table 14-1. Recommendations to modify dietary components associated with reducing the risk of cancer (1989–1996)[a]

Report	Veg/fruit	Starch/grains	Meat	Fiber (g/d)	CHO	Fats/oils	Sat/unsat	Refined sugar	Salt (g/d)
	(servings/d)	(servings/d)				(% energy)			
U.S. NAS '89	≥5	≥6	lean	yes	>55	<30	<10	ind	<6
WHO '90	400 g	ind	ns	16–24	50–75	15–30	0–10	0–10	<6
U.S. DHHS '91	≥5	≥6	nc	ind	ind	<30	<10	nc	mod
CCS '92	yes	yes	nc	ind	ns	<30	ns	nc	mod
SO '93	3+	ind	→	>16	<40	<35	<11	<10	4
ESO '94	5	6	nc	ind	ind	<30	<10	ns	6
U.S. ACS '96	5	3+	lean	ns	nc	→	→	nc	ns
U.S. HR '96	>5	ind	<1/wk	ns	↑ complex	no	↓ animal	→	mod

ACS, American Cancer Society; CCS, Canadian Cancer Survey; DHHS, Department of Health and Human Services; ESO, European States Organization; HR, Harvard Report on Cancer Prevention; ind, restriction/increase indicated but not quantified; NAS, National Academy of Science; nc, not asked; ns, not stated; SO, Scotland; WHO, World Health Organization.

[a] The U.S. reports offer recommendations for individuals. The European reports offer percentages of population limits.

Adapted from National Research Council, Commission on Life Sciences, Food and Nutrition Board, Committee on Diet and Health. *Diet and health implications for reducing chronic disease risk.* Washington, DC: National Academy Press, 1989.

serum vitamin levels, all within the normal range. Intervention trials with these vitamins have not demonstrated a protective effect to date (see Chapter 6). Sources are liver (vitamin A); dark green and yellow vegetables, including spinach, carrots, and tomatoes (β-carotenes); cruciferous vegetables, such as broccoli, brussels sprouts, cabbage, and cauliflower (vitamins A and C); and citrus fruits, berries, green peppers, peaches, melons, tomatoes, and green and leafy vegetables (vitamin C).

3. **Drink alcoholic beverages only in moderation.** The carcinogenic effect of alcohol is associated with a large intake, especially when combined with cigarette smoking.

4. **World Cancer Research Fund/American Institute for Cancer Research recommendations.** These private organizations have compiled their own guidelines for individuals based on many of the population-based recommendations (3) (Table 14-2). These recommendations are more focused on cancer than the general recommendations for healthy populations, especially regarding food preparation and preservation, but the general restrictions regarding the composition of the diet are very similar.

Additional information for patients regarding diets and cancer can be obtained from the American Cancer Society, 90 Park Avenue, New York, New York 10016, and from the American Institute for Cancer Research, Washington, D.C. 20069.

B. **Cancer prevention by dietary components**

1. **Available components.** Although epidemiologic data may suggest an association between overall diet/environment and the risk for cancer morbidity and mortality, it is difficult to identify prospectively the dietary components that may influence such risks. Table 14-3 summarizes much of the data associating dietary components with risks for cancer. It is clear that only a few of the associations are convincing. When components of the diet are tested prospectively, some of the data suggest prevention, but in general the data are negative, especially when specific interventions are attempted (see Chapter 6 for information on vitamins and Chapter 11 for a discussion of fiber). Some cohort studies continue to suggest a role for vitamin intake, but most do not (5–8). Even when premalignant endpoints are examined, such as colorectal polyps, the data for the role of increased fiber, prospectively provided, are negative (7).

2. **Future possibilities.** Current research is examining the development of specific natural compounds in the diet that appear promising for chemoprevention (9). These include green and black tea polyphenols (10), soy isoflavones, protease inhibitors, curcumin, lycopene, vitamin D, vitamin E, selenium, and calcium. For each, a possible mechanism has been identified that is fueling further studies (Table 14-4). However, none of the compounds has yet proved useful in preventing cancer. Some synthetic compounds (e.g., retinoids) are being developed in the hope of obtaining a chemical with uniquely anticancer properties (11). Research on these dietary compounds is worth watching for future developments (see Chapter 15 for further discussion of some of these compounds).

C. **Diagnosis of nutritional abnormalities in cancer patients**

1. **Nonspecific findings.** A number of findings in patients with advanced cancer are related to nutrition but are often difficult to treat with specific nutritional intervention. The most prevalent of these are weight loss and a decreased intake of food (12). Abnormal carbohydrate metabolism is characterized by glucose intolerance and insulin resistance. Body fat tends to become more depleted relative to protein loss, and lipolysis is increased. Protein turnover in the entire body increases as the disease progresses, with a reduced fractional synthetic rate in muscle. The protein kinetics in cancer patients with weight loss resemble those in persons with trauma and infection; patients with these clinical conditions cannot easily be brought into positive nitrogen balance, even

Table 14-2. WCRF/AICR goals for public health and advice to individuals

Factor	Public health goals	Advice to individuals
Food supply	Adequate, varied diet based on foods of plant origin	Choose mostly plant-based foods, few processed starchy foods.
Body weight	BMI ranging from 18.5 to 25	Limit weight gain in adulthood to <5 kg (11 lb).
Physical activity	Active lifestyle, with periods of vigorous activity	If daily activity is low, take 1-h brisk walk/d, + vigorous activity 1/wk.
Vegetables/fruits	≥7% of total energy	Eat 400–800 g (15–30 oz), ≥5 servings/d.
Other plants	Starchy, protein-rich foods; processed sugar, 45–60% of energy; refined sugar, <10% of energy	Eat 600–800 g (20–30 oz) of cereals, legumes, roots, tubers; limit refined sugar.
Alcohol	Not recommended, or limit to <5% total energy for men, <2.5% women	If consumed, limit to <2 drinks/d for men, <1 for women.
Meat	Red meat <10% of total energy	Limit to <80 g (3 oz) daily, especially fish, poultry, nondomesticated animals.
Fats/oils	15–30% of total energy	Limit fatty foods, especially of animal origin, use moderate amounts of vegetable oils.
Salt	<6 g/d	Limit salted foods, use of table salt.
Preservation	Keep frozen or chilled	Don't eat foods liable to be contaminated with mycotoxins.
Additives	Monitor safety limits for additives	Must be alert to unregulated uses.
Preparation	Use low temperatures for cooking meat, fish	Avoid charred food, cured or smoked meats.
Supplements	Not recommended	Not recommended, some may harm.
Tobacco	Discourage use	Don't smoke or chew.

AICR, American Institute for Cancer Research; BMI, body mass index; WCRF, World Cancer Research Fund.
Adapted from National Research Council, Commission on Life Sciences, Food and Nutrition Board, Committee on Diet and Health. *Diet and health implications for reducing chronic disease risk.* Washington, DC: National Academy Press, 1989.

with total parenteral nutrition (TPN). When sepsis develops, serum levels of tumor necrosis factor (TNF) increase, but high levels, such as are seen in childhood leukemias, have not been reproducibly found in patients with solid tumors (13). The hormones synthesized by some tumors cause clinical syndromes that appear to be nutritionally based (e.g., weight loss, bone disease) but are not. These include carcinoid syndrome, Zollinger–Ellison syndrome, hypercalcemia, and oncogenic osteomalacia secondary to renal phosphate wasting and decreased levels of plasma dihydroxyvitamin D, parathyroid hormone, and calcium. These syndromes must be identified and the manifestations of increased hormone production treated with available (non-nutritional) methods.

2. **Cachexia.** Anorexia frequently accompanies the cachexia of cancer. Proposed mediators have included hypothalamic serotonin, leptin, proinflammatory cytokines, prostaglandins, and tumor-specific products. However, none of these has been documented to be causative in the anorexia of cancer (13). Starvation is characterized by an excessive loss of nutrients, but cachexia is associated with the acute-phase responses that are part of underlying inflammatory or malignant conditions. Thus, feeding does not reverse the macronutrient deficiency. Body compartment analysis in cachexia, in contrast to starvation, shows increases in resting energy expenditure, protein degradation, and serum insulin and cortisol levels (14). These changes lead to increases in urinary nitrogen loss, skeletal protein breakdown, and lipolysis and to glucose intolerance. Despite aggressive caloric replacement, lean body mass decreases in critically ill patients with underlying infection or tumor (14).

Many attempts have been made to alter anorexia and cachexia pharmacologically with steroids, antiserotoninergics (cyproheptadine), and hydrazine sulfate, but these have not been successful. The progestational agents megestrol acetate and dihydroxyprogesterone acetate inconstantly improve appetite (13) (see later discussion of their use in AIDS) and increase weight, but the weight gain represents increases in fat, not fat-free tissue. Both these agents produce side effects, including venous thrombosis and peripheral edema, the latter finding supporting the observation that the weight gain does not represent an increase in lean tissue mass. Growth hormone has not yet been shown to be useful in managing cachexia. However, anabolic steroids (e.g., 20 mg of oxandrolone per day in conjunction with a high intake of protein and physical therapy) do increase fat-free mass (14). Although inhibition of proinflammatory cytokines has not been shown to increase weight, such treatment may decrease protein breakdown and be clinically useful. For example, the use of thalidomide in HIV-infected patients being treated for tuberculosis can promote weight gain (14). Preliminary studies of a combination of a progestational agent and nonsteroidal antiinflammatory drugs have reported some success, but no recommendation can be made from such early data. The administration of 6 g of eicosapentaenoic acid per day or 2 g of fish oil per day appeared to stabilize the weight of patients with pancreatic cancer in a few studies (13).

3. **Nutritional management of patients with specific cancers.** Nutritional intervention is sometimes appropriate when a specific cancer causes a clinical syndrome or problem that can be reversed. Most often, calories or fluid is provided when oral intake becomes limited, either by the cancer itself or by the side effects of medication. In such situations, nutritional intervention may resolve the immediate problem, but in most instances, the effect on the eventual outcome is small. The metabolic alterations caused by the tumor usually blunt or prevent the effects of nutritional intervention. Thus, nutritional intervention must be undertaken with a full understanding on the part of both patient and physician of the limited goals of such therapy. Table 14-5 outlines some of the more common nutritionally related problems that develop in cancer patients.

A frustrating situation is created when decreased food intake, vomiting, weight loss, and chronic fluid loss develop in a patient undergoing chemotherapy. With a malnourished patient, there is often little choice but to intervene, provided the intervention does not create a distasteful situation (e.g., gastrostomy) that will continue after the course of chemotherapy is over. A metaanalysis of 12 randomized studies of normally nourished patients receiving chemotherapy showed no benefit of TPN (15). Even though enteral feeding causes fewer complications than

(*text continues on page 542*)

Table 14-3. Nutrition, food, and cancer prevention

Nutrient	Evidence for relationship to cancer		
	Convincing/probable	Possible	Insufficient
Energy			
↓ Risk	Physical activity: colon	Physical activity: lung, breast	—
None	—	↑ Body mass: pancreas, prostate	—
↑ Risk	↑ Body mass: breast, kidney, endometrium	↑ Intake: pancreas ↑ Height: colorectal ↑ Mass: GB, colon	↑ Intake: prostate ↑ mass: thyroid
Carbohydrate			
↓ Risk	—	Starch: colorectal	Resistant starch: colorectal Fiber: breast
None	—	NSP/fiber: pancreas, colorectal, breast Sugar: stomach	—
↑ Risk	—	Starch: stomach Sugar: colorectal	Sugar: pancreas
Fat and cholesterol			
↓ Risk	Cholesterol: breast	Monounsaturated fat: breast Polyunsaturated fat: breast	—
None	—	—	Total fat: endometrium, ovary, bladder Saturated fat: ovary Cholesterol: endometrium
↑ Risk	—	Total fat: lung, breast, colorectal, prostate Saturated fat: lung, breast, colorectal, endometrium, prostate Cholesterol: lung, pancreas	

Protein			
↓ Risk	—	—	—
None	—	—	—
↑ Risk	—	—	Animal fat: breast
Vitamins			
↓ Risk	Vitamin C: stomach	Carotene: esophagus, colorectal, breast, cervix Vitamin C: pharynx, lung, esophagus, pancreas, cervix Vitamin E: lung, cervix Folate: breast	Carotene: larynx, lung, ovary, bladder, endometrium, stomach Vitamin C: larynx, colorectal, breast, bladder Vitamin E: colorectal Folate: colorectal
None	—	Vitamin C: prostate Vitamin A: lung, stomach, breast, cervix Vitamin E: stomach, breast Folate: cervix	—
↑ Risk	—	—	—

GB, gallbladder; NSP, nonstarch polysaccharides.
Adapted from World Cancer Research Fund. *Food, nutrition and the prevention of cancer: a global perspective.* Washington, DC: World Cancer Research Fund, American Institute for Cancer Research, 1997, and from National Research Council, Commission on Life Sciences, Food and Nutrition Board, Committee on Diet and Health. *Diet and health implications for reducing chronic disease risk.* Washington, DC: National Academy Press, 1989.

Table 14-4. Possible mechanisms for future diet-derived compounds in cancer prevention

Mechanism	Possible target	Examples of compounds
↓ Carcinogen uptake	Bind bile acids	Calcium
↓ Carcinogen formation	Inhibit cytochrome P-450	PEITC, tea, soy isoflavones
	Inhibit PG synthase	Curcumin
	↓ Natural bile acids	Ursodiol
Detoxify carcinogen	Enhance GSH	NAC, garlic/onion disulfides
↓ Carcinogen–DNA binding	Inhibit cytochrome P-450	Tea
↑ DNA repair fidelity	Enhanced poly-ADP transferase	NAC, protease inhibitors
Modulate growth factors	Inhibit estrogen receptor	Soy isoflavones
	Inhibit IGF-1	”
Inhibit oncogene activity	Inhibit farnesyl protein translation	Perillyl alcohol, DHEA
Inhibit polyamine metabolism	↓ ODC induction	Retinoids, tea, curcumin
↑ Differentiation	Induce TGF-β	Retinoids, vitamin D, soy isoflavones
Induce apoptosis	Activate caspase	Curcumin, tea, retinoids
	Induce TGF-β	Retinoids, vitamin D, soy flavones
	Inhibit telomerase	Perillyl alcohol, DHEA
Inhibit angiogenesis	Inhibit tyrosine kinase	Soy isoflavones
	Inhibit thrombomodulin	Retinoids

ADP, adenosine diphosphate; DHEA, dehydroepiandrosterone; GSH, reduced glutathione; IGF, insulin-like growth factor; NAC, N-acetyl cysteine; ODC, orotidine 5'-phosphate decarboxylase; PEITC, phenethyl isothiocyanate; PG, prostaglandin; TGF-β, transforming growth factor-β.
From Kelloff GJ, Crowell JA, Steele VE, et al. Progress in cancer chemoprevention: development of diet-derived chemopreventive agents. *J Nutr* 2000;130:467S.

TPN does, it is unlikely that enteral nutrition would produce a different long-term result. In severely malnourished patients who are undergoing major surgery, analysis of the available data suggests a very modest improvement in survival (~10%) when TPN is given perioperatively (16).

II. HIV infection

A. Body composition. AIDS and its complications remain a national concern and a major priority in health care management. Patients infected with HIV are frequently malnourished, and the causes of protein–energy malnutrition in patients with AIDS are multiple. Wasting is usually defined according to weight loss as mild (<5%), moderate (6% to 10%), or severe (>10%). However, weight loss can represent loss of lean tissue or loss of fat stores, and the severity of malnutrition can be underestimated in severely ill patients if they have large fat stores. At all stages of the HIV-mediated wasting syndrome, women lose more body fat than men, but lean mass is also lost (17). Measurements of body composition can be used to detect fat stores (e.g., triceps skin folds), but these are not usually helpful for routine clinical management (see Chapter 6). Antiretroviral therapy stabilizes weight and lessens the severity of malnutrition (18,19). However, body cell mass is decreased even in patients on protease inhibitors; some patients do not respond optimally, and some gain weight on treatment even though their lean body mass does not increase (19). Residual nutrition-related abnormalities in HIV-infected patients treated with pro-

Table 14-5. Nutritional consequences of cancer and its treatment

Problem	Pathophysiology	Nutritional intervention
Weight loss	Decreased intake	Table foods, calorie supplements
Nausea	Multifactorial	Encourage oral intake, antiemetics limited except at chemotherapy
Enterocutaneous fistula	Fluid/electrolyte loss	Replacement, orally if possible
Protein-losing enteropathy	Lymphatic blockage	Low-fat diet
Anemia	Blood loss (iron), ↓ intake (folate)	Iron, folate supplements, orally if possible
Abdominal radiation	Diarrhea, malabsorption	Opiates as needed
Oral/mediastinal radiation	Ulcers, dysphagia, stricture	Full liquid diets, avoid TPN or gastrostomy, if possible
Vagotomy	Steatorrhea	Limit fat intake
Gastrectomy	Loss of reservoir, intrinsic factor, dumping syndrome	Small meals, antidumping diet, vitamin B_{12} supplement
Ileal resection	↓ Bile salt pool, bile salt/fatty acid diarrhea	Low fat intake, Ca/Mg supplements, ? cholestyramine
Ileostomy/colostomy	↓ Salt, fluid absorption	Replace orally, if possible
Pancreatectomy	↓ Pancreatic enzymes	Limit fat intake
Corticosteroids	Salt retention	Limit salt intake
Chemotherapy	Nausea, diarrhea, anorexia	None, use serotonin-receptor antagonists
Surgery	↑ Catabolism in severely malnourished patients	Limited benefit (up to 10% ↑ survival) of TPN given perioperatively

TPN, total parenteral nutrition.

tease inhibitors include subcutaneous and visceral accumulation of fat, hypertriglyceridemia and hypercholesterolemia, and peripheral insulin resistance (20). These effects were initially considered to be caused by protease inhibitors, but clearly they can occur in patients not taking protease inhibitors (21). The optimal management of these patients requires the same working knowledge and skillful management of nutrition that is required in the management of others, plus a knowledge of the numerous symptoms, complications, and infections associated with progressive HIV infection.

B. Etiology of nutritional deficiency in patients with HIV infection. A person's nutritional status represents a balance of caloric and nutrient intake, absorption or malabsorption, and energy expenditure, which are altered by hormonal and metabolic factors. Weight loss is the most frequent finding associated with HIV infection. A weight loss of 10% is generally considered to have a significant impact on a patient's functional status. Weight loss may be caused by inadequate oral intake, intestinal malabsorption, altered metabolism, or a combination of these factors.

    1. Causes of decreased intake of nutrients

        a. Anorexia. A loss of appetite may be caused by myriad reasons, including systemic infection and fever, depression, and side effects of medication. Alterations in taste sensation resulting from medications or oral infections may decrease salivation and appetite. Ulcerative gastritis or duodenitis also may cause anorexia. Nausea, vomiting, anorexia, abdominal discomfort, or diarrhea may compound the loss of appetite. These symptoms may be secondary to drugs or to the underlying medical process. The intake of food may be decreased by a complete loss of appetite, early satiety, or fear of pain or diarrhea. An early recognition of these concerns is important in preventing malnourishment in these patients.

b. **Oral and esophageal pain and/or dysphagia.** Oral pain and discomfort can be secondary to oral candidiasis, oral herpes, cytomegalovirus (CMV) infection, aphthous ulcers, oral hairy leukoplakia, or oropharyngeal bulky tumors of Kaposi's sarcoma or non-Hodgkin's lymphoma. HIV-associated gingivitis and HIV-associated periodontitis can be rapidly destructive and may resist therapy. Esophageal odynophagia and dysphagia may be caused by ulceration from CMV, herpes simplex virus (HSV), or candidal infection. Pharyngeal or esophageal lesions of Kaposi's sarcoma may cause dysphagia through obstruction.

c. **Nausea and vomiting.** Nausea and vomiting may be secondary to gastrointestinal (GI) or central nervous system (CNS) malignancies or infections. Symptoms also may be exacerbated by any of the commonly used therapeutic agents.

d. **Neurologic causes of decreased nutritional intake.** HIV-associated dementia, CNS pathogens, weakness, debilitation, and depression also may contribute to a decreased oral intake. CNS disease processes include CMV infection, HIV encephalitis, cryptococcal meningitis, primary lymphomas, and progressive multifocal leukoencephalopathy.

e. **Cytokines.** Cytokines such as TNF may cause anorexia by decreasing GI motility. Interleukin-1 and α- and γ-interferons have been shown to contribute to anorexia. TNF and α- and γ-interferons have been reported to induce nausea and vomiting during therapeutic trials, although their precise role in causing anorexia in clinical disease is not known.

2. **Causes of diarrhea and malabsorption.** With improved diagnostic capabilities and a greater awareness of the spectrum of diarrheal pathogens in AIDS, an increasing number of causes of chronic diarrhea are being identified.

a. **Infections of the GI tract.** Parasitic causes include *Cryptosporidium parvum, Giardia lamblia, Isospora belli,* and *Enterocytozoon bieneusi* (microsporidia). Viral causes include CMV and HSV. Bacterial agents include *Campylobacter* and *Mycobacterium avium-intracellulare.* Cryptosporidiosis and microsporidiosis are associated with decreased jejunal disaccharidase activity and D-xylose absorption. The pattern of injury is similar to that in tropical and nontropical sprue, with rapid turnover and functional immaturity of villus enterocytes.

b. **Bacterial overgrowth.** Bacterial overgrowth has been reported and may be related in part to the high frequency of gastric achlorhydria seen in HIV infection, especially with enteropathogenic strains of *Escherichia coli.*

c. **Malabsorption.** Malabsorption may be present, even in the absence of diarrhea. Lactase deficiency is common and causes lactose intolerance. Abnormal findings on D-xylose absorption studies, Schilling tests, or [^{14}C]glycocholate absorption studies suggest small-bowel dysfunction. Fat malabsorption secondary to small-bowel disease or pancreatic insufficiency may lead to caloric and fat-soluble vitamin depletion. Vitamin B_{12} deficiency occurs in at least 15% of patients with HIV infection. An abnormal Schilling test result in some patients despite the coadministration of intrinsic factor and pancreatic enzymes suggests small-bowel disease as the cause of malabsorption (22).

  d. **Kaposi's sarcoma.** In approximately 40% of HIV-infected patients with Kaposi's sarcoma, GI lesions are detected on endoscopy. Kaposi's sarcoma in the GI tract is rarely symptomatic, but when involvement is extensive, it may contribute to malabsorption and diarrhea.

 3. **Role of concurrent infection.** Hypermetabolism was considered a significant contributor to the wasting syndrome in the past. However, when caloric intake and resting energy expenditure were examined in HIV-infected patients with weight loss at various stages of disease, only the patients with secondary infections lost weight (23). In patients without infection, only those with a decreased intake lost weight, and only in those patients was total energy expenditure decreased (24). Thus, it now appears that weight loss in HIV-infected patients is caused by decreased food intake, not hypermetabolism. A similar observation has been made in cancer patients (12). Although the metabolic rate can be extremely high (e.g., because of fever), food intake is invariably diminished in such patients.

   These observations translate into practical considerations. When the provision of calories was increased (by TPN) in patients with AIDS wasting, the increased caloric intake led to weight gain (25). When weight loss was secondary to malabsorption or GI disease, the administration of TPN increased body cell mass (26). However, patients with AIDS wasting who had infection but not malabsorption continued to lose weight on TPN therapy (26).

C. **Effects of malnutrition**
 1. **Protein–calorie malnutrition.** In AIDS patients, body cell mass depletion is increased out of proportion to total weight loss. Body cell mass, measured by total body potassium, is more depleted than body fat mass in immunodeficient patients (27). A linear relationship can be found between the degree of body mass depletion and time to death. The loss of body cell mass correlates with time to death when the body cell mass is depleted by about 50% and the body weight is decreased by about 33%. The time to death does not correlate with body fat depletion. Thus, it has been surmised that the time to death in AIDS patients with wasting may be more closely related to the degree of body cell mass depletion than to its underlying cause (28).
 2. **Nutrition and the immune system.** Both malnourishment and overnourishment affect immune status. Nutritional deficiencies, seen most commonly in some Third World countries, are linked with decreased immune function and increased rates of infection. However, no solid scientific data are available to prove that malnutrition *per se* predisposes HIV-infected patients to AIDS. Body cell mass correlates better than immune function (assessed by CD4+ lymphocyte count) with physical performance (29).
 3. **Individual micronutrients**
  a. **Vitamin B$_6$.** Pyridoxine deficiency may result from decreased food intake or from treatment with pyridoxine antagonists such as isoniazid or hydralazine. Symptoms of peripheral neuropathy, seborrheic dermatitis, and oral lesions, including glossitis, angularis stomatitis, and cheilosis, may be present.
  b. **Vitamin B$_{12}$.** Deficiency is present in 16% to 33% of patients with AIDS. Vitamin B$_{12}$ deficiency may be secondary to malabsorption resulting from ileal dysfunction, bacterial overgrowth with bacterial binding of vitamin B$_{12}$, or intrinsic factor deficiency (21). Symptoms include anorexia, loss of taste, glossitis, diarrhea, hair loss, impotence, and anemia, which may result in weakness, fatigue, and dyspnea. Neurologic symptoms include paresthesias, loss of sensory

and motor function, irritability, and memory disturbances. Many of these patients do not have megaloblastic changes; however, when deficiency is suspected, it should be documented with elevated serum methylmalonic acid and homocysteine levels (see Chapter 7). If the diagnosis remains in doubt, treatment should not be withheld.

c. **Folate.** Folate levels are low in one-third of patients. Absorption may be decreased by inhibition of the dihydrofolate reductase enzyme by drugs, including methotrexate, trimethoprim, pyrimethamine, and triamterene. Supplements should be administered when a deficient state is suspected or when these drugs are used. It is essential to include vitamin B_{12} replacement when deficiencies of both vitamins are expected.

d. **Vitamin D.** Excess amounts of vitamin D have been shown to decrease T-cell function. It is important to monitor for additional regimens that patients may be taking, including megadoses of certain vitamins and minerals.

e. **Iron.** Deficiency favors *Candida* and *Salmonella* infections. The prevalence of iron deficiency is higher in adults with recurrent HSV infections than in matched controls. However, current data do not indicate that correction of this deficiency protects against infection. Deficiency results in depletion of storage iron, a decrease in circulating iron, and a hypochromic, microcytic anemia. Iron-containing substrates such as muscle myoglobin and mitochondrial cytochromes are also affected, which may account for symptoms of weakness.

f. **Zinc.** Deficiency is secondary to decreased absorption and increased losses in chronic diarrhea. Zinc deficiency itself may cause diarrhea in addition to poor wound healing, dysgeusia, skin rashes, and apathy.

g. **Selenium.** Selenium deficiency is common in HIV-infected patients and may play a role in the pathogenesis of cardiomyopathy. It also is an independent factor associated with decreased survival (30).

D. **Evaluation of malnutrition in patients with AIDS.** The assessment and evaluation of the nutritional status of patients with AIDS follow the general nutritional principles discussed in detail in Chapter 5. Evaluation for individual micronutrient deficiencies is covered in Chapters 6 and 7.

1. **Anthropometric parameters** provide the most reliable overall assessment of nutritional status. These include weight and height. A body mass index below 20 and an involuntary weight loss of more than 10% are most often seen in late stages of disease. Other measurements of body composition, such as skinfold thickness, bioimpedance analysis, and dual x-ray absorptiometry, can sometimes be helpful in earlier disease but are more useful for clinical studies (19).

2. **Further investigations**

   a. **Intercurrent disease.** If the history does not suggest a significantly decreased intake of food, a careful search for oral pathology, infection, or CNS disease should be undertaken.

   b. **Laboratory tests.** Serum albumin is the most readily available and commonly performed test. A serum protein such as retinol-binding protein is a more reliable index of short-term changes in nutritional status, given the short half-life in comparison with that of albumin. Both measurements may be affected by extracellular fluid status. Anemia with abnormal red blood cell indices may indicate low levels of folate, vitamin B_{12}, or iron.

   c. **Protein–calorie malnutrition.** Parameters such as a low lymphocyte count or a diminished delayed-type hypersensitivity reaction, which are used in patients without AIDS, may not be valid in patients with immunodeficiency resulting from HIV infection.

E. **Treatment for specific complications of HIV infection contributing to malnutrition.** Table 14-6 outlines the nutrition-related treatment recommendations for HIV-infected patients. No standard of nutritional man-

Table 14-6. Nutrition-related treatment recommendations for AIDS patients

Clinical evaluation	Resulting action
Normal weight, food intake, body composition (if used)	Ensure that intake of protein, fat, and carbohydrate is adequate, including ≥1 g protein/kg body weight.
Normal weight, food intake	Provide adequate amounts (about two or three times the DRI or RDA) for each nutrient.
Weight loss, decreased food intake	Give appetite-stimulating drugs.
Decreased stores of micronutrients	Treat with larger doses of appropriate nutrients.
Laboratory evidence of hypogonadism	Give testosterone (parenteral) in men.
Severe weight loss failing other treatments	Growth hormone (0.1 mg/kg/d) can be tried.

DRI, dietary reference intake; RDA, recommended dietary allowance.
From Corcoran C, Grinspoon S. Treatments for wasting in patients with the acquired immuno-deficiency syndrome. *N Engl J Med* 1999;340:1740.

agement in AIDS is universally accepted. In general, patients who are not malnourished do not require nutritional supplements. However, they do need an adequate intake of macronutrients and micronutrients from a balanced diet of table foods.

1. **Dietary recommendations**
   a. Optimal oral and dental hygiene is essential to prevent infections, oral discomfort, and changes in taste.
   b. Patients who are at risk for aspiration because of oropharyngeal dysfunction should be evaluated by a speech pathologist or ear, nose, and throat specialist.
   c. Meals and the administration of medication should be timed to avoid anticipatory vomiting. Drugs that induce nausea or vomiting should be administered long before meals.
   d. Foods should be thoroughly cooked and stored with adequate refrigeration. Leftover foods should be completely reheated. Bacterial food contamination can be fatal in the immunocompromised patient. Raw or undercooked shellfish and seafood, meat, poultry, and unpasteurized milk products (e.g., steak tartare and sushi) should be avoided because they may lead to enteric infections with *Salmonella, Campylobacter, Listeria,* and *Escherichia coli.* Separate cutting boards should be used for uncooked meats, fruits, and vegetables. Neutropenic diets, in which uncooked fruits and vegetables are avoided, are advisable for patients whose white blood cell counts are low.
   e. Avoidance of significant alcohol consumption is advisable. Ethanol abuse decreases function in multiple components of the immune system and further compromises nutrient absorption, utilization, storage, and secretion (31).
   f. Patients with diarrhea or fat malabsorption should avoid fatty foods.
   g. For anorectic patients, meals should be served in an appetizing fashion in a well-lit environment free from distractions. Frequent small meals served on small plates are often best tolerated. Providing nutrient-dense foods may help in these situations. Variety in the temperatures of food is welcomed by some. Offering favorite foods in a pleasant atmosphere in the presence of family members or companions may help.

h. Foods served at cool temperatures may be more soothing. Foods with strong aromas and spices should be avoided.

i. Fluid intake during meals, which causes early satiety, should be avoided. The remainder of the fluid requirement should be ingested between meals.

j. For patients with dysgeusia, serving liquids at meal time and altering the texture and temperatures of foods may stimulate sensory feedback. Serving foods with small amounts of liquids may aid chewing and swallowing. Sour candy may stimulate salivation in patients with dry mouth.

k. Enteral nutritional supplementation is best given at times other than meal times, such as just before bedtime, to allow for optimal appetite during meals. Iso-osmolar formulas with an increased fat content may be better tolerated by patients with sepsis who are glucose-intolerant. Patients with malabsorption may benefit from low-fat diets or diets containing medium-chain triglycerides. The use of these supplemental diets may be limited because of their potentially adverse effects of hyperosmolarity and diarrhea. The intake of carbohydrate and fat in both table foods and enteral supplements should be adjusted to reduce symptoms of diarrhea.

2. Appetite stimulants and anabolic agents. These should be reserved for patients with weight loss and decreased food intake (Table 14-7).

a. Megestrol acetate. The progestational agent megestrol acetate may increase appetite and promote weight gain in AIDS patients without any clear underlying cause of weight loss. Similar benefits have been seen in some cancer patients. In two trials in which 800 mg of megestrol acetate was given daily for 12 weeks to AIDS patients with anorexia and cachexia, a weight gain of 3 to 4 kg was reported (32,33). The optimal dosing of megestrol acetate remains to be determined. No significant side effects were observed during the course of therapy. Long-term effects on weight gain, repletion of body cell mass, and quality of life are not yet known. Consistent with its glucocorticoid action, the drug can exacerbate diabetes (34) and cause adrenal insufficiency on withdrawal. Fat deposition may be the major component of weight gain.

Table 14-7. Anabolic treatments for patients with AIDS wasting

Treatment	Usual dose	Demonstrated result
Appetite-stimulating drugs		
Megestrol acetate	800 mg/d	Improved appetite, weight gain
Dronabinol	5 mg/d	(mostly fat)
Testosterone and analogues		
Testosterone, IM	300 mg q3wk	↑ lean body mass
Testosterone, transdermal	5 mg/d	"
Oxandrolone, oral	20 mg/d	Weight gain, ↑ lean body mass
Nandrolone, IM	100 mg q2wk	
Recombinant human growth hormone	6 mg/d	Weight gain, ↑ lean body mass (short-term)
Exercise training	Individualized	↑ Lean body mass
Cytokine modulators		
Thalidomide	200–400 mg/d	Weight gain

From Corcoran C, Grinspoon S. Treatments for wasting in patients with the acquired immunodeficiency syndrome. *N Engl J Med* 1999;340:1740.

    b. **Dronabinol (δ-9-tetrahydrocannabinol).** The active agent in marijuana has been shown to enhance appetite, but weight gain is very slight (35). The body composition of this weight gain has yet to be evaluated. Side effects include drowsiness, anxiety, poor coordination, and confusion.

    c. **Anabolic steroids** have been useful only in men, producing a modest increase in lean body mass and a weight gain of about 1 kg over control during 12 to 14 weeks (19).

    d. **Growth hormone.** Patients with weight loss may have some resistance to endogenous growth hormone, perhaps related to malnutrition or underlying HIV infection. In an uncontrolled 3-month study, an increase in weight of 3 kg was achieved by giving 5 mg SC every other day. Other studies showed an improved exercise capacity and a confirmed modest weight gain in comparison with controls (19). However, the recombinant drug is very expensive, and side effects include edema, arthralgias/myalgias, and decreased glucose tolerance.

    e. **Thalidomide.** The data supporting use of this drug are very preliminary, and weight gain is modest, as with the other drugs. Somnolence and rash are frequent side effects, and the drug is contraindicated in women because it is teratogenic, even in very small doses. The best data are for adjunctive therapy in patients being treated for tuberculosis (14).

  3. Accompanying disorders. The causes of weight loss must be evaluated. Treatment of any underlying infection is imperative when feasible. Evaluation of diarrhea should begin with stool studies for culture and toxins of *Salmonella, Campylobacter, Shigella,* and *Clostridium difficile.* These patients may have accompanying fever and abdominal pain, and the diarrhea is often bloody. Bacteremia is common, and parenteral antibiotics should be administered empirically to severely ill patients pending the results of stool culture. The stool should also be examined for ova and parasites. Duodenal aspiration may be useful to identify *Cryptosporidium, Giardia lamblia,* and *Entamoeba histolytica* and may be better tolerated than endoscopy by some patients. However, endoscopy with biopsy is useful to diagnose *M. avium-intracellulare* infection, microsporidiosis, and CMV infection. It is important to keep in mind that multiple pathogenic processes may exist concurrently in these immunocompromised hosts.

    Gastrointestinal Kaposi's sarcoma can be diagnosed histologically by endoscopic biopsy. When these lesions are symptomatic or interfere with nutrition, they can be treated with chemotherapy and radiation.

    AIDS and other chronic, incurable diseases frequently precipitate anxiety, fear, and depression. These symptoms alone can contribute significantly to a decline in adequate nutritional intake. Appropriate measures should be taken to address these primary problems, both for nutritional purposes and to optimize the quality of the patient's remaining life.

III. Nutritional support in patients with wasting disorders (cancer, AIDS). Many studies have shown that a loss of body weight or lean body mass is associated with an increase in mortality. However, no data indicate that wasting is the cause of death or that nutritional support reverses wasting. It is just as likely that wasting is a measure of disease severity. The use of nutritional support does not improve the condition of patients with cancer (36–38) or AIDS (16). A conference examining the current evidence concluded that the routine use of short-term enteral or parenteral feeding does not decrease complications or mortality in patients with cancer, and that it does not reverse wasting syndrome in patients with HIV infection if decreased food intake alone is not the cause of wasting (16). However, these conclusions are not meant as guidelines for individual patients. The use of nutritional support can be considered for patients with documented or probable deficiencies who require nutrition if other treatments are to proceed. However, no clear indication for the use of nutritional support as primary therapy can be found in the literature.

References

1. Chief Medical Officers' Committee on Medical Aspects of Food. *Nutritional aspects of the development of cancer.* London: Stationery Office, 1998 (Department of Heath report on health and social subjects No. 48).
2. World Cancer Research Fund. *Food, nutrition and the prevention of cancer: a global perspective.* Washington DC: World Cancer Research Fund, American Institute for Cancer Research, 1997.
3. National Research Council, Commission on Life Sciences, Food and Nutrition Board, Committee on Diet and Health. *Diet and health implications for reducing chronic disease risk.* Washington DC: National Academy Press, 1989.
4. de Logeril M, Salen P, Martin J-L, et al. Mediterranean dietary pattern in a randomized trial. *Arch Intern Med* 1998;158:1181.
5. Zhang S, Hunter DJ, Hankinson SE, et al. A prospective study of folate intake and the risk of breast cancer. *JAMA* 1999;281:1632.
6. Cummings JH, Bingham SA. Diet and the prevention of cancer. *BMJ* 1998; 317:1636.
7. Janne PA, Mayer RJ. Chemoprevention of colorectal cancer. *N Engl J Med* 2000; 342:1960.
8. Biasco G, Paganelli GM. European trials on dietary supplementation for cancer prevention. *Ann N Y Acad Sci* 1999;889:152.
9. Kelloff GJ, Crowell JA, Steele VE, et al. Progress in cancer chemoprevention: development of diet-derived chemopreventive agents. *J Nutr* 2000;130:467S.
10. Yang CS, Chung JY, Yang G, et al. Tea and tea polyphenols in cancer prevention. *J Nutr* 2000;130:472S.
11. Lippman SM, Lotan R. Advances in the development of retinoids as chemopreventive agents. *J Nutr* 2000;130:479S.
12. Shils ME, Shike M. Nutritional support of the cancer patient. In: Shils ME, Olson JA, Shike M, et al., eds. *Modern nutrition in health and disease,* 9th ed. Baltimore: Williams & Wilkins, 1999:1297.
13. Barber MD, Ross JA, Fearon KCH. Disordered metabolic response with cancer and its management. *World J Surg* 2000;24:681.
14. Kotler DP. Cachexia. *Ann Intern Med* 2000;133:622.
15. American College of Physicians. Position paper. Parenteral nutrition in patients receiving cancer chemotherapy. *Ann Intern Med* 1989;110:734.
16. Klein S, Kinney J, Jeejeebhoy K, et al. Nutrition support in clinical practice: review of published data and recommendations for future research directions. *JPEN J Parenter Enteral Nutr* 1997;21:133.
17. Grinspoon S, Corcoran C, Miller K, et al. Body composition and endocrine function in women with acquired immunodeficiency syndrome wasting. *J Clin Endocrinol Metab* 1997;82:3360.
18. Flexner C. HIV-protease inhibitors. *N Engl J Med* 1998;338:1281.
19. Corcoran C, Grinspoon S. Treatments for wasting in patients with the acquired immunodeficiency syndrome. *N Engl J Med* 1999;340:1740.
20. Kotler DP. Nutrition and wasting in HIV infection. In: *HIV clinical management* (vol 8). Available at: *www.medscape.com/home/topics/internalmedicine/internal medicine.html.* Accessed November 4, 1999.
21. Lo JC, Mulligan K, Tai VW, et al. Buffalo hump in men with HIV-1 infection. *Lancet* 1998;351:867.
22. Harriman GR, Smith PD, Horne MK. Vitamin B_{12} malabsorption in patients with acquired immunodeficiency syndrome. *Arch Intern Med* 1989;149:2039.
23. Grunfeld C, Pang M, Shimizu L, et al. Resting energy expenditure, caloric intake, and short-term weight change in human immunodeficiency virus infection and AIDS. *Am J Clin Nutr* 1992;55:455.
24. Macallan DC, Noble C, Baldwin C, et al. Energy expenditure and wasting in human immunodeficiency virus infection. *N Engl J Med* 1995;333:83.

25. Melchior J, Chastang C, Gelas P, et al. Efficacy of 2-month total parenteral nutrition in AIDS patients: a controlled randomized prospective trial. *AIDS* 1996;10:379.

26. Suttmann U, Ockenga O, Selberg O, et al. Incidence and prognostic value of malnutrition and wasting in human immunodeficiency virus-infected outpatients. *J Acquir Immune Defic Syndr Hum Retrovirol* 1995;8:239.

27. Kotler DP, Wang J, Pierson RN. Body composition studies in patients with the acquired immunodeficiency syndrome. *Am J Clin Nutr* 1985;42:1255.

28. Kotler DP, Tierney AR, Wang J, et al. Magnitude of body-cell-mass depletion and the timing of death from wasting in AIDS. *Am J Clin Nutr* 1989;50:444.

29. Ott M, Fischer H, Polat H, et al. Bioelectrical impedence analysis as a predictor of survival in patients with human immunodeficiency virus infection. *J Acquir Immune Defic Syndr Hum Retrovirol* 1995;9:20.

30. Baum MK, Shor-Posner G, Lai S, et al. High risk of HIV-related mortality is associated with selenium deficiency. *J Acquir Immune Defic Syndr Hum Retrovirol* 1997;15:370.

31. Watzl B, Watson RR. Role of alcohol abuse in nutritional immunosuppression. *J Nutr* 1992;122:733.

32. Von Roenn JH, Armstrong D, Kotler DP, et al. Megestrol acetate in patients with AIDS-related cachexia. *Ann Intern Med* 1994;121:393.

33. Oster MH, Enders SR, Samuels SJ, et al. Megestrol acetate in patients with AIDS and cachexia. *Ann Intern Med* 1994;121:400.

34. Henry K, Rathgaber S, Sullivan C, et al. Diabetes mellitus induced by megestrol acetate in a patient with AIDS and cachexia. *Ann Intern Med* 1992;116:53.

35. Beal JE, Olson R, Laubenstein L, et al. Dronabinol as a treatment for anorexia associated with weight loss in patients with AIDS. *J Pain Symptom Manage* 1995;10:89.

36. Klein S, Koretz RL. Nutrition support in patients with cancer: What do the data really show? *Nutr Clin Pract* 1994;9:91.

37. Klein S, Simes J, Blackburn GL. Total parenteral nutrition and cancer clinical trials. *Cancer* 1986;58:1378.

38. McGeer AJ, Detsky AS, O'Rourke KO. Parenteral nutrition in cancer patients undergoing chemotherapy: a meta-analysis. *Nutrition* 1990;6:233.

15. ALTERNATIVE NUTRITIONAL THERAPY

Alternative nutritional therapy includes the use of a wide variety of dietary supplements: herbal products, vitamins, minerals, amino acids, and biochemical intermediates such as carnitine and creatine. Dietary supplements are consumed widely in the United States and elsewhere; in the United States alone, more than $13 billion is spent on dietary supplements each year.

For some dietary supplements, good scientific data are available to support safety and efficacy, whereas for others, no such data exist. Few large, controlled clinical trials have assessed the safety and efficacy of dietary supplements. In contrast, large, controlled trials are required by law for the approval of prescription drugs. For this reason, far less information is available to assess the safety and efficacy of dietary supplements than to assess prescription drugs. To address this lack of data, the National Institutes of Health Office of Dietary Supplements (ODS) and the Consumer Healthcare Product Association (CHPA) have jointly developed a bibliography of original research papers recommended by the editors of peer-reviewed journals. Their first publication highlights 25 articles based on scientifically sound research in the area of dietary supplements. It is hoped that the bibliography will serve as a useful reference source for nutrition and health care professionals, educators, and scientists. It is posted on the Internet at *http://ods.od.nih.gov/publications/publications.html,* and copies are available from the ODS at 301-435-2920 or *ods@nih.gov.*

I. Regulation of dietary supplements

- **A.** The Food and Drug Administration (FDA) requires that prescription drugs have been proved safe and effective for their labeled use before they are marketed; however, no such requirement applies to dietary supplements provided they are not marketed as a treatment for a specific disease. Dietary supplements are regulated under the Dietary Supplement Health and Education Act of 1994 (DSHEA). These regulations, which are largely favorable to the manufacturers of dietary supplements, were enacted by Congress in response to an effort by the FDA to remove some herbal products from the market. The negative public response to this effort caused the government to relax the regulations on dietary supplements.

- **B.** Under the DSHEA, the labels of dietary supplements can include "statements of nutritional support," but not claims of their efficacy in the treatment of specific diseases. Statements of nutritional support may describe the ability of a supplement to affect the function or structure of an organ, or promote general well-being. Thus, the label of a dietary supplement can claim that the supplement "improves memory," "supports cardiovascular health," or "enhances mental well-being," but it cannot claim that the supplement is effective in the treatment of Alzheimer's disease, coronary artery disease, or depression. The standards for the evidence required as a basis for the statements of nutritional support are quite lax.

- **C.** Drug manufacturers are required by the FDA to prove that their products are safe before they can be marketed. The manufacturers of dietary supplements are not required to demonstrate safety; instead, the FDA has the burden of demonstrating that a dietary supplement is unsafe before it can restrict or ban the product. Moreover, it is difficult for the FDA to demonstrate safety problems with dietary supplements because no uniform system is in place for reporting adverse events.

- **D.** The FDA does require that the labels of dietary supplements include an "information panel," similar to the "nutrition facts" panel required on food labels. The information panel must describe the part of the plant used, the suggested serving size, and the amount of specific nutrients included (e.g., vitamins and minerals). For herbal products in particular, such labeling is not informative because herbs contain many different compounds, the levels of which vary according to the soil and climate conditions where the herbs are grown. Moreover, for many herbs, the specific active ingredient is unknown and therefore the amount present in a product cannot be stated.

E. In Germany, where herbal products are widely used, a government agency, the German Federal Institute for Drugs and Medicinal Devices, formed a commission to evaluate the safety and efficacy of a large number of herbal remedies. The report of that commission was translated into English and published as *The Complete German Commission E Monographs: Therapeutic Guide to Herbal Medicines* (Blumenthal M, ed. Austin, Texas: American Botanical Council, 1998). This publication is a comprehensive and objective guide to the efficacy and safety of herbal medicines.

II. Dietary supplements. In this chapter, we review a few of the hundreds of alternative nutritional products that are available commercially (Table 15-1). Vitamins (the B vitamins and vitamins A, C, and E) and minerals (potassium, calcium, magnesium, zinc) are covered in Chapters 6 and 7. The nutritional products presented in this chapter were chosen because of wide use (e.g., ginkgo biloba, *Echinacea*), good evidence of efficacy (e.g., fish oil, phytosterols), or significant safety issues (e.g., Ma huang). A larger range of dietary supplements is reviewed in *The Health Professional's Guide to Popular Dietary Supplements* (Sabourin A. Chicago: American Dietetic Association, 2000).

A. Acidophilus/lactobacillus acidophilus. *Lactobacillus acidophilus* is a lactic acid bacterium normally found in the human gastrointestinal tract. Lactic acid bacteria convert carbohydrates to lactic acid. Lactobacilli are found in yogurt, where they produce lactase, which hydrolyzes lactose to glucose and galactose. The addition of lactobacilli to milk (acidophilus milk) results in the hydrolysis of lactose. This is one of a group of additives referred to as *probiotics*.

1. Claims and supporting evidence

a. Decreases lactose intolerance. If *Lactobacillus* is added to milk, up to 50% of the milk lactose is hydrolyzed. In most affected persons, lactose intolerance is the result of a decreased amount rather than a complete absence of intestinal epithelial lactase, and symptoms are related both to the amount of lactose ingested and to the degree of intestinal lactase activity. By reducing the amount of lactose in milk, treatment with lactobacilli increases the quantity of milk that a lactose-intolerant person can ingest without symptoms. However, even with the use of lactobacilli, most lactose-intolerant persons will have symptoms if they consume a sufficiently large amount of milk.

b. Decreases antibiotic-associated diarrhea, recurrent *Clostridium difficile* colitis, and *Candida* vaginitis. A few studies, most with small numbers of patients, suggest that treatment with lactobacilli reduces the incidence of antibiotic-associated diarrhea and prevents the recurrence of *C. difficile* colitis (1). Treatment with lactobacilli also appears to prevent candidal vaginitis and pouchitis.

2. Dosing. *L. acidophilus,* in addition to occurring naturally in yogurt, is available in tablets, capsules, and powders. It is often sold in combination with other *Lactobacillus* species and with *Bifidobacterium*. Typical dosing for *L. acidophilus* is 1 billion to 10 billion live bacteria per day.

3. Safety issues. None.

B. Chondroitin sulfate and glucosamine. Chondroitin sulfate and glucosamine are sold separately but are more commonly sold in combination. Both of these agents are produced endogenously in joints. Chondroitin sulfate, a glycosaminoglycan that is formed from repeating disaccharides of galactosamine sulfate and glucuronic acid, is found in articular cartilage, where it is secreted by chondrocytes. It inhibits the enzymes that degrade cartilage and holds water in cartilage, thereby increasing its elasticity. Glucosamine is an aminosugar found in cartilage, tendons, and synovial fluid; it stimulates the synthesis of proteoglycans and glycosaminoglycans.

(*text continues on page 556*)

Table 15-1. Summary of selected alternative medicines

Supplement	Proposed mechanisms	Disease claims	Safety issues
Lactobacillus acidophilus	Reestablish flora	**Antibiotic diarrhea (B)** Lactose intolerance (B)	None
Chondroitin/glucosamine	Inhibits cartilage degradation, increases synthesis	Arthritis (A)	None
Creatine	Role in energy storage	High-intensity exercise (C)	Muscle cramping, dehydration; avoid with renal disease
Echinacea	Immune stimulant	**Common cold (C)**	Allergy, hepatic toxicity
Fish oil	Eicosanoid synthesis Plt aggregation (TXA_2) Blood flow, edema (PGE_2) Chemotaxis (LTB_4)	TG, plt aggregation (A) Improves symptoms in RA (A) IBD treatment (A)	Bleeding time
γ-Linolenic acid (GLA)	Blocks eicosanoid synthesis, provides GLA	RA (A) PMS (C)	Drug interactions, potentiates hepatotoxicity
Ginkgo biloba	Flavonoids improve memory, blood flow	Alzheimer's (A) Peripheral vascular disease (A)	Potentiate antiplatelet agents

Ginseng	Saponins	Improves exercise (C) Enhances cognition (C)	CNS excitation, hypertension, nervousness, drug interactions, hypoglycemia
Ma huang	Sympathomimetic	Bronchodilator (B) Weight loss (B)	Stroke, MI, death, tremors, dizziness, urinary retention
γ-Oryzanol	↓ Phytosterols, cholesterol absorption	Serum cholesterol (B)	None
Saw palmetto	5-α-Reductase activity	BPH symptoms (A) Prostate enlargement (C)	Hepatic toxicity (1 case)
Soy protein	Isoflavonoids are weak estrogens	Menopause (A) Serum cholesterol (A)	Very large amount needed for effect
St. John's wort	5-HT levels	Depression (A)	Photosensitivity, allergy, fatigue, dyspepsia, sleep disturbance

Support for claims:
A, placebo-controlled, randomized trials support.
B, inadequate support.
C, negative studies.
CNS, central nervous system; IBD, inflammatory bowel disease; LTB_4, leukotriene B_4; MI, myocardial infarction; PGE_2, prostaglandin E_2; PMS, premenstrual syndrome; RA, rheumatoid arthritis; TG, triglycerides; TXA_2, thromboxane A_2; 5-HT, serotonin.

1. **Claims and supporting evidence of efficacy in the treatment of arthritis.** In a 6-month, double-blinded, placebo-controlled trial of 93 patients with osteoarthritis of the knee, those who received glucosamine (2,000 mg/d) and chondroitin sulfate (1,600 mg/d) had both a lower arthritis score and a lower requirement for pain medication (2). A metaanalysis of 17 studies of chondroitin sulfate and glucosamine in osteoarthritis concluded that they are effective in improving outcomes, but that the magnitude of their effect is unclear because of inconsistencies in the study methods and dependence on industry support for execution of the studies (3).

2. **Dosing.** Typical dosing for chondroitin sulfate is 1,200 mg/d; for glucosamine, it is 1,500 mg/d.

3. **Safety issues.** None.

C. **Creatine.** Creatine is synthesized from arginine, glycine, and methionine in a two-step process. It is synthesized endogenously in skeletal muscle and other organs, and dietary creatine is not required. Exogenous creatine is taken up into muscle and increases muscle levels of creatine. Creatine and phosphocreatine are involved in the storage and transmission of phosphate bond energy; phosphocreatine is an important reservoir of chemical energy in muscle. It has been suggested that increased amounts of phosphocreatine can shorten the recovery time of muscle adenosine triphosphate levels after exercise.

1. **Claims and supporting evidence that creatine enhances performance in high-intensity exercise.** A large number of blinded, placebo-controlled studies of the effect of creatine on athletic performance have been performed. In a typical study, 32 swimmers were timed in sprints and then received placebo or creatine (20 g/d) for a week. No difference in performance was observed between the placebo and creatine-treated groups after a week of therapy (4). A review of creatine supplementation and exercise performance concluded that creatine supplementation has not consistently proved to enhance exercise performance (5).

2. **Dosing.** Creatine is available in pills and powders as creatine monohydrate. Many formulations combine creatine with carnitine and amino acids. Typical dosing is a loading dose of 20 g/d for 5 or 6 days followed by a maintenance dose of 2 g/d.

3. **Safety issues.** Creatine holds water in muscle; increases in intramuscular water may contribute to muscle cramping and dehydration. Creatine should not be given to patients with renal disease. Some athletes consume doses of creatine that are higher than recommended; whether excessive doses lead to additional adverse events is unclear.

D. **Echinacea.** Three of the nine species of the genus *Echinacia* are commonly found in herbal preparations. The most commonly used is *Echinacea purpurea,* the purple coneflower. Both the above-ground parts and the root have been used as herbal medicines. *Echinacea* has been used to treat or prevent the common cold and influenza and as a stimulant to the immune system. In one *in vitro* study, *Echinacea* stimulated the production of interleukins-1, -6, and -10 and tumor necrosis factor-α by human macrophages (6); whether an *in vivo* counterpart of this effect exists is unknown.

1. **Claims and supporting evidence that *Echinacea* prevents or treats the common cold and influenza.** The ability of *Echinacea* to prevent colds in persons with a history of frequent colds has been studied in a placebo-controlled trial. In this trial, no benefit of *Echinacea* in reducing the number of colds was seen in comparison with placebo (7). The symptoms of patients treated with *Echinacea* who did catch colds may have been less severe.

2. **Dosing.** *Echinacea* is available as the root or the herb; some formulations contain both. Commercial products include tinctures, tablets, capsules, lozenges, and teas. Typical daily dosing is 300 to 900 mg of dried

extract, but dosing is difficult to analyze because of the wide range of formulations available.

3. **Safety.** Allergic reactions and asthma have been reported with *Echinacea*. Hepatotoxicity has been seen after prolonged use; *Echinacea* should be used cautiously by persons taking potentially hepatotoxic drugs. One anaphylactic reaction to an *Echinacea* extract has been reported.

E. **Fish oil.** Fish oil contains large amounts of highly unsaturated fatty acids, including docosahexaenoic acid (DHA), which has six double bonds, and eicosapentaenoic acid (EPA), which has five. In these fatty acids, the last double bond is located three carbons from the end (ω-3), whereas in the polyunsaturated fatty acids from plants, the last double bond is typically located six carbons from the end (ω-6). EPA and DHA can serve as substrates for cyclooxygenase, the rate-limiting step in prostaglandin production, and for lipoxygenase, the rate-limiting step in leukotriene production. The metabolic products of EPA and DHA derived through these pathways are less biologically active than the metabolites of arachidonic acid, the more typical substrate for these enzymes. Thus, one effect of fish oil is to diminish the production of conventional eicosanoids, including thromboxane A_2, prostaglandin E_2, and leukotriene B_4. By blocking the synthesis of thromboxane A_2, fish oil inhibits platelet aggregation and so acts as an antithrombotic agent. By blocking the synthesis of prostaglandin E_2, fish oil reduces the increased blood flow and edema associated with inflammation. Finally, by reducing the synthesis of leukotriene B_4, fish oil reduces the neutrophil infiltration associated with inflammation.

1. **Claims and supporting evidence**

   a. **Beneficial effects in heart disease.** Fish oil supplementation beneficially affects persons with cardiovascular disease by at least three mechanisms. It reduces plasma triglycerides by about 30% (8) and reduces blood pressure by a small but statistically significant amount (9). Fish oil also has antithrombotic properties; it reduces platelet aggregation by decreasing thromboxane production.

   b. **Treatment of chronic inflammatory diseases, including rheumatoid arthritis and inflammatory bowel disease.** Eicosanoids have been identified as mediators of the inflammatory response in chronic inflammatory diseases, so it is not surprising that an agent that reduces eicosanoid production may be of therapeutic value in these diseases. After prolonged treatment (>3 months) with fish oil, joint tenderness and morning stiffness were decreased in patients with rheumatoid arthritis (10). Fish oil has also proved useful in the therapy of acute disease and in maintaining remission in inflammatory bowel disease (11,12).

2. **Dosing.** Fish oil is available in gelatin capsules and as liquid oil. Supplements typically contain 180 to 300 mg of EPA and 120 to 200 mg of DHA. Dosing in either cardiovascular or chronic inflammatory disease studies is 4 to 5.4 g/d (total of EPA and DHA). Most trials of fish oil in either cardiovascular or inflammatory disease lasted at least 3 months. Thus, the benefits of fish oil were largely seen when high doses were taken for a long period of time.

3. **Safety.** The FDA has declared fish oil to be GRAS (generally recognized as safe) at doses up to 3 g/d. The major toxic effect is a prolonged bleeding time secondary to inhibition of platelet aggregation. Fish oil should be used cautiously by patients who have bleeding disorders or are taking anticoagulants. Patients taking large amounts of fish oil complain that they acquire a fishy odor.

F. **γ-Linolenic acid (evening primrose oil, borage oil, black currant oil).** γ-Linolenic acid (GLA) is a fatty acid that is endogenously synthesized in humans (13,14). Linolenic acid is converted to GLA by δ-6-desaturase. GLA is also available from the diet. Evening primrose oil (8% GLA), borage oil (23% GLA), and black currant oil (15% GLA) are especially rich dietary sources. GLA can be metabolized to a biologically inactive prostaglandin (prostaglandin E_1) and to a lipoxygenase product, 15-S-hydroxy-8,11,13-eicosatrienoic acid, that blocks the synthesis of biologically active arachidonic acid metabolites. In certain disease states, including diabetes and hypercholesterolemia, the conversion of linoleic acid to GLA by δ-6-desaturase may be impaired. In addition, impaired synthesis of GLA has been associated with advanced age, alcoholism, and a variety of vitamin and mineral deficiencies. It has been suggested that supplying dietary GLA may compensate for impaired endogenous conversion of linoleic acid to GLA.

1. **Claims and supporting evidence**
    a. **Treatment of rheumatoid arthritis.** In a 24-week, double-blinded study, 37 patients with rheumatoid arthritis received placebo or GLA (1,400 mg/d) in borage oil. In the patients who received GLA, disease activity decreased during the 24 weeks, whereas in those receiving placebo, it did not change or increased (15).
    b. **Treatment of premenstrual syndrome (PMS).** It is possible that serum levels of certain fatty acids are altered in PMS. Levels of arachidonic acid and dihomo-γ-linolenic acid (DGLA), a metabolite of GLA, are decreased in PMS. However, a series of trials in which evening primrose oil was given to patients with PMS failed to reveal compelling evidence of a clinical benefit (16).

2. **Dosing.** Evening primrose oil, borage oil, and black currant oil are all available in capsules or as liquid oil. The rate of endogenous synthesis of GLA in normal humans is 250 to 1,000 mg/d. Typical dosing of GLA is 500 to 3,000 mg/d.

3. **Safety.** Drug interactions with anticonvulsants and tricyclic antidepressants may occur. Patients taking potentially hepatotoxic drugs should not use GLA.

G. **Ginkgo biloba.** Ginkgo biloba, an extract of the leaves of the ginkgo tree, is used to improve memory and increase peripheral blood flow. Ginkgo leaves contain flavonoids, sesquiterpenes, and terpenes called *ginkgolides*. Which of these is the active ingredient is unknown, although flavonoids are scavengers of free radicals and ginkgolides may be platelet-activating factor antagonists.

1. **Claims and supporting evidence**
    a. **Improves memory.** In a double-blinded, placebo-controlled study of older persons with mild to moderate memory impairment, ginkgo biloba extract (120 mg/d) improved results on some but not all tests of memory (17).
    b. **Alzheimer's disease.** In a 52-week, double-blinded, placebo-controlled trial of 309 patients with Alzheimer's disease or multi-infarct dementia, the condition of patients receiving ginkgo biloba extract (120 mg/d) stabilized on the Alzheimer Disease Assessment Scale, whereas the condition of those on placebo deteriorated (18).
    c. **Peripheral vascular disease.** In a 24-week, double-blinded, placebo-controlled trial of 111 patients with peripheral vascular disease, superior, pain-free walking and maximal walking distance were noted in those who received ginkgo biloba extract (120 mg/d) (19).

2. **Dosing.** Ginkgo biloba extract is available as a tincture, tablets, and capsules. Typical dosing is 40 to 80 mg three times a day.

3. **Safety.** Ginkgo is thought to be a platelet-activating factor antagonist and may potentiate the effects of antiplatelet drugs and anticoagulants.

H. **Ginseng.** The term **ginseng** includes American ginseng *(Panax quinquefolius)* and Asian ginseng *(P. ginseng* and *P. japonicus)*. Siberian ginseng *(Eleutherococcus senticosus)* is not a true ginseng but is promoted and sold as ginseng. *Panax* ginseng is the species most widely available in the United States and also the most widely studied. The plant part used is the root. Air-dried root is "white ginseng"; steam-treated root is "red ginseng." Saponins (ginsenosides) are thought to be the active ingredients, although their mechanism of action is unknown.

1. **Claims and supporting evidence**
   a. **Enhances exercise performance.** In a 3-week, double-blinded, placebo-controlled trial of 28 normal volunteers, exercise time, work load, plasma lactate, and hematocrit did not differ between those who received *Panax* ginseng (200 mg/d) and those who received placebo (20). A review of studies of ginseng and exercise performance concluded that compelling evidence that ginseng improves exercise performance is lacking (21).
   b. **Enhances cognitive function.** In an 8-week, double-blinded, placebo-controlled trial of 60 elderly patients, no difference in cognitive function was noted between those receiving *Panax* ginseng extract (40 mg/d) and those receiving placebo.
   c. **Enhances sexual function.** No blinded studies of the effect of ginseng on sexual function have been performed.
2. **Dosing.** The Asian, American, and Siberian forms of ginseng are available as tablets, capsules, powders, teas, and tinctures. Most commercial products contain 100 to 400 mg of extract (equivalent to 0.5 to 2.0 g of root). The levels of ginsenosides vary widely among different commercial products.
3. **Safety.** High doses of ginseng are associated with central nervous system excitation, hypertension, sleeplessness, and nervousness. Drug interactions may occur with corticosteroids, estrogens, and digitalis preparations. *Panax* ginseng produces hypoglycemic effects, perhaps by accelerating hepatic lipogenesis, and should be used cautiously in patients with diabetes.

I. L-Carnitine is a short-chain carboxylic acid formed from lysine and methionine. It serves as a carrier molecule for the transport of fatty acids across the mitochondrial membrane into the mitochondria, where they undergo oxidation. Carnitine is found primarily in skeletal and cardiac muscle, which contains large numbers of mitochondria. Humans can synthesize carnitine from lysine and methionine. The major dietary source of carnitine is meat. Carnitine is sold as L-carnitine, propionyl-L-carnitine and L-acetylcarnitine in capsules or tablets.
1. **Claims and supporting evidence**
   a. **Benefits in heart disease.** In one study, patients with angina were randomized to propionyl-L-carnitine or placebo. The incidence of angina and the consumption of nitroglycerin were not affected by carnitine (22). In another study, patients with claudication were given propionyl-L-carnitine or placebo for 6 months; a small improvement in walking distance was noted in those who received carnitine (23). This study is difficult to interpret because of a high dropout rate.
   b. **Improvements in exercise performance.** It has been suggested that carnitine may improve exercise performance by enhancing fatty acid oxidation and decreasing lactic acid production. When carnitine was given to athletes immediately before exercise, serum carnitine levels increased, but no improvements in respiratory exchange ratios, muscle lactate accumulation, plasma lactate levels, or exercise performance were noted (24,25).
2. **Dosing.** Carnitine is available in capsules or tablets as L-carnitine, propionyl-L-carnitine, and L-acetylcarnitine. Dosing is 2 to 4 g/d in two or three divided doses.
3. **Safety.** Very high doses can cause diarrhea and nausea.

J. **Ma huang *(Ephedra sinica).*** Ma huang, the dried root of the herb *E. sinica,* has been used in Chinese medicine for centuries. It contains the alkaloids ephedrine and pseudoephedrine and is used as a bronchodilator in asthma, a nasal decongestant, and an aid to weight loss. Ephedrine, which is used to treat asthma, is a sympathomimetic agent that can induce tachycardia, raise blood pressure, and cause urinary retention and restlessness. Pseudoephedrine is found in many over-the-counter cold medicines.

1. **Claims and supporting evidence**
   a. **Bronchodilation and nasal decongestion.** Ephedrine is an effective bronchodilator, and pseudoephedrine is an effective nasal decongestant. The ephedrine and pseudoephedrine in ma huang provide no advantage over the same substances in prescription drugs and over-the-counter medications. Because of the inability to quantify the alkaloid content of ma huang, both underdosing and overdosing (with toxicity) are possible; the use of prescription drugs or over-the-counter medications poses no such risks.
   b. **Weight loss.** Ephedrine, frequently in combination with caffeine, has been used in a number of weight loss programs. When ephedrine and caffeine are combined with a low-calorie diet, a marginally greater weight loss is achieved than with a low-calorie diet alone, but at the expense of a high incidence of insomnia, tremors, and dizziness (26).
2. **Dosing.** Ma huang is available as teas, tinctures, capsules, and tablets. The alkaloid content of commercial ma huang products varies from 0.3 to 56 mg. In comparison, prescription asthma medications contain 24 mg of ephedrine, and over-the-counter cold preparations contain 60 to 120 mg of pseudoephedrine.
3. **Safety.** Ma huang has been associated with stroke, myocardial infarction, and death (27). More common side effects include tremors, insomnia, and urinary retention. The risk for adverse events associated with ma huang is increased when it is given to patients with preexisting hypertension, coronary artery disease, thyroid disease, and benign prostatic hypertrophy (BPH). The FDA recommends that everyone avoid ma huang.

K. **Phytosterols (γ-oryzanol).** Plants contain sterols that are structurally similar to cholesterol but are poorly absorbed from the gastrointestinal tract. These plant sterols (which include sitosterol, sitostanol, and campesterol) are collectively called *phytosterols.* Vegetable oils contain significant levels of phytosterols. In general, vegetable oils containing large amounts of polyunsaturated fatty acids (e.g., corn oil) have more phytosterols than oils containing smaller amounts of polyunsaturated fatty acids (e.g., palm oil, coconut oil). Purification and processing can remove phytosterols from vegetable oils. γ-Oryzanol, which is prepared commercially from rice bran oil, is a mixture of ferulic acid esters of phytosterols. Sitosterol esters are available as an additive to margarine (Benacol).
   1. **Claims and supporting evidence that phytosterols lower serum cholesterol.** The evidence that phytosterols lower serum cholesterol levels is excellent (28,29). The mechanism of this effect is not definitely known, but it may be that phytosterols diminish cholesterol absorption from the intestine. The poor absorption of phytosterols from the intestine supports the suggestion that they act in the intestinal lumen to impair cholesterol absorption. No blinded studies of the effects of γ-oryzanol on serum cholesterol levels have been performed.
   2. **Dosing.** γ-Oryzanol is available in tablets and capsules in doses of 100 to 500 mg/d. Sitosterol esters are available as an additive to margarine (Benacol).
   3. **Safety issues.** None.

L. **Saw palmetto.** Saw palmetto berry is the ripe dried fruit of *Serenoa repens,* a dwarf palm tree that grows in the southern United States. Commercial preparations are extracts containing phytosterols and polysaccharides from these berries. Saw palmetto has been used to treat BPH. Some evidence indicates that it inhibits 5-α-reductase, the enzyme that converts testosterone to dihydrotestosterone, a steroid that promotes prostate growth.
   1. **Claims and supporting evidence that saw palmetto is an effective treatment for BPH.** Saw palmetto is promoted as an agent that reduces symptoms associated with BPH. A series of double-blinded, ran-

domized, placebo-controlled trials have demonstrated decreases in noc-
turia, increases in peak urine flow, and decreases in residual volume in
patients with BPH who receive saw palmetto (30). Although the evidence that saw palmetto relieves the symptoms of BPH is reasonably
good, no evidence has been found that it reduces an enlarged prostate
or prevents prostatic cancer.

2. **Dosing.** Saw palmetto, prepared as whole berries or as a lipophilic extract, is available as capsules, tablets, and tinctures. Typical dosing is
1 to 2 g of berries or 160 to 320 mg of lipophilic extract per day. A number
of commercially available formulations provide subtherapeutic doses.

3. **Safety.** A single case of hepatic toxicity has been ascribed to saw
palmetto.

M. **Soy protein and isoflavones.** Plant products with estrogen-like effects
are called *phytoestrogens.* Isoflavones, which are found primarily in soy
products, are weak estrogens. The major isoflavones in soy proteins are
genestein, daidzein, and glycetein. Because of their estrogenic effects, soy
products containing isoflavones have been used to relieve hot flashes and
other menopausal symptoms. It has been suggested that phytoestrogens relieve menopausal symptoms without causing the adverse effects seen with
hormone replacement therapy, particularly the increased risk for breast
cancer. The reasoning behind this suggestion is difficult to grasp because
only one estrogen receptor is known; if isoflavones bind to the estrogen receptor in other organs, there is no reason to believe that they do not also bind
to the estrogen receptor in breast tissue. Soy protein also lowers serum cholesterol; whether or not the effects of soy proteins on serum cholesterol are
mediated through isoflavones is not known.

1. **Claims and supporting evidence**
   a. **Relieves menopausal symptoms.** In a 12-week trial, postmenopausal women received placebo or 40 g of soy protein isolate
   containing 76 mg of isoflavones. In the women who received soy, hot
   flashes were reduced by 45%, where in those receiving placebo, they
   were reduced by 30% (31). This is clearly a large amount of soy protein, and the consumption of this amount of soy protein would require a major change in dietary habits.

   b. **Reduces serum cholesterol.** A metaanalysis evaluated the results
   of 38 controlled trials of the effects of soy protein (average intake of
   47 g/d) on serum cholesterol. Soy protein was associated with decreases in total cholesterol (9.3%), low-density-lipoprotein (LDL) cholesterol (12.9%), and triglycerides (10.5%) (32). In all these trials,
   large amounts of soy protein were consumed, amounts so large that
   major reductions of other dietary components would be needed to accommodate the increase in soy protein. The FDA allows commercial
   products containing at least 6.25g of soy protein to carry a label claim-
   ing a role for soy protein in reducing the risk for coronary artery disease when combined with a diet low in cholesterol and saturated fat.

2. **Dosing.** Soy proteins are available as soy flour, soy milk, soy protein iso-
lates, natto (fermented soy beans), tofu, and textured soy protein. These
preparations contain 1 to 10 mg of isoflavones per gram of protein. The
dosage of isoflavones used to treat menopausal symptoms is 76 mg/d or
more. Genestein supplements are also available.

3. **Safety issues.** None.

N. **St. John's wort,** the dried, above-ground parts of *Hypericum perforatum,*
has been used extensively to treat depression and as a mood elevator. Several
mechanisms of action have been proposed, including increases of serotonin
levels and monoamine oxidase activity, but little evidence is available to
support any specific mechanism.

1. **Claims and supporting evidence that St. John's wort is an effective treatment for depression.** In a double-blinded, placebo-controlled

trial, an extract of St. John's wort was superior to placebo in relieving depressive symptoms as assessed by the Hamilton Rating Scale for Depression (33). In a metaanalysis of 23 randomized, controlled trials of St. John's wort in the treatment of mild to moderate depression, it was superior to placebo (34). A more recent review came to the same conclusion (35). Three trials comparing St. John's wort with tricyclic antidepressants showed no obvious advantage of either therapy. The daily dose of St. John's wort varied greatly in these trials; some trials based the dose of St. John's wort on the content of a single component, usually hypericin, whereas other trials based the dose on the total extract. The authors of the metaanalysis suggested a comparison of different doses and different extracts of St. John's wort and comparisons with other antidepressants in defined patient groups. No evidence has been found that St. John's wort improves the mood of persons without clinical depression.

2. **Dosing.** St. John's wort is available as tablets, capsules, tinctures, powders, and teas. Typical daily dosing is 900 mg of standardized extract.

3. **Safety.** St. John's wort may induce photosensitivity; allergic reactions with hives and skin rash have occurred. Common side effects include fatigue, dyspepsia, and sleep disturbances. No evidence is available that St. John's wort can be safely combined with prescription antidepressants.

References

1. Elmer GW, Surawicz CM, McFarland LV. Biotherapeutic agents. A neglected modality for the treatment and prevention of selected intestinal and vaginal infections. *JAMA* 1996;275:870.
2. Das AK, Eitel J, Hammad T. Efficacy of new class of agents (glucosamine hydrochloride and chondroitin sulfate) in the treatment of osteoarthritis of the knee. *Abstracts of American Association of Hip and Knee Surgeons,* 8th Annual Meeting, Dallas, November 6–8, 1998.
3. McAlindon TE, LaValley MP, Gulin JP, et al. Glucosamine and chondroitin for treatment of osteoarthritis: a systematic quality assessment and metaanalysis. *JAMA* 2000;283:1469.
4. Burke LM, Pyne DB, Telford RD. Effect of oral creatine supplementation on single-effort sprint performance in elite swimmers. *Int J Sport Nutr* 1996;6:222.
5. Williams MH, Branch JD. Creatine supplementation and exercise performance: an update. *J Am Coll Nutr* 1998;17:216.
6. Burger RA, Tores AR, Warren RP, et al. *Echinacea*-induced cytokine production by human macrophages. *Int J Immunopharmacol* 1997;19:371.
7. Grimm W, Muller HH. A randomized controlled trial of the effect of fluid extract of *Echinacea purpurea* on the incidence and severity of colds and respiratory infections. *Am J Med* 1999;106:138.
8. Harris WS, Ginsberg HN, Arunakul N, et al. Safety and efficacy of Omacor in severe hypertriglyceridemia. *J Cardiovasc Risk* 1997;4:385.
9. Morris MC, Sacks F, Rosner B. Does fish oil lower blood pressure? A metaanalysis of controlled trials. *Circulation* 1993;88:523.
10. Fortin PR, Lew RA, Liang MH, et al. Validation of a metaanalysis: the effects of fish oil in rheumatoid arthritis. *J Clin Epidemiol* 1995;48:1379.
11. Stenson WF, Cort D, Rodgers J, et al. Dietary supplementation with fish oil in ulcerative colitis. *Ann Intern Med* 1992;116:609.
12. Belluzzi A, Brignola C, Campieri M, et al. Effect of an enteric-coated fish-oil preparation on relapse in Crohn's disease. *N Engl J Med* 1996;334:1557.
13. Fan YY, Chapkin RS. Importance of dietary gamma-linolenic acid in human health and nutrition. *J Nutr* 1998;128:1411.
14. Horrobin DF. Nutritional and medical importance of gamma-linolenic acid. *Prog Lipid Res* 1992;31:163.
15. Leventhal LJ, Boyce EG, Surier RB. Treatment of rheumatoid arthritis with gamma-linolenic acid. *Ann Intern Med* 1993;119:867.
16. Budeiri D, Li Wan Po A, Dornan JC. Is evening primrose oil of value in the treatment of premenstrual syndrome? *Control Clin Trials* 1996;17:60.

17. Rai GS, Shovlin C, Wesnes KA. A double-blinded, placebo-controlled study of Ginkgo biloba extract ("tanakan") in elderly outpatients with mild to moderate memory impairment. *Curr Med Res Opin* 1991;12:350.
18. Le Bars PL, Katz MM, Berman N, et al. A placebo-controlled, double-blinded, randomized trial of an extract of Ginkgo biloba for dementia. *JAMA* 1997;278:1327.
19. Peters H, Kieser M, Holscher U. Demonstration of the efficacy of Ginkgo biloba special extract EGb 761 on intermittent claudication—a placebo-controlled, double-blinded multicenter trial. *Vasa* 1998;27:106.
20. Allen JD, McLung J, Nelson AG, et al. Ginseng supplementation does not enhance healthy young adults' peak aerobic exercise performance. *J Am Coll Nutr* 1998; 17:462.
21. Bahrke MS, Morgan WP. Evaluation of the ergogenic properties of ginseng. *Sports Med* 1994;18:229.
22. Bartels GL, Remme WJ, den Hartog RF, et al. Additional antiischemic effects of long-term L-propionylcarnitine in anginal patients treated with conventional antianginal therapy. *Cardiovasc Drugs Ther* 1995;9:749.
23. Brevetti G, Perna S, Sabba C, et al. Effect of propionyl-L-carnitine on quality of life in intermittent claudication. *Am J Cardiol* 1977;79:777.
24. Colombani P, Wenk C, Kunz I, et al. Effects of L-carnitine supplementation on physical performance and energy metabolism of endurance-trained athletes: a double-blinded crossover field study. *Eur J Appl Physiol* 1996;73:434.
25. Brass EP, Hoppel CL, Hiatt WR. Effect of intravenous L-carnitine on carnitine homeostasis and fuel metabolism during exercise in humans. *Clin Pharmacol Ther* 1994;55:681.
26. Astrup A, Breum L, Toubro S, et al. The effect and safety of an ephedrine/caffeine compound compared to ephedrine, caffeine, and placebo in obese subjects on an energy-restricted diet. A double-blinded trial. *Int J Obes Relat Metab Disord* 1992; 16:269.
27. Haller CA, Benowitz NL. Adverse cardiovascular and central nervous system events associated with dietary supplements containing ephedra alkaloids. *N Engl J Med* 2000;343:1833.
28. Yoshino G, Kazumi T, Amano M, et al. Effects of gamma-oryzanol and probucol on hyperlipidemia. *Curr Ther Res* 1989;45:975.
29. Rong N, Ausman LM, Nicolosi RJ. Oryzanol decreases cholesterol absorption and aortic fatty streaks in hamsters. *Lipids* 1997;32:303.
30. Wilt TJ, Ishani A, Stark G, et al. Saw palmetto extracts for treatment of benign prostatic hyperplasia: a systematic review. *JAMA* 1998;280:1604.
31. Albertazzi P, Pansini F, Bonaccorsi G, et al. The effect of dietary soy supplementation on hot flushes. *Obstet Gynecol* 1998;91:6.
32. Anderson JW, Johnstone BM, Cook-Newell ME. Meta-analysis of the effects of soy protein intake on serum lipids. *N Engl J Med* 1995;333:276.
33. Laakmann G, Schule C, Baghai T, et al. St. John's wort in mild to moderate depression: the relevance of hyperforin for the clinical efficacy. *Pharmacopsychiatry* 1998;31[Suppl 1]:54.
34. Linde K, Ramirez G, Mulrow CD, et al. St. John's wort for depression—an overview and metaanalysis of randomized clinical trials. *BMJ* 1996;313:253.
35. Gaster B, Holroyd J. St. John's wort for depression: a systematic review. *Arch Intern Med* 2000; 160:152.

APPENDIXES

Appendix A. FACTS AND FORMULAS COMMONLY USED IN NUTRITIONAL THERAPEUTICS

Caloric Value of Macronutrients

1 g dietary fat = 9 kcal
1 g carbohydrate = 4 kcal
1 g protein = 4 kcal
1 g ethanol = 7 kcal
1 g medium-chain triglycerides = ~8 kcal
1 g IV dextrose monohydrate = 3.4 kcal
1 mL 10% fat emulsion = 1.1 kcal
Caloric value of alcohol-containing beverage:

$$0.8 \times \frac{\text{Proof of Beverage}}{2} \times \text{Volume of Beverage (dL)} = \text{Weight of Alcohol (g)} \times 7 = \text{kcal}$$

Estimation of Nitrogen Content in Dietary Protein

$$\text{Nitrogen (g)} = \frac{\text{Protein (g)}}{6.25}$$

Estimation of Basal (Resting) Energy Needs (kcal/d)

Harris–Benedict method for calculating basal metabolic rate

BMR (women) $= 665 + (9.6 \times W) + (1.8 \times H) - (4.7 \times A)$

BMR (men) $= 66 + (13.7 \times W) + (5 \times H) - (6.8 \times A)$

where W = weight (kg)
H = height (cm)
A = age (y)

World Health Organization/Food and Agriculture Organization of the United Nations equations for estimating resting energy expenditure

Age (y)	Male	Female
0–3	$(60.9 \times W^a) - 54$	$(61.0 \times W) - 51$
3–10	$(22.7 \times W) - 495$	$(22.5 \times W) + 499$
10–18	$(17.5 \times W) + 651$	$(12.2 \times W) + 746$
18–30	$(15.3 \times W) + 679$	$(14.7 \times W) + 996$
30–60	$(11.6 \times W) + 879$	$(8.7 \times W) + 829$
>60	$(13.5 \times W) + 987$	$(10.5 \times W) + 596$

[a] Weight in kilograms.

Estimate of energy requirements for patients based on body mass index[a]

| | Energy requirements (kcal/kg per day) | |
BMI (kg/m^2)	Critically ill patients (RMR)	Other patients (RMR + TEF + TEA)
<15	35–40	35–40 + 20%
15–19	30–35	30–35 + 20%
20–29	20–25	20–25 + 20%
≥30	15–20[b]	15–20

[a] Use the Harris–Benedict or World Health Organization equation to estimate the requirement for patients whose estimate by this method is less than 1,200 kcal/d.
[b] Do not exceed 2,000 kcal/d.
RMR, resting metabolic rate; TEF, thermal energy of food; TEA, thermal energy of activity.

Estimation of Recommended Daily Protein Intake

Clinical condition	Protein requirements (g/kg IBW/d)*
Normal	0.75
Metabolic "stress/illness/injury"	
Mild/moderate	1.0–1.25
Moderate/severe	1.25–1.5
Severe with extra losses (e.g., skin, urine)	1.5–*
Renal failure, acute (undialyzed)	0.8–1.0
Hemodialysis	1.2–1.4
Peritoneal dialysis	1.3–1.5
Hepatic encephalopathy	0.4–0.6

IBW, ideal body weight.

* Upper limit determined from measured losses.

Estimation of Ideal Body Weight for Adults

Woman with medium frame: 120 lb for first 5 ft of height + 3 lb/in.
Man with medium frame: 130 lb for first 5 ft of height + 3 lb/in.
Small frame: Subtract 10 lb from above.
Large frame: Add 10 lb to above.

Approximate Calorie Equivalent of 1 lb of Body Weight

1 lb = 3,400 kcal

Body Mass Index

$BMI = W \text{ (kg)}/H^2 \text{ (m)}$, or $= W \text{ (lb)}/H^2 \text{ (in)} \times 703$

Conversion Factors for Major Minerals

1 mEq Na = 1 mmol Na = 23 mg Na
1 g Na = 43 mEq Na = 43 mmol Na
1 mEq K = 1 mmol K = 39 mg K
1 g K = 26 mEq K = 26 mmol K
1 mEq Ca = 0.5 mmol Ca = 20 mg Ca
1 g Ca = 50 mEq Ca = 25 mmol Ca
1 mEq Mg = 0.5 mmol Mg = 12 mg Mg
1 g Mg = 82 mEq Mg = 41 mmol Mg
1 mmol P = 2 mEq HPO_3 = 31 mg P
1 mEq Cl = 1 mmol Cl = 35 mg Cl
1 g Cl = 29 mEq Cl = 29 mmol Cl

Major Mineral Content in Various Compounds and Solutions

1 g NaCl = 393 mg Na = 17 mEq Na
1 g $NaHCO_3$ = 273 mg Na = 12 mEq Na
1,000 mL saline solution = 9 g NaCl = 3.5 g Na = 154 mEq Na
1,000 mL lactated Ringer's solution = 3 g Na = 130 mEq Na
1 ampule (50 mL) 7.5% $NaHCO_3$ = 1 g Na = 44 mEq Na
1 g KCl = 524 mg K = 13 mEq K
1 g $CaCl_2$-$2H_2O^a$ = 273 mg Ca = 13.6 mEq Ca
1 g calcium gluconate[b] = 93 mg Ca = 4.6 mEq Ca
1g $MgSO_4$-$7H_2O^a$ = 99 mg Mg = 8.1 mEq Mg
1 g Mg gluconate-$2H_2O^a$ = 54 mg Mg = 4.4 mEq Mg
1 g $CaCO_3$ = 400 mg Ca = 20 mEq Ca
1 g $FeSO_4$-$7H_2O^a$ = 201 mg Fe
1 g Fe gluconate-$2H_2O^a$ = 116 mg Fe
1 mL Fe dextran = 50 mg Fe

[a] When weighed in hydrated forms, as indicated.
[b] Small amounts of calcium D-saccharate may be added for stabilization and contribute to the total calcium content.

Liquid Measure Equivalents: Volume

Apothecary	Metric	Household
1 fluid gram	4 milliliters (mL)	1 teaspoon (tsp)
½ fluid ounce (oz)	15 mL	1 tablespoon (tbs) (3 tsp)
1 oz	30 mL	2 tbs (⅛ cup)
4 oz	118 mL	8 tbs (½ cup)
8 oz	237 mL	16 tbs (1 cup)
16 oz	473 mL	1 pint (pt)
32 oz	947 mL	1 quart (qt) (2 pt)
128 oz	3,785 mL	1 gallon (gal) (4 qt)

Appendix B. RECOMMENDED DIETARY ALLOWANCES

The National Academy of Sciences will release new data on macronutrients in late 2001. Please consult the NAS web site (www.nas.edu) for further information.

Table B-1. Dietary reference intakes: recommended intakes for individuals

Life stage group	Calcium (mg/d)	Phosphorus (mg/d)	Magnesium (mg/d)	Vitamin D (μg/d)[a,b]	Fluoride (mg/d)	Thiamine (mg/d)
Infants						
0–6 mo	210*[1]	100*	30*	5*	0.01*	0.2*
7–12 mo	270*	275*	75*	5*	0.5*	0.3*
Children						
1–3 y	500*	**460**	**80**	5*	0.7*	0.5
4–8 y	800*	**500**	**130**	5*	1*	0.6
Males						
9–13 y	1,300*	**1,250**	**240**	5*	2*	**0.9**
14–18 y	1,300*	**1,250**	**410**	5*	3*	**1.2**
19–30 y	1,000*	**700**	**400**	5*	4*	**1.2**
31–50 y	1,000*	**700**	**420**	5*	4*	**1.2**
51–70 y	1,200*	**700**	**420**	10*	4*	**1.2**
>70 y	1,200*	**700**	**420**	15*	4*	**1.2**
Females						
9–13 y	1,300*	**1,250**	**240**	5*	2*	**0.9**
14–18 y	1,300*	**1,250**	**360**	5*	3*	**1.0**
19–30 y	1,000*	**700**	**310**	5*	3*	**1.1**
31–50 y	1,000*	**700**	**320**	5*	3*	**1.1**
51–70 y	1,200*	**700**	**320**	10*	3*	**1.1**
>70 y	1,200*	**700**	**320**	15*	3*	**1.1**
Pregnancy						
≤18 y	1,300*	**1,250**	**400**	5*	3*	**1.4**
19–30 y	1,000*	**700**	**350**	5*	3*	**1.4**
31–50 y	1,000*	**700**	**360**	5*	3*	**1.4**
Lactation						
≤18 y	1,300*	**1,250**	**360**	5*	3*	**1.4**
19–30 y	1,000*	**700**	**310**	5*	3*	**1.4**
31–50 y	1,000*	**700**	**320**	5*	3*	**1.4**

Riboflavin (mg/d)	Niacin (mg/d)[c]	Vitamin B6 (mg/d)	Folate (μg/d)[d]	Vitamin B12 (μg/d)	Pantothenic acid (mg/d)	Biotin (μg/d)
0.3*	2*	0.1*	65*	0.4*	1.7*	5*
0.4*	4*	0.3*	80*	0.05*	1.8*	6*
0.5	6	0.5	150	0.9	2*	8*
0.6	8	0.6	200	1.2	3*	12*
0.9	12	1.0	300	1.8	4*	20*
1.3	16	1.3	400	2.4	5*	25*
1.3	16	1.3	400	2.4	5*	30*
1.3	16	1.3	400	2.4	5*	30*
1.3	16	1.7	400	2.4[g]	5*	30*
1.3	16	1.7	400	2.4[g]	5*	30*
0.9	12	1.0	300	1.8	4*	20*
1.0	14	1.2	400[h]	2.4	5*	25*
1.1	14	1.3	400[h]	2.4	5*	30*
1.1	14	1.3	400[h]	2.4	5*	30*
1.1	14	1.5	400	2.4[g]	5*	30*
1.1	14	1.5	400	2.4	5*	30*
1.4	18	1.9	600[i]	2.6	6*	30*
1.4	18	1.9	600[i]	2.6	6*	30*
1.4	18	1.9	600[i]	2.6	6*	30*
1.6	17	2.0	500	2.8	7*	35*
1.6	17	2.0	500	2.8	7*	35*
1.6	17	2.0	500	2.8	7*	35*

continued

Table B-1. (*Continued*)

Life stage group	Choline[e] (mg/d)	Vitamin C (mg/d)	Vitamin E[f](mg/d)	Selenium (µg/d)	Vitamin A (µg/d)[j]	Vitamin K (µg/d)
Infants						
0–6 mo	125*	40*	4*	15*	**400**	2.0
7–12 mo	150*	50*	6*	20*	**500**	2.5
Children						
1–3 y	200*	**15**	**6**	**20**	**300**	30
4–8 y	250*	**25**	**7**	**30**	**400**	50
Males						
9–13 y	375*	**45**	**11**	**40**	**600**	60
14–18 y	550*	**75**	**15**	**55**	**900**	75
19–30 y	550*	**90**	**15**	**55**	**900**	120
31–50 y	550*	**90**	**15**	**55**	**900**	120
51–70 y	550*	**90**	**15**	**55**	**900**	120
>70 y	550*	**90**	**15**	**55**	**900**	120
Females						
9–13 y	375*	**45**	**11**	**40**	**600**	60
14–18 y	400*	**65**	**15**	**55**	**700**	75
19–30 y	425*	**75**	**15**	**55**	**700**	90
31–50 y	425*	**75**	**15**	**55**	**700**	90
51–70 y	425*	**75**	**15**	**55**	**700**	90
>70 y	425*	**75**	**15**	**55**	**700**	90
Pregnancy						
≤18 y	450*	**80**	**15**	**60**	**750**	75
19–30 y	450*	**85**	**15**	**60**	**770**	90
31–50 y	450*	**85**	**15**	**60**	**770**	90
Lactation						
≤18 y	550*	**115**	**19**	**70**	**1,200**	75
19–30 y	550*	**120**	**19**	**70**	**1,300**	90
31–50 y	550*	**120**	**19**	**70**	**1,300**	90

[1] This table presents recommended dietary allowances (RDAs) in bold type and adequate intakes (AIs) in ordinary type followed by an asterisk (*). RDAs and AIs may both be used as goals for individual intake. RDAs are set to meet the needs of almost all (97–98%) individuals in a group. For healthy breast-fed infants, the AI is the mean intake. The AIs for other life-stage and gender groups are believed to cover the needs of all individuals in the group, but lack of data or uncertain data make it impossible to specify with confidence the percentage of individuals covered by these intakes.
[a] As cholecalciferol. 1 µg cholecalciferol = 40 IU vitamin D.
[b] In the absence of adequate exposure to light
[c] As niacin equivalents (NE). 1 mg niacin = 60 mg tryptophan; 0–6 mo = preformed niacin (not NE).
[d] As dietary folate equivalents (DFE). 1 DFE = 1 µg food folate = 0.6 µg of folic acid from fortified food or as a supplement consumed with food = 0.5 µg of a supplement taken on an empty stomach.
[e] Although AIs have been set for choline, few data have assessed whether a dietary supply of choline is needed at all stages of the life cycle, and it may be that the choline requirement can be met by endogenous synthesis at some of these stages.
[f] As α-tocopherol. α-Tocopherol includes *RRR*-α-tocopherol, the only form of α-tocopherol that occurs naturally in foods, and the *2R*-stereoisomeric forms of α-tocopherol (*RRR*-, *RSR*-, *RRS*- and

Chromium (μg/d)	Copper (μg/d)	Iodine (μg/d)	Iron (mg/d)	Manganese (mg/d)	Molybdenum (μg/d)	Zinc (mg/d)
0.2	**200**	110	**0.27**	0.003	**2**	**2**
5.5	**200**	130	**11**	0.6	**3**	**3**
11	**340**	90	**7**	1.2	**17**	**3**
15	**440**	90	**10**	1.5	**22**	**5**
25	**700**	120	**8**	1.9	**34**	**8**
35	**890**	150	**11**	2.2	**43**	**11**
35	**900**	150	**8**	2.3	**45**	**11**
35	**900**	150	**8**	2.3	**45**	**11**
30	**900**	150	**8**	2.3	**45**	**11**
30	**900**	150	**8**	2.3	**45**	**11**
21	**700**	120	**8**	1.6	**34**	**8**
24	**890**	150	**15**	1.6	**43**	**9**
25	**900**	150	**18**	1.8	**45**	**8**
25	**900**	150	**18**	1.8	**45**	**8**
20	**900**	150	**8**	1.8	**45**	**8**
20	**900**	150	**8**	1.8	**45**	**8**
29	**1,000**	220	**27**	2	**50**	**13**
30	**1,000**	220	**27**	2	**50**	**11**
30	**1,000**	220	**27**	2	**50**	**11**
44	**1,300**	290	**10**	2.6	**50**	**14**
45	**1,300**	290	**9**	2.6	**50**	**12**
45	**1,300**	290	**9**	2.6	**50**	**12**

RSS-α-tocopherol) that occur in fortified foods and supplements. It does not include the 2S-stereoisomeric forms of α-tocopherol (SRR-, SSR-, SRS-, and SSS-α-tocopherol), also found in fortified foods and supplements.

[g] Because 10–30% of older people may poorly absorb food-bound vitamin B_{12}, it is advisable for those older than 50 years to meet their RDA mainly by consuming foods fortified with vitamin B_{12} or a supplement containing vitamin B_{12}.

[h] In view of evidence linking folate intake with neural-tube defects in the fetus, it is recommended that all women capable of becoming pregnant consume 400 μg from supplements or fortified foods in addition to intake of food folate from a varied diet.

[i] It is assumed that women will continue consuming 400 μg from supplements or fortified food until their pregnancy is confirmed and they enter prenatal care, which ordinarily occurs after the end of the periconceptional period—the critical time for formation of the neural tube.

[j] As retinol activity equivalents (RAE). 1 RAE = 1 μg all-trans-retinol, 12 μg β-carotene, 24 μg α-carotene, or 24 μg β-cryptoxanthin.

From the National Academy of Sciences. Reprinted courtesy of the National Academy Press, Washington, DC, 2000.

Table B-2. Recommended dietary allowances[a] for protein and energy, revised 1989 (abridged)[1]

Category	Age (y) or condition	Weight[b] (kg)	Weight[b] (lb)	Height[b] (cm)	Height[b] (in)	Protein (g)	Resting energy expenditure (kcal/d)[d]	Average daily energy allowance (kcal)[c] Per kg	Average daily energy allowance (kcal)[c] Per day[d]
Infants	0.0–0.5	6	13	60	24	13	320	108	650
	0.5–1.0	9	20	71	28	14	500	98	850
Children	1–3	13	29	90	35	16	740	102	1,300
	4–6	20	44	112	44	24	950	90	1,800
	7–10	28	62	132	52	28	1,130	70	2,000
Males	11–14	45	99	157	62	45	1,440	55	2,500
	15–18	66	145	176	69	59	1,760	45	3,000
	19–24	72	160	177	70	58	1,780	40	2,900
	25–50	79	174	176	70	63	1,800	37	2,900
	51+	77	170	173	68	63	1,530	30	2,300

Females								
11–14	46	101	157	62	46	1,310	47	2,200
15–18	55	120	163	64	44	1,370	40	2,200
19–24	58	128	164	65	46	1,350	38	2,200
25–50	63	138	163	64	50	1,380	36	2,200
51+	65	143	160	63	50	1,280	30	1,900
Pregnant					60			+300
Lactating 1st 6 months					65			+500
Lactating 2nd 6 months					62			+500

[1] This table does not include nutrients for which dietary reference intakes have recently been established. See *Dietary reference intakes for calcium, phosphorus, magnesium, vitamin D, and fluoride* (1997); *Dietary reference intakes for thiamine, riboflavin, niacin, vitamin B6, folate, vitamin B12 pantothenic acid, biotin, and choline* (1998); *Dietary reference intakes for vitamin C, vitamin E, selenium, and carotenoids* (2000); and *Dietary reference intakes for vitamin A, vitamin K, arsenic, boron, chromium, copper, iodine, iron, manganese, molybdenum, nickel, silicon, vanadium, and zinc* (2001).

[a] The allowances, expressed as average daily intakes over time, are intended to provide for individual variations among most normal persons as they live in the United States under usual environmental stresses. Diets should be based on a variety of common foods to provide other nutrients for which human requirements have been less well defined.

[b] Weights and heights of reference adults are actual medians for the U.S. population of the designated age, as reported by NHANES II. The median weights and heights of those under 19 years of age were taken from Hamill PPV, Drizd TA, Johnson RB, et al. Physical growth: National Center for Health Statistics Percentiles. *Am J Clin Nutr* 1979;321:607. The use of these figures does not imply that the height-to-weight ratios are ideal.

[c] In the range of light to moderate activity, the coefficient of variation is ±20%.

[d] Figures are rounded.

From the National Academy of Sciences. Reprinted courtesy of the National Academy Press, Washington, DC, 2000.

Table B-3. Dietary reference intakes: tolerable upper intake levels[a]

Life stage group	Calcium (g/d)	Phosphorus (g/d)	Magnesium (mg/d)[b]	Vitamin D (µg/d)	Fluoride (mg/d)	Niacin (mg/d)[c]
Infants						
0–6 mo	ND[e]	ND	ND	25	0.7	ND
7–12 mo	ND	ND	ND	25	0.9	ND
Children						
1–3 y	2.5	3	65	50	1.3	10
4–8 y	2.5	3	110	50	2.2	15
Males, females						
9–13 y	2.5	4	350	50	10	20
14–18 y	2.5	4	350	50	10	30
19–70 y	2.5	4	350	50	10	35
>70 y	2.5	3	350	50	10	35
Pregnancy						
≤18 y	2.5	3.5	350	50	10	30
19–50 y	2.5	3.5	350	50	10	35
Lactation						
≤18 y	2.5	4	350	50	10	30
19–50 y	2.5	4	350	50	10	35

Vitamin B_6 (mg/d)	Folate (μg/d)[c]	Choline (mg/d)	Vitamin C (mg/d)	Vitamin E (mg/d)[d]	Selenium (μg/d)	Vitamin A (μg/d)
ND	ND	ND	ND	ND	45	600
ND	ND	ND	ND	ND	60	600
30	300	1.0	400	200	90	600
40	400	1.0	650	300	150	900
60	600	2.0	1,200	600	280	1,700
80	800	3.0	1,800	800	400	2,800
100	1,000	3.5	2,000	1,000	400	3,000
100	1,000	3.5	2,000	1,000	400	3,000
80	800	3.0	1,800	800	400	2,800
100	1,000	3.5	2,000	1,000	400	3,000
80	800	3.0	1,800	800	400	2,800
100	1,000	3.5	2,000	1,000	400	3,000

continued

Table B-3. (*Continued*)

Life stage group	Copper (μg/d)	Iodine (μg/d)	Iron (mg/d)	Manganese (mg/d)	Molybdenum (μg/d)	Zinc (mg/d)
Infants						
0–6 mo			40			4
7–12 mo			40			5
Children						
1–3 y	1,000	200	40	2	300	7
4–8 y	3,000	300	40	3	600	12
Males, females						
9–13 y	5,000	600	40	6	1,100	23
14–18 y	8,000	900	45	9	1,700	34
19–70 y	10,000	1,100	45	11	2,000	40
>70 y	10,000	1,100	45	11	2,000	40
Pregnancy						
≤18 y	8,000	900	45	9	1,700	34
19–50 y	10,000	1,100	45	11	2,000	40
Lactation						
≤18 y	8,000	900	45	9	1,700	34
19–50 y	10,000	1,100	45	11	2,000	40

ND, not determined because of lack of data for adverse effects in this age group and concern with regard to lack of ability to handle excess amounts. Source of intake should be food only to prevent high levels of intake.

[a] The tolerable upper intake level (UL) is the maximum level of daily nutrient intake that is likely to pose no risk of adverse effects. Unless otherwise specified, the UL represents total intake from food, water, and supplements. Because of a lack of suitable data, ULs could not be established for thiamine, riboflavin, vitamin B_{12}, pantothenic acid, or biotin. In the absence of ULs, extra caution may be warranted in consuming levels above recommended intakes.

[b] The ULs for magnesium represent intake from a pharmacologic agent only and do not include intake from food and water.

[c] The ULs for niacin and folate apply to synthetic forms obtained from supplements, fortified foods, or a combination of these.

[d] As α-tocopherol; applies to any form of supplemental α-tocopherol.

From the National Academy of Sciences. Reprinted courtesy of the National Academy Press, Washington, DC, 2000 and 2001.

I. **New regulations.** Both the Food and Drug Administration (FDA) and the U.S. Department of Agriculture Food Safety and Inspection Service (FSIS) have established regulations for food labeling (*Code of Federal Regulations*; Title 21, Vol. 2, Parts 100 to 169, 4/1/99). The FDA rules comply with the provisions of the Nutrition Labeling and Education Act of 1990, and the FSIS rules are coordinated with the FDA rules. The FDA rules became effective May 8, 1994, and apply to most processed foods. Nutritional information is also available for fresh fruits and vegetables and raw fish at the point of purchase. The FSIS rules became effective July 6, 1994, and apply to meat and poultry products.

II. **Nutrition panel.** The new food label has a revised nutrition panel that is now headed "Nutrition Facts." A new set of dietary components appears on the nutrition panel (Table C-1). These mandatory and voluntary components are the only ones allowed on the nutrition label and must be presented in the order given. "Voluntary" nutrients can be included if the manufacturer chooses; however, if a claim is made about them, or if a food is fortified or enriched with them, then they must be listed. This list of nutrients has been chosen because it reflects health concerns in the population. Nutrients are listed in the order of priority of current dietary recommendations. Thiamine, riboflavin, and niacin, which were required elements on the old nutrition label, are not required on the new nutrition label because they are no longer considered to be of public health significance; however, they can be listed voluntarily.

Data for each of the nutrients must be presented as grams (or milligrams) per serving and as percentage of daily value (Fig. C-1). Daily values are a new way of presenting nutritional information. Percentage of daily value expresses the amount of a nutrient in a serving of a particular food as a percentage of the amount of the nutrient that would be consumed in a 2,000-cal balanced diet. Daily values are based on two sets of new dietary standards, daily reference values (DRVs) and reference daily intakes (RDIs); however, only the term *daily value* appears on the label. DRVs have been established for fat, carbohydrate, protein, cholesterol, sodium, and potassium. DRVs for the energy-producing nutrients (fat, carbohydrates, and protein) are based on the number of calories consumed per day. The daily values that appear at the top of the nutrition label are based on a 2,000-cal diet. Adjustments for other caloric intakes are included at the bottom of the label.

A. The DRVs for macronutrients are calculated as follows:

1. Fat is based on 30% of calories.
2. Saturated fat is based on 10% of calories.
3. Carbohydrates are based on 60% of calories.
4. Protein is based on 10% of calories.
5. Fiber is based on 11.5 g/1,000 cal.

B. The DRVs for some nutrients represent the upper limits of the desirable range based on public health recommendations:

1. Total fat should be less than 65 g.
2. Saturated fat should be less than 20 g.
3. Cholesterol should be less than 300 mg.
4. Sodium should be less than 2,400 mg.

C. The RDIs are reference values for vitamins and minerals; *RDI* replaces the term *U.S. recommended dietary allowance (RDA)*. The values for the RDIs are the same as those for the old U.S. RDAs. The required data for vitamin A, vitamin C, calcium, and iron are presented as a percentage of the RDI. Voluntary data for other vitamins and minerals are presented in the same way.

Daily values may be confusing for consumers because some of the data, such as those for vitamin A, vitamin C, iron, and calcium, are presented as a percentage of the smallest desirable daily intake, whereas other data, such

Table C-1. **Mandatory** and voluntary dietary components of the nutrition panel

---

Total calories
Calories from fat
Calories from saturated fat
Total fat
Saturated fat
Polyunsaturated fat
Monounsaturated fat
Cholesterol
Sodium
Potassium
Total carbohydrate
Dietary fiber
Soluble fiber
Insoluble fiber
Sugars
Sugar alcohol (e.g., the sugar substitutes xylitol, mannitol, and sorbitol)
Other carbohydrates (difference between total carbohydrate and the sum of dietary
   fiber, sugars, and sugar alcohol if declared)
Protein
Vitamin A
Vitamin C
Calcium
Iron
Other essential vitamins and minerals

---

as those for fat, cholesterol, and sodium, are presented as a percentage of the maximum recommended daily allowance. Thus, consumers may misinterpret the labels as indicating that at least 300 mg of cholesterol and at least 2,400 mg of sodium should be consumed, rather than no more than 300 mg of cholesterol and no more than 2,400 mg of sodium.

All the data in the new nutrition label are presented in relation to a defined serving size (which is presented in both household and metric measures); the same serving sizes must be used by all manufacturers. Under the old regulations, serving sizes were defined by the food manufacturer; under the new regulations, the serving sizes are defined by the FDA and represent amounts that people actually consume.

  III. **Nutrient content descriptors.** The new regulations define terms that may be used to describe the level of a nutrient in a food.

    A. Free. The term *free* means that a product does not contain the nutrient, or contains only a trivial or "physiologically inconsequential" amount. *Calorie-free* means less than 5 cal per serving. *Sugar-free* and *fat-free* both mean less than 0.5 g per serving.

    B. Low. The general definition for *low* is that it is possible to consume a food low in a nutrient frequently during the course of a day without exceeding the dietary guidelines.

      1. *Low in fat* means 3 g or less per serving.

      2. *Low in saturated fat* means 1 g or less per serving.

      3. *Low in sodium* means less than 140 mg per serving.

      4. *Very low in sodium* means less than 35 mg per serving.

      5. *Low in cholesterol* means less than 20 mg per serving.

      6. *Low in calories* means 40 cal or less per serving.

2% MILKFAT LOWFAT MILK

Nutrition Facts
Serving Size 1 cup (236 mL)
Servings Per Container 16

Amount Per Serving

Calories 130 Calories from Fat 45

	% Daily Value*
Total Fat 5g	**8%**
Saturated Fat 3g	**15%**
Cholesterol 20mg	**7%**
Sodium 125mg	**5%**
Total Carbohydrate 13g	**4%**
Dietary Fiber 0g	**0%**
Sugars 12g	
Protein 8g	**17%**

Vitamin A 10% • Vitamin C 4%

Calcium 30% • Iron 0% • Vitamin D 25%

* Percent Daily Values are based on a 2,000 calorie diet. Your daily values may be higher or lower depending on your calorie needs:

	Calories:	2,000	2,500
Total Fat	Less than	65g	80g
Sat Fat	Less than	20g	25g
Cholesterol	Less than	300mg	300mg
Sodium	Less than	2,400mg	2,400mg
Total Carbohydrate		300g	375g
Dietary Fiber		25g	30g
Protein		50g	65g

INGREDIENTS: GRADE A LOWFAT MILK, VITAMIN A PALMITATE AND VITAMIN D3 ADDED.

1 GALLON (3.78 L)

FIG. C.1. Representative nutrition panel.

C. **Lean and extralean.** These terms are used to describe meats, poultry, and seafood. *Lean* means less than 10 g of fat, less than 4 g of saturated fat, and less than 95 mg of cholesterol per serving and per 100 g. *Extralean* means less than 5 g of fat, less than 2 g of saturated fat, and less than 95 mg of cholesterol per serving and per 100 g.

D. **High.** *High* means that a single serving of a food contains 20% or more of the daily value for a particular nutrient.

E. **Good source.** The term *good source* means that one serving of a food contains 10% to 19% of the daily value for a particular nutrient.

F. **Reduced.** The term *reduced* means that a nutritionally altered product contains 25% less of a nutrient or 25% fewer calories than the regular (unaltered) product. A claim that a product is *reduced* cannot be made if the reference food already meets the requirements for a *low* claim.

G. **Less.** The term *less* means that a food contains 25% less of a nutrient or 25% fewer calories than the reference food. Pretzels with 25% less fat than potato chips can carry the *less* claim.

H. **Light.** The term *light* can mean that an altered product contains one-third fewer calories or half the fat of the reference item. If more than 50% of the calories in a food are derived from fat, then the fat must be reduced by 50% if the food is to qualify for a *light* claim. *Light* can also mean that the sodium content of a low-calorie, low-fat food has been reduced by 50%. A claim of *light in sodium* may be used on foods in which the sodium content has been reduced by 50%. The term *light* also can be applied to color and texture, in such terms as *light brown sugar,* as long as the meaning is clear.

  I. More. The term *more* means that the quantity of a nutrient in a serving of food is at least 10% greater than the daily value of the reference food. The terms *enriched, fortified* and *added* also can be used if the quantity of a nutrient is at least 10% greater than the daily value of the reference food, and in this case, the food must be altered.

  J. Percentage fat-free. To qualify for this claim, a product must meet the definition for *low in fat* or *fat-free.* In addition, the value for *percentage fat-free* must reflect the amount of fat in 100 g of the food. Thus, if a claim is to be made that a food is *95% fat-free,* 100 g of the food must contain no more than 5 g of fat.

  K. Implied. Claims cannot be made when they wrongfully imply that a food contains or does not contain a meaningful level of a nutrient. Thus, one cannot claim that a food is "made with oat bran," implying that the food is a good source of fiber, unless the product contains enough oat bran to meet the definition for a *good source* of fiber.

  L. Meals and main dishes. Claims for the amount of sodium or cholesterol in a meal or main dish must meet the same requirements as those for individual foods. Some other definitions are more relaxed; *low-calorie,* when applied to a meal or main dish, means that the meal or main dish contains no more than 120 cal/100 g.

  M. Healthy. The term *healthy* can be used to describe a food that is low in fat and saturated fat and that contains no more than 480 mg of sodium and no more than 60 mg of cholesterol per serving.

  N. Fresh. When the term *fresh* is used to suggest that a food is raw or unprocessed, it can be used only to refer to a food that has never been frozen or heated and that contains no preservatives (irradiation at low levels is allowed). The term *fresh frozen* can be used for foods that are quickly frozen while still fresh. Brief scalding before freezing (blanching) is allowed.

IV. Health claims. The FDA allows health claims for relationships between several nutrients and risk for a particular disease. The claims for the food product must meet the requirements for authorized health claims. They cannot state the degree of risk reduction and must use the word *may* or *might* in discussing the relationship between the nutrient and the disease. The claims also must phrase the relationship between the nutrient and the disease in a way that the consumer can understand. An example of an appropriate claim is the following: "While many factors affect heart disease, diets low in saturated fat and cholesterol may reduce the risk for heart disease." Claims for the following nutrient–disease relationships are allowed on food labels:

  A. Calcium and osteoporosis. A food must contain 20% or more of the daily value for calcium (200 mg) per serving, as much or more calcium than phosphorus, and a form of calcium that is readily absorbed. The claim must name the target groups most in need of an adequate calcium intake (teenagers and young-adult white and Asian women) and state the requirement for exercise and a healthy diet to prevent osteoporosis. A product that contains 40% or more of the daily value for calcium must state on the label that a total dietary intake of more than 200% of the daily value for calcium ($\geq$2,000 mg) is not known to be of additional benefit.

  B. Fat and cancer. To carry this claim, a food must meet the requirements for *low in fat* or, if the food is fish or a game meat, for *extralean.*

  C. Saturated fat and cholesterol in coronary heart disease. This claim may be used if the food meets the requirements for the descriptors *low in saturated fat, low in cholesterol,* and *low in fat,* or, if the food is fish or a game meat, for *extralean.* It may mention the link between a reduced risk for coronary heart disease and lower intakes of saturated fat and cholesterol to lower blood cholesterol levels.

  D. Fiber-containing grain products, fruits, and vegetables and cancer. To carry this claim, a food must be or contain a grain product, fruit, or vegetable, meet the requirements for the descriptor *low in fat,* and be a *good source* of dietary fiber without fortification.

E. Fruits, vegetables, and grain products that contain fiber and risk for coronary heart disease. To carry this claim, a food must be or contain fruits, vegetables, or grain products. It also must meet the requirements for the descriptors *low in saturated fat, low in cholesterol,* and *low in fat* and contain, without fortification, at least 0.6 g of soluble fiber per serving.

F. Sodium and hypertension. To carry this claim, a food must meet the requirements for the descriptor *low in sodium.*

G. Fruits and vegetables in cancer. This claim may be made for fruits and vegetables that meet the requirement for the descriptor *low in fat* and that, without fortification, are a *good source* of at least one of the following: dietary fiber, vitamin A, or vitamin C. This claim relates diets low in fat and rich in fruits and vegetables (and thus vitamins A and C and dietary fiber) to a reduced risk for cancer.

H. Folate and neural tube defects. When pregnant women consume a diet containing a minimum of 400 µg of folate per day, the risk for neural tube defects in the fetus is reduced. Foods containing 400 µg of folate can make this claim.

I. Sugar alcohols and dental caries. Between-meal consumption of foods high in sugars promotes tooth decay. Foods containing sugar alcohols, such as sorbitol, can claim an association with a reduced risk for tooth decay.

J. Soluble fiber from oats or psyllium and coronary artery disease. Foods that provide 3 g or more of B-glucan soluble fiber from whole oats per day or 7 g of soluble fiber from psyllium seed husk per day can claim an association with a reduced risk for coronary artery disease.

K. Soy protein and coronary artery disease. Foods containing at least 6.25 g of soy protein per serving can claim an association with a reduced risk for coronary artery disease.

Appendix D. DIETARY GUIDES FOR PATIENT USE

The diets outlined on the following pages are meant to be practical guides for patients. They should be given to patients along with explanations by the physician and individualized according to need. In some instances, the diet is sufficiently complex that referral to a dietitian will be needed. Those diets that require such expertise (e.g., diabetic, low-cholesterol, gluten-free diets; diets with strict sodium restrictions) are not included here.

Table D-1. Patient's guide to a clear liquid diet

The unsupplemented clear liquid diet does not provide adequate calories, protein, vitamins, or minerals. It is not designed to be used for prolonged periods. Supplementation with commercial products (see below) can provide adequate nutrition.

Food item	Foods allowed	Foods not allowed
Beverages		
Milk	None	All
Milk-free beverages	Carbonated beverages, coffee, iced tea, Kool-Aid, tea	Lemonade, orangeade
Available supplements	Citrotein, Polycose, Precision LR, Vivonex, Ensure	All other supplements
Soups	Broth, bouillon, consommé	All others
Animal protein sources		
Meat	None	All
Poultry	None	All
Fish	None	All
Nonmeat protein sources	None	All
Vegetables	None	All
Potato and substitutes	None	All
Breads and cereals	None	All
Fruits	Strained fruit juice	All others
Fats	None	All
Combination dishes	None	All
Snacks	None	All
Desserts and snacks	Flavored gelatin, hard sugar candy, honey, plain sugar	All others
Miscellaneous	None	Spices, condiments, seasonings

Supplementation: One liter of clear liquid diet (fruit juices) plus three 8-oz servings of Ensure plus three 8-oz servings of Citrotein provide 1,760 cal with 58 g of protein and adequate vitamins and minerals.

Modified from *Barnes-Jewish Hospital Nutrition Guide.*

Table D-2. Dietary preparation for occult blood testing

1. Avoid these drugs: iron supplements, aspirin, nonsteroidal antiinflammatory drugs, vitamin C supplements.
2. Avoid these foods for 72 hours before the test: rare red meat, broccoli, turnips, cantaloupe, cauliflower, red radishes, bean sprouts, cucumber, green beans, parsley, zucchini, lemon rind, mushrooms, horseradish.
3. Chicken, turkey, and fish are low in peroxidase activity and may be eaten.

Table D-3. Patient's guide to a restricted-fat diet

General guidelines
1. Meats should be baked or broiled, not fried.
2. The skin of chicken and turkey should be removed.
3. Avoid most desserts (cakes, cookies, pies, pastry, candy).
4. Avoid sauces and gravies.

Food item	Foods allowed	Foods not allowed
Beverages		
Milk	Skim milk and the following products if prepared with skim milk: buttermilk, Instant Breakfast	Chocolate milk, cocoa, eggnog, malted drinks, milkshakes, Ovaltine, 2% or whole milk
Milk-free beverages	Any	None
Available supplements	Casec, Citrotein, MCT oil, Polycose, Precision LR, Vivonex	Ensure, Portagen
Soups	Bouillon, consommé, fat-free broth, soups prepared with allowed foods	Cream soups
Animal protein sources		
Meat (any of the following foods or a combination of these foods must be limited to 7 oz/d)	Any whole or ground lean cuts of meat: beef, lamb, organ meats, pork, rabbit, squirrel, veal, venison	Creamed or fried meats, frankfurters, heavily marbled and fatty meats, luncheon meats, mutton, sausages, spare ribs
Poultry	Chicken, Cornish hen, turkey	Creamed or fried poultry, duck, goose
Fish	Fish, shellfish	Salted mackerel and the following fish if packed in oil: salmon, sardines, tuna; any creamed or fried fish
Nonmeat protein sources		
Any of these may be substituted for animal sources of protein	Boiled, poached, or scrambled egg; any cheese or yogurt	Fried eggs; canned pork and beans
Total protein must not exceed 7 oz/d	Dried beans, lentils, meat extenders, peas	Nuts, nut butter, peanut butter, soybeans
Vegetables	Canned, fresh, or frozen vegetables	Au gratin or creamed vegetables; avocado
Potato and substitutes	Any	Au gratin or creamed potato or pasta
Breads and cereals	All breads except those not allowed; any cereals prepared with skim milk; bread sticks, croutons, graham crackers, matzoh, melba toast, saltines, zwieback	Barley, biscuits, buns, cereals prepared with whole or 2% milk, cheesebread, cornbread dressing, crackers, dumplings, French toast, muffins, pancakes, rolls, waffles, except those allowed

Table D-3. (*Continued*)

Food item	Foods allowed	Foods not allowed
Fruits	Any canned, dried, fresh, or frozen fruit	None
Fats	None	All (margarine, butter, salad oil, mayonnaise)
Combination dishes	Any combination dish prepared with allowed foods	Any combination dish prepared with foods not allowed
Snacks	Unbuttered popcorn popped without oil	All other snacks
Desserts and sweets	Angel food cake, honey, plain flavored gelatin, plain sherbet or ices, sponge cake, sugars	Pies, other cakes and cookies, custard, Danish, doughnuts, ice cream
Miscellaneous	Baking powder, baking soda, brewer's yeast	Gravy, olives

Modified from *Barnes-Jewish Hospital Nutrition Guide.*

Table D-4. Patient's guide to a minimal lactose diet

What is lactose?

Lactose is a sugar found in milk and milk products. When the body is unable to digest this sugar, it causes gas, bloating, and diarrhea. The best way to prevent this is by eliminating lactose-containing foods from the diet.

General instructions

1. Avoid milk and liquid milk products.
2. Read labels carefully. Products containing milk, milk products, milk solids, whey, curd, casein, lactose, galactose, skim milk powder, skim milk solids, or milk sugar contain lactose. Many patients can tolerate small doses of lactose and need not be so cautious with restricting their intake of prepared foods containing small amounts of lactose. Often, however, the amount of lactose is not stated on the label.
3. Milk or cream should not be used in cooking.
4. Small amounts of cheese and butter may be tolerated.
5. Commercially available fermented milk products (buttermilk, yogurt) are sweetened by adding cream or milk and are not low in lactose. Homemade yogurt is lower in lactose content, but considerable amounts of lactose remain. Nearly complete fermentation would produce an inedible product. However, natural yogurt is allowed in moderate amounts because the bacteria in the yogurt digest the lactose after it is eaten.

continued

Table D-4. (*Continued*)

Food item	Foods allowed	Foods not allowed
Meat, fish, poultry, cheese	Beef, veal, lamb, pork, fish, poultry, cold cuts (check labels for nonfat dry milk)	Creamed or breaded fish, meat, or poultry; sausage, frankfurters, and cold cuts containing nonfat dry milk; all cheese and cheese products
Eggs	Any prepared with allowed foods	Eggs prepared with milk products
Bread	Any bread or crackers that do not contain milk or milk products	All bread products, crackers, cereals containing milk or lactose
Cereals	Any that do not contain milk or milk products (e.g., oatmeal, puffed rice, shredded wheat, grapenuts, cornflakes, puffed wheat)	
Vegetables and vegetable juices	All vegetables and vegetable juices	Vegetables prepared with butter, margarine, milk, or cheese
Fruits and fruit juices	All except those listed to avoid	Canned or frozen fruits and fruit juices prepared with lactose
Beverages	Coffee, tea, carbonated beverages and cereal beverages, soy milk substitutes	All milk and milk drinks (skim, dried, evaporated, condensed), powdered soft drinks, whey, casein
Soups	Broth-based soups prepared with meat and vegetables only	All other soups
Fats	Bacon, lard, peanut butter, pure mayonnaise, vegetable oils, some cream substitutes (check labels), milk-free margarine	Butter, margarine, cream substitutes with added milk solids, salad dressings, sour cream
Desserts	Angel food cake; cakes made with vegetable oils; gelatin, puddings prepared with fruit juices, water, or allowed milk substitutes; fruit ices	Desserts prepared with milk and butter or margarine, commercial desserts and mixes, yogurt, sherbet
Potatoes or substitutes	White or sweet potato, hominy, macaroni, rice, spaghetti, noodles	Commercial potato products; any substitutes with milk, cheese, or butter

Table D-4. (*Continued*)

Food item	Foods allowed	Foods not allowed
Miscellaneous	Corn syrup, honey, nuts, nut butters, olives, pickles, pure seasonings and spices, pure sugar candies, some cream substitutes, sugar, popcorn made with allowed fats	Ascorbic acid and citric acid mixtures, butterscotch, caramels, chewing gum, chocolate candy, cordials, liqueurs, dried soups, frozen cultures, health and geriatric foods, molasses

Caution: This diet may be deficient in calcium; check with your physician to see if calcium supplements are required.

Enzyme replacement: Lactose-depleted milk can be prepared by hydrolysing the lactose with a yeast enzyme preparation (Lactaid, Sugarlo Company, Atlantic City, NJ 08404). When one packet containing lactase from the yeast *Kluveromyces lactis* is mixed with 1 qt of milk at 4°C, lactose is 70% hydrolysed in 1 day and 90% hydrolysed in 2 or 3 days. Patients with limited tolerance can use this milk, which is sweeter than regular milk but well accepted in cooking or on cereal. Dairy products other than milk cannot be treated in this way.

Milk substitutes: A few chemically defined products are now available that simulate milk and use corn solids as the carbohydrate source. These products (e.g., Coffee Rich, Vita Rich) can be used as milk substitutes if the taste is acceptable, but their sugar content is high.

Modified from *Barnes-Jewish Hospital Nutrition Guide*.

Table D-5. Patient's guide to a low-oxalate diet

Foods high in oxalate (>10 mg per serving). Avoid completely.
Beans in tomato sauce, beets, celery, chard, collards, dandelion greens, eggplant, escarole, leek, okra, parsley, green pepper, sweet potatoes, spinach, summer squash, blueberries, blackberries, black and red raspberries, strawberries, currants, Concord grapes, lemon and lime peel, rhubarb, draft beer or stout, Ovaltine, tea, chocolate, cocoa, nuts (especially peanuts and pecans), wheat germ, tomato soup, tofu, juices containing berries

Foods moderately high in oxalate (2–10 mg per serving). Limit to two ½-cup servings per day.
Sardines, asparagus, broccoli, carrots, corn, cucumber, canned peas, lettuce, lima beans, parsnips, tomato, turnips, apples, apricots, oranges, peaches, pears, pineapple, prunes, cornbread, sponge cake, chicken noodle soup (dried), pepper (>1 tsp/d), coffee (8 oz), orange or tomato juice (4 oz), cola beverage (12-oz limit per day), bottled beer (12-oz limit per day)

Foods low in oxalate (0–2 mg per serving). Eat as desired.
Avocado, brussels sprouts, cauliflower, cabbage, mushrooms, onions, peas (fresh), radishes, milk, yogurt, eggs, cheese, lean lamb, beef or pork, poultry, seafood, bananas, Bing cherries, grapefruit, green grapes, melons, nectarines, plums, rice, spaghetti, white bread, noodles, oatmeal, bacon, oils, salad dressing, jellies or preserves, apple juice, wine, lemonade or limeade (without peel).

Table D-6. Patient's guide to a higher-fiber diet

A high-fiber diet contains 30 to 45 g of fiber per day. Dietary fiber can be increased by increasing the consumption of high-fiber foods or by supplementing the diet with commercial fiber supplements.

1. High-fiber foods

   Five grams of total dietary fiber

   Baked beans (¼ cup)
   Split peas (½ cup)
   Butter beans, cooled (½ cup)
   Blackberries (¼ cup)
   Grapes, white (12)
   Raspberries (½ cup)

   Bran wheat (¼ cup)
   All-Bran (⅓ cup)
   Shredded wheat (2 biscuits)
   Almonds (15)
   Grapenuts (1 cup)
   Prunes, stewed (½ cup)

   Four grams of total dietary fiber

   Peas, fresh or canned (½ cup)
   Turnip greens (½ cup)
   Broccoli (1 cup)
   Apricots (5)
   Apple (1 large)

   Cranberries (1 cup)
   Prunes, dried (3)
   Pear (1 medium)
   Figs, dried (2)

   Three grams of total dietary fiber

   Beets, boiled (½ cup)
   Potato with skin, baked (one 2½-in diameter)
   Rye crackers (4)
   Fruit pie (9-in diameter, ⅙ of pie)
   Corn flakes (1 cup)

2. Commercial supplements

Product	Fiber source	Dose	Dietary fiber (g)
Bran, wheat	Wheat	1 tbsp	1.6
Citrucel	Methylcellulose	1 tbsp	2.0
Fiberall	Psyllium	1 tsp	3.4
FiberCon	Calcium polycarbophil	2 tablets	1.0
Hydrocil Instant	Psyllium	1 tsp	3.5
Konsyl	Psyllium	1 tsp	6.0
Maalox fiber therapy	Psyllium	1 tbsp	3.4
Metamucil			
Regular	Psyllium	1 tsp	3.4
Water	Psyllium	water	3.0
Mylanta fiber supplement	Psyllium	1 tsp	3.4
Perdiem plain	Psyllium	1 tsp	4.0
Serutan toasted granules		1 tsp	2.5
Syllact	Psyllium	1 tsp	3.3

Table D-7. Patient's guide to a minimal-fiber diet

This diet does not provide the minimal requirements for some nutrients and is not intended for long-term use. It can be used as a preoperative or postoperative diet for patients undergoing certain abdominal procedures or during some attacks of acute diverticulitis. It is not appropriate for the long-term management of diverticular disease or intestinal strictures.

Food item	Foods allowed	Foods not allowed
Beverages		
Milk	Any	None
Milk-free beverages	Any	None
Available supplements	Any	None
Soups	Any creamed or broth-based soups without vegetables	Soups with vegetables
Animal protein sources		
Meat	Any	None
Poultry	Any	None
Fish	Any	None
Nonmeat protein sources	Any cheese, yogurt made without fruit or seeds, any eggs, meat extenders, smooth peanut butter	Yogurt with seeds or fruit, chunky peanut butter, dried beans, lentils, nuts, peas, seeds
Vegetables	None	All vegetables
Potato and substitutes	Potato without skin	Kasha
Breads and cereals	Bagels, biscuits, bread crumbs, bread sticks without seeds, cornbread, croutons, enriched white or whole grain rolls made from finely milled flour, French toast, graham crackers, matzoh, pancakes, refined cereals, rusk, saltines, waffles	All-Bran, barley, bran flakes, cracked wheat bread and rolls, grapenut flakes, Pettijohns, shredded wheat, Wheat Chex
Fruits	Strained fruit juices	All fruits
Fats	Any fat	None
Combination dishes	Those made with cheese, fish, meat, pasta, or rice	Any made with fruits, vegetables, or other foods not allowed
Snacks	Corn chips, plain crackers without seeds or cracked grain, potato chips, pretzels	Any made from foods not allowed
Desserts and sweets	Any without seeds or fruit	Any made with cracked wheat, fruit, or seeds

Modified from *Barnes-Jewish Hospital Nutrition Guide.*

Table D-8. Patient's guide to the caffeine content of foods

Sensitivity to caffeine is usually proportional to the amount consumed. Some people who cannot tolerate a cup of percolated coffee (97 to 125 mg of caffeine) tolerate a 12-oz Coca-Cola (65 mg), but others cannot tolerate even that much. This table can be used to identify caffeine-containing foods and their relative caffeine content.

Food	Unit	Caffeine content (mg/unit)
Prepared coffee	6-oz cup	
Instant, freeze-dried		61–72
Percolated		97–125
Drip		137–174
Decaffeinated coffee	6-oz cup	
Ground		2–4
Instant		0.5–1.5
Tea, bagged or loose	6-oz cup	15–75
Black, 5-minute brew		40–60
Green, Japanese, 5-minute brew		20
Cocoa	6-oz cup	10–17
Chocolate bar	Bar	60–70
Carbonated drinks	12-oz can	
Coca-Cola		65
Dr. Pepper		61
Mountain Dew		55
Diet Dr. Pepper		54
Tab		49
Pepsi-Cola		43
RC Cola		34
Diet RC		33
Diet Rite		32
Drugs	Tablet	
Cold tablets		30–32
Cafergot		100
NoDoz		100–200

Table D-9. Patient's guide to mild sodium restriction

No special foods are needed unless one prefers to substitute a low-sodium product for a high-sodium food, such as low-sodium tuna for canned tuna, low-sodium crackers for regular salted crackers.

Foods allowed with mild sodium restriction
Meat: poultry, fresh pork, fresh fish, fresh beef
Eggs: no more than two per day
Vegetables: fresh or frozen
Natural cheese (examine label carefully)
Fruits and fruit juices
Bread: white, rye, whole wheat
Milk: whole, 2%, skim
Butter or margarine
Desserts
Salt foods lightly during preparation and *do not add salt at the table.*

High-sodium Foods (one food from this list may be used daily)
Canned vegetables
Meats: cured or smoked meats such as ham, lunch meat (bologna, salami, Braun-schweiger), chipped or corned beef, frankfurters, meats koshered by salting, sausage, smoked tongue, canned meats, canned tuna and salmon packed in oil
Processed cheese, cheese spreads, or Roquefort, Camembert, blue cheese
Salted crackers, cornbread, biscuits
Buttermilk

Foods too high in sodium to be included in your diet
Sauerkraut, pickles
Anchovies, caviar, salted and dried cod, herring, sardines
Snack foods: salted potato chips, pretzels, salted popcorn, salted nuts, Fritos, corn curls, Cheez-Its
Salt pork, ham hock, smoked jowl
Miscellaneous: bouillon, commercial canned and dried soups, olives, soup base, pickles, relishes
Convenience meals: Hamburger Helper, TV dinners, canned chili, canned hash, others
Flavorings: salt and combination salts, such as celery salt, onion salt, garlic salt, seasoned salt; Worcestershire sauce, A-1 sauce, chili sauce, Accent (monosodium glutamate), horseradish (prepared with salt), meat extracts, meat sauces, meat tenderizers, soy sauce
Medications: most antacids, Alka-Seltzer, Rolaids (check with your doctor about over-the-counter medications)
Here is a list of the most common sodium compounds added to foods: When any of these compounds are listed on the label of a food, the food has some sodium. The word *soda* or the abbreviation *Na* on the label will often help you recognize a product that contains a sodium compound. More than one sodium compound indicates a high-sodium food.

Salt	Sodium saccharin
Sodium chloride	Sodium citrate
Baking soda	Sodium alginate
Bicarbonate of sodium	Sodium propionate
Sodium bicarbonate	Sodium benzoate
Baking powder	Sodium sulfite
Brine	Sodium hydroxide
Disodium phosphate	

Modified from *Barnes-Jewish Hospital Nutrition Guide.*

Table D-10. Patient's guide to a weight loss diet

These are guidelines to diet changes for persons who are presently eating a balanced diet and want to lose a small to moderate amount of weight (10 to 20 lb). Weight loss with this program will be slow, about a pound a week. These guidelines are suggested modifications of your present diet rather than an entirely new diet.

1. Eliminate or markedly limit concentrated sources of calories. Foods with a high caloric content and little additional nutritive value include the following: sugar, jelly, syrup, potato chips, crackers, fried foods, gravy, cream sauces, regular soft drinks, ice cream, candy, regular chewing gum, cakes, pastries, and doughnuts.

   Alcoholic beverages also have a high caloric content. A 12-oz beer contains 168 cal, and 2 oz of whiskey contains 172 cal. Many people consume 10%–20% of their calories as alcoholic beverages. Eliminating alcoholic beverages without other dietary changes would lead to significant weight loss in these people.
2. Change methods of food preparation. The caloric content of food can be greatly affected by the method of preparation. Fried chicken has a higher caloric content than baked chicken. The caloric content of French fries is much greater than that of a baked potato. Similarly, the way food is treated at the table affects caloric content. The salad dressing may have more calories than the salad, the gravy may have more calories than the biscuit, and the sour cream may have more calories than the baked potato.
3. Reduce the portion sizes of foods of high caloric content. Fats have a higher caloric content than carbohydrates or protein. Reducing the portion size of foods high in fat (meat, butter, margarine, salad oil) will reduce caloric intake more than will reducing the portion sizes of foods high in carbohydrates (fruits, vegetables, breads, potatoes, pasta).
4. Add high-fiber, low-calorie foods to the diet. A number of foods contain few calories. These include celery, cucumbers, lettuce, carrots, cauliflower, green peppers, bean sprouts, mushrooms, and onions. A plate of raw vegetables with meals or as a snack can satisfy the desire for food without contributing much to caloric intake.
5. Be aware of calories. Successful weight loss with a low-calorie, nutritionally balanced diet requires that the dieter be aware of the caloric content of foods. Buy and use one of the pocket calorie counters that are available at all major bookstores.

SUBJECT INDEX

Page numbers followed by a *t* refer to tables; those followed by an *f* refer to figures.

A

Absorptiometry
single-photon, 178
Acanthosis nigricans
niacin and, 135
Accucheck, 373
Acesulfame-K, 424–425, 474
Acetaminophen
nutrient effect on, 46t
Acetate
in parenteral nutrition solutions,
356t–357t
in TPN solution, 353
Achalasia, esophageal, 300
Acidophilus/lactobacillus acidophilus, 553,
554t
Acidosis
electrolyte depletion and, 212t
hyperkalemia and, 483
metabolic, 213
potassium deficiency and, 221
renal tubular, 221, 237
Acids/bases, 14t
Acne vulgaris, 172
Acquired immunodeficiency syndrome
(AIDS), 542–550
breast-feeding and, 66
malnutrition in, 545–549
nutritional support in, 113t, 549–550
nutrition in
deficiencies in, 543–544
management of, 546–548
oral and esophageal pain in, 544
Acrodermatitis enteropathica, 266–267,
267t
zinc in, 269
Activity
food intake balanced with, 33
in noninsulin-dependent diabetes
dietary modification in, 475
Addison's disease
hypermagnesemia in, 239
Additives
cancer prevention and, 538t
definition of, 12–13, 14t
sensitivity or intolerance to
diets for, 448–451
uses, toxicity, current status of, 14t, 16
Adenosine triphosphate (ATP)
thermic effect of foods and, 71
urinary creatinine excretion and, 102
Adolescence. *See also* Children
diabetes in, 465, 476–477
energy requirement in, 91
pregnancy in, 62
vitamin A in, 165
Age. *See also* Adolescence; Aging; Children
basal metabolic rate and, 73–77
body mass index and, 509

Aggregation in emulsions, 363
Aging
definitions of, 40
pathophysiologic consequences of, 41–42
theories of, 41, 41t
Alanine
as dietary supplement, 457t
in parenteral solutions, 358t, 359t
Alanine aminotransferase
serum, during parenteral nutrition therapy, 385
Albumin
in forced enteral nutrition
monitoring of, 337t
parenteral nutrition compatibility of, 371t
serum, 103–104, 104t
interpretation of, 104–105
in malnutrition, 546
Alcohol
carcinogenicity of, 537, 538t
consumption of
in pregnancy, 35, 63
in young adults, 35, 37
in diabetic diet, 475–476
effect on nutrients, 44t
folate levels and, 143
food intake and, 29t
intake guidelines for, 4t
mineral loss with, 284t
teratogenicity of, 63
vitamin A effect on, 28t
Alcoholism
calcium absorption in, 180
enteral therapy in, 326
folacin and, 142, 143, 147
hypomagnesemia in, 180, 236
osteoporosis and, 180
in pregnancy, 63
thiamine deficiency in, 126
vitamin D deficiency in, 162, 180
vitamin deficiency in, 20t–21t
zinc and, 267, 267t
Aldosterone
potassium and, 221
AlitraQ, 314–315, 316t–317t, 320t
glutamine in, 327–328, 328t
Alka-2, 233t
Alkaline phosphatase, 242
in calcium deficiency, 229
serum
vitamin D and, 178
in TPN, 385
Alkalosis
electrolyte depletion and, 212t, 213
hypokalemia and, 220
Alka-Mints, 233t
Alka-Seltzer
sodium content in, 210t
Allergy. *See also* Intolerance
to additives and, 448–451